The Path

Book I: Origins

Dedicated with love, respect and gratitude to four beautiful, brilliant,
loving and self-actualized women who, for better or for worse,
helped make me who I am today:

Ann P. Teszler
Essie J. Price
Nancy M. Smith
and
Sheila Robin Smith

Contents

BOOK I: Origins

Long ago, it's said, a Cherokee elder told his grandson,
"Two wolves battle inside each of us.
One is Evil: anger, jealousy, regret, greed,
arrogance, self-pity, guilt, resentment, & lies.
The other is Good: joy, peace, love, hope, serenity,
humility, empathy, generosity, truth, compassion and faith."

Asked the boy, "Which wolf wins?"
To which the elder replied, "The one you feed."
– John Bisagno, 1965

Serendipity

"These are the things, like Saturn V rockets, and Sputnik, and DNA, and literature and science –
these are the things that hydrogen atoms do when given 13.7 billion years."
– Dr. Brian Cox, lecture, "CERN's supercollider", April 2008, TED Talks

"The nitrogen in our DNA, the calcium in our teeth, the iron in our blood, the carbon
in our apple pies were made in the interiors of collapsing stars.
We are made of star stuff." – Carl Sagan, Cosmos, 1980

Consider for a moment the staggering alignment of circumstances that have led to your existence: 13.7 billion years ago – give or take some pocket change – the universe was born in a primal blast of plasmic energy that rocketed outwards with incomprehensible force and speed, expanding trillions upon trillions of times from a single point within the space of 10^{-32} seconds. At the outset, the universe was so superhot that no stable particles could emerge, and fundamental forces such as gravity and electromagnetism were merged into a single, tremendously powerful unified force, which blasted all of space outward. Gradually this plasma cooled, allowing the separation of the fundamental forces, and the first particles began to form.

The cooling of this great plasma cloud allowed the formation of particles such as those which make up our present-day universe, primarily the simplest of elements, hydrogen. Over billions of years, giant *molecular clouds* of superhot gases called *stellar nurseries* would give birth to successive generations of supermassive primeval stars. Hot gases and stardust ejected from these blazing primeval stars clustered in great swirling clouds, forming galaxies and planets.

The Milky Way Galaxy is among them, 100,000 light years in diameter and about 1,000 light years thick on average, containing somewhere on the order of 100 billion stars, with possibly 300 billion more tiny *dwarf stars* we are not yet able to detect. At its core, a light-devouring *supermassive black hole* seems to lurk, some four and a half million times the mass of our Sun.

The Solar System itself lies on the edge of the galaxy's spiral *Orion arm*, some two-thirds of the way out from the core. It formed 4.6 billion years ago, as a region of molecular cloud underwent gravitational collapse. Gravity, pressure, rotation and magnetic fields flattened and contracted its mass, creating a dense, hot protostar at its core. This core condensed and grew even hotter, causing hydrogen atoms to fuse together, giving birth to our Sun, while the outer reaches of the disk cooled and condensed into mineral grains. Dust and grains collided and clumped, growing by stages into ever-larger forms – *chondrules, meteoroids, planetesimals, protoplanets* and finally *planets*, as gravitational attraction swept up additional fragments encircling the Sun.

Formed 4.54 billion years ago, once every 365 days Earth itself faithfully orbits that tremendous ball of blazing hydrogen and helium 93 million miles away. Our home is a rather unlikely object – a massive, spinning sphere of liquid, rock, metal and gas, fluid layers and plates surrounding a molten, iron-rich core, all held in delicate suspension within a great void by the invisible, binding force of gravity.

Some nine billion years after the universe's explosive birth, the first forms of life began to swim about this watery, star-born mass of rock. A very precise sequence of events occurred, allowing these fragile organisms to gradually grow in ever-greater complexity, to the point where they became self-aware, able for the first time to stare into the vast, cold reaches of the cosmos and wonder what miracle begat them.

Even today, far from the distant past, when those first glimmers of consciousness formed in the minds of mankind's early ancestors, the questions have remained unchanged – *Why am I here? What's the meaning of all of this? Is there a God? What happens after I die? Does my consciousness continue?*

Believers say evidence for a Creator can be found in the sheer number of "lucky" events which allow human life. As Sir Stephen Hawking, the world's most famous cosmologist, and heir to Sir Isaac Newton's chair at Cambridge University, put it:

> *How could such an astounding chain of events, which resulted in us, be an accident? Perhaps science has revealed that there is some higher authority at work, setting the laws of nature so that our universe, and we, can exist.*
>
> *On the face of it, life does seem to be too unlikely to be just a coincidence. Think about it: the Earth lies at exactly the right distance from the sun to allow liquid water to exist on its surface. And the sun just happens to be the right size to burn for billions of years – long enough for life to have evolved. The solar system is littered with all the elements needed for life. These elements themselves are only possible because of older stars that have burnt out. These older stars only existed because of a tiny unevenness in the early primordial gas, which was itself produced by a one in a billion imbalance in the sea of particles that came from the Big Bang.*

The extraordinary coincidences pile up, one upon another, to a spine-tinglingly profound degree. Your ability to exist at this very moment rests upon a stunning set of very precise circumstances, which, if thrown just the slightest bit out of balance, would render the planet completely barren, or even cause the universe itself to vanish in an eyeblink.

In the end, Professor Hawking says he doesn't believe a god could have created the universe, for two reasons: mathematically, at the instant of the Big Bang, the ratio of energy and matter to negative energy and antimatter balance out, equaling zero – nothingness. And physicists routinely observe subatomic particles popping in and out of existence from nothing. In other words, says Hawking, mathematics proves that nothing outside the universe existed, and physics proves that you can indeed get something from nothing.

What's more, his own groundbreaking work on black holes demonstrates that when sufficient gravity exists to create a black hole, that gravity warps space and time, to the point at which *time itself stops*. This means that, since the Big Bang began from a single infinitesimally tiny point of concentrated gravity, *there was no time outside the universe before the Big Bang.*

Time did not exist until the actual explosive release of energy and space-time that resulted in the present-day universe; and, Hawking concludes, if there was neither time nor space before the Big Bang, there couldn't have been a god or moment of creation to set events in motion. On the other hand, says Hawking, the trade off is that the existence of the universe is an "inevitability of matter", and our Universe is likely to be teeming with life.

The Goldilocks Engima

The probability that all the precise conditions allowing you to exist occurred by chance alone is, according to many, overwhelmingly low. As in the famous children's fairy tale, conditions are neither too hot nor too cold, neither too big nor too small; the universe is "just right" – for life, that is.

This has long been the central argument in support of an intelligent force behind the universe's birth. A huge number of conditions are in just the precise, delicate balance to allow us to live and ponder the question of our origin. Were even one of them to go the slightest bit awry, it would wipe us instantly and utterly out of existence. Chief among these variables are the four fundamental forces of physics:

- **gravity**, *the space- and time-bending force attracting objects toward one another;*

- **electromagnetism**, *the force behind charged particle behavior, upon which most energy exchanges are based;*

- **the weak force**, *which involves radioactivity and radioactive decay;*

- **the strong (nuclear) force**, *which binds together protons and neutrons in an atomic nucleus.*

These forces, among other things, keep us and our atmosphere bound to the planet's surface, govern the *nuclear fusion* powering our sun and other stars; they also keep fundamental particles bound together instead of flying apart, and ensure consistent, predictable results from chemical reactions.

If the strong force (nuclear binding energy) varied only slightly, carbon – the very basis of life – could never have formed inside the raging heart of a star.

What's more, the delicate balance of elements in our atmosphere filters out deadly high-energy radiation from the sun, and allows us to breathe. This atmosphere is held in place by precise gravitational force. Meanwhile, the sun's mass is precisely sufficient to hold earth in a constant orbit at a life-sustaining distance, with a gravitational pull neither too strong – to pull us in and incinerate us – or too weak – to send us hurtling out into the cold vastness of space.

Scientists refer to this mix of favorable circumstances as the *Goldilocks Enigma*, a case of "not too hot, not too cold, but just right". Earth's conditions are all so precisely perfect for spawning and supporting intelligent life that it all seems to argue for the existence of a creator.

British physicist and bestselling author Paul Davies says this suitability of our planet for life isn't necessarily evidence for an invisible "hand of God", but the puzzling question still remains: why is the universe so perfectly suited for the emergence of intelligent life?

Somehow, the universe has engineered, not just its own awareness, but its own comprehension. Mindless, blundering atoms have conspired to make, not just life, not just mind, but understanding. The evolving cosmos has spawned beings who are able not merely to watch the show, but to unravel the plot.

Creationists believe a deliberate, active hand designed the universe, but it's also been suggested that perhaps the universe "becoming" *is* such a Grand Design unfolding through a simple act of will – the will of a *conscious* universe to simply Be.

Modern string theorists also propose that ours is only one of a number of parallel universes, in which the laws of physics differ wildly; in other words, we just got lucky. Perhaps, given a sufficient number of universes, galaxies, stars, planets and eons, the emergence of life is an inevitability.

I would contend that, rather than the universe being attuned to us, through billions of years of hit-and-miss adjustment (natural selection), we've become attuned to it. But even if that's true, why does anything exist at all?

The University of Colorado's Dr. Victor Stenger say it's possible to create artificial states of complete nothingness, but these states are extremely unstable, and matter and antimatter *spontaneously pop into existence* to break this void: complete nothing-ness is too perfect, too symmetrical, an exceedingly unnatural state. In other words, says Dr. Stenger, "...something is the more natural state than nothing". Nature abhors a vacuum.

Prevailing scientific theories do generally agree that before the universe began there was nothing. The greatest physicist in history – Stephen Hawking – says that in fact, all space and time exist within an expanding bubble – and *all points in space and time (past, present and future) co-exist simultaneously*. This, he says, may also explain such phenomena as ghosts and precognition. Our brains understand time moving forward, from past to future, but he says some people may be unusu-ally sensitive, able to perceive people and events in a past or future *which still exist alongside the present day most of us perceive*. These areas of space-time remain, he says, and are still – and always *will* be – every bit as "real" as the present most of us perceive.

All this, of course, leads to another profound realization. As Kurt Vonnegutt, Jr. wrote in Slaughterhouse Five:

The most important thing I learned... was that when a person dies he only ap-pears to die. He is still very much alive in the past, so it is very silly for people to cry at his funeral. All moments, past, present and future, always have existed, always will exist.... It is just an illusion we have here on Earth that one moment follows another one, like beads on a string, and that once a moment is gone it is gone forever.

Get Real

So what *is* reality? It's certainly constancy – the fact that the Earth's rotation will bring sunrise and sunset predictably every day at approximately the same time, and that, if you knock over a glass of milk, it will fall to the floor, shattering and spilling milk. This predictability means the book you placed on the shelf in the living room before going to sleep will still be there when you awaken in the morning. And the sun will rise and set every 24 hours, moving from the eastern to the western horizon. There's also the principle of *entropy* – the tendency for disorder to increase with the (apparent) passage of time.

While it's tempting to say reality is the sum of what our senses take in, the fact that one can hallucinate shows that perceptions aren't always reliable. They're subjective – filtered by individual experiences, sensory sensitivity and personal biases. Nor can reality be defined as something upon which the majority agrees – mass hallucinations and delusions are common. So reality must be something that remains constant, independent of human perception and biases. It has fundamental laws – gravity, the speed of light, etc. – and common constituent elements – atoms, subatomic particles and *electromagnetic radiation* like light, radio waves, etc. But what's at the very bottom of it all – the fundamental unit of "stuff" that makes up reality at its smallest level?

Well, one could start by asking the question "Is *anything* real?" The answer seems absurdly simple – "of course!" Should one harbor any doubt, try walking through a brick wall. Your nose will painfully answer the question.

So what is actually *in* that wall? Brick is typically composed of clay, dried in a special oven called a *kiln*, and joined to its neighbors with *mortar*, a paste of mixed sand, cement, and water that hardens as it dries. In other words, your wall is made of various types of dried, hardened soil, with trapped air pockets.

The chemical elements within that soil include *silicates* – minerals which make up 90% of the Earth's crust – oxygen, nitrogen, iron, calcium and sodium, as well as a number of trace metals. Go down a level further, and a single brick contains about 1.5 octillion atoms, $15 * 10^{27}$, or about 1,500 trillion trillion atoms (see chapter appendix for this calculation). These atoms, in turn, will be made up of subatomic particles – a nucleus of protons and neutrons, orbited by electrons.

But *matter is almost entirely empty space.* Between each nucleus and its orbiting electrons is a vast amount of empty space. To illustrate, in a hydrogen atom at a normal (*ground*) energy state, the distance between the nucleus and electron shell is, on average, one *angstrom* (about 4 billionths of an inch). In a scale model, the atomic nucleus would be represented by a grape seed, and the electron's orbit would be a sphere the length of three football fields end-to-end; the electron itself would be a speck of dust.

What this means is that *every atom in your body is 99.99% nothing, as is every atom in the brick wall,* just as, on a massive scale, the universe is also largely comprised of nothingness, interspersed with threads of clumped matter much like a sponge. Most of that is hydrogen – 75% and helium – 25%.

So why *can't* you walk through that wall? The answer lies in one of the four fundamental forces of physics – the *electromagnetic force*, the interaction of charged particles, positive particles attracting negative ones and vice versa. Since two identical charges repel each other, this ensures two electrons can't be crammed into the same space.

Since the nuclei of atoms are never close enough to interact, *chemical reactions* – the combining or breakdown of molecules – is solely determined by electrons in the outermost shells of atoms. This means electrons function as the "workhorses" of reality, giving form and bulk to everything around you. So the short explanation is that electromagnetic repulsion between atoms in the wall and those in your body prevent your walking through.

Psst – It's Only a Model

Physicists explain how the universe works through the *Standard Model of Physics*, which describes fundamental particles and forces. In the Standard Model, there are twelve building blocks of matter, grouped into three progressively more massive generations. It was long held that the tiniest subatomic particles were protons, neutrons and electrons, but particle accelerator experiments have proven that smaller fundamental particles exist.

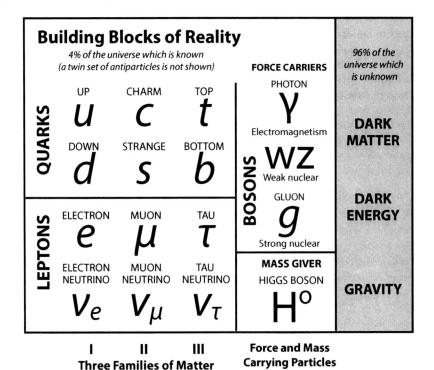

12 fundamental particles of matter are acted upon by four forces of nature. **Quarks** *combine into protons and neutrons.* **Leptons** *include electrons and* **neutrinos***, particles cast off by the sun (about 60 billion of which pass through every square centimeter of your body every second).* **Bosons** *are force-carrying particles, such as the gluons which hold together quarks into protons and neutrons and the* **Higgs Boson***, which gives mass to matter; 2012, Polyglot Studios, KK*

All ordinary matter is made up of these *fermions* – quarks and leptons. There are six of each – six *quarks*, and six *leptons*, and each has a corresponding *antiparticle*. Quarks, named after a passage in the novel *Finnegans Wake*, are always found in combinations – physicists have tried to break them apart, without success. In triplets, they form protons and neutrons, bound together in the atomic nucleus by the *strong force*.

Leptons are the second class of matter. Three are charged particles – electrons, *muons* and *taus* – and three are electrically-neutral *neutrinos*. Quarks and electrons appear to be the smallest units into which normal matter can be broken down. Everything you see in the "normal" world is composed of just two types of quarks in the atomic nucleus, around which electrons orbit.

Only first-generation particles (electrons and the products of up and down quarks) are observed in "normal" matter. The purpose of the additional, more massive generation particles is not yet fully understood, but they very rapidly decay into first generation particles, and are thus found only under special conditions. None of these particles can interact without the four fundamental forces working upon them, however – *gravity*, *electromagnetism*, and the *strong* and *weak forces* – acting upon fundamental particles by an exchange of force-carrying particles called *bosons*. Fermions thus communicate through space using bosons, packets of energy which include *photons*.

Gluons are another type of boson, which holds quarks together according to *color*, a special attractive-repulsive property described as red, green, or blue. Just as mixing these three colors equally on a computer monitor creates pure white, equal mixtures of red, green and blue quarks creates stable particles with no net color value. Protons and neutrons each contain three quarks – one red, one green, and one blue, held together by gluons, which also bind them within the atomic nucleus. Quarks can, however, change color by emitting or absorbing gluons.

The Standard Model of Physics predicts 61 elementary particles:

- *24 fermions (six quarks of three possible colors and six leptons)*

- *24 antiparticles (antiquarks, positrons, antineutrinos, etc.)*

- *13 bosons, including photons, eight gluons, the Higgs Boson, and the weak force carriers W-, W+, and Z*

In the atom, electron clouds orbit clusters of protons and neutrons, each of which is made up of triple-quark sets which are normally inseparable. Although particles with the same charge normally repel each other, in an atomic nucleus, multiple protons cluster together with neutrons. This is due to the strong force, which holds quarks together, and secondarily holds sets of protons and neutrons together in the nucleus.

This force doesn't decrease with distance – if quarks are pulled apart, the strong force "stretches" like a rubber band, its energy gradually increasing. Eventually, the energy reaches a point where it converts into matter – a quark/antiquark pair. The field's energy is converted into mass, and the strong force returns to a relaxed state. This arrangement keeps quarks from existing individually.

11

There are six types of quarks: up, down, charm, strange, top and bottom. Up and down quarks are the lightest, first-generation quarks, found in the atomic nucleus, and making up ordinary matter. *Charm* and *strange* quarks make up the second heavier generation, and *top* and *bottom* quarks are the third and heaviest.

Quark clusters are all classified as *hadrons* – the source of the name for the Large Hadron Collider. There are over 200 combinations of hadrons, in configurations of two (*mesons*) or three (*baryons*), though only the baryons called protons and neutrons are stable and constitute "normal" matter.

THE QUIRKS OF QUARKS

THE PROTON

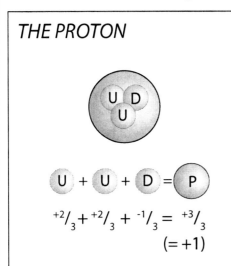

$$^{+2}/_3 + {}^{+2}/_3 + {}^{-1}/_3 = {}^{+3}/_3$$
$$(= +1)$$

THE NEUTRON

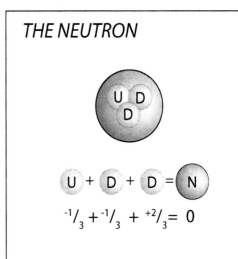

$$^{-1}/_3 + {}^{-1}/_3 + {}^{+2}/_3 = 0$$

Quarks are *elementary particles* which combine to form composite particles called *hadrons*, the most stable of which are protons and neutrons. Together these two particles form atomic nuclei. Quarks are never found separately in nature; they are only found combined into protons or neutrons. Together with electrons, they form all "normal" (baryonic) matter in the universe.

There are six "flavors" of quarks: *up, down, strange, charm, bottom,* and *top*. Up and down quarks have the lowest masses; heavier quarks quickly decay into up and down quarks, transforming from a higher mass state to a stable, lower mass state. Because of this natural tendency to decay, up and down quarks are the most stable and plentiful in the universe, while strange, charm, top, and bottom quarks are only produced by high energy collisions (like those which involve cosmic rays or in particle accelerators).

Every quark has special properties, including a "color", mass, spin, and fractional electric charge. They are also the only particles known to be affected by all four fundamental forces: electromagnetism, gravitation, and the strong and weak interactions. Every quark has a corresponding *antiquark* which differs from its counterpart with the opposite sign. All six quark flavors have been observed in accelerator experiments.

Up quarks have a *positive* charge of +2/3 and *down* quarks have a *negative* charge of -1/3. When two *up* quarks combine (+4/3) with a *down* quark (-1/3), it creates a positive charge of +1 (+3/3). When two *down* quarks combine (-2/3) with an up quark (+2/3), they cancel each other, creating a charge of 0. Although quarks with the same charge repulse each other, this repulsion is overcome by the strong force provided by *gluons*, which hold the nucleus together.

One flavor of quark can transform into another through the *weak interaction*, one of the four fundamental forces of particle physics. Here, an up quark (up, charm, or top quarks) can change into a down quark (down, strange, or bottom quark) or vice versa, by absorbing or emitting a W boson. This change in states is the radioactive process called *beta decay*, in which a neutron splits into a proton, electron and antineutrino.

Scientists have also discovered more massive versions of electrons: second-generation *muons* and third-generation *taus*. These particles are highly unstable, quickly decaying into first-generation electrons. *Neutrinos*, which are nearly massless and barely interact with other particles, also exist in three generations. A fourth generation of even more massive particles may exist, but none have yet been discovered.

Higgs Boson

The Standard Model doesn't work mathematically without the addition of *mass* – requiring a special boson to impart that property upon particles. This is the famous *Higgs boson*. In 1964, physicist Peter Higgs first proposed that an energy field permeating the entire universe – the *Higgs field*. Particles interacting with the Higgs field acquire energy and, therefore, mass, this energy-mass equivalence shown in Albert Einstein's famous equation $E = mc^2$. Particles like top quarks are strongly affected by interaction with the Higgs field, making them massive, while particles like electrons are not.

The universe is full of Higgs bosons – a Higgs field which surrounds subatomic particles, giving them mass. The Higgs field can be thought of as a medium in empty space, through which particles move, much as things move through air or water, media which are in turn made up of tiny particles themselves. Some particles moving through the Higgs boson field are affected by the medium's particles (Higgs bosons), while others aren't. Particles which are affected acquire mass, while those which pass through unaffected are massless and able to travel at the speed of light.

If one envisions the Higgs field as an ocean, a barracuda can zip through the water very quickly, while a manatee moves much more sluggishly. The medium – water – completely surrounds both creatures, but its molecules slow one creature more than another. If the ocean represents the Higgs field, the ocean's water molecules represent Higgs bosons, which "cling to" objects in the field, imparting varying degrees of mass. Greater mass requires more energy to move than lesser mass, and gravity acts more strongly upon more massive particles.

Electromagnetic force is created when the bosons called *photons* – normally thought of as packets of light – are exchanged between charged particles. Photons themselves have no electric charge, so they don't experience electromagnetic force and don't interact directly with one another. However, photons do carry energy and momentum, and, by transmitting these properties between charged particles, they produce the effects of electromagnetism. For example, as electrons draw close together, they exchange photons between them, causing a mutual repulsion.

Just as an electromagnetic field is created by photons, the Higgs field is created by Higgs bosons woven into space. Using CERN's *Large Hadron Collider*, researchers managed to blast one of these bosons out of space, and into a brief, isolated existence.

The degree of certainty that CERN researchers actually detected a Higgs boson is at a *5.9 sigma level of significance*. Usually, a five-sigma result is considered the "gold standard" for confidence in an experimental result, equal to one-in-a-million that the findings are simply due to random chance, while six sigma is only one chance in a half-billion the result is a random fluke.

Statistical Significance: *The traditional method for deciding if a statistical finding is meaningful is through significance testing. Results are "significant" if the probability of their occurring purely by chance is under five percent.*

*Some scientists argue this is not strict enough; if a sample size is small, it can skew the results. An alternative method called **Bayesian analysis** updates the probability with the accumulation of new evidence. It combines additional probabilities from outside the main study to evaluate the believability of a finding.*

This much more cautious, skeptical approach weighs findings against real-world experience, so if someone says, "My study demonstrates that drinking tap water twice a day reduces the risk of diabetes by 40%", Bayesian analysis brings other related studies into play before such a statement can be considered conclusive.

*In physics there is a stricter accepted definition of "certainty": the **five-sigma standard**. The number of **standard deviations** from the mean – called **sigmas** – measures how unlikely it is an experimental result is simply due to chance. Five-sigma is a **p-value** (probability), of 3×10^{-7} – approximately 1 in 3.5 million. For example, tossing a coin and getting several heads in a row may just be because of chance instead of, say, a faulty or deliberately "loaded" coin. The "five sigma" level of certainty, however, represents approximately the same chance of tossing over 21 heads in a row.*

***Correlation** (two events which share a relationship) often resembles **causation** (one event causing a second event), but it's easy to draw mistaken conclusions this way; two events may be related, but more information may be needed to show that one caused the other. For example, violent people often enjoy violent video games, television programs and movies. But does the entertainment trigger their violence, or do violent people just prefer violent entertainment? Further information is necessary before any conclusions can be drawn.*

Says Dr. Virginia Campbell, who runs the Brain Science psychology podcast interview series, "Our brains are wired to jump to conclusions, because we evolved in a world where making rapid decisions based on incomplete data was often a matter of life or death. We see cause and effect everywhere, even when it doesn't exist. Ironically, the more intelligent you are, the more prone you are to see correlations and to mistake them for causes."

The God Damned Particle – The Large Hadron Collider – the most complex engineering feat and largest scientific experiment ever – is the joint effort of over 10,000 international physicists from over 80 countries. Here, 100 meters underground, between the Swiss and French borders, pressurized hydrogen gas is fed into a source chamber, where the electrons are stripped away, leaving only hydrogen nuclei - positively-charged protons. Their positive charge allows them to be propelled through a vacuum tube by an on-off pulsing electrical field and trajectory-bending "steering magnets", which speed them ever faster through a circular booster chamber, before release.

By the time they reach full velocity, twin proton beams are hurtling at 99.9% the speed of light in opposite directions, circling the 27-kilometer ring over 11,000 times a second. The pipes cross over at four intersection points where the beams can be directed by magnets into a collision, and tracks from the impact debris can be analyzed by computers. Cameras capture the instant these particles smash into one another in "mini-Big Bangs", disintegrating into fundamental particles under conditions which recreate those present at the birth of the universe. The types of particles produced by the collision can be classified by the distances, directions and patterns in which they scatter.

After nearly 50 years of searching, the Large Hadron Supercollider discovered what it was specifically designed to find – the so-called "God Particle", which gives mass to matter. On September 12, 2012, CERN, the European Organization for Nuclear Research, officially confirmed the discovery after the findings passed two stringent peer reviews. The find has been hailed as the greatest scientific breakthrough since DNA's discovery. In physics, the Standard Model has long held up, explaining how the world as we know it is made up of a finite number of specific fundamental particles, each with a specific function. This model fits together beautifully and is at the heart of much modern technology.

But a problem with the Standard Model that has long bothered physicists is that the equations only work if the fundamental particles have no mass - a situation that made no sense. Therefore, it was reasoned, mass somehow emerges from interacting with something else that gives them mass. This is where the Higgs boson comes in.

The Higgs, like other bosons, applies force to fundamental particles; in this case, Higgs bosons exist in a universal field, a medium like water, in which matter is immersed. When particles come in contact with the bosons in this Higgs field, it gives them energy and, with it mass (thanks to Albert Einstein's famous equation $E = mc^2$, we know that with one comes the other).

To observe a Higgs boson, it has to be physically "blasted out" of the vacuum. This is what researchers at the Large Hadron Collider believe they have done - with 99.99999% (over "five-sigma") certainty. The standard model is now complete.

The mass that the Higgs boson gives to other particles was responsible for the formation of the universe as we know it - without it, particles ejected from the Big Bang would never have coalesced into the galaxies, stars, planets and other matter we see today.

While Nobel Prize-winning physicist Leon Lederman is credited with originally coining the term for his 1993 book The God Particle, it's said his real nickname for it was the "God Damned Particle", because it was so difficult to find evidence of it, despite how mathematical equations repeatedly showed it must exist. His publishers, it's said, edited the name to a more public-friendly version. Physicists call it the Higgs boson, after Peter Higgs, who first hypothesized its existence in 1964. The Higgs boson has helped to maintain the Standard Model of Physics, upon which much of our modern technology is built.

Aside from discovering the Higgs boson, the CERN collider has also succeeded in producing larger amounts of antimatter than ever before, which may someday be the basis of the non-bulky energy needed for interstellar travel.

Speed Demons

One of the strangest particles to have been proposed out of mathematical models is the *tachyon*, a subatomic particle able to travel faster than the speed of light. While it seems that this violates the "universal speed limit" of light (infinite energy is required to accelerate matter to the speed of light), this limit wouldn't necessarily apply to a particle which has *always* traveled faster than light. If a tachyon was "born" traveling at the speed of light, that would become its minimum speed limit, and infinite energy would be required to slow it down to less than light speed.

A Matter of Some Gravity

Other more exotic particles seem to exist, though they have not yet been confirmed. Among them is the *graviton*, a theoretical boson which imparts gravity upon matter. While we have a fairly extensive understanding of the effects of gravity, and can use it to calculate space flight trajectories and celestial mechanics, we still don't know where it comes from. If it does exist, this hypothetical particle transmits the force of gravity, attracting objects to one another. Its existence would also enable physicists to unite the theories of general relativity – physics on a cosmic scale – with those of quantum mechanics – physics on a subatomic scale.

While it looks tremendously powerful, gravity is comparatively very weak – for example, it keeps your feet anchored to the ground, but with minimal effort you can jump in the air, overcoming the gravitational pull of six sextillion tons of planetary mass. The other forces of nature are comparatively far stronger.

One explanation for gravity's comparative weakness is that we experience only a fraction of its force, the rest acting upon microscopic, curled up extra dimensions of space. According to Cambridge Professor Andy Parker, "The gravitational field we see is only the bit in our three dimensions, but actually there are lots of gravitational fields in the fourth dimension, the fifth dimension, and however many more you fancy. It's an elegant idea. The only price you have to pay is that you have to invent these extra dimensions to explain where the gravity has gone."

Bang On

The Universe's origin was first explained in 1925 by the Belgian priest Georges Lemaître, who was also an astronomer and professor of physics at the Catholic University of Louvain. His model has since even been accepted by the Pope. But for the record, the Big Bang is now more than just a hypothesis. Lingering microwave radiation found throughout the universe corroborates the theory – showing the Big Bang's afterglow.

Scientists have also been able to deduce more of the story from mathematical models and astronomical observations: the Universe began as an infinitely dense, tiny point – a "primeval atom" which exploded in the Big Bang 13.7 billion years ago. Matter then formed in four stages. Says Dr. N. R. Das of the Saha Institute of Nuclear Physics:

At the beginning, the universe was extremely hot, dense and filled with radiation and elementary particles – a hot quark-gluon plasma, with evenly-distributed energy.

On November 8, 2010, scientists recreated these conditions on a much smaller scale: researchers at the Large Hadron Collider accelerated a beam of lead ions (atoms from which the electrons have been stripped) up to 0.9999 times the speed of light (670 million miles an hour) – in opposite directions through a 17-mile tunnel deep underground near Geneva, Switzerland.

By focusing the particles into a tight beam and sending them hurtling through the tunnel in opposite directions at near-light speed, the team was able to smash them together, resulting in an explosion 10 trillion degrees centigrade, recreating conditions like those during the birth of the universe. The force of the collision was sufficient to liquefy matter into a plasma of subatomic particles such as those which existed immediately after the Big Bang.

It's from such plasma that all matter in the Universe was formed through the process known as *nucleosynthesis*:

> *Several important stages [were] the crucial period of formation of baryonic matter, that is the nucleons (elementary particles) required for nucleosynthesis after the Big Bang.... The Plank era (when all four forces, namely, matter, energy, space and time, are thought to have been united during this 10^{-43} seconds), the GUT era (particles including leptons, quarks, lepto-quarks, etc., came into existence during 10^{-8} s), the Inflation era (the Universe began to expand, exchange of particles occurred, the gluon appeared, matter became more abundant than antimatter during 10^{-35} to 10^{-33} s), the Electroweak era (exchange of particles occurred, electrons, positrons, neutrinos and antineutrinos came into existence in 10^{-6} s) and the Quark Confinement era (protons and neutrons appeared and matter became dominant over antimatter).*

When the Universe had cooled sufficiently for the first heavy combinations of particles to stabilize, it was over three minutes old, and had expanded by a factor of about a billion. From this point, protons and neutrons began to fuse.

But it was about 250 million years before the first stars and galaxies appeared out of the plasma cloud that filled the early Universe, growing in number during the half billion years of the *Epoch of Reionization*. According to University of Portland theoretical astrophysicist Ethan Siegel:

> *This is where all the matter today eventually comes from... including things like you and me, made primarily out of carbon, oxygen, hydrogen and nitrogen, where most of the elements in our body did not exist at the beginning of the Universe. In order to create them — in fact, in order to create nearly all of the*

elements on our planet — it took generations of stars burning through their nuclear fuel, fusing light elements into heavier ones, and recycling those elements back into the interstellar medium to form new and subsequent generations of stars, now enriched with these heavy elements.

Because of this, astrophysicists long predicted the existence of "pure" stars dating from the birth of the Universe, stars containing nothing but undiluted hydrogen and helium, and gas clouds which had not yet collapsed to form stars. In 2011, their predictions were borne out with the discovery of two such clouds with the exact proportions of Hydrogen and Helium predicted, and a year later, with the discovery of a 13-billion-year-old "first generation" star.

Fade Away and Radiate

Today's universe is alive with *electromagnetic radiation,* from radio and microwaves through the light spectrum, X rays and gamma rays. These are all streams of photons, vibrating at different rates as they streak out from their source at the speed of light.

The vibration – or *oscillation* – of a photon depends upon the energy it contains, while the number of times it vibrates per second is its *frequency,* measured in *Hertz* (cycles per second). The distance a photon travels as it oscillates through one cycle is its *wavelength,* measured in *nanometers* (billionths of a metre).

The lowest energy photons – those which vibrate slowest – are radio waves, oscillating at 3 kHz (3,000 cycles per second) to 300 GHz (300,000,000,000 cycles per second). Microwaves are slightly more energetic, infrared light still more so, and then there are visible and ultraviolet light, X-rays, and gamma-rays, the most energetic of all photons, with a typical frequency of 10 *exahertz* (10^{19} Hz or more).

THE ELECTRO MAGNETIC SPECTRUM

Electromagnetic Spectrum, University of Oregon, 1994. Used with permission.

What's Cooking? Unstable *isotopes* are atoms with an unbalanced nucleus which *decays*, ejecting particles to become more stable. These particles are classified as *alpha*, *beta* or *gamma*, according to their size. A stream of these particles constitutes harmful *ionizing* (electron-stripping) radiation.

While radio waves and visible light are harmless, *non-ionizing* forms of radiation (lower-energy *photon emissions*), high doses of ionizing radiation can kill quickly, causing major organ failures, while low levels can disrupt DNA, triggering genetic mutations with cancer-causing or hereditary consequences, including sterilization.

During *alpha decay*, a nucleus with too many protons contains excessive repulsive forces. To relieve this and reach stability, the nucleus ejects an *alpha particle* (the nucleus of a helium atom, with two protons and two neutrons), resulting in a new element at a lower atomic number.

The weak force drives *beta decay*, the process which maintains a balance of protons and neutrons in an atomic nucleus. If there are too many neutrons, a neutron decomposes into a proton and emits a high-speed beta particle (electron), and a non-interacting antineutrino. Conversely, if there are too many protons-to-neutrons, an up quark changes into a down quark, transforming the proton into a neutron, and ejecting a positron and neutrino. A third type of beta decay called *electron capture* can also occur, when the proton-to-neutron ratio is too large, so the nucleus captures an electron, using it to transform a proton into a neutron, emitting a neutrino.

Gamma decay results when an atomic nucleus is in a state of excessive energy. The nucleus sheds a high-energy photon called a gamma particle, thereby returning the nucleus to a more stable, lower-energy *ground state*. This gamma particle release is the highest-energy form of *electromagnetic radiation*, which ranges from radio waves to visible light, x-rays and high-energy gamma radiation.

The high-speed emission of these particles can tear apart molecular bonds, with deadly effects upon living tissue. While alpha radiation cannot penetrate deeply into human skin, it is particularly deadly if inhaled or ingested, mutating DNA and usually leading to cancer. The most dangerous, however, is gamma radiation, which can penetrate most deeply into living tissue.

Next Year's Model

Interestingly, mathematical models show there's a *lot* more matter in the universe than what we've been able to see, which adds up to a paltry four percent – the other 96% is thought to be mysterious *dark matter* and *dark energy*.

Mathematical measurements and calculations show that as one recedes in time toward the Big Bang, the four fundamental forces of nature change: the electromagnetic force (which uses proton and electron charges to bind atoms into large-scale matter), grows stronger at higher temperatures; meanwhile the strong nuclear force (which binds protons and neutrons in the nucleus) grows weaker. Three of the fundamental forces – all but gravity – almost converge into a single kind of merged "super-force", back at the birth of the universe. Almost.

But relatively new theories of *super-symmetry* double the number of fundamental particles by adding a second set of *supersymmetric particles*, which may account for dark matter, dark energy and gravity. Adding these particles allows all four of the changing fundamental forces to mathematically converge neatly at the point of the Big Bang. It's hoped that the Large Hadron Collider will discover these supersymmetric particles, thus filling in the missing pieces of the puzzle for modern physics.

Still, while the mathematics may fit neatly together, the space-bending, time-slowing force of gravity seems to insist on remaining the "odd man out", stubbornly refusing to mesh with existing quantum theory. This is where *string theory* comes in, which says, in a nutshell, that on an even smaller scale, all subatomic particles are simply strands of energy vibrating at different frequencies.

Our current technology makes it impossible to detect objects on such a minute scale, but on paper at least, string theory manages to reconcile gravity with the laws of quantum mechanics, something that has eluded physicists until now.

In the Dark

According to NASA, only about 5% of the universe is composed of ordinary matter. Six to seven times more mass seems to exist in the form of invisible *dark matter*. In other words, the universe is primarily made up of matter which sheds no electromagnetic radiation – emitting no light of any sort, from infrared to gamma rays. Dark matter particles apparently carry no electric charge, and thus don't interact with ordinary matter via electromagnetic forces. But they appear to be everywhere in the universe, including where you are, surrounding you and even passing through you constantly.

So, while scientists can observe "luminous matter" like stars, gas and dust, dark matter can't be observed directly because it doesn't emit or absorb light or any other kinds of energy (hence its name). Instead, it reveals itself through the pull it exerts on galaxies.

Spinning galaxies rotate at such high speed that they would tear themselves apart if it weren't for a large amount of invisible matter holding them together through gravity. This clearly shows there is much more matter in galaxy clusters than just detectable *baryonic* matter (stable triple-quark particles) – unless our understanding of gravity is incorrect, which is doubtful considering our theories have held true for over 300 years of experimentation and innovation, including successful space flight.

Evidence of dark matter is growing. NASA's Hubble Space Telescope announced the discovery of a giant filament of dark matter for the first time in October, 2012. Stretching 60 million light-years between two galaxy clusters, the dense *MACS*

J0717 filament is said to be part of a cosmic web upon which the fabric of the Universe is strung, a structure resulting from the very first moments after the Big Bang.

Theoretical models and computer simulations show that variations in the density of matter during the universe's birth caused the cosmos to condense into a web of long, tangled filaments, which seem to connect at the locations of massive galaxy clusters. The finding seems to confirm the *lambda cold-dark-matter (ΛCDM)* model of the universe, which says that, in the early universe, dark matter spread out in a web of filaments, while baryonic matter clumped together in the regions where those filaments intersected.

Physicists aren't quite sure what dark matter is, though they say it's not the "normal" baryonic matter of which visible stars and planets are composed. It doesn't seem to be made up of clouds of ordinary matter, because such clouds absorb radiation passing through them. Dark matter isn't made up of antimatter either, because the gamma rays produced by antimatter-matter annihilations aren't observed to a high enough degree.

It's been proposed that dark matter may be highly compressed conventional matter in the form of ultradense *brown dwarf stars* or chunks of extremely dense heavy elements, aggregates which physicists call *Massive Compact Halo Objects*, or *MACHOs* for short.

Such ordinary matter would emit little to no detectable electromagnetic radiation. Other MACHO candidates include neutron stars and black holes. MACHOs have been observed, and while they probably contribute to the dark matter equation, they seem to be far too few to account for all the dark matter in the universe. Because of this, astronomers believe dark matter consists of entirely new types of elementary particles, exotic particles they're calling *WIMPS (Weakly Interacting Massive Particles)*. These theoretical particles "weakly interact" because they pass through ordinary matter without any effects.

If WIMPs exist, they are tens or hundreds of times more massive than protons, but like neutrinos, lack charges, and thus interact so weakly with ordinary matter that they're difficult to detect. These include *neutralinos* – theoretical massive forms of neutrinos not accounted for in the Standard Model.

Another WIMP candidate is the hypothetical *axion* – a tiny neutral particle under a millionth the mass of an electron, possibly produced in tremendous abundance during the Big Bang. *Photinos* have also been suggested – particles which resemble photons, but with a mass 10 to 100 times that of a proton. If they exist, photinos lack charges, and like other WIMPs, would interact with normal matter weakly.

Dark matter may be a mixture of MACHOs and WIMPs, but NASA physicists believe it's primarily composed of some type of slow-moving WIMP, because fast-moving particles would be unable to clump sufficiently to create such strong gravitational effects.

Galaxies provide other hints of dark matter. Albert Einstein's theory of General Relativity predicts that large masses curve space-time around them. This means the gravitational force of a massive object also curves the path of light rays around it, much like a lens. When a massive object is in front of a more distant star or galaxy, astronomers can observe this effect through "lensing events" – the galaxy clusters act as a gravitational lens, similar to an optical lens.

The greater an object's mass, the greater the distortion that occurs. By measuring the curvature of light, astronomers can use this effect to calculate the mass causing the distortion. Using these calculations, astronomers have discovered additional evidence that galactic clusters have an invisible mass far exceeding that which we can see.

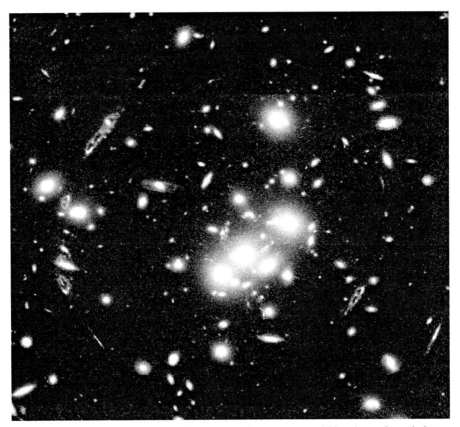

A lensing event captured by the Hubble Space Telescope. Several blue, loop-shaped objects are multiple images of the same galaxy, duplicated by the gravitational lens of the cluster of galaxies near the photograph's center. The cluster's gravitational field bends light to magnify, brighten and distort the image of a more distant object. Source: NASA, October 14, 1994, public domain.

On the Dark Side

Physicists Brian Schmidt, Saul Perlmutter and Adam Reiss shared a 2011 Nobel Prize for demonstrating that the universe's expansion is accelerating rather than slowing down, as was previously believed. If "normal" matter comprises 4% of the Universe, and dark matter 24%, the remaining 72% of the universe is thought to be comprised of *dark energy*, the force driving this acceleration of the universe's expansion.

Right now, physicists are searching for it in the form of a mysterious new boson called a *chameleon particle*. If they're correct, this will add a fifth force and a new particle to the Standard Model. Columbia University astrophysicists Dr. Justin Khoury and Amanda Weltman first suggested a chameleon particle in 2003 as a possible explanation for dark energy, the mysterious force pushing the universe apart. Like their namesake, chameleon particles are thought to "adjust" to their surroundings, scaling their mass up or down in response to nearby matter. With the reduction in mass comes a proportionate increase in the propulsive force they exert upon ordinary matter.

This means that in the great emptiness of space, the force chameleons exert would theoretically be huge – and growing, as the universe continues to expand. Here on Earth, however, chameleons would be too heavy to exert any noticeable force, explaining why none have yet been detected. Dr. Weltman and colleagues ran a series of experiments at Fermi National Accelerator Laboratory which failed to detect a chameleon particle, but two additional approaches are currently underway.

Theoretically, photons travelling through intense magnetic fields can decay into chameleons, reducing the amount of light reaching Earth from distant sources. This reduction in photon intensity will vary depending upon the light's frequency. In late 2012, a team of astrophysicists at Queen Mary University of London compared light emissions from the luminous centers of 77 galaxies across a range of frequencies, and announced "good evidence" that some photons went missing in transit. The detected photons showed they had acquired a polarization (change in the direction of oscillation as a photon travels) which matched the magnetic fields they had passed through, something which should only occur if the chameleon model is true.

However, these observations alone aren't enough to prove the existence of chameleon particles. 2014 is the launch of the French Space Agency CNES's *MicroSCOPE microsatellite*, which will engage in a variety of tests, including a search for chameleon particles in outer space.

Much Ado About Nothing

Dark matter and dark energy may well decide the universe's ultimate fate. We know that the universe is expanding, and at an accelerated rate, but the question is whether or not that expansion will continue infinitely. Gravity will ultimately determine the limits of that expansion, and gravity depends upon the density of the universe.

The ratio of that density – the universe's total matter and energy – versus the density required for an endlessly expanding *flat universe* is referred to as "omega" (Ω). According to conventional calculations, the universe has only 30% of the matter necessary to continue expanding. However, according to Arizona State University's Dr. Lawrence Krauss, the energy found in empty space alone is sufficient to account for the acceleration of the universe's expansion.

Empty space, he says, is alive with *zero point energy*, quantum fluctuations spontaneously creating matter and energy. This, he says, is the cosmological constant that Einstein had first proposed, then retracted in embarrassment – 70% of the energy in the universe residing in empty space.

According to this theory, so-called empty space is far from empty. Even after all the matter and energy in a space have been removed, this vacuum never remains empty, but is instead "...a boiling, bubbling brew of virtual particles popping in and out of existence on a timescale so short you can't see them", according to Dr. Krauss, best-selling author of *A Universe From Nothing*.

Nothingness – empty space – is "teeming with" particles and electromagnetic fluctuations which spontaneously wink in and out of existence in a matter of *femtoseconds* (10^{-15} seconds). 90% of the mass in protons, he says, comes not from the quarks themselves, but *from the empty space between the quarks* – from fields popping in and out of existence. This sub-atomic activity may be the source of dark energy, existing at the same level throughout the universe.

Thus, zero-point energy is what remains after all the other energy has been removed from a system. The phenomenon can be observed in liquid helium: as the temperature drops to absolute zero, helium condenses into liquid form, but doesn't freeze because of the zero-point energy of atomic motion, which cannot normally be removed (although pressurizing it to 25 atmospheres causes helium to freeze).

Unfortunately, calculations for zero point energy show it to be overwhelmingly huge – 120 orders of magnitude more powerful than it could possibly be and still allow the universe to exist. However, if that energy is balanced with the negative energy produced by gravity, the equation balances out. As Dr. Krauss puts it:

> It turns out empty space weighs something, and we don't understand why. But 70 per cent of the energy in the universe is contained in empty space, the biggest surprise in the history of physics in the last century, and that empty space energy is even weirder because it's gravitationally repulsive, a kind of cosmic antigravity, and it's causing the expansion of the universe to speed up, and all of that is totally unexpected.

This, he says, is a *cosmological constant* that Einstein had first proposed, then retracted in embarrassment – 70% of the energy in the universe residing in empty space. Albert Einstein had suggested this cosmological constant allowed the universe to remain static. Later, it was discovered that the universe was expanding, and Einstein recanted, calling the cosmological constant "his biggest blunder." Without the addition of this number, known physics produces a model which is over 10 to the power of 60 times too large, which is why physicists introduced the concept of a dark energy driving the accelerated expansion. However, says Dr. Thompson, inputting a different value for Einstein's "fudge factor" does produce the universal acceleration that has been observed, showing that Einstein may have been right all along.

Not everyone is in agreement over dark energy, however. University of Arizona astronomer Dr. Rodger Thompson says his calculations show this theory doesn't fit with the proton-to-electron mass ratio, a fundamental constant.

In The End

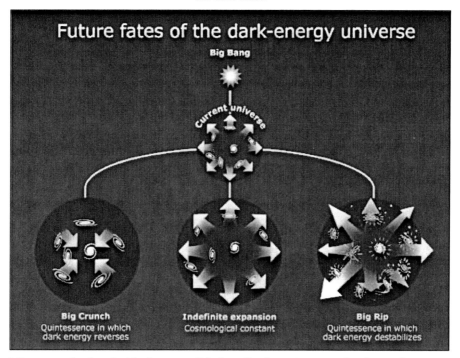

We seem to be faced with three possible fates for the universe in the distant future:

1) The Big Crunch: if the Universe has greater than critical mass density, it will expand, then eventually slow, stop and collapse back on itself;

2) The Big Chill: if the Universe has critical mass density, it will continue to expand forever, but the expansion will slow, and the universe will eventually grow cold.

3) The Big Rip: Recent observations indicate the universe is expanding at an accelerated rate. If this expansion continues to accelerate, eventually all matter will fly apart. The cause of this apparent acceleration is currently unknown, so physicists have proposed the force driving it is dark energy. *Image: NASA, public domain, 2010.*

Ghost Particles

Neutrinos, from the Italian for "small neutral one", are by-products of nuclear fusion in the core of stars, subatomic particles with a mass of nearly zero that carry no electrical charge. Because they lack any charge, they're unaffected by the electromagnetic forces attracting and repelling electrons and protons. This means that they can travel tremendous distances at near light-speed, even through solid matter, without slowing.

Produced in great numbers when stars die in supernova explosions, neutrinos are one of the most abundant particles in the universe, able to move as easily through lead as you can move through air. Hold out your hand in direct sunlight, and about a billion neutrinos from the sun will pass through in a single second.

There are three known neutrinos. Each "flavor" is associated with a charged particle, giving the neutrino its name – the *electron neutrino* is associated with electrons, while the other two are associated with special, heavier versions of electrons called the *muon* and *tau*. It's possible that neutrinos also "oscillate" – changing between the three varieties, though this is something current technology hasn't allowed us to determine yet.

A byproduct of *nuclear fusion* – the explosive merging of hydrogen atoms into helium, that also releases light packets called photons – neutrinos are the only particles capable of penetrating the very dense material produced by collapsing stars; they've been referred to as "ghost particles" because they're almost nothing – having no electric charge and nearly no mass. Because they interact so weakly with other particles, neutrinos are extremely hard to detect.

But they appear to have played a central role in the birth of the universe. According to mathematical models, during the early stages of the Big Bang, equal amounts of matter and antimatter existed. Most of these particles annihilated each other as the universe expanded and cooled, but a slight imbalance existed between the two, giving rise to the universe as we know it – a universe comprised of matter. Physicists believe neutrinos were at the heart of that fortunate imbalance. and that the universe's mysterious "dark matter" may consist of neutrinos with special properties left over from the early stages of the Big Bang.

A Breathing Universe

Most physicists today believe that, as dark energy drives the universe apart, eventually it will all expand across immeasurable distances, and the stars burn out one by one in a "Big Chill" – or perhaps a "Big Rip", as dark energy eventually tears the fundamental particles of matter apart.

But some physicists concur with a thousand-year-old idea first proposed by Eastern mystics: that the universe is *cyclical* – appearing and disappearing endlessly, a Big Bang which culminates, after billions of years, in a Big Crunch, as gravity slows expansion and pulls everything back inward for a great collapse. This is followed by yet another Big Bang and Crunch, etc. – an eternal "Breathing Universe" model.

In 2012, Penn State physicists used *loop quantum cosmology* to construct a new mathematical model of the universe. The approach allowed researchers to extend quantum physics further back in time than ever before – to the very moment of the universe's birth. What the model shows is that, after the universe's initial expansion 13.7 billion years ago, small variations in space-time settled into the large-scale structures of our current universe.

Had space-time been completely "smooth", the universe could not have evolved, but very minor fluctuations at the moment of the universe's conception expanded into seed-like structures found in cosmic microwave background radiation. By coupling Einstein's equations with inflation theories of how the universe expanded from a single point, the model shows how seed-like clumps scattered across the cosmos to evolve into galaxy clusters and other massive structures observable in the universe.

The theory's borne out by observations of specific patterns of irregularities in cosmic background radiation, and the model – with research backed by the American National Science Foundation – has the added advantage of being testable against observations from cutting-edge modern telescopes.

This mathematical model also lends growing support to the theory that the universe has been through multiple incarnations, dubbed by the Penn State team a "Big Bounce" – which says our universe "bounced back" from the collapse of a pre-existing universe into a super-compressed mass.

Haverford College theoretical physicist Dr. Stephon Alexander – recipient of both the National Science Foundation CAREER award and National Geographic's Emerging Explorer status – says mathematics proves the "Big Bounce" theory, echoing the idea that our universe's current incarnation is just one in an infinite cycle of expansion and contraction phases, like the beating of a cosmic heart.

According to Dr. Alexander, when the universe collapses, neutrinos condense into a unique state called a *neutrino condensate*, which acts as a "superfluid", which doesn't lose energy to friction. (If you were able to stir superfluid milk into your superfluid coffee, it would never stop swirling about in your coffee cup). But this superfluid state has an intense repulsive pressure, that builds and eventually results in an explosive expansion, which then continues until there is insufficient energy to counter matter's gravitational mass, and the entire cosmos once again contracts.

Physicists have long sought an explanation for the driving force behind *inflation* – the universe's post-Big Bang expansion – and Dr. Alexander says such a compressed neutrino condensate would unquestionably provide the necessary force. An interesting side note, he adds, is that a collapsing star, en route to becoming a black hole, could theoretically produce just such a neutrino condensate. If this is true, it may well mean that black holes are the birth sites of universes everywhere. What's more, Dr. Alexander believes that we might exist within such a neutrino condensate, which could explain the baffling acceleration of the universe's expansion, typically attributed to unknown dark energy.

Fellow theoretical physicist at the Perimeter Institute for Theoretical Physics, Dr. Lee Smolin, believes this theory points to a *cosmic natural selection*, producing new universes which branch off from our own within the unique physics of black holes. And universes which produce the greatest number of offspring – via black holes – are most likely to proliferate.

To produce black holes, says Dr. Smolin, what's required are massive stars – on the order of twenty times the magnitude of our sun. The formation of such massive stars requires great clouds of cooling gases, and the coolant is carbon monoxide – in turn requiring large amounts of carbon and oxygen – the two most vital constituents of life as we know it. Thus he says, *the abundance of life's most critical ingredients throughout the universe is simply an inevitable byproduct of a universe capable of reproducing itself.*

This also implies that parallel universes may be everywhere: between December 2009 through February 2011, NASA's Wide-field Infrared Survey sky-mapping telescope recorded about three times as many undiscovered black holes than had ever before been found in visible light surveys. While scanning the entire sky in infrared, the telescope recorded a massive cache of information, data which astronomers are still sifting through.

These newly-discovered black holes aren't the typical tiny, dense objects created by collapsing stars, but are instead the *supermassive black holes* that create *quasars*, the brightest objects in the universe, caused by the light and friction energy of entire galaxies being sucked into oblivion.

As for evidence of a higher being, some physicists suggest the entire universe may be a single, living *superorganism*. Particle physicist Dr. Jeffrey West founded and heads the high energy physics group at Los Alamos National Laboratory in New Mexico. A Fellow of the American Physical Society, West has lectured at the World Economic Forum, won the Oxford University and the Glenn Award for research on Aging and was named one of Time magazine's 2006 *100 Most Influential People in the World*, and his work has been selected as one of the breakthrough ideas of 2007 by the Harvard Business Review.

West and his team have been collaborating with biologists, asking questions like "Why is it that we die?" and "What sets the scale of human lifetime at 100 years?" The answers have filled books which describe *biological scaling*, the mathematical relationships between a creature's size and the rate at which life processes occur, such as the speed at of its heartbeat or its energy consumption.

These formulas govern universal principles of structure and function, including cell size, *metabolism* (food-to-energy conversion and molecular assembly), growth and DNA modification rates, and even the structures and dynamics of ecosystems. They are also helping to answer long-running questions at the forefront of medical research about aging, sleep, and illnesses such as cancer. West and his colleagues believe the entire universe follows these same laws, and that the universe may well be a living, conscious superorganism, on an incomprehensibly massive scale.

MIT mechanical engineering professor Seth Lloyd has a slightly different take, maintaining that the universe is indisputably a massive quantum computer. He says this is simply the fundamental nature of reality – it's an inarguable, self-evident fact that elementary particles comprising the entire cosmos are computing on a massive parallel scale, and that nature, while it appears to be *analogue* – continuous, flowing states – is actually *digital*, comprised of discrete particles, processes and states. This is analogous to how a printed image looks smooth from a distance, but closer examination reveals its individual pixels.

Grains of Sand on a Beach

String theorists and others suggest our reality is only one within a multiverse, where our bubble of space-time is perhaps only one among an infinite number of universes, as plentiful as grains of sand on a beach, each with unique laws of physics and a uniquely unfolding reality. The fundamental constants we know would have very different values in these other universes.

If this is so, each of these realities will be tremendously different, operating under a cosmic natural selection, in which universes which cannot be sustained arise and then quickly wink out of existence, collapsing upon themselves and leaving only stable ones such as ours remaining. A number of physicists say mathematics does predict such a multiverse, in which the laws of physics vary widely. At this point, however, because it's not *falsifiable*, we can only use mathematics to try and understand the possibility.

Falsifiability is a basic underpinning of science. For any theory to be accepted, there must be a means of disproving it if it's incorrect. If a theory is not demonstrably false, it may be the truth, and if it's repeatable, eventually it can be accepted as true. But if it's impossible to show if something is false, it's also impossible to show if it's true.

Science is based upon testing theories with measurements that can be repeated, among independent groups, with different equipment and analytical methods. Such measurements and methods are constantly evolving and improving, increasing the statistical certainty of what can be accepted as "fact". Progress occurs when new evidence is gathered which further strengthens this mathematical certainty, or which disproves the original hypothesis.

Professor Laura Mersini-Houghton at the University of North Carolina believes we've already found "real-world" evidence for parallel universes. Deep in the southern hemisphere of the *celestial sphere* – a hypothetical globe with the Earth as its central reference point – lies the constellation *Eridanus*, named after a Greek legend. The myths tell of how young Phaëton, son of the sun-god Helios, borrowed his father's sky chariot, but wasn't strong enough to control the twin horses dragging the sun across the sky. As the solar chariot wheeled out of control, it pulled the sun along a fiery, destructive path, scorching the sky and earth.

To prevent the complete destruction of heaven and earth, Zeus, the god-king of Mt. Olympus, struck the boy dead with a thunderbolt, sending him hurtling downward to the Earth. The constellation Eridanus, a great river of stars, is said to be the fiery afterglow of Phaëton's final, fatal fall.

Within the heart of the Eridanus constellation lies a compelling mystery – an apparent massive expanse of space devoid of galaxies, stars or other matter. Nearly a billion light-years across, it's one of the largest voids in the known universe, and seems to defy the laws of nature because of its great emptiness.

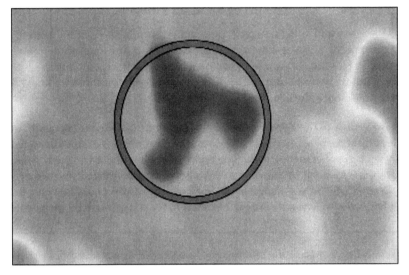

Discovered in 2007, the Eridanus Supervoid has been suggested as a window into another reality, one with eventually testable evidence of a parallel universe. Lawrence Rudnick, 2007, NASA, public domain

Matter always naturally disperses into a state of randomness; because of this, an area of nothingness a billion light years across should be impossible. But the Eridanus Supervoid may be, says professor Mersini-Houghton, one point at which another universe with a completely different set of fundamental laws converges upon our own.

Drs. Ray Zhang and Dragan Huterer of the University of Michigan in Ann Arbor and Kendrick Smith of the University of Cambridge say this cold spot may just be an *artifact* (defect) in the statistical method used to analyze the data, though there are other undisputed supervoids, including the *Boötes* and the *Northern* and *Southern Local Supervoids.*

Still other researchers with the Institute for Astronomy at The University of Hawaii reject the notion that this supervoid is merely an artifact, saying instead that supervoids and the opposite, highly-compressed *galaxy superclusters* – are the stretching and flattening effects of dark energy upon space.

Stringing Us Along

Physicists have long sought a *grand unifying theory* – a master equation to tie together the logic of all the laws of physics in our universe. Thus far, they have only been able to agree upon four fundamental forces, briefly mentioned earlier:

- *Electromagnetism*, the attraction between particles of opposite charges, binds molecules together, attracts electrons into orbit around atomic nuclei, and repels particles with the same charge, creating the apparent solidity of objects, which can't pass through one another because their electrons repel one another.

- *The strong nuclear force*, which holds the nuclei of atoms together. Without this, all matter would fly apart, unable to exist in stable forms.

- *The weak nuclear force*, responsible for subatomic particle decay and allowing *hydrogen fusion* in stars. In unstable atoms, neutrons stabilize by undergoing *beta negative decay*, emitting an electron and an *antineutrino* to become protons. The process is caused by the emission or absorption of W and Z bosons, which changes a neutron's quarks from one form into another. In the reverse (*beta positive decay*), protons decay into neutrons, emitting *positrons* and neutrinos.

  When a particle decays, it disintegrates into tinier particles whose combined energy equals that of the original particle. This is like getting change for a dollar. While a dollar bill isn't physically composed of coins, its value is equal to that of the change. And, just as several different coin combinations add up to one dollar, many particle combinations can contain the energy of one massive particle.

  This weak nuclear force controls the first stage of the sun's fusion cycle, where two hydrogen nuclei fuse into helium. In the process, some of the nuclear mass is converted into energy, in a tremendous energy release (an amount determined by Einstein's famous equation $E=MC^2$). The weakness of this force, however, allows star energy emission to continue for billions of years. Had this force been stronger, the sun would have burnt out long before life evolved.

  Beta positive decay is the basis of *PET* (*Positron Emission Tomography*) scanners, which measure emissions of an antimatter particle – the positron – the antimatter opposite of an electron, which is emitted from special *marker chemicals* injected into a patient's body. Positrons are identical to electrons, save for a positive rather than negative charge. PET scanners are used to search for abnormalities in cells and tissues.

- *Gravity*, the force attracting large bodies of matter to one another. Gravity, by far the weakest of these four forces, was once thought to instantaneously affect matter across any distance. But, according to everything we know, that would be faster than the speed of light, which is theoretically impossible; light itself isn't even instantaneous, taking eight minutes to travel the 93 million miles from the Sun to Earth.

Gravity explains the behavior of large objects, while the other three forces explain the behavior of small objects, but a single explanation for how all four fit together has been elusive.

However, Columbia University Professor Brian Greene believes he may have the solution in *string theory*: everything in the universe is, he says, composed of tiny vibrating stands of energy – and varying frequencies of those vibrations results in the different kinds of matter and energy.

In *The Elegant Universe, The Fabric of the Cosmos* and *The Hidden Reality,* he outlines his theories, which he believes unify the four fundamental forces. He also contends that the deepest levels of physics – including string theory – appear to confirm the existence of multiple universes.

Not just string theory, but many aspects of cosmology, relativity, and quantum mechanics all point to parallel universes. The problem with proving it, he says, is in the impossibility of falsification – the ability to prove a theory wrong – making such theories "beyond science". Thus, for now, string theory must remain in the realm of mathematics; however, mathematics has often proven invaluable in exploring ideas beyond current testing capabilities, which were later proven true.

Six Numbers

As for the question of consciousness, most scientists now maintain it's simply a matter of biology – an inward-focused energy-monitoring and management system; without physical substance to house it, most say consciousness has no means of existing. In other words, there is no room in such logic for a spiritual reality, including a creator.

Nonetheless, it is truly humbling to consider the incredibly fragile balance of conditions which allow conscious life to exist: In the year 2000, England's Royal Astronomer and Cambridge Professor Sir Martin Rees published *Just Six Numbers*, which describes six values necessary for the existence of the universe and life as we know it. These *fundamental constants* – unvarying, basic laws of the universe – fall within a very narrow range. If they varied in the slightest degree, life – and even the universe itself – could not exist. Two of these are related to the fundamental forces; two determine the universe's overall "texture", size, and longevity; and two more determine the properties of space. As Sir Rees puts it:

> *These six numbers constitute a 'recipe' for a universe. Moreover, the outcome is sensitive to their values: if any one of them were to be 'untuned', there would be no stars and no life. Is this tuning just a brute fact, a coincidence? Or is it the providence of a benign Creator? I take the view that it is neither. An infinity of other universes may well exist where the numbers are different.*
>
> *Most would be stillborn or sterile. We could only have emerged (and therefore we naturally now find ourselves) in a universe with the 'right' combination. This realization offers a radically new perspective on our universe, on our place in it, and*

on the nature of physical laws. It is astonishing that an expanding universe, whose starting point is so 'simple' that it can be specified by just a few numbers, can evolve (if these numbers are suitably 'tuned') into our intricately structured cosmos.

N The ratio of *electromagnetism* (which attracts oppositely-charged subatomic particles) to *gravity* (which bends space-time to "attract" large objects to one another) is approximately 10^{36}. This is the strength of the forces holding atoms together, divided by the strength of gravity between them.

Had N been smaller "*by a few less zeros, only a short-lived miniature universe could exist: no creatures could grow larger than insects, and there would be no time for biological evolution.*" The value is, says Rees, the reason the universe is so vast. It also determines, among other things, the minimum and maximum sizes of stars.

Stars, which make up most of the universe's visible matter, are primarily composed of hydrogen and helium. They act as massive nuclear furnaces, transforming matter through *nuclear fusion*, the forced compression of two or more atomic nuclei into a heavier nucleus, with a massive release of energy in the form of heat and light. Through fusion, stars convert the simplest element hydrogen into helium, lithium, beryllium, and so on through the periodic table of elements. This process, *nucleosynthesis*, creates chemical elements six (carbon) through 26 (iron). Elements heavier than iron are the products of stars which explode into supernovae. A supernova explosion releases a huge amount of energy, with much higher temperatures, allowing fusion into heavier elements – usually within the first few seconds. In these first few seconds, a shock wave blows off a star's outer layers and compresses its core.

Most of Earth's elements – iron, silicon, carbon, etc. – and its atmosphere are all matter cast off from the Sun as it cooled over billions of years. These elements, in turn, have been "recycled" from early stars which gave birth to our third-generation Sun. That's why the lyrics of Joni Mitchell's *Woodstock* are so poignant – they're true. We really are "stardust"; everything on Earth, including you, is a product of cosmic "dust" cast off by the Sun and similar celestial bodies. In a very real sense, you were born from the death of an exploding star.

But an object has to reach a certain mass so that its gravity can force atomic nuclei together, overcoming the repulsion of electromagnetic forces. If the ratio between gravity and electromagnetism were significantly smaller, the stars would burn too hot, exhausting all their fuel much too quickly. Life would never have a chance to develop.

ε (Epsilon), is the proportion of mass which gets converted into energy when hydrogen atoms fuse within a star, becoming helium. The value, says Dr. Rees, is 0.007. If this number were smaller, nuclear fusion could not occur, and hydrogen atoms would never be able to fuse into helium.

(Epsilon) defines how firmly atomic nuclei bind together and how all the atoms on Earth were made. Its value controls the power from the Sun and, more sensitively, how stars transmute hydrogen into all the atoms of the periodic table.

Carbon and oxygen are common, whereas gold and uranium are rare, because of what happens in the stars. If Є were 0.006 or 0.008, we could not exist.

This is a measure of nuclear efficiency. If it were 0.006, the only matter in the universe would be hydrogen gas. Hydrogen couldn't fuse to form helium, and stars would have been unable to create carbon, iron, and other heavier elements which ultimately allowed life to form. Had that number been 0.008, protons would have fused during the Big Bang, leaving no hydrogen to fuel the stars.

Ω (Omega), is the amount of matter in the universe. This density is approximately 0.3. Were it higher, it would have long ago reached *critical density,* overcoming expansive energy and causing the universe to collapse upon itself. Omega also sets limits on the speed at which the universe expands. If ordinary matter's density were too high, the universe would have collapsed early, but if its density were lower, the universe would have expanded far too quickly for stars or galaxies to have formed.

λ (Lambda), represents the cosmological constant, the energy present in seemingly empty space. This may be the source of the cosmic "antigravity" or repulsive force physicists are referring to as dark energy, driving the universe's expansion at an observable, accelerating rate. The force is said to be about 0.7. If the number were smaller, itwould not be much of an issue, but if it were much larger, again the universe would have expanded much too rapidly for stars or galaxies to have formed.

This is the cosmological constant first proposed by Einstein as a means of explaining the relative stability of the universe. When Caltech astronomer Edwin Hubble announced in 1929 discovery of a "red shift" of light from distant stars, evidence that the universe is expanding, Einstein called his idea the "biggest blunder of his life". History, however, has shown that he was likely correct after all, and in fact, this value may well decide the ultimate fate of the universe itself.

Q represents a ratio between the energy stored in matter at its resting state versus the force of gravity. The value, which is constantly about 1/100,000, allowed the formation of everything in the known universe. Were it a lot smaller, gases would have never condensed to form galaxies. Were it slightly smaller, galaxies would be formless and *inert* (incapable of action, motion, or resistance); too large, and stars would swiftly collapse into black holes, bathing the universe in deadly gamma radiation.

D is the number of dimensions in normal space – height, width and depth. There are only three. If there were more (on a large scale), planetary orbits would be unstable; if there were only two, life could not exist.

Those are the minimal conditions for the universe to exist as it is. But life as we know it has five additional very specific requirements:

- *A very narrow range of pH (acid to alkaline balance)*
- *A very narrow range of temperatures*
- *Water*
- *A constant energy source*
- *A very narrow range of ion concentrations*

In Earth's environment, all of these conditions vary from moment to moment, hour to hour, day to day, and season to season, and the adaptability of creatures to these changes is the heart of *natural selection,* the main process underlying evolution.

Living organisms maintain internal stability by adjusting to these variations – the process American physiologist Walter Cannon first called *homeostasis* (biological balance). Homeostasis is the critical balance regulated primarily by your liver, kidneys, and central nervous system (in turn controlled by the *hypothalamus, autonomic nervous system* and hormone-driven *endocrine system,* about which you'll learn later).

These internal conditions are not absolutely stable, but fluctuate to a slight degree above and below *set points.* For the human body, those set points include a temperature of 99.4 degrees F (37.4 degrees C) and a blood pH between 7.35 and 7.45.

So what *is* pH? Combining two Hydrogen atoms with one Oxygen atom creates water, vital to life on Earth. Water covers 70% of the planet's surface, and comprises about 60% of the human adult body. In other words, you are mostly water – a combination of hydrogen and oxygen. Because it dissolves substances better than any other liquid, it is very useful for the transport of chemicals and nutrients between and within living cells.

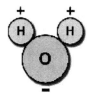 Within a water molecule, positively-charged hydrogen atoms are on one side of the oxygen atom, so water molecules are slightly positively charged on the hydrogen side and negatively charged on the oxygen side. Because opposite electrical charges attract, water molecules are therefore attracted to each other, creating a sort of molecular "stickiness".

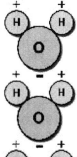 However, a water molecule can also separate into a single positively-charged *hydrogen ion* (H+) and a negatively-charged *hydroxide ion* (OH-). The concentration of hydrogen ions is called *pH*, short for *potential Hydrogen.* The greater the concentration of hydrogen ions, the more *acidic* a liquid is; the fewer the hydrogen ions, the more *alkaline* (base) a liquid is. Acids add hydrogen protons, while bases absorb them.

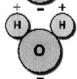 Thus, the pH scale measures a liquid's degree of positively-charged hydrogen ions, its acidity or alkalinity on a scale from zero to fourteen – zero is pure acid, fourteen is pure alkaline, and seven is neutral, the pH of pure water. Alkaline substances will absorb hydrogen ions, while acid substances will not.

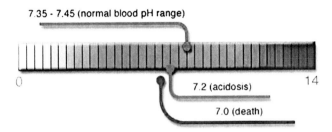

pH. US Geological Survey, 2009, public domain

The pH scale is *logarithmic*, meaning each unit in the scale represents an increase or decrease by a factor of ten. This means, for example, a substance with a pH of 6 is a thousand times more acidic than one with a pH of 3 (10x10x10).

Blood pH is one of the most critical balances the human body needs to maintain. If it's between 7.35 and 7.45, it allows an adequate supply of oxygen in the blood to feed the body's cells. But even slight decreases in pH can cause blood oxygen levels to drop, starving the cells of oxygen.

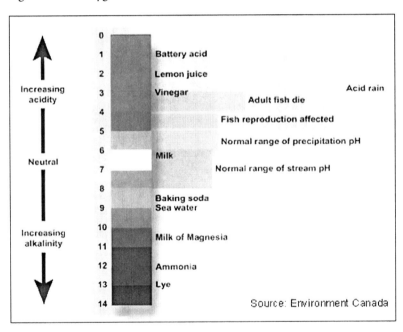

pH below 7.35 is the life-threatening state of *acidosis*, and pH above 7.45 is the equally dangerous condition called *alkalosis*. In both conditions, *proteins* (molecules that are the building blocks of life) *denature* (fall apart), and *enzymes* (special reusable proteins which control chemical reactions) lose the ability to function. Humans can only live a few hours if blood pH falls below 7.0 or rises above 7.7; greater deviations are very quickly fatal.

The huamn brain and body keep blood pH within a strict range of 7.35 to 7.45 (slightly alkaline), and most other living organisms depend upon a similar pH balance to sustain life. Because of this vulnerability, unfortunately, human fossil fuel consumption is a serious danger to the Earth's ecosystem: burning fossil fuels like coal releases gases into the upper atmosphere; these gases combine with rainwater, changing its composition to *acid rain*. Governments have instituted antipollution laws to protect the air and drinking water supply, but cleaner energy sources – such as solar power – are always a better option (as Spain has demonstrated with its five-unit *Solnova Solar Power Station*, currently supplying nearly half a million homes with clean, emission-free energy).

Temperature

Although clothing, shelter and modern heating allow us to maintain our core body temperature within about one degree of 99.4 degrees F, if that temperature falls below 91 degrees F (33 Celsius), *hypothermia* and death can quickly result; if it rises above 108 degrees (42 degrees Celsius), *hyperthermia* will quickly kill the victim.

The shape and flexibility of protein *enzyme* molecules usually dictates their function. They work like chemical keys upon chemical locks called *substrates* (the substances they chemically change). When temperatures drop, energy drops, and enzyme processes slow to a halt. Extremely low temperatures have a more dramatic larger-scale effect, ripping membranes, cells and tissues apart, because water expands as it freezes.

When temperatures grow too high, the rate of enzyme reactions increases, and at extremely high temperatures, these enzymes eventually *denature,* completely losing their structure. In other words, enzymes, the chemical structures which are the basis of all life, require an extremely narrow temperature range, which is neither too hot nor too cold, so the balance between shape, flexibility and molecular function can be maintained. Extremely high temperatures also eventually rupture cell membranes, and tissue damage results.

The Earth maintains stable temperatures in a most novel and serendipitous way: when temperatures become too high, tiny ocean algae called *zooxanthellae* remove greenhouse gases from the air, providing energy for growing coral reefs. When temperatures drop too far, these coral reefs die, and volcanoes circulate more carbon dioxide into the atmosphere. These systems ensure the stable temperatures that allow the presence of liquid oceans over the billions of years needed to incubate life.

4.5 billion years ago, the Earth was struck by an object the size of Mars, which tilted its *axis* (the point upon which it rotates), giving us our seasons and the Moon. The Moon slowed Earth's rotation from a six-hour day to a 24-hour one and stabilized Earth's axial tilt. This was most fortunate for us, because, without seasons, modern civilization almost certainly couldn't have arisen.

In a world without seasons, we wouldn't have been able to grow staple crops such as wheat. Humans would never have advanced past small, scattered settlements, scrounging for survival and often dying of horrific insect-borne diseases.

Earth without an axial tilt would be divided into climate bands which become progressively colder further from the equator, creating permanent ice ages in the poles, and a permanent band of global desert at the equator. Humanity would be forced to live within the tropical and temperate midbands. The humid tropics would be continuously beaten down by rainfall, which would wash away any fertile soil, forcing a nomadic life of ever-shifting agriculture upon unfortunate survivors.

To worsen matters, pathogens and tropical insects which thrive in warm, humid conditions would run rampant, unchecked by the winters which keep them at bay in our world today. This would be devastating not just to humans, but also to any crops and livestock. *Human mortality and morbidity rates (due directly to disease and indirectly to hunger) would go through the roof*, according to McGill University ecological anthropologist Don Attwood.

Cool or cold winters are essential for many of mankind's most important staple crops, including wheat, corn, maize, potatoes, oats and barley.

Water

As Earth was forming, Jupiter's and Saturn's gravitational influence propelled nearby icy bodies toward Earth, supplying it with water for its oceans.

This water is essential to life. It's used internally by all life forms to transport nutrients, and to cool tissue through evaporation. Plants, fungi and bacteria also use water to maintain *turgor,* the interior pressure that holds cell shape, and animals use water to remove waste and enable *cellular respiration* (the extraction of energy from food). Too little water results in dehydration and death within a matter of days.

Earth is just the right distance from the sun to allow water to exist without evaporating or freezing. If we were 50% closer or farther away, Earth would probably be unable to sustain life – at least as we know it.

Energy

In the sun's core, tremendous gravity and temperatures of hundreds of millions of degrees overcome the mutually repellent forces between protons, which carry the same positive charge. This compresses hydrogen atoms, which fuse to form *deuterium*, then *helium-3*, and finally *helium-4* atoms in a three-step process, releasing massive bursts of energy in the form of *gamma rays* – high-energy *oscillating* (vibrating) packets of light called photons.

These gamma rays push outward from the sun's core, their energy being absorbed and re-ernitted from atom to atom as they travel through the sun. This gradually saps gamma ray energy, until what escapes, streaming off the solar surface, are primarily lower-energy photons oscillating at much lower frequencies – constituting the visible light spectrum.

These photons reach Earth's atmosphere approximately 8.33 minutes later, where a thin layer of ozone (O_3 molecules) absorbs the highest-energy portion of sunlight radiation, preventing photons oscillating in the ultraviolet range from reaching the surface of the planet. Were it not for this thin layer of protection, intense radiation from the sun would quickly sterilize the planet of all life.

The remaining portion of sunlight – photons oscillating between the rapid, visible blue, and the slow, invisible infrared light range – powers nearly all life on Earth. Through *photosynthesis*, plants trap energy from the sun's photons in large chained molecules called *polysaccharides*, better known as *plant starch*, the basis of nutrition supplied from the bottom of the food chain. In other words, with the exception of *extremophiles* (microorganisms which can derive life energy from volcanic heat or chemical reactions), all life on Earth is run by solar power.

This is the most critical element driving the development of life – a steady energy source. For life on Earth, that energy source is the sun. Animals on Earth transform food into a molecule called ATP, a fuel which drives all the complex functions of living cells. ATP is continuously recycled throughout the day, with humans churning through 70 to 100 kilograms of ATP a day.

This ATP production is driven by special proteins called enzymes, biological catalysts which have been fine-tuned over billions of years to the point at which they can extract every last *joule* of usable energy from chemical reactions.

Photosynthesis – the trapping of light energy in the bonds of complex plant starch molecules – is much too complex a process to have powered the first primitive life forms. But by examining the DNA of simple cells, we can deduce that the earliest life forms harvested energy and carbon from hydrogen and carbon dioxide – H_2 reacts with CO_2 with an energy release to produce organic molecules. Such chemical reactions are common in geothermal vents, which were the most likely birthplaces of Earth's first life forms.

Extraordinary Luck

Were the Earth's orbit only slightly different, or the sun too large or small, life could not exist here. Were we without a *magnetosphere* (a protective shield formed by solar winds and the Earth's magnetic fields) and an *ozone layer* (a thin blanket of triple-oxygen molecules in the upper atmosphere that filters out highly-energized ultraviolet light) to protect us, solar radiation would quickly destroy all life. Additionally, our gravity is just sufficient to hold both us and our atmosphere to the planet's surface without crushing us.

Stars with the chemical composition of our sun are born cool, only gradually warming through chemical changes. This means our sun's output was originally 25 to 30 percent lower than today, and Earth should have spent the first half of its life as a frozen ball of rock. However, fossil and geological records clearly show Earth was watery and habitable from the outset, giving organic molecules and single-celled organisms billions of years to evolve within a hospitable climate. This mystery of Earth's warm early years is known as the *faint young sun paradox*. Exotic theories exist to explain it, though the majority believe greenhouse gases insulated the early Earth's surface.

Today, Earth's atmosphere has a balance of Nitrogen (78%), Oxygen (21%), and Carbon Dioxide (1%) in the right proportions to sustain complex life, providing a hospitable climate, liquid water, and protection against radiation from the Sun.

Galaxy centers are host to supermassive black holes, which devour space-time, and throughout the universe, dying stars are collapsing and exploding into supernovas, emitting ozone-destroying and life-eradicating bursts of gamma rays, and incinerating everything for hundreds of millions of miles around, before burning out or collapsing into superdense *neutron stars*. Fortunately, the nearest known candidate to Earth is *IK Pegasi*, 150 light years away.

In fact, Earth is in a very favorable location about halfway from the galaxy's core; if we were closer, radiation or a massive black hole could destroy us. We are also sufficiently far from the spiral arms of the Milky Way Galaxy so that deadly supernovas and star formations cannot destroy us.

It takes an enormous amount of time for organisms to evolve into, for example, velociraptors or pterodactyls. During these billions of years, Earth has suffered remarkably few large asteroid impacts. This is because of its proximity to the gas giant Jupiter, whose enormous gravitational field pulls in most wayward asteroids and comets; it's been estimated that, without Jupiter, Earth would have been struck at a 10,000-fold higher rate. In other words, Jupiter's proximity has ensured Earth's relative stability for the billions of years needed for the evolution of intelligence from single-celled life.

That evolution really began in earnest about two billion years ago, when a simple bacterial cell ended up being absorbed within a larger host, then growing and dividing. These inner cells-within-cells went through a natural selection process, becoming gradually more and more efficient as tiny ATP power generators, known as *cellular mitochondria*.

The highly efficient, mutually-beneficial accident allowed the "host cell" to grow in sophistication, accumulating more complex DNA, the genetic raw material which would lead to the evolution of complex multicellular life. The genetic record shows this symbiotic fusing only occurred once on Earth – all multicellular organisms share DNA from a common ancestor. Thus, complex life apparently arose as the result of a single extraordinary event – a single host cell absorbing another.

Our luck seems so extreme, one cannot help but wonder if a deliberate force may be behind it. Then again, it could be argued that if the universe HADN'T developed in this manner, we wouldn't be here to observe it. Thus, no matter how improbable a life-accommodating universe might be, it happened, and that's why we're able to observe it. In fact, many scientists believe life cannot *help* but arise naturally. Among them is Dr. Nick Lane of University College London, who suggests that primitive life forms are almost certainly plentiful throughout the universe, noting that:

Simple cells are built from the most ubiquitous of materials – water, rock and CO_2
– and they are thermodynamically close to inevitable. Their early appearance on
Earth, far from being a statistical quirk, is exactly what we would expect.

But the fact that *humans* are here at all appears to be a particularly extraordinary stroke of luck: 99% of all species that have ever lived have gone extinct. In fact, the Earth has undergone at least five mass extinction events that destroyed 75% of all species alive at the time.

So does all this mean a great "hand of God" has been at work to set things in motion and assure your personal survival? The evidence wouldn't seem to support it, though a purely speculative case could be built for a *universal consciousness*, a matter to be addressed later in this chapter.

It's Alive!

What are the odds of life arising – here or elsewhere?

To attempt to answer that question, in 1961, the founder of *SETI – the Search for Extraterrestrial Intelligence* – astronomer Frank Drake devised the *Drake Equation* to estimate the number of technological civilizations in the Milky Way galaxy (N) with whom we could make contact.

It's written as $N = R^* \bullet f_p \bullet n_e \bullet f_l \bullet f_i \bullet f_c \bullet L$

   R = *rate of stars formed per year*

   f_p = *fraction of stars with planets*

   n_e = *average number of habitable planets per star system*

   f_l = *fraction of planets on which life actually begins*

   f_i = *fraction of life forms that develop intelligence*

   f_c = *fraction of life forms that develop communications technology*

   L = *longevity of civilizations (during which they send detectable signals)*

Based on Hubble Telescope observations, astronomers conservatively estimate the number of *exoplanets* (planets beyond the solar system) lying within the habitable zones of their parent stars (a product of the first three terms $R^* \bullet f_p \bullet n_e$) to be about *500 million in our galaxy alone*. In fact, at the American Association for the Advancement of Science, Kepler chief scientist William Borucki announced in 2011, "...there is a rich ocean of planets out there to explore. For every two stars we are seeing a candidate planet."

The latter four terms in the Drake Equation – the percentage of planets with life, intelligence, and currently operating communications technology – are still open to debate. Discovering life elsewhere within our solar system, however, will mean that life arises easily, and that it is abundant in the universe.

Related to the Drake Equation is the *Fermi Paradox*, which asks the question "So where are they?" – in other words, there's a contradiction between the apparently high number of possible candidates for intelligent civilizations and the complete lack of conclusive evidence for those civilizations.

The age of the universe and the huge number of stars indicate that unless Earth is unique to an amazingly profound degree, extraterrestrial life should be common, and among it, intelligent life. In our galaxy alone, there are billions of stars likely to have Earth-like planets, and if Earth is typical, intelligent life should have evolved and developed interstellar travel on at least some other planets. Interstellar travel would naturally be followed by rapid colonization of entire galaxies. Thus, Earth should have already been colonized, or at least visited.

However, there is no convincing evidence of such visitation or colonization, in our galaxy or over 80 billion other galaxies in the observable universe. This led Fermi to pose the question "Where is everybody?"

Some suggest alien life may well exist without our knowledge, even in forms we cannot currently recognize. It's also been suggested that the window of time in which intelligent civilization exists is so small that it either occurred long before or will occur long after human civilization. Intelligent life may be either very rare, or very short-lived. Others argue that human civilization is alone, and that the conditions necessary to give rise to intelligent life are unique to Earth. Perhaps life is indeed abundant, but the evolutionary "accidents" which specifically gave rise to complex multicellular life and intelligence may be very rare.

Some believe technological civilizations inevitably destroy themselves shortly after developing advanced space flight and communications technology, or are so potentially threatened by others that alien life may wish to hide its existence. Radio signals may even be an entirely inappropriate, primitive signalling method.

Then again, SETI has only been searching for signs of extraterrestrial life since 1984 – a mere eyeblink in the 13.7-billion-year life of the universe. Still, over the last decade, NASA has been quietly assembling compelling evidence that life probably exists scattered across the cosmos. They've discovered a lake buried under Antarctic ice for the last 2,800 years that's "teeming with bacteria", and they've found life flourishing in near-boiling water so acidic it eats through metal. They've discovered amino acids – the building blocks of proteins – in meteorites and comet debris here on Earth.

Meanwhile, the number of exoplanets in the habitable zone of distant stars we've found is growing daily – As of January, 2013, 854 exoplanets within 673 planetary systems had been confirmed. Another 2,320 were awaiting confirmation. In the Milky Way galaxy alone, every star may have at least one planet, resulting in an estimated 100-400 billion in total, including an Earth-sized planet orbiting Alpha Centauri, our nearest stellar neighbor.

Researchers have also found tremendous caches of water on Mars, traces of it in moon rocks, and even evidence of water and organic molecules in the permanently shadowed polar regions of Mercury, the barren ball of rock orbiting closest to the sun. In fact, water, a primary prerequisite for life (at least as we know it) turns out to be "...one of the most abundant molecules in the universe".

One of the most startling discoveries of 2011 was the universe's largest known water reservoir in a quasar 12 billion light years from Earth. This titanic mass of water vapor is estimated to hold at least 140 trillion times the water of all Earth's oceans combined, bound up in the *APM 08279+5255 quasar* – a superbright galaxy cluster being consumed by a supermassive black hole at its core.

In August 2012, Chilean astronomers also discovered the sugar compound *glycolaldehyde* in orbit about a sunlike star approximately 400 light-years from Earth. Two months later, Parisian astronomers discovered over 2,000 Earth oceans' worth of water vapor in the Taurus constellation.

While none of these findings necessarily add up to the existence of *intelligent* aliens, they definitely suggest an abundance of life likely exists throughout the universe.

Spooky

"Those who are not shocked when they first come across quantum theory cannot possibly have understood it." – Niels Bohr, Nobel winner, Physics and Beyond, 1971

"Curiouser and curiouser!" cried Alice (she was so much surprised, that for the moment, she quite forgot how to speak good English). – Lewis Carroll, Alice's Adventures in Wonderland, 1865

"A human being is a part of the whole, called by us "universe", a part limited in time and space. He experiences himself, his thoughts and feelings as something separated from the rest – a kind of optical delusion of his consciousness. The striving to free oneself from this delusion is the one issue of true religion. Not to nourish the delusion, but to try to overcome it is the way to reach the attainable measure of peace of mind." – Albert Einstein, letter to Robert S. Marcus, whose son had died of polio, 1950

Within the last 40 years, modern physics has repeatedly demonstrated some surprising things about the nature of reality; for example:

- The fabric of reality is essentially "fuzzy" – at the level of sub-atomic particles, the location of objects can only be estimated, described in terms of probabilities.

- Subatomic particles appear able to exist in multiple states *simultaneously*, (e.g. spinning in opposite directions and/or existing in two different energy states at the same time).

- At times, a single particle appears to exist in two – or more – locations at the same time

- Formerly paired particles can influence the state of their "partners" over any distance when moved apart. This *quantum entanglement* defies known laws of space and time.

Albert Einstein called such quantum entanglement *spooky action at a distance* – two objects influencing each other's behavior across space, without communicating through any known means.

This aspect of quantum theory has bothered physicists since its initial discovery, with its predictions of seemingly impossible things – two or more entangled particles instantly influencing each other after separation.

The behavior violates logic: when measuring one entangled particle with a magnetic 'spin' pointing up, quantum physics predicts its partner will point in the opposite direction, wherever this partner may be. Logically, such seemingly coordinated behavior must stem from either an advance "arrangement" or synchronization via a signal between both particles.

Bell Inequality Tests have consistently shown since the 1960s that no "prior arrangements" determine the fate between two entangled particles, so physicists still hoping for a logical answer are searching instead for some sort of entangled-particle communication.

Any such signals, however, would need to travel at over 10,000 times the speed of light to account for this mutual simultaneous influence on spin direction. Einstein's equations, however, say that nothing can travel faster than the speed of light, a constant that has been repeatedly demonstrated in real-world applications.

So either quantum entanglement requires faster-than-light communication, violating a long-standing successful model of reality (upon which much of modern technology is built), or quantum entanglement's remote mutual influence is infinitely fast – unaffected by time itself. This would require a universe which is *nonlocal* – with every bit of matter in the universe constantly and instantly connected to every other bit, no matter where.

Dr. Dean Radin, psychologist, engineer and author of *Entangled Minds,* says that quantum entanglement means the fabric of reality is bound by entangled threads that are nonlocal – interconnections through space and time that bind all things to one another. This causes everything in the universe to act together *holistically* – as a unit.

Duality

About 25 years ago, I had the chance to interview Sir Roger Penrose, one of the modern giants of science, who, together with Steven Hawking co-developed the theories that led to the discovery of black holes. As Sir Penrose puts it, "The maddening part of that problem is that the ability of particles to exist in two places at once is not a mere theoretical abstraction. It is a very real aspect of how the subatomic world works, and it has been experimentally confirmed many times over. One of the clearest demonstrations comes from a classic physics setup called the double-slit experiment."

In this often-repeated experiment, physicists at the Weizmann Institute of Science demonstrated that an electron beam can behave as either a stream of matter or waves of energy, and that it apparently changes its behavior depending on whether it is being observed or not.

In 1927, Nobel Prize-winning physicist Werner Heisenberg, and his former teacher Niels Bohr arrived at the conclusion that quantum-level particles don't exist in a single state at any given moment, but in all possible states simultaneously. The total of all possible states in which a quantum object can exist is called its *wave function*, and an object existing in multiple possible states at once is in its *superposition*.

Bohr said when we observe a quantum particle, we alter its behavior, through this observation *collapsing* its superposition and forcing it to exist in one from among all possible states contained in its wave function.

The experiment to which Penrose was referring demonstrates this principle at work: While an observer is watching, an electron will pass through a single opening, but, when unobserved, it will move as an energy wave, "vibrating" through the opening. The BBC has filmed a demonstration of the experiment, available online at Youtube.

The Cat That Was and Wasn't Dead

One of the most puzzling problems facing modern quantum physics theories is this central paradox of how elementary particles like photons can simultaneously exist in multiple states until the point of being observed.

In 1935, Austrian physicist Dr. Erwin Schrödinger illustrated the improbability of the situation with a famous thought experiment: a cat is placed into a box with a radioactive particle, a Geiger counter, and a vial of poisonous gas. If the particle decays, shedding radioactive energy, the Geiger counter triggers a release of poison gas, killing the cat. If there is little or no nuclear decay, the poison-gas vial remains intact, and the cat survives. The question is, when the box is opened, do you find a live cat or a dead one? According to accepted theories of physics, you could have both – at the same time.

This absurd paradox illustrates the central problem with quantum mechanics theory – forcing us to either conclude that A) matter works much differently on the subatomic scale than it does in the observable world; or B) something is wrong with the theory itself, even though it has led to many scientific advances over the last century.

Most physicists resolve the paradox by saying that observation "collapses" particles into a single state, but this still raises troubling questions, such as: if there is more than one observer, which one is entitled to cause the collapse? and where does the border lie between the laws of the subatomic world, in which these paradoxical states (superpositions) can exist, and the observable world, in which they cannot?

In other words, at the quantum level, it seems that objects are not really definable until they're observed – it seems particles don't actually resolve themselves into a single, measurable state unless they're being observed, and return to a multiple set of *potential* states when they're not.

In 1996, Dr. Christopher Monroe and colleagues Dawn Meekhof, Brian King and David Wineland at the National Institute of Standards and Technology in Boulder, Colorado cooled a single beryllium ion to near absolute zero, trapping it in a magnetic field and bringing it to a near motionless state. Stripped of two outer electrons, the ion's single remaining outer electron could be in two quantum states, having either an "up" or "down" spin. Using lasers, the team applied a tiny force one way to induce an "up" state in the electron, then in the opposite direction to induce rapid oscillation between both the "up" and "down" spins.

The electron was induced to spin in both orientations simultaneously – in what physicists call a "superposition". The team then used lasers to gently nudge the two states apart physically, without collapsing them to a single entity, so that the two states of the single electron were separated in space by 83 nanometers, 11 times the size of the original ion.

In other words, while the old proverb says "You can't have your cake and eat it, too", or perhaps, "You can't be in two places at the same time", it appears that, at least on the quantum scale, you certainly can. Schrödinger's cat is alive and well... dead. Simultaneously.

We Can't Be Certain

In 2010, in a darkened laboratory at the University of California Santa Barbara, a tiny metal paddle the width of a human hair was refrigerated, and a vacuum created in a special bell jar. The paddle was then plucked like a tuning fork and observed, as it simultaneously moved and stood still. Superposition was being directly observed – objects in the visible world existing in multiple places and states simultaneously.

In quantum mechanics, there is an inherent uncertainty to reality; the location of an electron can never be precisely pinpointed at any moment in its orbit. Instead, its position can only be predicted in terms of probability.

According to some physicists, if there are a thousand possibilities, eventually all thousand possibilities will occur, and so, at the quantum level, the outcome of experiments cannot be 100% predicted. All things are only based on probabilities.

A great deal of modern technology works upon the paradoxical principles of quantum physics, but this seems to contradict everyday common sense – when we observe objects in the real world, they always exist in only one place and one state at a time. Quantum physicists call this paradox the *measurement problem*, and have long resolve it by saying that particles collapse into single states at the time of observation. But in the 1950s, some physicists first began to hypothesize that in fact *all possible states exist, separating into different realities at the moment of change.*

Infinite Realities

Wave function collapse is the point at which a particle existing in several potential states resolves into a single state. Some physicists now believe that at this moment, reality branches off into every one of these potential states, and our path of reality simply continues along the path we've observed. And this *Many-Worlds theory* means that an infinite number of alternate realities exist.

Quantum physicist Hugh Everett says that this is because a quantum particle doesn't collapse into a measurable state, but actually causes a split in reality, with a universe existing for every possible state of the object. Superposition, he asserts, actually means parallel worlds exist – one arising anew out of each of a particle's states.

For example, photons beamed through double-slits strike an opposing surface in both single streams and in spread-out wave patterns, depending upon whether or not they're being observed. When the particle is observed, it functions as a particle; but when it's not observed, it acts like a wave. At the moment of observation, according to Dr. Everett's Many-Worlds theory, the universe splits, and both results occur, but in different realities.

Objects you can observe can thus exist simultaneously in parallel universes – the reality in which *you* continue, and those alternate ones in which the *other yous* exist. This implies that anytime alternative actions can be taken, the universe splits into alternate realities, where each decision was taken.

According to Berkeley's Dr. Raphael Bousso and Stanford's Dr. Leonard Susskind (among others), this means an infinitely expanding range of multiple universes exists, some with distinctly different laws of physics than the ones governing ours. Our reality is one *causal patch* among an infinite number of others.

Every conceivable possibility eventually comes to pass in one of these infinite realities and perhaps information from separate causal patches of reality can *leak across* between universes. Although the specifics of parallel universes are still in question, a great deal of evidence suggests their existence, reality splitting into an infinite number of paths for every event occurring in space-time. Every possibility is thus eventually realized.

The Matter of Consciousness – and Vice Versa

"We cannot live for ourselves alone. Our lives are connected by a thousand invisible threads, and along these sympathetic fibers, our actions run as causes and return to us as results." – Herman Melville, Moby Dick, 1851

"All things by immortal power,
Near and Far
Hiddenly
To each other linked are,
That thou canst not stir a flower
Without troubling of a star."
– Francis Thompson, New Poems, 1897

Drifting away from the realm of science into speculation about things that cannot be falsified, it's been suggested that the Universe contains energy linking you, the Sun, ice crystals trailing comets in the Oort Cloud at the edge of our Solar System, and the clouds of stellar gas and dust some 13 billion light-years away at the very edge of what Stephen Hawking says is the great bubble of space and time that makes up our universe.

The evidence, it could be speculated, lies in the demonstrable principle of quantum entanglement. The measurable phenomenon of quantum entanglement (two formerly-paired particles changing in harmony nearly instantaneously – no matter what the distance) seems to demonstrate quite clearly that very real connections outside of normal time and space can exist between particles.

If entangled particles have been repeatedly shown to have connections outside of normal space-time in this manner, it's not much of a stretch to suggest that particles everywhere have a similar fundamental, underlying connection.

In fact, in 1927, French physicist Louis de Broglie, one of the founders of modern quantum physics, first developed a solution to the measurement problem with his *pilot wave theory*. The same theory was later developed independently by physicist David Bohm in 1952. Many contemporary physicists believe the measurement problem – the demonstrable property of subatomic particles to collapse into one state or the other when observed – has always been satisfactorily solved by pilot wave theory.

According to pilot wave theory (also known as Bohmian Mechanics), a universal connecting energy called a *pilot wave* is instantly everywhere in the universe at once, guiding subatomic particle movement. This theory applies to the entire universe, positing that a pilot wave guides the motion and behavior of all particles in the universe simultaneously at every instant – and the motion of every single particle depends on the positions and behavior of every other particle in the universe.

This leads to an astonishing conclusion: every particle in the universe affects every other particle in the entire universe, and, conversely, the whole configuration of the universe affects and is affected by the behavior of any one particle – an interdependence that, on a personal level, implies that everything you do has an effect on everyone and everything else in the universe.

British theoretical physicists Dr. Antony Valentini and Dr. Mike Towler of Cambridge University organized a physics conference in 2010 to discuss these theories, which they believe to be very much correct.

Rejection of pilot wave theory, say Dr. Valenti and many of his peers, has limited our understanding of the fundamental nature of reality. This guiding wave would explain the troubling *Copenhagen Interpretation* – which says that elementary particles are both – and neither – particles and waves, suddenly collapsing into one of the two states at the moment of being observed. Perhaps, if there is indeed such a thing as a universal consciousness, its secret lies within the principles of pilot wave theory.

Reality – Or a Reasonable Facsimile Thereof

"Reality is merely an illusion, albeit a very persistent one." – Albert Einstein

Here are a few final things to consider about the nature of what we collectively define as reality:

- *Gravity doesn't pull objects together. According to Einstein, massive objects actually curve space and time. Objects aren't pulled by an instantaneous invisible force, but follow the curves massive objects create in space-time.*

- *Relativity shows that even time itself is "relative" to one's point of reference, capable of speeding up or slowing down, depending upon such things as one's subjective gravity and the speed at which one is moving.*

- *All time may exist simultaneously – past, present and future, although we see it as progressing from the past into the future*

- *We never see actual objects, only the light reflected from them.*

- *None of us sees colors exactly the same way – your interpretation of "red" is going to be different from mine.*

- *Seemingly solid objects are, at the fundamental level, in constant motion and flux, and quite possibly nothing more than energy at the tiniest level.*

So if *reality itself* is so tenuous and subjective, upon what standard *can* we rely?

The Platonic Ideal

2,500 years ago, across the sea, in the ancient Greek capital of Athens, lived a teacher named Plato. A formidable visionary of his time, he founded the Academy, the first university in history, and wrote of the teachings of his mentor Socrates, and his own thoughts about those teachings.

His philosophy later came to be known as *Platonism*, which teaches that what we see, hear and feel – what people collectively call reality – is not the highest form of what is real. Paradoxically, the ultimate destiny of what we believe to be real – material items – is that they erode, decay, rust, fall to pieces, and their elements scatter randomly.

On the other hand, mathematics is eternal, unchanging (one plus one will always equal two), and exists outside of time and space, in human consciousness. In this sense, it can be said to occupy a "higher reality". Thus, the desk beneath your hands feels solid, but because it cannot last forever, it's arguably less real than the perfect Truth of human thought.

Consider the matter another way: think about your commute today. Think of the people around you. They looked bored, tired, and probably not a single one of them was memorable in any way. The key word is that they are uninspired.

The sad truth is that 99.99% of the human race spends every waking moment blindly, ignorantly sleepwalking. The things to which most people attach importance are a shiny new car, fancy new clothes, the approval of peers, making the boss happy, meeting the next deadline.

Most people have thus fallen into a trap from which they will almost certainly – sadly – never escape. They are slaves to what pioneering psychologist Karen Horney called *the tyranny of the shoulds*, doomed to live out their lives in trying to meet expectations placed upon them, often by themselves.

Think about David Cross in the Sales Department, whose boss says "You've GOT to get that report on my desk by MONDAY at 9 am!" That deadline becomes David's world. He believes (unnecessarily) that if he doesn't meet that deadline, a disaster will ensue.

In truth, that sales report, and in fact all of David's work is utterly, completely meaningless in the great, long view of time. If David misses his deadline, his boss may lose his temper, and poor David may feel horrible stress. But by next week, do you think either one will spend much time thinking about this?

And in a year, it's quite likely everyone will have forgotten the matter. In thirty years, there's an excellent chance the company will no longer exist. And in two hundred, nobody will even remember the company's name. All that intense worry and effort was wasted energy, serving no truly significant purpose.

Now please look down at your desk. At this moment in time it's solid, hard, and substantial. If you rap it hard with your knuckles, you can confirm this. But the very matter within it is mostly empty space, and in constant flux. What's more, in twenty years, it will likely be in pieces. In a thousand, it will have been buried, and in perhaps ten thousand years, your desk will be dust. So what outlasts the material world of cars, shoes, desks, factories?

It's the power of human thought. A vision, a dream holds the power to launch an army that changes the face of history, or to build a monument that lasts four thousand years. As Plato taught, the realm of the ideal – of thought – is the higher reality – the only reality able to transcend time and space.

❖ *A typical brick has a mass of 2.3 kg, a volume of 1,230 cubic centimeters and a density of 1.84 grams per cubic centimeter. If we say the molar mass of the clay is 258, we can multiply it by Avogadro's constant – the number of atoms in a mole of any substance is 6.022 x 10^23 atoms. We find 1553.7 * 1,000,000,000,000,000,000,000,000 or 1.5 octillion atoms in a typical brick.*

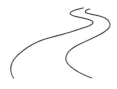

Origins

"The amino acid glycine, a fundamental building block of proteins, has been found in
a comet for the first time, bolstering the theory that raw ingredients of
life arrived on Earth from outer space, scientists said on Monday."
—Steve Gorman, Reuters News Agency, Aug 18, 2009

"We are a way for the cosmos to know itself. We are creatures of the
cosmos and always hunger to know our origins, to understand our
connection with the universe." – Carl Sagan, Cosmos, 1980

"...it is clear that you, like many others, view God as the Creator of the Universe. I respect that
view. I find it baffling, however, that someone can worship God as the all-mighty Creator while,
at the same time, denying even the possibility (not to mention the overwhelming evidence)
that God's Creation involved evolution. It is as though a person thinks that God
must have the same limitations when it comes to creation as a person
who is unable to understand, or even attempt to understand, the
world in which we live. Isn't that view insulting to God?"
– Richard Lenski, rebuttal, 2008

"Although the vast majority of evolutionary change took place before any human being was born,
some examples are so fast that we can see evolution happening with our own eyes during
one human lifetime." – Richard Dawkins, "The Greatest Show on Earth", 2009

Stardust

Astronomers sometimes call comets "dirty snowballs" – chunks of frozen gases and water, dust and rock ten miles or more in diameter. They usually orbit the Sun within the distant *Oort cloud*, a spherical band of comets surrounding the solar system a light-year out from the Sun. Periodically, one breaks free and hurtles inward toward the Sun.

Much closer is the massive asteroid ring called the *Kuiper belt*, a region of the solar system extending 30 *astral units* – 30 times the average distance between Earth and the Sun – from the orbit of Neptune to 50 astral units out from the Sun.

Most scientists now agree that it was these wayward cosmic missiles that jumpstarted life on Earth, seeding its primordial oceans with the precursors to life. In 2011, NASA laid out its strongest case to date for the theory that cosmic bombardment deposited the key ingredients for life on Earth billions of years ago:

Amino acids are the building blocks of *proteins*, the workhorse molecules of life, used in everything from skin cells to the *enzymes* which speed up or regulate chemical reactions in living organisms. One – the amino acid *glycine* – was found in comet samples from NASA's Stardust mission in 2009. But this wasn't the first time signs of life from outer space had been found. 50 years earlier, scientists had discovered amino acids in *meteorites*, remnants of asteroids which fall to Earth. That early discovery opened the field of *astrobiology*, which seeks to answer the age-old question of whether life exists elsewhere in the Universe. By 2011, amino acids had been found in over a dozen meteorites.

In 2012, NASA exobiologist Dr. Jennifer G. Blank ran a series of experiments to determine whether or not these amino acids could realistically have survived the searing heat and pulverizing shock waves of a descent through the Earth's atmosphere.

Her team employed powerful gas guns and computer models to recreate the effects of a comet entering the Earth's atmosphere at nearly 25,000 miles per hour, and then slamming into its surface.

Her team bombarded mixtures of amino acids, water and other materials with supersonic, high-pressure blasts of gas. Not only did the amino acids survive the heat and shock, they began to form the *peptide bonds* which link amino acids into proteins.

Dr. Blank adds that there were probably multiple deliveries of such biological precursors over billions of years from comets, asteroids and meteorites:

> *Our research shows that the building blocks of life could, indeed, have remained intact despite the tremendous shock wave and other violent conditions in a comet impact. Comets really would have been the ideal packages for delivering ingredients for the chemical evolution thought to have resulted in life. We like the comet delivery scenario because it includes all of the ingredients for life – amino acids, water and energy.*

3.8 billion years ago, a *late heavy bombardment* of comets and asteroids repeatedly struck the planets of the early solar system, including the Earth, forming visible craters like those we see on the moon today.

Prior to this era, the Earth's surface had been too hot for known life forms to survive, but fossils show life began to appear right around the era of bombardment.

Related experiments at Princeton, the University of Arizona and the Centro de Astrobiología (CAB) in Spain add further weight to the *panspermia* scenario, in which Earth was "seeded" with life from space.

The international team believes that alien microorganisms embedded in fragments of distant planets sprouted life on Earth. They say life probably arrived on Earth – and then spread to other planets – during the infancy of the solar system, when Earth and planetary neighbors orbiting other stars were close enough to exchange solid material.

This is the *lithopanspermia* theory, which says that primitive life forms are distributed throughout the Universe by planetary fragments hurled into space by volcanic eruptions and planetary collisions. Fragments are propelled into space, drifting until they are pulled in by the gravity of another planetary system, where they deposit their living cargo.

Using the star cluster in which our sun was born as a model, the team has simulated lower speed transfers of solid material to show that, out of the boulders ejected from the solar system and its closest neighbor, about nine out of every 10,000 could have been captured by the other.

During the first hundreds of millions of years of the universe, our Sun was one of a tight-knit star cluster full of planetary systems. The research team says the solar system and our nearest planetary-system neighbor may have swapped rocks *100 trillion times* well before the sun migrated from its native star cluster.

Existing biological finds on meteorites show that basic life forms could indeed date back from the time of the sun's birth cluster and have been tough enough to survive interstellar travel and impact.

Computer simulations show microorganisms can survive from 12 to 500 *million years*, depending upon the mass of the object hosting them, and that, given the calculated distance, mass and velocities of the ancient stars and planets, about 300 million lithopanspermia events may have occurred between the solar system and its closest ancient planetary neighbors. This also suggests, of course, that Earth may have seeded life on other planets.

Ideal lithopanspermia conditions existed for several hundred million years, when the early solar system and Earth resided within the sun's birth cluster, and rock evidence suggests Earth contained surface water at a time when weak gravity boundaries existed between the sun and its closest cluster neighbors. Such low gravity and early slow orbits allowed "weak transfer" of materials between planetary systems. This also coincides with high meteorite activity in the solar system, because of the early sun's weak gravity.

Everywhere

In July 2011, a very special meteorite landed in the Moroccan desert. The *Tissint meteorite*, discovered by the University of Alberta's Dr. Chris Herd, contained traces of gases which matched samples of the Mars atmosphere collected by the 1976 NASA Viking lander mission.

It's a plum-sized chunk of 600-million-year-old volcanic rock, struck from the surface of the Red Planet by an asteroid close to a million years ago. Tiny cracks and fissures in the rock were instantly sealed shut by the impact's heat, trapping tiny pockets of ancient Martian atmosphere within.

Most remarkably, however, weathering on the rock shows that water was present on the Mars surface sometime within the past few hundred million years.

And that water appears to have been rather balmy at one time. A joint research project by the University of Leicester and The Open University found additional evidence of water on Mars, at temperatures ranging from 50 to 150°C – warm enough to support life. Even at the upper extreme, these are temperatures such as those around volcanic thermal vents in Yellowstone National Park, where terrestrial microbes currently thrive.

According to lead investigator Dr. John Bridges, numerous Mars rocks have been retrieved which contain small mineral veins formed by hot water near the Martian surface. This is but one of several recent analyses showing the amount of water which existed on Mars is much larger than previously realized, similar to Earth's. Which of course means that, whether or not it actually did, Mars could well have supported life. Which in turn means that, out of the dizzyingly huge numbers said to exist in the Universe, countless other planets must have been able to as well.

Setting the Record Straight

It's both interesting and disturbing to watch the reaction that the mere mention of evolution evokes in Western fundamentalists. It's also sad – the American fundamentalist war on science only serves to hold back progress and weaken the country's global competitiveness.

Such animosity toward science is also surprising, considering so much science, including evolution, is based upon the findings of devout clergymen. Take for example Georges Lemaître, the priest, astronomer and professor of physics who first realized and taught that the universe began with the Big Bang. Others include Nobel prizewinner Max Planck, the father of Quantum mechanics; Nobel Prizewinner Robert Millikan, who advanced the study of evolution; and Gregor Mendel, the Czech abbot who launched the science of modern genetics through his observations of trait inheritance in pea plants.

Evolution is just the mechanism through which populations adapt to their environments – maximizing their chances of survival. If a chance mutation results in a physical or behavioral trait that helps a creature better adjust to its environment, that creature stands a better chance of surviving and passing its genes on to future generations.

In the 1830s, Charles Darwin first noted how Galapagos Island finches, sometimes separated by only a few hundred meters, developed distinctly different beaks. Their shapes had physically altered over generations in response to environmental and dietary changes.

Darwin wasn't the first to propose evolution as the force driving life's diversity and complexity; 19th century French soldier-aristocrat Jean-Baptiste Lamarck had earlier outlined a theory of the transmutation of species. But Darwin's *On the Origin of Species* brought the ideas to the mainstream public.

So what is the evidence that life on Earth evolved through a series of gradual structural and biological modifications? Visually, the most immediately striking evidence is provided by *homologies* – characteristics shared between widely divergent animal species because of common ancestry. There are three types:

- *morphological homologies* – shared anatomical structures

- *ontogenetic homologies* – shared stages of embryonic development

- *molecular homologies* – shared DNA, RNA and proteins

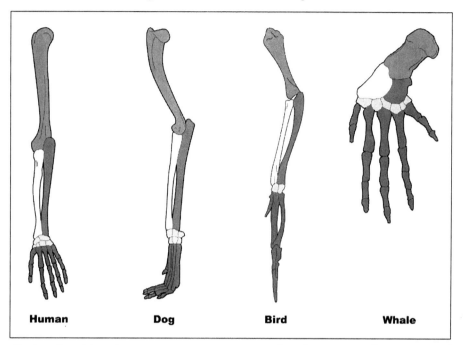

Human   **Dog**   **Bird**   **Whale**

Charles Darwin's primary argument in support of evolution was the existence of **homologous structures** *between species. These striking similarities are particularly easy to spot in skeletal formation: throughout the animal kingdom, forelimbs consist of a long* **humerus** *bone extending from the shoulder, connecting to two parallel arm bones – the* **radius** *and* **ulna** *– which bend at the elbow. Homologous bone structures are also found in the wrists and digits, all signs pointing to a common ancestry. Such common ancestry is represented in* **phylogenetic** *diagrams (evolutionary trees). The tree's root is the ancestor, the branch tips represent its descendants and moving from the root to the tips represents the progression of time. This occurs as the result of* **speciation events**, *when an organism with distinctly different new traits emerges from the split of an ancestral lineage into branches.*

Not only are limbs among *vertebrates* (spined, skeleton-bearing animals) similar, but the same fundamental genetic, neural and physiological structures appear everywhere in nature, in a very clear progression of biological sophistication– from worms and molluscs through fish, amphibians, reptiles, birds and mammals.

By comparing embryonic development, the evolutionary relationships between animals becomes even clearer. This study of *ontogeny* (from the Greek words for *beginning* and *existence*) is quite convincing; as evolutionary biologist Ernst Mayr first pointed out in *What Evolution Is*, if evolution is untrue, "why should the embryos of birds and mammals develop gill slits, like fish embryos?"

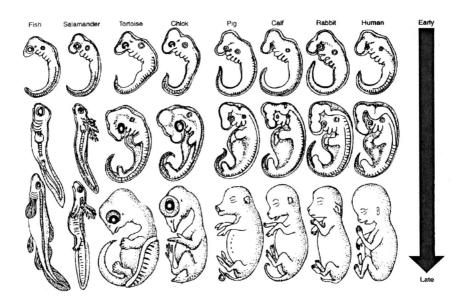

Comparative embryonic development, J. G. Bach after Haeckel, Anthropogenie, October 1, 1874.

On a molecular level, hemoglobin is a blood protein common among many animals, which transports oxygen to cells. Like all proteins, it's built of polypeptides, chained amino acids. Many hemoglobin amino acid sequences are shared between species, and the closer the relationship, the greater the similarities become, in a clear progression:

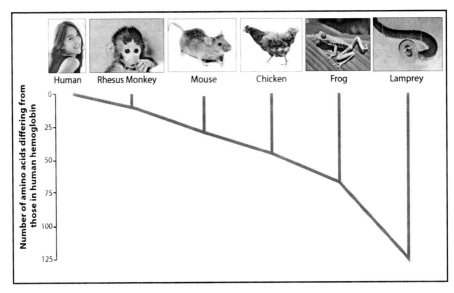

A much more sobering recent example of rapid natural selection is found in the disastrous consequences of corporate *factory farms* feeding antibiotics to their livestock. An estimated 70 to 80% of antibiotic use in the US is attributed to feeding livestock.

Corporate agricultural interests claim this practice is to prevent the spread of infections among severely overcrowded pens and cages (euphemistically referred to as *concentrated animal-feeding operations* or CAFOs), but in 2001, the Union of Concerned Scientists said that 70 percent of the antibiotics were used simply to boost profits; for reasons yet unclear, antibiotics fatten up livestock.

The consequences have been deadly; bacteria have very quickly evolved antibiotic resistance, resulting in deadly *superbugs* immune to our strongest medical defenses. When consumers eat the meat of animals fed these antibiotics, it creates the perfect incubation conditions for a bacterial resistance.

According to the Food and Drug Administration, approximately *100,000 Americans die yearly from antibiotic-resistant bacterial infections contracted in hospitals, and an even greater number die from superbug infections contracted outside hospitals.*

Although the FDA has been trying to ban the use of certain critical antibiotics in agriculture, American corporate agribusiness has formidable financial muscle with which to leverage federal politicians. To date, the FDA's efforts at ensuring public safety have been met with frighteningly little success.

Evolution in Action: The Lizards of Pod Mrcaru

Two small islands lie just to the northeast of Croatia, called *Pod Kopiste* and *Pod Mrcaru*. Pod Kopiste originally had a population of common Mediterranean wall lizards (*Podarcis sicula*), while Pod Mrcaru, just 4.2 km away, had none.

In 1971, Israeli biologist Eviatar Nevo transported five wall lizard male-female pairs from Pod Kopiste to Pod Mrcaru for experimentation. On their native island of Pod Kopiste, these lizards dined on insects which were easily found scurrying about the bare rocks, but on Pod Mrcaru, scrubs and grasses are abundant, making insects much harder to find.

Nevo's field observations were abruptly interrupted when civil war broke out in Yugoslavia, but 33 years later, a separate Belgian research team returned to an electrifying discovery: the lizards of Pod Mrcaru had evolved completely new digestive systems to accommodate the local diet within just three decades, breeding by the thousands, and wiping out the indigenous lizard population.

Their jaws had also transformed, allowing for stronger biting, and their territorial defense behaviors had vanished. They had completely adapted, both physically and behaviorally, within the span of just three decades. When the new Pod Mrcaru lizard descendants were compared with the original Pod Kopiste lineage, striking anatomical differences were observed: Longer, wider and taller heads, with much stronger jaw muscles, necessary for a stronger bite to accommodate a plant-based diet.

Animals typically can't digest the tough cellulose fiber of plant cell walls, so herbivorous animals have evolved a digestive pouch called a *cecum* at the entry to the large in-

57

testine. The cecum houses digestive bacteria, acting as a fermentation chamber which breaks down plant cellulose for digestion. In humans, the *appendix* is a vestige of the cecum from our early, more vegetarian human ancestors.

Prior to being transplanted, the wall lizards were insectivores, with digestive systems unsuited for plant diets, but because their new habitat offered few easily obtainable edible insects, they developed a completely new evolutionary feature – cecal valves, special muscles which slow digestion, allowing time to ferment the cellulose fiber of plant cell walls.

Peppered Moths

Another classic example of lightning-fast natural selection came from Darwin's own era. As 19th century England ushered in the industrial age, giant factories sprang up everywhere across the countryside. With no anti-pollution laws, great clouds of toxic, coal-burning smoke and other pollutants soon boiled over the skies of London and Manchester, and soot began to cover surfaces everywhere, including the trees.

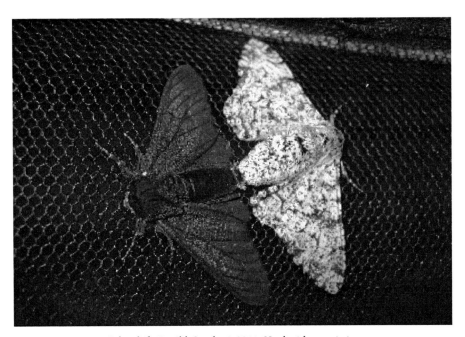

Color shift, Dr. Ilik Saccheri, 2011. Used with permission

Peppered moths had long ago evolved to camouflage themselves against the region's indigenous lichen and tree trunks, offering protection from being eaten by birds. But as soot began to turn everything black, some peppered moths adapted incredibly rapidly, their wings turning the color of soot-covered trees. Those moths which were darkest survived and bred, while those that were still light-colored stood out starkly against the sooty trees and were soon eaten by birds.

The first sightings of soot-colored peppered moths began in 1848 near Manchester. Within 50 years, 98 percent of all England's peppered moths had adapted new colors. The same phenomenon was soon noticed in America and continental Europe, as moths everywhere adapted to the widespread pollution of the Industrial Revolution.

For the peppered moth, the color change was triggered by a single mutation. In 2007, Liverpool geneticist Ilik Saccheri found the gene responsible for the color change in the DNA region which programs *melanism*, an increase in dark pigmentation. This single, special region of DNA exists in every butterfly and moth species, leading to thousands of different colors and patterns which mimic everything from false eyes to the colors of nastier-tasting bugs.

Amazingly, with the advent of clean air laws, when air quality was restored in Britain, sooty peppered moths have nearly vanished. Peppered moths have reverted back to their former speckled white, to once again blend in with the natural surroundings.

Australian three-toed skinks

These lizards normally lay eggs, but some living in mountainous regions have begun giving live birth – researchers think this protects their young from predators in the comparatively treacherous mountain environments.

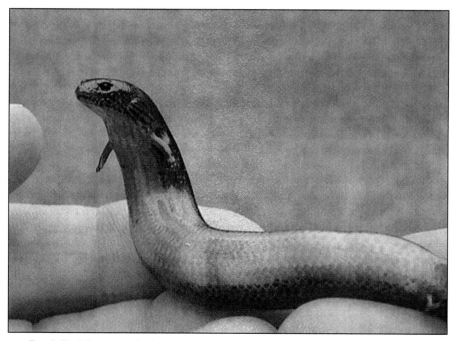

A yellow-bellied three-toed skink carries embryos, light areas visible from within its body. Rebecca A. Pyles; used with permission.

*What constitutes a **science**? According to the US National Academy of Sciences, science is "...the use of evidence to construct testable explanations and predictions of natural phenomena, as well as the knowledge generated through this process".*

***Paleontology**, the scientific study of prehistoric life, began soon after Danish Catholic bishop and scientist Nicolas Steno realized in 1666 that so-called "tongue stones" embedded in rock were actually ancient shark's teeth. This discovery helped revolutionize thinking about ancient Earth. Soon after, in the 1700s, Swedish biologist Carl Linnaeus began his life's work of systematically naming, ranking, and classifying animals by species.*

Recipe for a Fossil

Most creatures' remains don't leave fossil traces because they're quickly eaten after death by scavenging animals, insects, bacteria and fungi; soft-bodied creatures simply dissolve, leaving no trace.

However, in some cases, carcasses are covered in sediment too quickly to decompose or be devoured. Water can seep into the pores of bone and shell, filling the spaces with mineral deposits. Over thousands of years, as sediment accumulates, layers build, weighing down the material underneath, pressing and compacting sediment particles together. Meanwhile, water passing through spaces between the particles helps cement them even more firmly together. Thus, through compacting and cementing, animal remains and the surrounding sediment all fossilize, hardening into rock.

By analyzing the fossil chemistry, researchers can determine an animal's diet and environment. Trace chemical deposits and signs of wear on fossilized teeth show what creatures fed upon. The size and shape of bones reveal additional facts – eating, locomotive and reproductive methods, as well as the age of the creature at death.

Additional traces of life are sometimes found in the form of tiny organic molecules which leave telltale signs after billions of years. While DNA decays, disappearing from fossils within about a million years, *lipids* – oily molecules used in cell membranes – are carbon chains studded primarily with hydrogen, oxygen and traces of nitrogen, which don't dissolve in water. When a creature dies, its cells rupture, spreading lipids into the sediment, where chemical reactions leach out the oxygen and hydrogen, leaving telltale carbon chains of a sort only produced by living cells.

Setting a Date

Layers of accumulated sediment are a one method of calculating fossil age, but geologists and paleontologists can also measure radioactivity levels to calculate the age of rocks and fossils. Carbon-12 is a "standard" form of carbon, accounting for 98.89% of the element on Earth. Carbon-12 has six protons, six neutrons and six electrons, and is thus a balanced, stable atom – not subject to radioactive decay from the weak force.

Heavier forms of carbon also exist – *isotopes* like carbon-14, which contain additional neutrons. Carbon-14 accounts for only about one-tenth of a percent of the Earth's carbon. It's formed when high energy charged particles called *cosmic rays* strike the nuclei of atoms in the Earth's atmosphere, knocking out high-energy neutrons. These neutrons are captured by nitrogen, the predominant gas in our atmosphere, causing a proton to be ejected, which creates carbon-14.

Carbon-14 naturally binds with oxygen, forming carbon dioxide, which plants breathe and incorporate into their tissues. When animals eat tissues containing carbon-14, they absorb a little with each meal. After death, the carbon-14 they have absorbed breaks down, returning into stable nitrogen at a known rate, over thousands of years.

Carbon-14 has six protons and eight neutrons, something of an imbalance, and undergoes beta decay, shedding an electron and an antineutrino to transform an "extra" neutron into a proton. The strength of this beta decay (electron emission) can be measured with special Geiger counters.

It decreases at a known rate, called a *half-life*. The half-life of carbon-14 is 5,730 years, so every 5,730 years, half the carbon-14 atoms decay into stable nitrogen-14, shedding measurable levels of beta radiation – electrons – in the process.

Carbon-14 testing is used to determine the age of organic material up to about 50,000 years old, including charcoal from ancient fires, wood used for building or tools, bones, seeds, cloth, hide, or leather. It doesn't work on inorganic matter like stone tools or ceramic pottery. This *radiocarbon dating* method can be used on fossils up to about 50,000 years – after which the electron emission levels become too low to detect.

To determine the age of the rocks in which *fossils* are found, scientists instead measure the radioactivity of an element which decays much more slowly – the soft greyish-white metal called *rubidium-87*, which decays into the stable element strontium-87, with a half-life of 49 billion years – over three times the age of the universe. (This, by the way, makes rubidium a *primordial isotope* – an element which has remained unchanged since the supernova explosion which gave birth to the solar system.

Weighing the Evidence

Dr. Michael Shermer, author of the bestseller *Why Darwin Matters*, was a devout evangelical Christian before becoming one of evolution's strongest proponents. In the online radio broadcast The Skeptical Perspective, he says half of Americans today completely refuse to accept the well-established science.

People, he points out, tend to form beliefs first, and then look for evidence to support it. And because the human brain has developed to organize information in patterns, people easily fall prey to *apophenia* – finding deceptively meaningful but completely imaginary patterns in randomness; and to *agenticity* – attributing those patterns they see to invisible forces or spiritual beings. Some fear that believing in natural selection means life has no meaning, or that death may be simply the end of one's existence.

Evolution is perhaps the most solidly substantiated natural process in all of science, knowledge about the process rests upon a deep and wide base of merging and mutually-confirming cross-disciplinary evidence – anatomical, chemical, genetic, paleontological and more. Through these separate disciplines, scientists have gradually pieced together biological origins to such a precise degree that it can now be said confidently that the science of evolution is established fact and to argue otherwise is nonsense. *

Genetics experiments alone can be used to turn specific genes on or off, thereby triggering the growth of specific limbs and organs from ancient ancestors, or from future descendants. Such processes are used on a daily basis in medicine and agriculture – confirming Darwin's theories beyond the shadow of a doubt.

Fundamentalists also argue that life is so complex and well-constructed it cannot have arisen through natural processes. However, it both can and does, as one famous experiment clearly demonstrates:

A Special Brew

For all the breathtaking diversity of life on Earth, its living organisms are built almost entirely from only four classes of *organic compounds* – chemicals which all share the element carbon: *carbohydrates, lipids, proteins,* and *nucleic acids.* These are formed from about 50 relatively simple organic *monomer* (subunit) molecules, strung into repeating chain molecules called *polymers.*

Monomers are linked by removing a water molecule in the process called *dehydration synthesis.* Here, a *hydroxyl group* (-OH ion) is removed from the end of one monomer, and a hydrogen ion (-H) from the end of the other, using *enzymes* (proteins which initiate or speed up chemical reactions). The exposed ends of the two monomers carry opposite charges, causing them to bond. In this way, monomers join into a growing polymer chain. To split polymers back into simpler monomers, a water molecule is added, in the process called *hydrolysis.* Hydrolysis is the first step in breaking down food for digestion, for example.

Thus, life processes consist of an ongoing cycle of breaking down polymers (*catabolic metabolism*), then using the extracted energy and monomers to build new polymers (*anabolic metabolism*).

Hydrocarbons are polymers made from energy-dense hydrogen/carbon bonds – combustible fuels like propane, butane and octane. These are the fuels which run our machines. Similarly, *carbohydrates* are polymers of energy-dense hydrogen/carbon bonds, but are more complex, with the addition of oxygen. Carbohydrates form multiples of the formula CH_2O, from the monomer *glucose* – plant sugar. Just as hydrocarbons fuel our machines, glucose fuels living organisms.

Plants manufacture glucose during photosynthesis, and stockpile what they don't immediately need. Unused glucose is linked into the polymer *starch (amylopectin).* This *polysaccharide* (multiple sugar molecule) is stored as granules in cellular containers called *amyloplasts.* Energy can be extracted from starch again later by hydrolysis – the addition of a water molecule – which again breaks the polymer down into glucose monomers.

Humans and other animals also digest plant cells, extracting the starch and breaking it down into glucose through hydrolysis. However, instead of starch, animals store the polysaccharide *glycogen* as granules in muscle and liver cells, where the cell's energy factories called *mitochondria* can break it back down again and convert it into energy as needed. The human body can only store enough glycogen to last for about 24 hours, after the supply must be replenished by eating.

Lipids are a diverse group of *hydrophobic* (water-repellent) organic molecules that share the common property of being unable to mix with water. Because the weakly negative hydrogen side and the weakly positive oxygen side of water molecules attract each other, they "push away" hydrogen atoms on the outer surface of lipid molecules.

Just like hydrocarbons and carbohydrates, lipids like *fats* and *oils* are very energy-dense molecules, with the energy stored in multiple hydrogen-carbon bonds. Because of the bonds within them, fat molecules can be packed densely together, and so become solid more easily than oils at room temperature.

Oils have a "kink" in their molecules, meaning they don't stack as easily, and stay liquid at room temperature. Because plants don't need to move, bulkier lipid molecules are not a problem, but animals need mobility, and so evolved the ability to store excess glucose as fat, a much more compact form of molecular storage.

Nucleic acids – DNA and RNA – also constitute storage molecules, in this case storing information on how to assemble living organisms. *Proteins* are the most complex molecules known, and their assembly and functions will be dealt with in the following section.

These organic compounds are typically created by living creatures, but on their own, they tend to be fragile in Earth's oxygen-rich atmosphere. This is because oxygen *oxidizes* molecules – leeching electrons, leading to a kind of molecular decomposition. This is why metals rust and fruits and vegetables spoil. This wasn't always true however – the early Earth atmosphere wasn't as oxygen-rich. It originally consisted of hydrogen, methane, ammonia and water vapor.

Abiogenesis is the science of how early life arose on ancient Earth. The most famous experiment related to its study was conducted in 1953 by University of Chicago graduate student Stanley Miller, under the guidance of Nobel Prize-winning biologist Dr. Harold Urey.

Miller and Urey wanted to find out whether or not life could spontaneously occur under the atmospheric conditions which existed on Earth 4 billion years ago. Their question was, "Could organic chemicals – those found in living creatures – be created from purely inorganic elements, given early-Earth conditions?"

To find out, they sealed water, methane, ammonia, and hydrogen inside a loop of sterilized glass tubes and flasks. One flask in the loop was half-full of water, which was heated to create atmospheric vapor. A second flask contained a pair of electrodes across which an electrical spark would simulate atmospheric lightning. The cooled water vapor would then condense and trickle back into the loop, where samples could be collected.

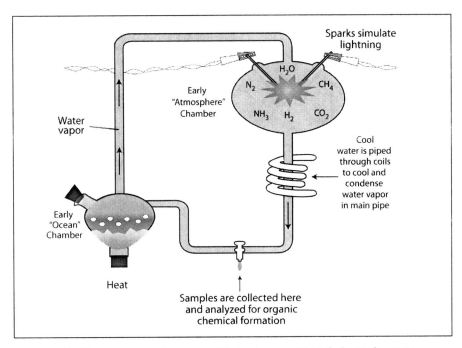

Miller-Urey experimental apparatus. Illustration copyright Polyglot Studios, 2011

Within just a matter of days, a full range of carbohydrates, lipids, amino and nucleic acids spontaneously formed in large quantities under these easily replicable conditions. Thus, under early-Earth conditions, organic compounds were shown to spontaneously form from inorganic materials. Numerous modern follow-up studies have duplicated the results, making it clear the chemical foundations of life can spontaneously emerge under atmospheric conditions which exist in abundance throughout the universe.

The Miller-Urey experiment proved the chemical basis of life can indeed be formed from inorganic elements, though critics argued that the atmosphere on early Earth may have been different from the gases used in the experiment.

Furthermore, to really approach what we normally define as *living systems*, organic compounds need to be organized, within a barrier protecting and separating them from inorganic compounds; this organization is the basis of a biological cell. However, notes Duke Biology Professor Dr. Stephen Nowicki, it isn't particularly difficult to coax such systems into existence; all it takes is the appropriate natural conditions.

Organic compounds, under relatively normal Earthlike conditions, naturally gather into primitive cell-like structures called *protobionts*. By simply placing them in water, lipids self-assemble into membrane-enclosed spaces, cell-like structures called *coacervates*, capable of housing organic molecules.

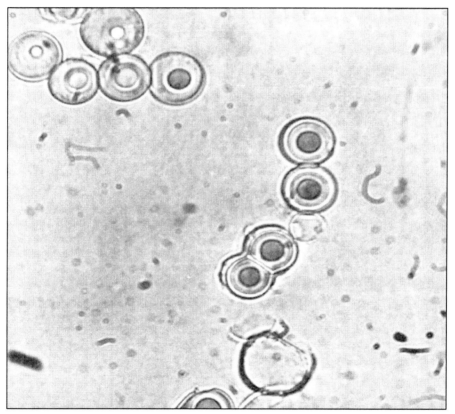

Coacervates, from In The Origin of Prebiological Systems and of their Molecular Matrices, Fox, et al, Academic Press, 1965, public domain image.

Since 2009, researchers at Cambridge University have also demonstrated that the building blocks of DNA – *nucleotides* – naturally assemble from simple molecules like the naturally-occurring three-atom combination of hydrogen, carbon, and nitrogen called *hydrogen cyanide*, found throughout the universe, including in outer space. Add two copper atoms and six cyanide molecules to water, flash it with ultraviolet light, and it triggers a series of spontaneous chemical reactions that produces key building blocks for RNA assembly. Other metals likely spur additional abiogenetic processes.

A Twist in the Tale

*"We have discovered the secret of life." – Francis Crick, Cambridge,
announcing his co-discovery of the structure of DNA, 1953*

Five simple chemicals – carbon, hydrogen, nitrogen, oxygen and phosphorous – combine to create the most interesting substances. Bonding these elements into fairly simple combinations creates four small molecules called *nucleotides – adenine, thymine, cytosine* and *guanine*.

These simple molecules pair up into interlocking units, connecting along a sugar-phosphate backbone in repeating combinations. These *polymers* – long, molecule chains of repeating subunits – are *Ribo-Nucleic acids: **ribose sugars*** in the **nucleus** of a cell inked into **acids**. *(Image: National Institutes of Health, 2012, public domain)*

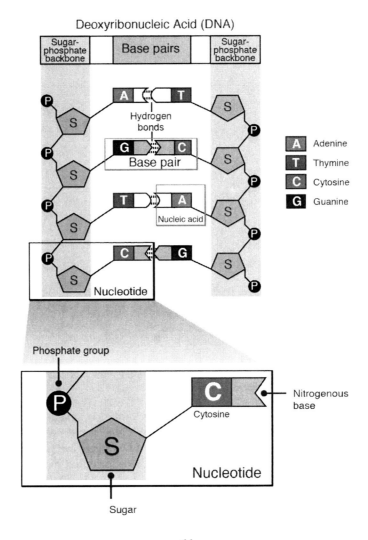

RNA is the single-strand nucleic acid, and DNA is the double-strand form. They differ in composition by one nucleotide subunit. *De-oxy* ribonucleic acid – DNA – has *deoxidized* ribose sugar – one oxygen atom missing from its ribose sugar molecule.

Ribose sugars linked by phosphate groups form RNA and DNA backbones. They join through dehydration synthesis – enzyme-driven removal of a water molecule. Polyglot Studios, 2011

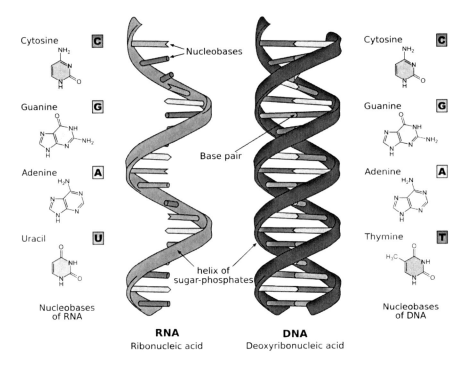

Cytosine **C**

Guanine **G**

Adenine **A**

Uracil **U**

Nucleobases
of RNA

Nucleobases

Base pair

helix of
sugar-phosphates

Cytosine **C**

Guanine **G**

Adenine **A**

Thymine **T**

Nucleobases
of DNA

RNA
Ribonucleic acid

DNA
Deoxyribonucleic acid

Wikipedia, 2009. Public domain

During *dehydration synthesis*, special proteins called *enzymes* remove a water molecule, exposing charged ends of the nucleotides, which bond together as subunits of a molecular chain called a *polymer*. These polymers can be *replicated* – copied into chains assembled from free-floating nucleotides, and then peeled away to make other special polymers called *proteins*.

Thus, nucleic acids DNA and RNA are information-carrying chemical blueprints found in cell nuclei for creating the proteins used to build every living creature from the most humble bacteria to humans.

If DNA is likened to a twisting ladder, its sides are the sugar-phosphate chains, and the rungs are nucleotide bases. These bases pair up with easily-broken hydrogen bonds, and the order in which they appear along the length is a genetic code used as instructions for creating RNAs, which in turn peel away and are used to assemble proteins.

DNA is a template for replicating itself as well as creating several kinds of RNA, the most important being mRNA, tRNA and rRNA, all used for making the tissue-building molecules called proteins.

Each DNA strand is one continuous molecule of nearly a billion nucleotide base pairs in different combinations, coiled tightly around protein spools – so tightly as to fit about one six-foot-long strand into the nuclear membrane of every cell. These coiled strands are called *chromatin*. When a cell divides and replicates, normally loosely-floating chromatin strands form gather into the microscopic configurations called *chromosomes*.

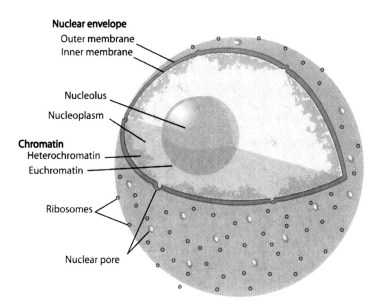

Nuclear envelope
Outer membrane
Inner membrane

Nucleolus
Nucleoplasm

Chromatin
Heterochromatin
Euchromatin

Ribosomes

Nuclear pore

Cell nucleus, Wikipedia, 2012, public domain. Once RNA has been transcribed, it leaves the nucleus through nuclear pores, and directs ribosomes in protein assembly. Heterochromatin is densely packed chromatin (DNA strands), while euchromatin is loosely packed. The nucleolus makes ribosomes from ribosomal RNA.

There are TWO DNA copying processes: *replication*, in which both strands of the DNA are separated by the enzyme *helicase* and then copied, and *transcription*, where RNA polymerase splits the DNA molecule and builds RNA, guided by a single *template strand*. Only one side of the DNA double helix holds the key information for creating customized RNA and its protein products; the other side "complements" it, closing the molecule so it remains in a stable state.

In replication, the entire molecule is copied – and only one time, but in transcription, only small regions of the length of the DNA molecule called *genes* are copied, hundreds or even thousands of times at once, depending on how much protein needs to be produced by a given gene.

The human genome is made up of about 23,000 genes – commonly-shared sequences of DNA nucleotides, all of which are made up of about 3 billion "letters" of DNA code (A, T, C, G). The *Human Genome Project* finished cataloguing all 23,000 "standard" human genes in 2003, and that data is being analyzed to help understand the causes of genetic diseases and other critical aspects of biology.

All of your DNA combined is your *genotype*, a unique code which varies individually from the standard human genome, and every nucleus of your cells contains this – all the information for creating the proteins and tissues your body needs to sustain life. Your unique variations in gene sequences make you completely different from any living organism that has ever existed before.

In 2006, Harvard University launched the **Personal Genome Project**, sequencing the genomes of 100,000 volunteers to advance the frontier science of personalized medicine, where medicines and treatments can be tailor-made specifically to treat each individual. Similarly, the **proteome** is a recently-completed database of every protein produced by human DNA; this project holds tremendous potential for the future of medicine. It's now used in several international open-access online databases.

Genes to Proteins

Genes are *expressed* when their instructions are used to build proteins. The nucleotide combinations of each gene specifies the order in which chemical subunits called amino acids are lined up and chemically bonded together to form proteins.

The smallest change in the order or expression of these genes – substituting a single base pair for another, omitting or repeating even the smallest segment – can radically change a gene's function, often resulting in developmental disorders, which arise from the production of faulty proteins.

Proteins are the most sophisticated molecules known, and all living creatures are built from them. They range from the *keratin* hardening your fingernails to the *hemoglobin proteins* carrying oxygen in 25 trillion red blood cells in your body. Proteins called *enzymes* split molecules in the food you eat, and others act as cell-to-cell or intracellular signallers.

Proteins vary in physical structure, their linear strands coiling, twisting and folding into three-dimensional molecules, with each protein's function largely dependent upon its shape. These shapes are determined by the amino acids in the chain, as they carry ionic charges which attract or repel other nearby amino acids.

Proteins are generally flexible, but at extreme temperatures, or in the presence of strong acid, alkaline or salt solutions, the molecules *denature* – losing their structure and eventually falling apart. Important proteins include:

- *Structural proteins* such as hair, skin and muscle

- *Enzymes* – chemicals ending in -*ase* which cause biochemical reactions in living cells, triggering reactions or the breakdown/formation of molecules

- *Insulin* – used by mammals for extracting energy from sugar

- *Hormones* – used to regulate balances, body functions and growth

- *Immunoglobulins* – infection-fighting proteins

- *Globins* – used by the blood to transport oxygen and carbon dioxide

- *Kinases and phosphatases* – The on-off chemical switches that regulate all cellular functions

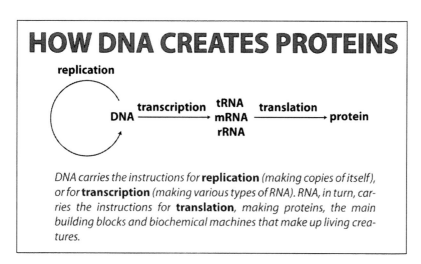

HOW DNA CREATES PROTEINS

replication

DNA —transcription→ tRNA mRNA rRNA —translation→ protein

DNA carries the instructions for **replication** *(making copies of itself), or for* **transcription** *(making various types of RNA). RNA, in turn, carries the instructions for* **translation**, *making proteins, the main building blocks and biochemical machines that make up living creatures.*

Transcription is the process in which short lengths of DNA's genetic code are copied into *messenger RNA* (mRNA); this messenger RNA moves out of a cell nucleus into the cell's *cytoplasm* (jellylike, semifluid contents). The mRNA is an information molecule made up of sequences of joined nucleotides which can be read like the tape in a cassette by cellular protein-assembly machines called *ribosomes*.

Thus, DNA and RNA molecules are cellular databases, storing the information needed to build all living creatures, from single-celled bacteria to blue whales.

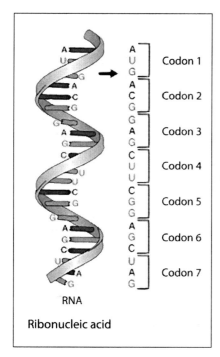

A U G | Codon 1
A C G | Codon 2
G A G | Codon 3
C U U | Codon 4
C G G | Codon 5
A G C | Codon 6
U A G | Codon 7

RNA

Ribonucleic acid

Your DNA – contained in the chromosomes of (nearly) every cell in your body – has 3 billion base pairs of the four nucleotides, in regions of varying sizes called **genes**, *each of which makes a specific RNA product.*

Triple-nucleotide combinations in the DNA sequence called **codons** *combine into genes. There are 23,000 genes, made up of 64 different possible codons, which act as genetic "words" in the "sentences" of the genes.*

The order in which codons and genes progress determines which proteins will be made, and to a large extent what type of cell will be created, such as bone, skin, nerve or tendon. A bone cell is different from a muscle cell because different genes have been switched on and off when creating them. Image: Codons, Human Genome Project, public domain

Step I: Transcription

Transcription is the synthesis of mRNA from a DNA template. The DNA strand is peeled apart, and a gene from one side, called the *template strand* (or antisense strand) is copied. This single gene may be transcribed thousands of times. After transcription, the DNA strands rejoin. This process is constantly occurring in almost every cell of your body, every moment of your life, and involves four main steps:

1. ***Preinitiation*** – A special nucleotide sequence called the *promoter* marks the starting point of a gene for transcription; it contains a sequence called a *TATA box* (named after the sequence of TATAAA nucleotide bases), located about 30 base pairs up from where transcription begins. This sequence indicates which strand will be copied, and in what direction. TATA-binding protein binds here, bending DNA, thus allowing the two strands of the double helix to separate more easily.

   An assembly of about 50 different proteins called *transcription factors* recognizes the TATA sequence, and binds to this DNA promoter region. This assembly attracts an enzyme called *RNA polymerase*, which binds to the transcription factor assembly on the DNA template strand at the region to be transcribed.

2. ***Initiation*** – The transcription factors next unwind the DNA double helix, as an enzyme called *helicase* breaks the weak hydrogen bonds joining the base pairs down the middle, unzipping the portion to be transcribed into two single strands. The protein complex then removes a molecular block in front of the RNA polymerase, enabling it to move forward.

3. ***Elongation*** – RNA polymerase moves down the template strand, reading the DNA sequence. As the polymerase travels down the template strand, nucleic acid subunits enter an intake hole in its other side, and they are matched to exposed base pairs on the DNA template strand.

   These nucleotides match up to the base pairs which they chemically compliment, and are inserted into the growing RNA chain. For every C on the DNA strand, a G is inserted in the RNA; for every G, a C; and for every T, an A. But every A on the DNA strand is matched with uracil (U) – There is no T in RNA.

   Sometimes RNA polymerase will insert an incorrect nucleotide. The enzyme will then back up, remove the incorrect nucleotide, as well as the one preceding it, and try again. As each nucleotide is added to the growing RNA polymer, phosphates acting as caps are removed, and this allows the nucleotides to bond. Sequences of As, Cs, and Gs nucleotide bases join to form a single-strand RNA molecule which snakes out of the RNA polymerase as it moves along the DNA strand. This creates a copy of the non-coding strand opposite the template, but in the RNA copy, the T (thymine) in the DNA sequence gets replaced by the closely-related nucleic acid subunit "U" (uracil).

   Multiple RNA polymerases can transcribe a single strand of DNA, and multiple rounds of transcription can take place, rapidly producing many mRNA molecules from a single gene.

Termination – The RNA polymerase moves down the DNA strand and stops after reaching the codon *termination sequence* – TAG, TAA, or TGA – codons which signal *"stop transcription"*. The newly-formed messenger RNA is then released, and the RNA polymerase molecule detaches from the DNA strand.

The newly-formed messenger RNA carries the genetic sequence needed to create one particular protein in the jellylike substance called cytoplasm that fills your cells. There, protein-assembly structures called *ribosomes* use it as a recipe to construct a protein in the process called *translation*.

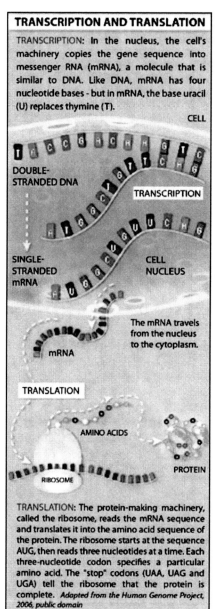

TRANSCRIPTION AND TRANSLATION

TRANSCRIPTION: In the nucleus, the cell's machinery copies the gene sequence into messenger RNA (mRNA), a molecule that is similar to DNA. Like DNA, mRNA has four nucleotide bases - but in mRNA, the base uracil (U) replaces thymine (T).

CELL

DOUBLE-STRANDED DNA

TRANSCRIPTION

SINGLE-STRANDED mRNA

CELL NUCLEUS

The mRNA travels from the nucleus to the cytoplasm.

mRNA

TRANSLATION

AMINO ACIDS

PROTEIN

RIBOSOME

TRANSLATION: The protein-making machinery, called the ribosome, reads the mRNA sequence and translates it into the amino acid sequence of the protein. The ribosome starts at the sequence AUG, then reads three nucleotides at a time. Each three-nucleotide codon specifies a particular amino acid. The "stop" codons (UAA, UAG and UGA) tell the ribosome that the protein is complete. *Adapted from the Human Genome Project, 2006, public domain*

National Institutes of Health, 2012, public domain.

Processing mRNA

Newly-transcribed mRNA has to be modified before use. *Introns*, regions which are not used to make proteins, are cut out; the remaining RNA regions are *exons*. After the intron regions are removed, the mRNA fragments are spliced together to form the final mRNA.

The *spliceosome* molecular machine usually controls splicing, but some introns are also self-splicing. In other words, RNA can act as an enzyme which cuts itself, deletes "junk" RNA sections and then splices together the remaining middle ends into new combinations.

The human genome only contains about 25,000 protein-encoding genes, but these can produce over 100,000 different proteins through *alternative splicing*, when RNA splices different combinations of exons together, creating a wide range of mRNAs. These are then translated into different proteins with different functions. *Alternative splicing* thus leads to changes in gene expression and the production of new proteins.

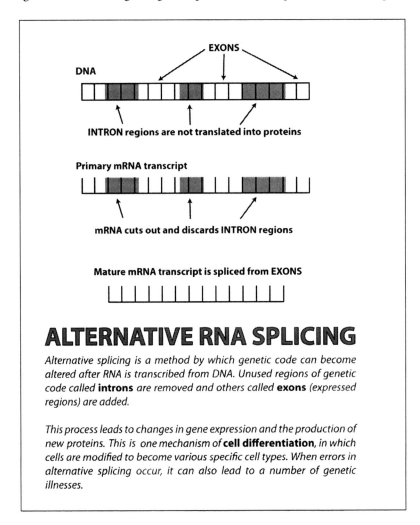

EXONS

DNA

INTRON regions are not translated into proteins

Primary mRNA transcript

mRNA cuts out and discards INTRON regions

Mature mRNA transcript is spliced from EXONS

ALTERNATIVE RNA SPLICING

Alternative splicing is a method by which genetic code can become altered after RNA is transcribed from DNA. Unused regions of genetic code called **introns** *are removed and others called* **exons** *(expressed regions) are added.*

This process leads to changes in gene expression and the production of new proteins. This is one mechanism of **cell differentiation**, *in which cells are modified to become various specific cell types. When errors in alternative splicing occur, it can also lead to a number of genetic illnesses.*

Types of RNA

Messenger RNA (mRNA) – after mRNA is copied from a gene on a DNA template strand, it carries this code out of the nucleus, into the cell's cytoplasm, where it's used as a blueprint to build a specific protein from amino acid subunits in the process called *translation*. The mRNA molecule directs assembly of the correct sequence of amino acids into the chain molecule of a specific protein.

Transfer RNA (tRNA) – tRNAs are 60 to 95 nucleotides in length. These clover leaf-shaped molecules transport amino acids to the ribosomes so they can be joined into proteins. The amino acids are joined by *dehydration synthesis* (enzyme removal of a water molecule) into a protein.

In a sense, tRNA is an interpreter which matches three-letter genetic codons of mRNA to the twenty-letter codes of amino acids. One arm of the tRNA cloverleaf is a loop of three nucleotides called the *anticodon*, which matches up to three bases of an mRNA codon. The opposite arm carries an attached amino acid "requested" by the mRNA codon.

Ribosomal RNA (rRNA) – rRNA is part of the ribosome, the protein-manufacturing organelle. Outside the nucleus, both in cytoplasm and lining the maze of membrane-covered tunnels of the *endoplasmic reticulum* are thousands of ribosomes, which automatically self-assemble when the component proteins and rRNA are present.

Step II: Translation

Outside the nucleus, mRNA is used to form proteins, so the language of RNA – nucleic acids – is *translated* into the language of proteins – amino acids. A codon of three mRNA nucleotide bases acts as a request for a specific amino acid. A cellular factory called a *ribosome* – a large assembly of proteins and rRNA – attaches to mRNA, and then slides along its strand, adding amino acids to a growing chain that eventually forms a full protein. Protein translation requires mRNAs, tRNAs, ribosomes, and energy. It occurs in three main steps:

1. *Initiation* – Proteins called *initiation factors* bind to the ribosome and align the mRNA molecule and the first tRNA carrying an amino acid into correct positions to start protein synthesis. A 3-letter anticodon on one arm of the tRNA molecule matches the 3-letter codon of the mRNA sequence. A specific tRNA carries each of the 20 different amino acids.

   An initiator tRNA molecule binds to the AUG "start" codon, delivering the first amino acid in the protein chain, and triggering the start of translation. The spent tRNA falls away, to be reused later.

2. *Elongation* – tRNAs with anticodon arms that match mRNA codons continue to deliver requested amino acids, which are lined up and bonded by enzymes in the ribosome. Enzymes then power mRNA to move through the ribosome.

3. *Termination* – The process of amino acid delivery and bonding continues until the ribosome reaches the "stop" codon on the mRNA strand (a UAA, UAG or UGA nucleotide sequence). Since no tRNA anticodons match stop codons, the process comes to a halt. A release factor protein cuts the completed protein loose, and the ribosome falls apart into subunits which can then be recycled.

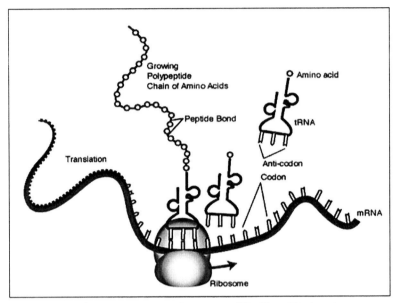

Translation, 2009, National Institutes of Health, public domain

Every cell in your body can create thousands of proteins simultaneously every second of your life. An amazing video of the process occurring in real-time can be seen in the 2003 PBS program *DNA: The Secret of Life*. The actual molecular structures, shapes and functions were programmed into a supercomputer for viewing at a visible size. It's amazing and well worth a watch – and includes the story of the race to discover DNA.

To create the animation, researchers used a technique called *electron cryomicroscopy* to capture a series of photographs of these molecules from different angles and moments in the cycle. These multiple images were then built into an animated 3D sequence of molecular activity at work in real time. You can view it online here: http://www.dnai.org/a/index.html

Mapping Life: ENCODE

There was an initial rush of excitement after the human genome was first mapped, but scientists were disappointed to discover that simply knowing which genes encoded "faulty" proteins usually wasn't enough to cure diseases; they needed to understand the controlling mechanisms involved in the process.

Multiple worldwide collaborative studies comparing the DNA of healthy people to those with specific illnesses often showed the problems weren't from "faulty" protein-

76

producing genes, but from something within the "non-coding", "junk" regions. Until recently, they had no idea why. Cutting-edge collaborative research within the EN-CODE project has revealed that, while "junk DNA" doesn't specifically express proteins, it regulates protein expression, is often the cause of illness, and helps determine physical traits like height.

If protein-expressing genes are the hardware of the DNA "computer", regulatory genes are its operating system – without these switches, the genome can't do anything. Small DNA regions – 'words' – function as docking sites for special gene-controlling proteins. These genetic operating instructions are scattered throughout the non-protein-expressing gene regions of the human genome, small chains of DNA 'words' that make up docking sites for special regulatory proteins involved in gene control. The human genome contains hundreds of genes which make such regulatory proteins.

This shouldn't have been terribly surprising, as nature tends to be rather frugal, never prone to waste precious resources like energy or complex organic molecules. The notion that 98% of the human genome served no purpose wasn't likely to stand the test of time: in 2000, when the Human Genome Project came to a close, out of the 3 billion nucleotide base pairs, researchers had identified just over 21,000 genes, of which a mere 2% contained instructions for building proteins. But a team of 442 scientists in 32 labs around the world participating in the international ENCODE project has demonstrated that between these regions, more than 10,000 of the "non-coding" genes control the protein-expressing genes, often by encoding single-strand "micro-RNAs" which help to regulate gene activity. The huge majority of our DNA doesn't encode proteins, but is instead devoted to the control of gene encoding.

This regulatory DNA affects every cell and organ in your body, throughout your lifetime, using over four million "switches", points where proteins called "transcription factors" bind to the DNA and help regulate gene expression. In this way, transcription factors determine which genes switch on or off, or act as "dimmer switches" – adjusting the "volume" of gene expression – the amount of protein created – up or down, depending upon a gene's specific function.

Such regulatory DNA also determines how a region of DNA is expressed, coaxing "undifferentiated" (uncommitted) stem cells within a developing embryo to become heart muscles, or prompting a pancreas cell to produce the blood-sugar-regulating protein called insulin after a meal, or producing a new skin cell to replace a dead one on the surface which has peeled away.

At this point, ENCODE is slowly cataloging the specific biochemical function of each switch into epigenomic maps. With a free online database available to anyone on the web, ENCODE functions as a sort of "Google Map" of these genetic switches, allowing scientists worldwide to learn what each of these variants does. This means that eventually the regulatory functions for all the key human genes will be mapped out, allowing us to manipulate them in treating any disease they may underlie. The possibilities are electrifying; 17 mutations from standard healthy human DNA affect the same two dozen transcription factors in 17 different varieties of cancer. This, says researchers, means many cancers seem to share the same cause – inherited, faulty genome control circuitry which increases the odds someone will eventually contract the disease. And learning how to manipulate these common regulatory genes may soon allow us to eradicate cancer.

As well as determining whether progenitor cells become, for example, muscle tissue or human hair, regulatory DNA can also determine your susceptibility to illnesses like diabetes, schizophrenia, autism, high blood pressure and many other conditions. In Crohn's disease, for example, a family of regulators cause the body's own immune system cells to turn upon and attack the host's own intestinal cells. Faulty regulatory genes leading to such autoimmune diseases, including lupus and rheumatoid arthritis, lie in DNA-regulating regions active only within immune cells. Those leading to cholesterol and metabolic diseases sit in DNA-regulating regions active in liver cells.

Dr. Eric Green, director of the National Human Genome Research Institute which initiated the ENCODE project, says, "By and large, we believe rare diseases may be caused by mutations in the protein [or gene-]coding region.... more common, complicated diseases may be traced to genetic changes in the switches."

The Encyclopedia for DNA Elements, or "ENCODE" for short, is a multinational, government-sponsored research project, in which scientists around the globe are sifting through the nucleotide sequences in human DNA to determine the specific function of each region.

Lead analysis coordinator Dr. Ewan Birney says, "we've shown that the human genome is simply alive with switches, turning our genes on and off and controlling when and where proteins are produced. ENCODE has taken our knowledge of the genome to the next level, and all of that knowledge is being shared openly.

"The ENCODE catalog is like Google Maps for the human genome. ENCODE maps allow researchers to inspect the chromosomes, genes, functional elements and individual nucleotides in the human genome in much the same way," according to Dr. Elise Feingold, who helped initiate the project on behalf of the US National Human Genome Research Institute.

The project allows researchers to search for which specific genes are expressed (or misexpressed) in diseases and in changing cellular functions. Researchers can then catalogue their functions, opening the door to unprecedented progress in treating and preventing diseases.

Many DNA regions linked to diseases aren't specifically used as templates for proteins, but instead act as regulatory sites. Researchers around the world are now able to freely access this database to examine how specific variants in these key regions contribute to diseases.

According to NHGRI program director Mike Pazin, Ph.D., "We expect to find that many genetic changes causing a disorder are within regulatory regions, or switches, that affect how much protein is produced or when the protein is produced, rather than affecting the structure of the protein itself. The medical condition will occur because the gene is aberrantly turned on or turned off or abnormal amounts of the protein are made. Far from being junk DNA, this regulatory DNA clearly makes important contributions to human health and disease."

By analyzing the nucleotide sequence in antibodies (natural immune responses built to "match" and destroy specific invading pathogens), researchers can purify specific matching sections of the genome, then key the nucleotide sequences into computers to find out where they're located on the DNA strand.

One of the techniques the team is using is to flash-freeze cells, enabling them to learn which specific regulatory proteins are moving to which specific regions of the DNA sequence at any given instance in a biological process they want to investigate.

ENCODE has already identified approximately 400,000 gene sequences, binding proteins and RNA segments which act as gene regulators, activating, enhancing or inhibiting genes. But this is just the beginning: Dr. Dirney estimates that only about 5% of the human genome's functions have thus far been discovered.

Expressive

Genes, as we've seen, are expressed by protein synthesis. Each gene is the template for a specific protein, which will take one of three forms: an enzyme, structural protein, or regulatory protein. The type and number of proteins expressed will determine how cells and whole creatures develop, physically and biochemically. This is a creature's *phenotype* – the observable, measurable traits that arise from the proteins its genes produce. The overall blueprint of all its genes is that creature's *genotype*.

Gene expression can be regulated at several points – during transcription of DNA into RNA, during translation of RNA into proteins, and by enzymes in the cell cytoplasm which alter mRNA after it exits the nucleus (in the case of eukaryotes). The longer mRNA remains before being dissolved by enzymes, the more proteins it can produce, and thus the greater that gene's expression. Regulatory proteins can also hasten, slow or stop translation, in this manner also influencing specific gene expression.

While geneticists previously dismissed most non-protein-producing DNA as useless artifacts – redundant genes accumulated over millions of years of evolution – now they know it regulates gene expression in ways we are only just beginning to understand. In fact, less than 1.2% of the DNA molecule is actually used to create proteins. Among the rest, some encodes tRNA, ribosomal RNA, and regulatory microRNAs. Much DNA also constitutes binding sites for regulatory components like transcription activators and repressors.

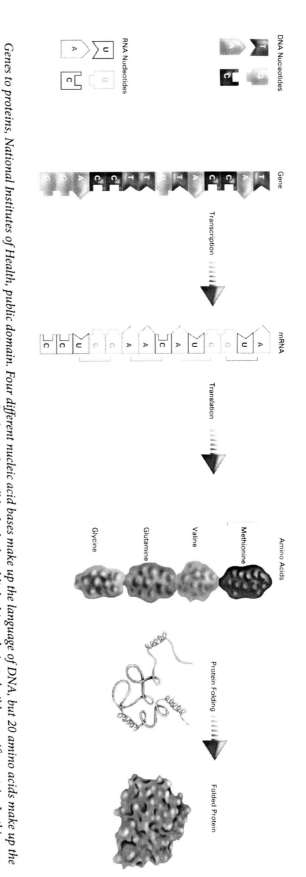

Genes to proteins, National Institutes of Health, public domain. Four different nucleic acid bases make up the language of DNA, but 20 amino acids make up the language of proteins. Each RNA codon "requests" a specific amino acid subunit that will be fetched and linked in a chain to build a specific protein. In this way, genes are the instructions that determine what proteins will be created. Special start codons (ATG in DNA, and AUG in RNA) and stop codons (TAG, TAA, or TGA in DNA and UAG, UAA or UGA in RNA) mark where each gene begins and ends. Computers are able to scan DNA base sequences and locate all these START and STOP codons — the beginnings and endings of all human genes. This is how the Human Genome Project was able to read all 23,000 genes in the human genome. We are now slowly testing how each of these functions, one by one.

Master Switches: Gene Regulation

Genes are the means by which living creatures pass down physical characteristics: DNA first synthesizes RNAs, and these RNAs direct the synthesis of proteins, the end products of genes. These proteins conduct all the biochemical processes required of living cells. But which regions of DNA are used or unused at any given moment must be strictly controlled through gene regulation. Like piano keys, genes contain the potential for creation, but must be activated in proper sequences, with precise timing, to make coherent music from chords and melodies which are harmonious.

Several hundred genes must be simultaneously regulated with precise timing, every one of them functioning perfectly for a cell to work correctly. Each gene must be activated at precisely the right moment, under the right conditions, and for the right duration – as little as 10% too much or too little protein production can result in malfunction or disease. Half of human DNA is tasked with regulating protein synthesis, over 11,000 genes involved in producing protein *transcription coregulators* which orchestrate this finely-tuned, complex process.

A complex network of these coregulators help control gene expression. Like a master pianist's hands, the "hands" which activate genetic sequences are these molecular machines, protein structures which temporarily bind to DNA, turning protein production on or off.

Since 1996, Drs. Bert O'Malley and Jun Qin of the Baylor College of Medicine have been identifying and classifying transcriptional coregulators, and found two types, *coactivators* and *corepressors*, which switch gene expression on or off. Among these are the molecular machine *Mot1*, which attaches to DNA and acts like a corkscrew, moving down the molecule's helix. As it progresses, it removes transcription factors – proteins like *TBP (TATA Box Binding Proteins)*, which bind to TATA boxes near the start of most genes.

TATA Box Binding Proteins form a kind of "kink" in the DNA chain, acting as a guidepost and platform which helps position the RNA polymerase enzyme into place. Various *initiating factor* proteins attach here and assemble into a complex that begins transcription. When these TBP positioning proteins are removed, transcription cannot proceed, and the gene is inhibited – the protein which that gene produces is not made. Thus, Mot1 regulates transcription, by removing TBPs from the DNA chain.

After Mot1 spots a TBP on the DNA strand, it attaches nearby, and begins to move downward, like a corkscrew being inserted. This detaches TBPs from the DNA, and, after this TBP removal, Mot1 then masks the spot where the TBP had been, preventing it from reoccupying the same position. Detached TBP is then free to be redistributed and bind to other gene sequences.

Looking Under the Hood

In the last decade, molecular biology has uncovered the genetic mechanisms at work in directing the physical development of animals – from which end is designated as a head or tail, to how hands are prompted to develop at the end of wrists rather than upon a creature's legs.

Such development is controlled by a genetic hierarchy, master genes at the top controlling the next level of genes, which in turn control the next, and so on. These gene hierarchies don't just give rise to certain favorable adaptations, they also inhibit the growth of others, determining not just what can and cannot emerge physically in a growing embryo, but also shaping the course of life itself.

For all its spectacular diversity, the animal kingdom evolved from a surprisingly small gene pool. Mice, for example share 80% of the same genes as humans, making them ideal for genetic studies. What drives this diversity is the group of proteins called *transcription factors* which bind to DNA and regulate gene expression.

The number of genes which encode proteins has remained fairly constant throughout evolution, but the number of regulatory DNA elements has increased dramatically.

The total number of genes in humans is about 30,000, regulated by an estimated 3,000 transcription factors, usually working in concert. This allows genes to be switched on to produce protein molecules or deactivated to suppress protein production. Activated genes can also be induced to express low levels of proteins in a limited area, or they can be "cranked up" to produce a lot of protein across multiple cells.

The genetic basis for the profound differences between species, even those with nearly identical genomes, has long puzzled scientists, but in December, 2012, a University of Toronto Faculty of Medicine research team uncovered an additional reason. After comparing hundreds of thousands of genetic sequences in *homologous organs* (organs with the same function appearing in different species) among ten different vertebrate species, ranging from humans to frogs, the team found that alternative splicing allows a single gene to produce a number of different proteins, dramatically changing the potential complexity and structure of cells, tissues and organs throughout evolution.

The very same process is thought to also underlie differences in susceptibility to disease. This, says lead author Nuno Barbosa-Morais, may one day help researchers understand why humans are prone to illnesses like Alzheimer's and cancers unknown among other species. Alternative splicing, it seems, is more complex among humans and other primates than in species like mice, chickens and frogs, providing one genetic basis for the complexity of such organs as the human brain.

A Newly-Discovered Level of Genetic Control

Another key mechanism controlling gene expression has only very recently been discovered, but it will forever change our understanding of biology.

Dr. Kohzoh Mitsuya of the University of Texas Health Science Center and Dr. Toshiaki Watanabe of the National Institute of Genetics in Japan and Yale University were the first to outline the mechanisms of *epigenetics* – the newly-emerging science of gene expression. While genes provide the code for producing proteins, chemicals called *epigenetic markers* sit atop genes and offer basic instructions to switch them on or off.

Every cell in your body – muscles, nerves, etc. – contains identical DNA. Epigenetic markers can silence certain genes and activate others, a means of controlling cell function. These chemical tags control which genes will be *expressed* (read and translated into proteins) and *suppressed* (unread and unused).

The organization of these master control patterns is like a second genetic code above the level of the DNA gene sequences themselves. Says Duke University's Dr. Randy Jirtle, a useful analogy might be to think of the genome (complete DNA code) as a computer's hardware, while the epigenome is the software that directs the hardware, telling it when, where, how and how much to work.

Through this mechanism, the DNA sequence itself doesn't change, but combinations of genes can be switched on and off, just like playing certain keys on a piano. This epigenetic modification is also reversible, making the DNA strand's instructions significantly more flexible.

Even though two creatures can share the same DNA, epigenetics can substantially alter how it is expressed. Particularly during embryonic development, environmental factors such as the mother's stress hormones and diet can radically affect the process.

DNA strands wrapped around protein spools called *histones* create tightly-packed, multiple coils resembling a length of macramé. Aside from tightly compacting the otherwise lengthy chain molecules, this coiling is another means of controlling genetic expression.

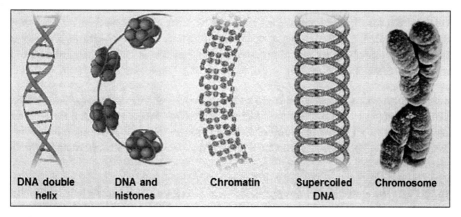

| DNA double helix | DNA and histones | Chromatin | Supercoiled DNA | Chromosome |

Multiple, tightly-wrapped lengths of DNA coils are the **chromatin** *which make up* **chromosomes** *– the structural groupings of all your DNA in the nuclei of your body's cells, which form when cells copy and divide (at other times the DNA is loose within cell nuclei). Image: NIH, public domain*

In eukaryotes, uncoiled DNA which would stretch out to about two meters in length is condensed about 20,000-fold to fit into the limited volume of the nucleus. It's bound to and winds around spool-shaped protein histones.

Eight histone proteins form a core called a *nucleosome*, around which the DNA winds. Since histone amino acids are positively-charged, they naturally bind to the negatively-charged phosphate groups along the DNA strand. When DNA is wound tightly around histones, transcription factors cannot access the genes, so protein production cannot proceed. Histone spools are positioned at regular points along the DNA strand, controlling how tightly or loosely wrapped the DNA strand is. When DNA is tightly coiled, that region of the DNA strand is inaccessible to transcription factors (a tightly-packed state of DNA organization called *heterochromatin*), and the gene cannot be transcribed until the coil loosens (a loosened state of DNA organization called *euchromatin*).

Histone proteins have long protruding tails, which can be modified by adding chemical groups. These chemical groups control whether a given gene is turned on or off, and how much it's expressed. There are several types of these groups, but three in particular with specific functions have been closely studied: *methyl, acetyl,* and *phosphate groups.*

To activate these regions, enzymes unwind them for transcription. Attaching a chemical phosphate group (*phosphorylation*) or acetyl group (*acetylation*) loosens the coiling, exposing the DNA and attracting RNA polymerase to promote RNA synthesis.

Conversely, attaching a methyl group (*methylation*) can stop transcription of that gene, either tightening DNA coils into compact, inactive regions of DNA heterochromatin or physically blocking the binding of transcription factors to the region.

In general, methylation silences genes, winding DNA tighter, so genes cannot be accessed, while acetylation promotes gene expression, uncoiling DNA, so genes are accessible to transcription factors. This allows gene expression to proceed, and proteins can be produced. Combinations of these modifications seem to constitute a complex histone code, involved not just in gene regulation, but also in DNA repair, mitosis and meiosis – forms of cell division.

Several enzymes can modify histones, adding a variety of chemical tags which control gene expression. For example, the tag added by enzyme *PRC2*, is essential for embryo development in all forms of multicellular life through *stem cell differentiation* – shutting genes off at appropriate times, thus helping decide which how a cell matures into a specific type.

In this way the *epigenome* (Latin for "over" and Greek for "*I am born*") helps maintain the types and functions of proteins (and ultimately cells) that are made. Will skin, blood, or muscle tissues continue to be formed, for example? All of these cells are created from the same DNA, but the epigenome uses patterns of expressed and suppressed genes to guide the continued creation of specific varieties.

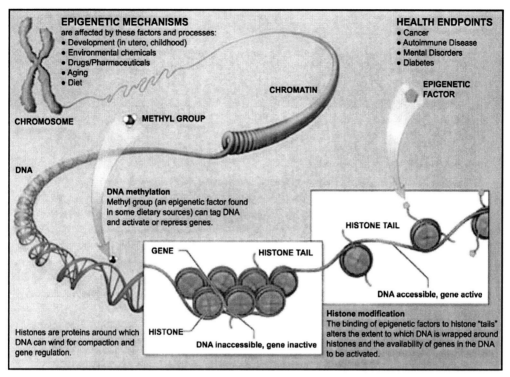

Epigenetic mechanisms, 2010, National Institutes of Health, public domain

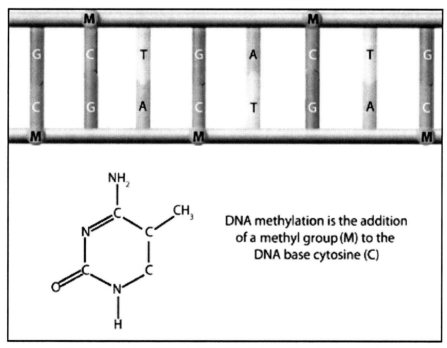

Methylation, Jen Philpot, 2004. The Science Creative Quarterly.
Reprinted with permission.

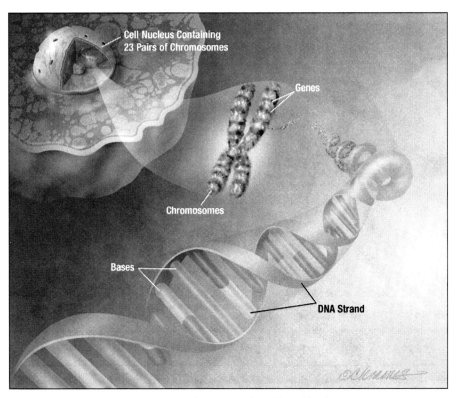

Cell Nucleus Containing
23 Pairs of Chromosomes

Genes

Chromosomes

Bases

DNA Strand

DNA, 2010, National Institutes of Health, public domain

Environment and Lifestyle Affecting Your DNA

Researchers are now studying how environmental and lifestyle factors influence gene expression via epigenetics: between identical twins, DNA can be identical at birth, but over time, various lifestyle and environmental factors radically change how their DNA functions.

Dr. Bruce Lipton, a developmental biologist and the author of *Spontaneous Evolution: Our Positive Future*, asserts that your personality – disposition and beliefs, positive or negative, manipulates your genetic expression – if you believe you're due for cancer or a heart attack because your parents had one, for instance, obsessively worrying about it will give rise to hormones that can change your body on an epigenomic level, and possibly bring your worries to reality. Poor diet, smoking and stress, particularly in childhood, have also all been shown to adversely affect epigenetic factors, with lasting consequences that even have the potential to be passed down to future generations.

The good news is that scientists are already finding ways to exploit epigenetics to enhance health and fight disease. Someday soon the science will be used to extend and enhance your lifespan.

Viruses are not true living cells – they're extremely primitive, comprised of only an outer protein shell and an inner core of nucleic acids – usually DNA, and some cases only RNA. They attach to cell walls and inject their nucleic acid into host cells. The viral genetic instructions then take over the host cell's protein-manufacturing machinery to create mass copies of the virus.

*The **flow of information** from DNA to proteins was long thought to be one-way, until the discovery of **retroviruses** – so-called because the transcription process is reversed, and RNA strands are used to create DNA, which is then injected by the virus into an infected creature's own DNA, thus changing the host creature's genetic code. The most famous of these is, of course, HIV.*

*Unfortunately, because the HIV virus' transcription factors (reverse transcriptase) are much less efficient than DNA's (DNA polymerase) at copying, a greater number of errors are introduced. These genetic "errors" include some which promote the survival of the HIV virus, such as granting eventual immunity to the drugs which treat HIV. In other words, the virus evolves within its host, providing a serious challenge to those seeking treatments. Because HIV specifically target's the human immune system, eventually the system breaks down, leaving the victim susceptible to diseases it would normally be able to fend off. This is the basis of the name **Acquired Immune Deficiency Syndrome**.*

Flipping the Switches

RNA Interference (RNAi) is yet another means of genetic manipulation, in which short RNA strands called *microRNAs* switch off a stretch of genetic code. Discovery of the process led to a 2006 Nobel Prize for Drs. Craig Mello and Andrew Fire of the Carnegie Institution of Washington. Since that time, microRNA strands have become a widely-used tool for gene suppression – turning off specific protein production.

RNA Interference is a natural defense mechanism living creatures evolved to combat viruses. Viruses operate by invading cells, producing RNA to copy themselves, and these copies eventually overwhelm the cell, leading to its rupture and the spread of the virus to other nearby cells.

Human cells have evolved special enzymes that destroy viral RNA, or RNA which acts like a virus. This defense mechanism is called *RNA interference* because it *interferes* with suspicious RNA production.

RNAi's power can also be exploited. To activate the defensive enzymes, RNA which carries the gene to be suppressed is paired up with its mirror image and injected into a cell nucleus. This tiny double-stranded nucleic acid registers as a dangerous *pathogen* (foreign threat) to the RNAi mechanism, which destroys production of the unwanted RNA throughout the host's body.

It's hoped that one day this innate gene-suppressing power can be used to cure a variety of diseases, including cancer. In the meantime, scientists are using it to turn off genes one at a time and study how organisms develop, slowly learning the function of every piece of code in the human genome.

Custom Messenger RNA

In 2011, University of Rochester researchers discovered an additional method of manipulating genetic code, likely of tremendous import for previously incurable genetic disorders. Frequent mistakes in transcription or translation can result in faulty proteins, with the potential for serious harm. For example, a common type of mutation occurs when mRNA molecules have premature "stop" codons – the RNA signals which halt protein production. It's believed that as much as 33% of all genetic diseases are derived from premature stop codons, which force ribosomes to stop reading genetic code before a protein has been completely synthesized.

The Rochester team was able to artificially modify messenger RNA, changing its protein-creating instructions. This modified mRNA can be injected into subjects for therapeutic purposes, providing a new means of both repairing faulty proteins and creating custom ones. Dr. Robert Bambara, chair of Biochemistry and Biophysics, calls this no less than a "miracle of modern medicine", destined to change lives.

Team leader Dr. Yi-Tao Yu created an artificial short-strand "guide RNA", programming it to change a stop codon into a normal codon. This enables ribosomes to finish translating genetic code to produce normal, full-length proteins. Dr. Yu believes the human body may use the same process to naturally alter RNA, a possibility his team is currently investigating.

Rise of the Mutants

DNA doesn't always accurately transcribe RNA, and these *RNA-DNA Differences* (RDDs) are much more common than previously realized. In 1988, Harvard biologists John Cairns, Julie Overbaugh and Stephan Miller discovered that mutations arise continuously, without any particular relevance to their usefulness, potentially leading to major evolutionary changes.

Ideally, DNA divides and copies identical genetic code. Sometimes, however, there are flaws in the process, and imperfect duplicates result. Spontaneous changes in nucleic acid sequences prompt genes to synthesize slightly altered proteins. Some of these mutations are harmless, some lead to disabilities or diseases, and some are beneficial. Mutations can be passed on through reproduction, leading to evolutionary changes.

In addition, DNA is quite fragile. Many common chemicals – including a number found in tobacco and in peanut molds – can cause extensive damage to cellular DNA, breaking apart the strands of the double helix, deleting or adding nucleotide base pairs. *Oxidation* is also common in nature, stripping electrons from DNA and increasing the chance of mutation.

Radiation can emit charged particles, often causing the formation of excess *free radical species*. These are atoms or molecules with unpaired electrons, which have extremely high chemical reactivity, explaining how they inflict damage on cells. Those of the greatest concern biologically are derived from oxygen, and are collectively called *reactive oxygen species*. Because oxygen has two unpaired electrons in its outer shell, it's especially susceptible to forming radicals. Radicals can ionize organic molecules, breaking molecular bonds, and potentially disrupting or altering normal genetic expression. In the case of ultraviolet radiation from the sun, high-energy (ultraviolet) photons can transfer energy to the electrons of organic molecules, thus also disrupting molecular integrity.

At worst, DNA-damaging agents commonly referred to as *carcinogens* can damage DNA, thus disrupting the function of tumor-suppressor genes and *oncogenes*, genetic on and off switches for normal cell division. When these genes no longer function properly, it leads to runaway cell division – the basis of tumor formation. Thus, mutations can be benign, dangerous, or, on occasion, beneficial. According to the late Carl Sagan, in his brilliant book *Cosmos*:

> *A mutation is a change in a nucleotide, copied in the next generation, which breeds true. Since mutations are random nucleotide changes, most of them are harmful or lethal, coding into existence nonfunctional enzymes. It is a long wait before a mutation makes an organism work better. And yet it is that improbable event, a small beneficial mutation in a nucleotide a ten millionth of a centimeter across, that makes evolution go.*

> *Evolution works through mutation and selection. Mutations might occur during replication if the enzyme RNA polymerase makes a mistake. But it rarely makes a mistake. Mutations also occur because of radioactivity or ultraviolet light from the Sun or cosmic rays or chemicals in the environment, all of which can change the nucleotides or tie the nucleic acids up in knots. If the mutation rate is too high, we lose the inheritance of four billion years of painstaking evolution. If it is too low, new varieties will not be available to adapt to some future change in the environment. The evolution of life requires a more or less precise balance between mutation and selection. When that balance is achieved, remarkable adaptations occur.*

> *A change in a single DNA nucleotide causes a change in a single amino acid in the protein for which that DNA codes. The red blood cells of people of European descent look roughly globular. The red blood cells of some people of African descent look like sickles or crescent moons. Sickle cells carry less oxygen and consequently transmit a kind of anemia. They also provide major resistance against malaria. There is no question that it is better to be anemic than to be dead. This major influence on the function of the blood, so striking as to be readily apparent in photographs of red blood cells, is the result of a change in a single nucleotide out of the ten billion in the DNA of a typical human cell.*

Specific varieties of mutations exist:

Frame shift mutations are usually severe, producing completely nonfunctional proteins. Nucleotide sequences are read three at a time in codons, but if one nucleotide is deleted, all the nucleotides in the codons that follow will shift over by one letter, resulting in a garbled sequence.

Point mutations have a single altered nucleotide, possibly resulting in a different requested amino acid. There are three kinds of point mutations:

- A *missense mutation* results in an amino acid substitution;

- A *nonsense mutation* results in a stop codon, producing an incomplete protein;

- A *silent mutation* produces a functioning protein.

All types of DNA are prone to mutations – errors during replication. As it's copied and passed down through generations, the DNA gradually accumulates more mutations.

Invasion of the Genetic Parasites

Transposons are DNA regions which are *transposed* into new positions, cut or copied and pasted back into different areas of the DNA strand from which they came. As they're reinserted elsewhere, it alters the code, which can then be replicated or transcribed, potentially altering gene expression.

Hundreds of thousands of copies of these *jumping genes* can exist in a single genome; in fact, over 45% of the human genome may have originated from these *transposable elements*.

The 1948 discovery of jumping genes in maize earned American biologist Barbara McClintock a 1983 Nobel Prize. Since then, researchers have developed techniques to alter DNA by injecting transposons into living organisms.

Animal genes are normally passed down from parent to offspring through reproduction – *vertical transmission* of genes within a species; but on rare occasions, snippets of genetic code can sometimes be transposed from the DNA of one species into that of another, a phenomenon called *horizontal transfer* (or lateral gene transfer).

After the transfer has taken place, this new combination of DNA is then passed down from parents to their offspring in the normal reproductive process, perpetuating the new genome. In this manner, viruses, bacteria and possibly other parasites are thought have contributed a great deal to the human genome through genetic transposition. Viral changes to DNA can be helpful or harmful, changing which and how many proteins are produced.

For example, in 2005, California geneticists Vladimir V. Kapitov and Jerzy Jurka discovered the *Rag1* and *Rag2* genes became part of vertebrate genome after a fish was infected by a virus some 500 million years ago. These two genes are largely responsible for the vertebrate immune response to infection.

And just as with epigenetics, lateral gene transfer provides a vehicle for extremely rapid evolutionary changes.

> **Rise of the Superbugs** – *Bacteria rapidly spread resistance to antibiotics by **lateral gene transfer**. If one bacterial strain possesses genes which grant resistance to a specific antibiotic, this DNA can be exchanged with a different bacterial strain by a protein **conjugation tube**, and the second strain of bacteria then also becomes immune to the antibiotic's effects.*
>
> *This is why the huge amount of antibiotics corporate agribusiness feeds to cheaply fatten commercial livestock is so hazardous to your health; it's giving rise to superbugs which are immune to conventional antibiotics, such as the deadly **CRKP bacteria**, said to kill 40% of those who contract it. There is currently no medicine available which can treat CRKP, and it has spread across the United States, appearing in major metropolitan hospitals, including in New York and Los Angeles.*

Bugs Getting in on the Game

In 2012, Harvard University's Dr. Jesse Shapiro used 20 complete genomes of the bacterium *Vibrio cyclitrophicus* to demonstrate how bacterial populations rapidly adapt to variations in the ecosystem, by engaging in frequent genetic exchanges.

Bacteria are the most populous organisms on Earth, thriving in nearly every known environment, able to adapt to diverse habitats via genetic variations which bestow survival advantages. These advantages can emerge very quickly via genetic exchanges, allowing bacteria to quickly take advantage of beneficial mutations. Adaptations which confer an advantage are quickly spread and incorporated into the DNA of a population.

A gene containing an advantageous mutation can spread from a single bacterium through an entire bacterial population on its own, and individuals can then replicate their genome many times over, forming a new, better-adapted population of identical clones extremely rapidly.

For the record, according to Princeton University molecular biologist Bonnie Bassler, your body is made up of about a trillion cells, but ten times as many bacteria – about ten trillon bacterial cells – are on you and inside you, covering you in an invisible armor, educating your immune system to protect you from dangerous pathogens, and helping you to digest your food. In a sense, you are more bacterial than human.

Jumping Genes

Upon completion of the Human Genome Project, in 2003, researchers were astonished to learn that the human genome is riddled with the remains of ancient viruses, called *Human Endogenous Retroviruses (HERVs)*. This discovery launched the new field of *paleovirology*, which attempts to shed light on modern illnesses through studying ancient viruses.

In fact, the human genome contains a huge amount of viral DNA, estimated to be at least 8%. This means about 100,000 viruses have become a permanent part of human DNA during its evolution. These lingering viral remnants were long considered junk DNA, but in 2006, French molecular geneticist Dr. Thierry Heidmann raised eyebrows by reassembling an ancient retrovirus back into its original infectious form.

The *Phoenix virus*, as he calls it, had long gone dormant because of mutation, but by comparing about a dozen genetic regions, Heidmann and his team were able to reconstruct the original virus which had originally infected our ancient human ancestors. This virus has only been found in humans, which means it became part of our genome sometime after our evolutionary split from the rest of the great apes.

The virus is now harmless because we long ago evolved an immunity to its effects, but he believes it may help with cancer research, as large numbers of similar retroviral components are associated with several varieties of tumors, so researchers believe they may contribute to cancer growth.

If a retrovirus is able to infect a gamete – a rare event – and if the embryo is able to survive – an even rarer event – the retrovirus has the power to influence the species by permanently becoming part of the genome. Heidmann says such endogenous retroviruses are simultaneously genes and viruses – viruses which helped shape modern humans just like other genes. In fact, he says, they may have been vital for the survival of the human race.

Viruses typically spread by injecting DNA copies of their genomes into host cells. This viral DNA is incorporated into the cell's native DNA, which creates new copies of the virus that can leave the cell and spread.

Normally, such viral infections cannot be passed down because *germline cells* – which produce sperm and eggs – have a special form of protection. Germline cells are the only cells which transmit genetic information to the next generation, and are therefore protected by the repression of RNA transcription.

However, in special cases when sperm or egg cells *do* become virally infected, if the embryo survives, the altered DNA becomes permanently integrated into the genome, and can be passed down to future generations. This is how the Phoenix virus appears to have spread. But after the sperm or egg cells were infected, the virus mutated in the developing embryo, and became unable to create viral copies of itself, instead becoming an integral part of human DNA.

One such viral infection, says Dr. Heidmann, gave rise to *placental birth* in mammals, encoding a protein called *syncytin*, found only in placental cells. The placenta is an organ connecting a growing embryo to the wall of its mother's uterus, allowing it to draw nutrients, eliminate waste, and exchange oxygen and carbon dioxide through the mother's blood supply.

Syncytin protein allows viruses to fuse host cells together to help spread infection. In mammals, however, it allows an embryo to fuse with its mother. A second version of the protein helps regulate high blood pressure during pregnancy, and suppresses the mother's immune system so it doesn't attack the developing baby as a foreign invader.

The placenta protects embryos, allowing them to mature slowly, and allowing live birth, a mammalian trait which gave a huge advantage over our egg-laying reptilian and amphibian competitors. Eggs don't have a means of providing the heavy nutritional demands of a large mammalian brain or of eliminating waste. Heidmann contends that without the beneficial influence of this virus, humans would probably be egg-laying animals.

Variety is the Spice of

Asexual reproduction creates duplicates through *mitosis* – cell division. This is how skin, heart, stomach, cheek, hair and other cells are constantly replenished, and how bacteria and other single-celled organisms reproduce. During mitosis, one cell splits into two, creating a new daughter cell with exactly the same genetic information as its parent.

Sexual reproduction, however, is the means by which animals reproduce. This process shuffles the genetic information of both parents, allowing for a tremendous variation in offspring. This means that each new generation will have variations that can be passed down, allowing a species to change over time.

Gametes (sperm and egg cells) are produced by *meiosis*, which begins with chromosome duplication, followed by two processes of cell divisions, and a final halving of the chromosomes. This gives *haploid* (half-style) gametes 23 chromosomes each, half the full *diploid* (double-style) chromosomes of all other adult cells.

Central to meiosis is the exchange of chromosome parts during the first round of division, called *crossing over*, or *recombination*. During recombination, fragments of each parents' chromosomes mix with their own corresponding partner, and that *haploid* (unpaired), mixed chromosome is contributed to match with the *other* parent's haploid, mixed autosome.

The double-round of cell division during *meiosis* eventually produces four daughter cells with half the normal chromosomes. In humans, each parent's gamete contributes half of 23 paired chromosomes to their child's genotype. 22 of these are *autosomes,* and the 23rd are sex chromosomes.

Both parents' gametes fuse into a single *zygote* cell during sexual reproduction, and in the process, the chromosome halves are shuffled and merge in a unique paired combination. The multiple shuffling of genetic code ensures tremendous variation between each generation: a single human couple's chromosomes can merge in over 8.3 million different combinations (2 to the power of 23). This genetic variation explains why we are all unique. For a visual illustration of the process, please see the illustration on the following page.

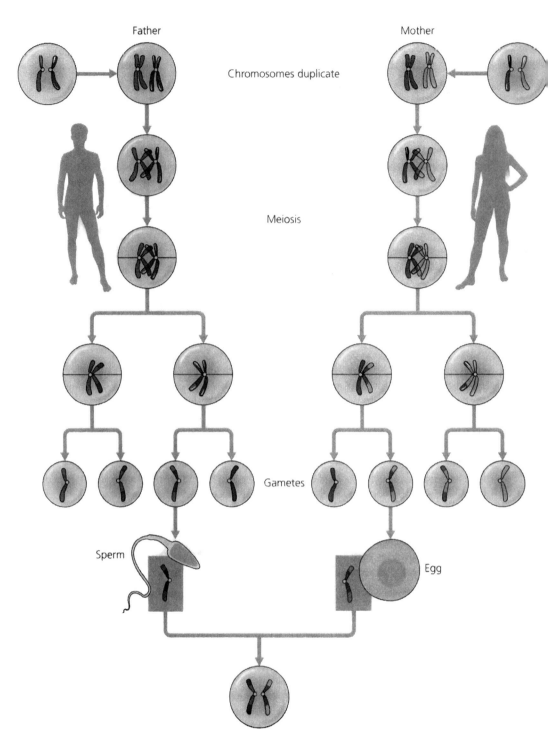

Figure 5.5 Among sexually reproducing organisms, like humans, males and females combine their gametes to reproduce. During the production of gametes, each pair of chromosomes cross over and exchange segments of DNA. Each gamete only receives one copy from each pair of chromosomes. As a result, each child carries a unique combination of the DNA of his or her parents. *Image: Copyright **The Tanged Bank: An Intro to Evolution** by Carl Zimmer (published by Roberts and Co. Publishers) Used with permission.*

Your Inheritance

99% of DNA is the same among humans. Among individuals, close relatives have fewer differences in their genomes, while more distant relatives have a greater number. Each strand of your DNA is a very long string of genes – about two meters in length. Long, clustered chains of these genes form chromosomes – long, tightly-coiled strands which form in the nuclei of every cell in your body except red blood cells.

The instructions required to make a human are crammed into 23 pairs (46 total) of chromosomes, and these pairs are a mixture of DNA from both your parents – one half from your mother, the other half from your father. Genes are thus the smallest logical unit of chemical code passed on from parent to child.

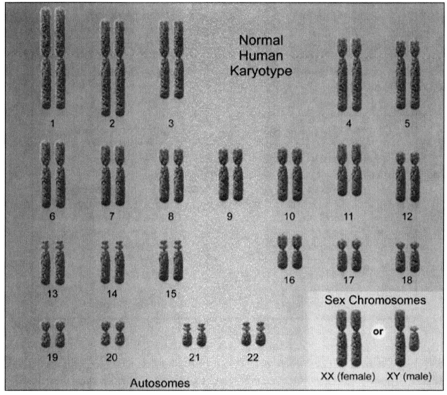

Image: NIH, public domain

While genes are DNA regions responsible for traits, *alleles* are different versions of those genes. *Dominant alleles* are always expressed, while recessive alleles aren't expressed unless a person has recessive alleles on both sides of his haploid chromosome.

An individual set of alleles across a stretch of DNA is called a *haplotype*, and people with similar haplotypes are closely related, look similar, and are members of the same *haplogroup*. Such haplogroups can be traced back to specific regions around the globe.

95

All the cells in your body (except red blood cells) contain the same DNA – wound into 23 pairs of chromosomes in your cell nuclei. Each of your parents contributed one half of your genes, creating your unique combination of traits.

Some of the traits your genes express, such as brown eyes, are *dominant*, so they will always be expressed, only needing the gene on one half of your DNA. If your father had brown eyes and your mother had blue ones, your eyes will be brown. Other traits, like green eyes, are *recessive*, so they're only expressed if the instructions aren't over-ridden by a dominant gene; both genes must contain code for green eyes to appear.

DOMINANT TRAITS	RECESSIVE TRAITS
Farsightedness	Nearsightedness
curly hair	straight hair
Dimples	no dimples
broad lips	thin lips
immunity to poison ivy	susceptibility to poison ivy
normal blood clotting	Hemophilia
brown eyes	grey, green, hazel, blue eyes
dark hair	blonde, light, red hair
full head of hair	baldness
Freckles	no freckles
double-jointedness	normal joints

If your father was *heterozygous* (possessing a different eye color gene on each half of his 15th chromosome), but has brown eyes, and your mother has blue eyes, you have a 50% chance of having blue eyes, but even if both your parents have brown eyes, there is still a chance you could have blue eyes, if both your parents have heterozygous genes.

Among the 23 paired chromosomes in nearly cell of your body are two specialized sex chromosomes, which hold the code that makes you male or female. Females have two X chromosomes, while males have one X and one Y.

While the number of chromosomes varies from species to species – cats have 38 and dogs 78 – the number of chromosomes is generally the same for every healthy member of a species. Rarely, a healthy creature might have extra chromosomes, such as a human with XYY sex chromosomes.

Might as Well Jump – *Sections of DNA called transposons often have no other obvious function than to copy and reinsert duplicates of themselves elsewhere in the genome.*

As much as half of all if human DNA has been shuffled via transposons during human evolution. There are several types of transposable elements (TEs), including **SINEs** (Short Interspersed Transposable Elements) and **LINEs** (Long Interspersed Transposable Elements). The human genome contains an estimated 850,000 LINEs and 1,500,000 SINEs – almost 30 percent of human DNA, passed down from generation to generation, but unique to each individual, who of course inherits a mixture of DNA from two parents. These are usually dormant, non-coding elements, but they can occasionally cause significant damage – or bring significant advantages. In organisms like bacteria, for example, they can confer antibiotic resistance.

Enzymes called **transposases** bind to the ends of a transposon, catalyzing its movement to another position in the genome, where it is inserted via cutting and pasting. In this way, genes can jump from one position or even one chromosome to another. Often these transposons will be found in sequences repeated dozens of times over, giving rise to completely novel traits.

Transposition is important for creating genetic diversity within species and adaptability to changing living conditions. In this way, transposons are a primary driver of evolution, causing mutations by inserting themselves into protein-encoding genes, or causing genome recombination. Gene jumping increases in response to environmental stresses, which thus trigger the mutations underlying evolution.

Epigenetic silencing may have evolved specifically as a defense mechanism to control the spread and silence the expression of transposons. Epigenetic mechanisms normally silence these regions, but in times of stress, this silencing is relaxed, and gene jumping increases. When the stressor has passed, epigenetic controls once again suppress the transposon regions.

Dr. Gershom Zajicek of the Hebrew University of Jerusalem believes transposon shuffling is a protective adaptation:

"There is", he continues, "an important biological law which ought to be considered when examining biological phenomena. A living entity under stress (perturbation) will restructure itself so as to maximize its survival". Thus, in a sense, says Dr. Zajicek, TEs are a creative mechanism meant to keep organisms alive, a means of reshuffling the genome in response to survival challenges.

"Transposons were instrumental in our evolution, contributing to our fitness more than all other traditional mutations. [They] constitute 50% of our genome, and continually move around. Hitherto we were told that the genome is static and nearly frozen, keeping its image from generation to generation. New studies reveal a dynamic and vibrant genome.... Stress initiates a barrage of genome changes.... When facing stress, TEs are turning over, some are born, others disrupted. I regard stress-induced TE changes and gene mutations as protective measures to keep a living entity alive."

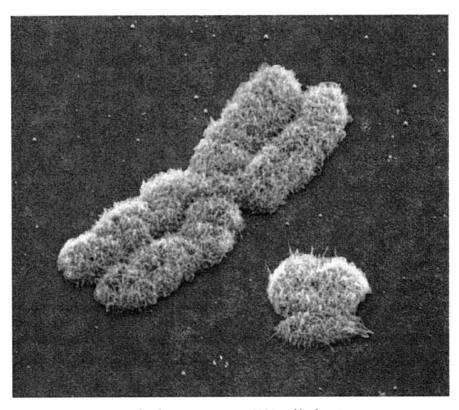

X and Y chromosomes, 2003, NASA, public domain

Interestingly, a joint 2006 study at Harvard, Cambridge and 11 other research centers worldwide discovered something predicted to "...change forever the field of human genetics": for some as yet unknown reason, large sections of genetic code get repeated within chromosomes, making individual differences much greater than previously realized. So among humans, each of us shares about 99% of the same DNA.

In other words, instead of only carrying two copies of every gene (one from each of your parents in each chromosome) some genes are multiplied many times over in a single chromosome. Not just "sentences" (codon sequences) vary from person to person, but chunks equivalent to entire genetic "pages" vary and repeat – a finding that has astonished biologists.

Variations in the number of these copies may lie at the heart of *Parkinson's disease* – a degenerative brain disorder which impairs movement, and *Alzheimer's disease* – a gradual buildup of plaques in the brain that leads to neural die-off and memory loss.

Divide and Conquer

Cell division occurs in three stages, beginning with *synthesis*, as cell components such as the nucleus and chromosomes are duplicated. Next, during *mitosis*, these two sets physically separate within the mother cell. Lastly, during *cytokinesis*, the mother cell splits into two daughter cells. More than a trillion rounds of this cell division occur as an organism develops from a single zygote into maturity.

The Backup Plan

In December 2012, researchers at the University of Wisconsin's Carbone Cancer Center discovered a new form of human cell division they believe acts as a natural backup in case of faulty cell division. They've called this newly-discovered form of cell division *klerokinesis*, and think it may be useful in preventing cancer.

Klerokinesis seems to be a fail-safe in the rare case that normal cytokinesis fails during the trillions upon trillions of cell divisions in an organism's lifetime. This backup strategy allows cells to recover from faulty division, and to proceed with normal growth.

Lead researcher Dr. Mark Burkard studies cancers that develop in cells with too many chromosomes, a condition known as *polyploidy*. Polyploidy is present in about 14 percent of breast cancers and 35 percent of pancreatic cancers, while many other forms of cancer involve cells with defective chromosomes instead of too many or too few.

His team's surprising discovery arose as they were attempting to artificially induce polyploidy in cells, chemically blocking the final cytokinesis stage of cell division, so that duplicated chromosomes remained locked inside a single cell. While they expected to find the experimental cells contained abnormal sets of chromosomes, instead they discovered 90% of the cells they harvested had managed to divide into normal daughter cells. To observe the effects, the team set up a microscope with video recording capabilities. They saw the cell components duplicate, leaving two nuclei in the mother call, and then the cell simply popped apart into two daughter cells without undergoing mitosis. Each of the two daughter cells had inherited an intact nucleus, with a complete set of chromosomes. Repeated experiments produced the same results. It's Dr. Burkard's hope that finding a way of inducing cells to divide through klerokinesis may someday lower the incidence of cancer.

Expression

As embryos mature, gene expression changes. Some genes trigger and guide development, while others produce proteins specific to each stage. For example, human blood contains *hemoglobin*, a protein which binds and transports oxygen throughout the body. But there are different forms of hemoglobin, produced by different genes. Since embryos need a high levels of oxygen, the form of hemoglobin expressed in the womb has the highest oxygen-carrying capacity. A mature human, however, requires less oxygen, so adult hemoglobin is expressed at a later stage.

Mammals have three categories of cells: germ cells, stem cells and *somatic cells*. Germ cells produce gametes – sperm and ova – while stem cells are the source of somatic cells, which comprise all other cells in the body, such as skin, blood, organs, muscle and bone cells.

Stem cells are derived from the original union of the sperm and egg, and are *pluripotent* – capable, when protein *receptors* are chemically triggered, to differentiate into whatever cells are needed, producing blood, brain, muscle, skin, bone, hair or internal organ tissue cells. The ambiguous stem cells are prompted by signalling molecules to permanently develop into specific cell types.

This *cell differentiation* is usually triggered by signal molecules – special cell-to-cell regulating proteins called *cytokines,* or *growth factors* like *steroid hormones.* Hormones are signalling proteins released by glands into the bloodstream, which act like general broadcasting messages affecting any cells which receive them.

Most animal cells aren't in open contact with the outer environment, but are instead surrounded by a liquid environment – blood in the case of humans. Signalling molecules like hormones circulate through the bloodstream, and lock onto matching protein receptors either embedded in cell membranes or within a cell's jelly-like cytoplasm. When hormones lock onto receptors, it triggers *chemical cascades* (chain reactions) that activate dormant transcription factors or structural (*cytoskeletal*) proteins within the target cell.

Whether a hormone can enter a cell or not depends upon its chemical structure. Cell membranes contain a fatty *hydrophobic* outer layer, which blocks water-friendly hormones, but allows fat-derived hormones to flow easily into a cell where they can bind to matching receptors. Fat-based *steroid hormones* like *testosterone* and *estrogen* are of this type, controlling processes like *metabolism* (the rate of energy use, tissue breakdown and synthesis), immune function, salt and water balance, and the development of sexual characteristics. Steroid hormones bind to receptors in the cell nucleus, and these activated receptors attach to promoter regions of DNA, triggering transcription of specific genes.

Similarly, *thyroid hormones* promote brain, skeletal, organ, and other body system development. The common factor among these hormones is that they alter gene expression.

Asymmetric cell division is another means of inducing cell differentiation, creating daughter cells which are given distinct developmental roles. Once a cell has "committed" to a specific role, its role is maintained through future divisions by epigenetic mechanisms like DNA methylation and histone modifications.

Let's Talk About Sex

Fetal divergence into either a female or male of the species is manifest in both the body and the brain. Initially, human fetuses all begin as females, but in the eighth week of *gestation* (fetal development), if the zygote contains a Y chromosome, the SRY (Sex-determining Region Y) gene on the Y chromosome expresses the *testis determining factor* (TDF) protein.

In 2012, German scientists at the Institute of Molecular Biology discovered the master control gene responsible for triggering the development of male sex organs. Switching off that single gene – *Gadd45g* – results in a complete sex reversal in male mice, giving them a fully female anatomy. The Gadd45g regulates chemicals that control the SRY gene, the master regulator of male sex development.

This transcription factor promotes the gene expression which produces testes. Testes, in turn, produce a steadily increasing surge of the steroid hormone *testosterone*, which triggers the conversion of the initially female fetus into a male one. In the second stage of male development, *antimüllerian hormone* is produced, which silences the genes that produce *müllerian ducts*, precursors to female genitalia.

In the absence of testosterone, a fetus will continue to develop into the default female state, with *follicle-stimulating hormone* (FSH) guiding the development of ovaries and the female genital tract. FSH is present in both male and female fetuses, but its effects are suppressed by testosterone.

Both testosterone and AMH also guide fetal brain development, helping guide specific neural development. Experiments show that exposure to low levels of testosterone in fetal brains during critical development phases triggers the development of a distinctive, physically recognizable female brain, whether the fetus is anatomically male or female. Conversely, high quantities of testosterone exposure during this window of development result in a distinctively male brain, again, independent of other anatomical development.

The regions of the brain that specifically differentiate into male or female nuclei govern mating, courtship and sexual behavior within the *hypothalamus* (which controls such behaviors through pituitary gland hormone releases into the bloodstream), and areas of the *limbic system* (hippocampus, amygdala and the orbitofrontal cortex), central to generating emotions, motivation, and memory.

This isn't just theoretical; neuroscientists can manipulate hormonal releases in developing rats and elicit female behaviors in males such as nest building and *lordosis* – the arching up of the pelvis in a receptive pose for sex, or male behaviors in female rats, such as sexual mounting.

Born That Way

In terms of natural selection, it seems illogical that homosexuality – emotional or sexual attraction and/or activity between two same-sex members – would be a heritable trait, because it decreases the likelihood of genes being passed on to future generations. But at least one in ten men and one in twenty women claim to be homosexual, and a 2006 study reported that one in five anonymous responders claimed to have experienced same-sex attraction, but hadn't acted upon the impulse.

Studies strongly suggest that homosexuality tends to run in families. Because of this, researchers have unsuccessfully sought a "homosexuality gene" for years. But a landmark 2012 study indicates that epigenetics – the regulation of genes via temporary switches called *epi-marks* – seems to underlie the development of same-sex preferences.

Epi-marks can control how instructions are carried out by genes, determining when, where and how much of a gene is expressed during development. Sex-specific epi-marks created during early fetal development protect each sex from extreme fluctuations in testosterone as the fetus continues to develop. This prevents unusually high testosterone levels from masculinizing female fetuses, and lower levels from feminizing male fetuses.

These *sexually antagonistic epi-marks* operate on various aspects of sexuality, such as genital formation, sexual identity, and sexual preferences.

Although epi-marks are usually unique to each generation, studies show they are sometimes passed down between generations, contributing to similarity between relatives, just like shared genes. When they are passed down from the opposite-sex parent – mother to son or father to daughter – they can result in reversed effects, for example causing feminized sexual preferences in sons, and masculinized sexual preferences in daughters.

The Miracle of a Single Cell

In the end, it's fascinating to realize that you began your journey on this planet as a single cell, formed from the union of a sperm and egg cell into a single hybrid *zygote*. This single cell contained a chemical chain which replicated many quintillion times over to form who you are at this very moment. And that DNA, in turn, is made from nothing more than combinations of five atomic elements in repeating patterns.

The incredibly complex arrangement of genes in your chromosomes came together perfectly, diversifying into the trillions of different cells that make you who you are today. And every second of your life, billions of these cells are duplicating and dying, renewing you in an ongoing, ever-changing, microscopic rebirth.

A Staggering Complexity

Until 2012, geneticists worked with the understanding that all a creature's somatic cells carry identical DNA within their nuclei, but a new Yale study of skin stem cells revealed genetic variations are actually widespread throughout the body's tissues, a finding with profound implications for modern medicine.

This means that when DNA is replicated from mother to daughter cells, deletions, duplications and sequence changes regularly occur, affecting entire groups of genes. The Yale team identified several deletions or duplications comprising thousands of DNA base pairs. Lead author Dr. Flora Vaccarino of the Yale Child Study Center said:

> We found that humans are made up of a mosaic of cells with different genomes. We saw that 30 percent of skin cells harbor **copy number variations** (CNV), which are segments of DNA that are deleted or duplicated. Previously, it was assumed that these variations only occurred in cases of disease, such as cancer. The mosaic that we've seen in the skin could also be found in the blood, in the brain, and in other parts of the human body.
>
> In the skin, this **mosaicism** is extensive and at least 30 percent of skin cells harbor different deletion or duplication of DNA, each found in a small percentage of cells. The observation of somatic mosaicism has far-reaching consequences for genetic analyses, which currently use only blood samples. When we look at the blood DNA, it's not exactly reflecting the DNA of other tissues such as the brain. There could be mutations that we're missing.

From Five to Nine

That wasn't the only discovery to completely shatter long-standing fundamental truisms in genetics. Since James D. Watson and Francis Crick first deduced the DNA double helix's structure in 1953, researchers have operated upon the premise that five nucleic acids (including uracil) link along a phosphate-sugar backbone to form ribonucleic acids.

This central gospel is at the heart of all our knowledge of genetics. But in 1999, researchers at the University of Paris discovered one of the bases – cytosine – is sometimes modified during natural gene regulation, resulting in a special sixth DNA base, *5-methylcytosine*, formed when a methyl group bonds to cytosine. Methylation can be involved in a number of processes, including gene silencing, causing the DNA's double helix to wind more tightly upon itself.

This discovery was followed up ten years later with the discovery of a seventh nucleotide, *5-hydroxymethylcytosine*, another modified form of cytosine used by the brain for the regulation of nuclear structure and in helping in the control of protein production.

In 2011, two more DNA base pairs were discovered – bringing the total to nine, with additional modifications of cytosine called *5-formylcytosine* and *5 carboxyl cytosine,* modified during natural stem cell reprogramming and regulation of gene expression.

This may give us the potential to reprogram normal cells into acting like stem cells – which can be programmed to develop into whatever is desired. They may also allow scientists to activate cancer-suppressing genes that have been silenced by DNA methylation.

To further complicate things, in 2013, a team at the University of Cambridge discovered that the human genome can contain four-stranded quadruple helix forms of DNA. These *G-quadruplexes* form in DNA regions rich in the nucleic acid guanine.

Over 10 years of searching for this hypothetical structure finally bore fruit with its discovery in living human cancer cells. G-quadruplexes seem to be concentrated at sites of intense DNA replication, central to cell division. The researchers think trapping these quadruplexes may block cell division and thus shut down the runaway cell growth at the heart of cancer. The next step is to determine how to target them in tumors.

Cancers are typically driven by *oncogenes,* genes which have mutated to increase DNA replication, causing runaway cell proliferation and tumor growth. By trapping the quadruplex DNA with synthetic molecules, the team is hoping to be able to block this runaway cell division.

Mix And Match – Your Hybrid DNA

Genetically, your own cells are *chimerae*, a hybrid fusion of genes inherited from two very diverse primitive, singled-celled ancestors. In 2011, Drs. James McInerney and David Alvarez-Ponce at the National University of Ireland matched the specific genes from still-surviving single-celled evolutionary ancestors to those found in human DNA.

Prokaryotes are organisms whose DNA clusters in a concentrated mass called a *nucleoid* or tiny rings called *plasmids*, without a true nucleus or surrounding membrane. This includes bacteria and *archaea*, a similar life form only discovered in 1990. Your hybrid genes arose one and a half billion years ago, when two types of these prokaryotes merged to create a novel life form: *eukaryotes* – creatures with cell nuclei. This genetic merger gave rise to an explosion in biological innovation. Cells were able to delegate life-sustaining tasks to tiny inner components called *organelles,* allowing specialization and the incredible diversity of life seen today, ranging from honey bees to great blue whales.

Human DNA is now comprised of three genetic groups: genes from archaea, genes from bacteria, and genes unique to eukaryotes. These still-segregated gene communities cooperate to keep your cells functioning. The proteins they encode interact, but with different functions. Archaeal genes are generally responsible for information processing, and have fewer mutations, suggesting they're particularly important for survival, and that changes to the DNA are likely to have greater consequences. Bacterial genes are generally involved in biochemical processes, and likely to be linked to risks of hereditary diseases.

Because multicellular organisms have many more different types of tissues, eukaryotes devote much more DNA to gene regulation than prokaryotes, requiring different sets of genes to be expressed for each cell type.

The Force

Evolution is driven by both genetics and environmental pressures – food availability, predators, competitors, climate, disease, etc. – which act as a filter weeding out organisms who don't possess the traits to adapt. Meanwhile, those with traits that help them survive can reproduce, thus increasing the spread of their favorable traits in a population.

Evolution is the accumulation of biological adaptations over time. This accumulation requires reproduction, so useful traits can be passed on to future organisms. The information is stored and transmitted to future generations via the biological recording devices of nucleic acids. Like video recorders or computers, they store information – in this case the information on how to build and operate specific living organisms. Over time, changes to this information result in what we call evolution.

Surprisingly, considering the large number of mutations that constantly occur, its role in evolution isn't as significant – this is because germ cells are sequestered from the rest of the body in multi-celled organisms. Research indicates the most powerful driving force of evolution is instead *genetic drift*: when a small population is isolated, it skews the odds of certain genes appearing which would otherwise be less prevalent in a normal-sized population.

If you were to flip a normal coin 1000 times, you can predict it would land on heads about 500 times and tails about 500 times. But if you only flip the same coin TEN times, you can expect a greater likelihood of skewed results – perhaps ten heads to two tails. I this way, among a tinier population, the gene pool is more likely to drift in the direction of genetic variations that wouldn't appear as often in a larger population.

The Ultimate Engineer

In a sense, evolution can be thought of as the ultimate engineer. Natural selection is at its heart a series of gradual design refinements, each generally requiring tens to hundreds of millions of years. The progress tends to be quite logical, and with single-minded purpose – to build an ever-more-efficient eating machine. To this end, natural selection has produced a staggering variety of methods for moving and eating. In most animals, various kinds of limbs and mouths evolved to accomplish these ends.

Biologists originally classified animal life according to variations and similarities in body plans – the *morphology*, or structural and functional design of the creature. Four criteria are used: the number of tissue types in the creature's embryo; the type of body symmetry and degree to which a head region has emerged; the presence or absence of a fluid-filled body cavity; and the progression of embryonic development.

But the last two decades have been a spectacular golden age of discovery in the life sciences. Most of our knowledge of evolution is no longer purely theoretical, having been bolstered not by simply comparing structural and developmental similarities between creatures, but by finding genes which still exist unchanged, passed down from ancient ancestors through several levels of evolution.

This final, most irrefutable proof of evolution is referred to as genetic *conservation* – organisms alive today still carry many of the same genes that were active in ancient ancestor species. While many of these genes have grown silent, no longer used in controlling or expressing traits necessary for creating humans or other creatures, evolutionary-developmental biologists are able to switch on some of these "redundant" genes again in, for example, chickens, resulting in their developing tails, teeth, etc. This dormant DNA also occasionally gets naturally reactivated, leading to *atavisms* – ancient evolutionary traits which spontaneously re-emerge, such as legs on whales and snakes, teeth in chickens, and occasionally a tail on humans.

Evolutionary-developmental biologists are able to recreate and test some of these specific ancient genes first by examining ancient physical traits (phenotypes), comparing them with those of modern descendants, hunting down the specific modern genes at work in the traits, and deducing how they have changed. They can then synthesize these ancient gene sequences in the laboratory and put them into living organisms, to observe what structures or functions emerge as a result.

Customized genes can also be introduced and observed, or specific genes can be *silenced* with the insertion of a stop codon, which brings translation to a halt on the RNA strand before the specific protein is expressed.

Geneticists accomplish this by using *restriction enzymes* to alter DNA sequences. Restriction enzymes only cut at specific, recognized DNA sequences, and geneticists can insert new DNA material into the separated region of the genome. After the new gene has been introduced, a second enzyme called *DNA ligase* reconnects the DNA fragments, including the new genetic material, now spliced into the organism's genome.

An alternative method is *transfection* – using a virus to inject customized genetic material into a host cell. These genes are then transcribed into RNA along with the host creature's original DNA.

A third method (*cationic liposome transfection*) uses liposome spheres called *micelles* (bubbles) placed in the cytoplasm inside of cells. The protective sphere protects DNA which is introduced to a host cell.

Three approaches are now available to modern researchers investigating evolution:

- **Paleontology** (fossils) for studying *morphology* (comparative anatomies)

- **Archaeology** (stones) for studying *behavior/habitat*

- **Genetics** (proteins/DNA) for studying *genealogy* (what genes and proteins have been *conserved* – passed on unchanged from ancestors)

Underpinnings of Evolution

People often mistake evolution as a movement toward some sort of perfection; in truth, evolution has no direction, but is instead a series of adaptations to the environment with the potential to provide survival advantages. However, as University of Delaware Anthropology Director Dr. Karen Rosenberg points out, what constitutes a survival advantage at one point in time might not in the future. As she puts it, "Evolution is a tinkerer, not a designer".

Natural selection results in species which have adapted to their environments. While a species will change very little while its environment remains stable, environmental changes can potentially trigger major changes, particularly when a portion of a species called a *population* becomes isolated and branches off into a new species. Such an environmental trigger occurred, for example, when the *supercontinent of Pangaea* split apart about 200 million years ago.

Beneficial traits can either help an individual organism survive, or help it to produce more offspring. These traits are then likely to be passed on to future offspring, becoming more common in a population through several generations.

Researchers have discovered additional core principles of evolution within the past five years. For example, it appears that there's an evolutionary trade off between longevity and fertility; whales, which appear to live over 200 years in some cases, produce few offspring, while insects and small mammals, which live short lives, produce many young.

Additionally, climate change seems to be a major driver of natural selection – for reasons as yet unknown, species diversity seems to decline with environmental warming and to increase with cooling.

In the process of evolving into present-day species, over 99% of the species that have existed on Earth have gone extinct. But the tremendous variety of species still in existence should come as no surprise, given the timescale over which they've developed.

It's also interesting to consider that, what we deem to be normal is entirely subjective. We see the Universe filtered through *anthropocentricity* – a human bias. But with just a few nucleotide shifts, we might all be sporting whiskered snouts and beaver-like incisors, considering them to be perfectly normal, indeed even the height of attractiveness.

Logical

Nature is *parsimonious* (stingy). Development tends to follow the path of least resistance, expending the least energy for the most efficient biological payoffs, in this case, successful adaptations. The progression is generally logical. Genes which help organisms survive and reproduce get passed on. This principle is seen at work in *conserved DNA* – nucleotide sequences passed down relatively unchanged to later species. And because DNA is conserved, anatomical structures are shared among many species.

Rather than being completely rebuilt from scratch, anatomical structures such as eyes, limbs, and antennae usually evolve from modifications to pre-existing body-pattern-regulating genes inherited from common ancestors. The evolution of limb function in particular has been critical to the adaptation of *tetrapods* (four-limbed animals), *arthropods* (animals with hard outer shells) and winged insects. By comparing the genes which produce fins, wings, limbs and other appendages, researchers can pinpoint the specific genetic modifications which give rise to these body structures. Modifications to the number and shape of appendages in each animal phylum correspond to changes in regulation of a core set of body-patterning *hox* genes, inherited from ancient common ancestors.

Nature, the ultimate engineer, builds living creatures in the same modular fashion as human engineers, combining distinct components into cohesive working units – living organisms. Biological systems, from protein-to-protein interactions to nervous systems to gene regulatory networks, are universally built from *modules* of dense clustered components connected within a wider network. This principle holds true for creatures as diverse as humans, insects and amoebas.

In 2012, a team of Cornell University engineers discovered why. A computer simulation of 25,000 evolutionary steps shows that using modules isn't because of adaptability, but because modularity is simply cost efficient. Component-driven designs require shorter and fewer network connections, which are expensive to create and maintain. Simply adding the concept of a *cost of wiring* pushes evolution naturally into a modular-based growth system. Cornell Professor Jeff Clune notes, "Once you add a cost for network connections, modules immediately appear. Without a cost, modules never form. The effect is quite dramatic".

The Big Tree

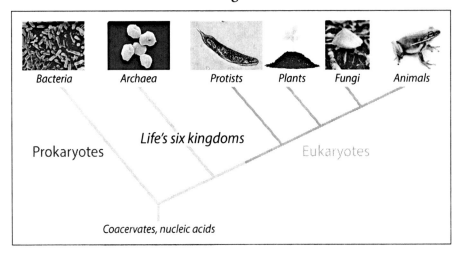

Bacteria   Archaea   Protists   Plants   Fungi   Animals

Prokaryotes

Life's six kingdoms

Eukaryotes

Coacervates, nucleic acids

There are three top level "domains" of life on Earth: Archaea, Bacteria and Eukaryotes. The Archaea and Bacteria are the oldest, single-celled micro-organisms.

Archaea have no nuclear membrane surrounding their genetic material, and are the oldest branch of Earth life, often living in extreme environments such as acids, extreme heat, cold or radiation, or thriving in salt.

Bacteria have more sophisticated, semi-rigid outer membranes and special RNA, but also lack nuclear membranes. They are the most abundant life form on the planet, able to quickly adapt to live in the most diverse conditions, and are found nearly everywhere on Earth, from the deep oceans, to lakes, rivers, on and under the Earth, and within other living organisms (such as you). They adapt and multiply extremely quickly, with generations as short as 10 to 30 minutes.

Eukaryotes include all other life forms, such as fungi, yeasts, plants, mosses, animals and insects. The feature which distinguishes eukaryotes is DNA enclosed within a nuclear membrane, rather than floating loosely within cells (hence the Greek *eu* for *good* and *karyon* for *kernel*).

Eukaryotes also have either an outer membrane or cell wall enclosing complex organelles – biological subunits which carry out specific life functions, such as *mitochondria*, which engage in energy production, or plant *chloroplasts*, which trap sunlight energy and incorporate it into energy-dense storage molecules (plant starch). Among multicellular eukaryotes, the most ancient animals still in existence are the sponges.

Taxonomy (from the Greek *method of arrangement*) is the system used to categorize living creatures, grouped by shared characteristics. Creatures are classified according to five criteria: the structure of their body, their body symmetry (sides which match), the presence or absence of a body cavity, number of tissues in the embryo, and developmental stages they undergo as embryos.

In order from the largest group downward, it's: Domain, Kingdom, Phylum, Class, Order, Family, Genus, Species. For a tiger, this would be broken down into:

Domain: Eukarya

Kingdom: Animalia

Phylum: Chordata

Class: Mammalia

Order: Carnivora

Family: Felidae

Genus: Panthera

Species: Tigris

And for humans:

Domain: Eukarya

Kingdom: Animalia

Phylum: Chordata

Class: Mammalia

Order: Primates

Family: Hominidae

Genus: Homo

Species: Homo Sapiens

As of 2013, there are about 1.9 million known species, over half of which are insects, and over 1.2 million of which are animals, and it's estimated that well over ten million species exist, most of which have not yet been discovered.

These creatures range in size and in complexity from the tiniest *sessile* (unmoving) sponges with no true tissues and only a few cell types, all the way to blue whales, roaming the oceans tens of thousands of kilometers every year in search of food, containing trillions of cells, dozens of different tissues, elaborate skeletons, and highly sophisticated brains, nervous systems and sensory organs.

The bad news is that human activity is killing species as fast as we discover them, to such a shocking degree that we're causing the sixth *extinction event* in the history of the planet. This is due to habitat destruction, pollution, global warming, and invasive species which we bring with us.

Our Story Begins

In the *Archean Age*, one billion years after Earth cooled from a spinning ball of fiery dust and gases cast off from our infant sun, the first traces of life began to appear in pools of water collecting on the planet's rocky, volcanic surface.

Life on Earth arose approximately 3.8 billion years ago from the humblest of beginnings – among volcanic mudpots and ocean slime drying along ancient coastlines.

The first complex organic molecules were amino acids, followed by the nucleic acid RNA, which could assemble proteins from the free-floating amino acids. Natural selection came into play even on this molecular level: those RNA molecules which were most efficient at copying themselves increased in number and complexity, forming a variety of proteins.

The first living organisms were nothing more than RNA strands and ribosomes enclosed by membranes formed from chains of easily-assembled, repeating organic molecules called *lipopolysaccharides*. Through natural hydrophobic (water-repellent) forces, these lipopolysaccharides formed spherical droplets, outer protective membranes which enclosed the replicating molecules inside. These protected forms of RNA were much hardier, and multiplied in increasingly greater numbers than their competitors. Living examples of these creatures still exist today.

110

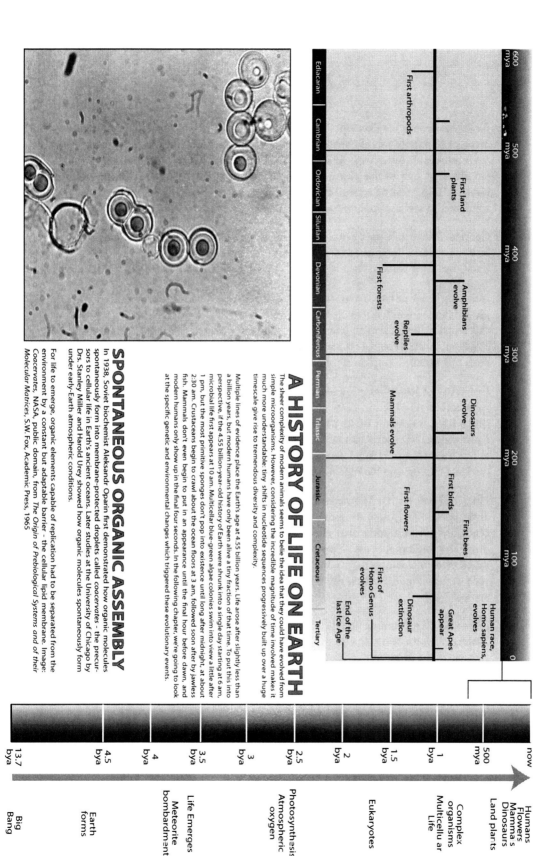

A HISTORY OF LIFE ON EARTH

The sheer complexity of modern animals seems to belie the idea that they could have evolved from simple microorganisms. However, considering the incredible magnitude of time involved makes it much more understandable. The tiny shifts in nucleotide sequences progressively built up over a huge timescale give rise to tremendous diversity and complexity.

Multiple lines of evidence place the Earth's age at 4.55 billion years. Life arose after slightly less than a billion years, but modern humans have only been alive a tiny fraction of that time. To put this into perspective, if the 4.55 billion-year-old history of Earth were shrunk into a single day starting at 6 am, microbial life first appears at 10 am. Multicellular blue-green algae colonies swim into view a little after 1 pm, but the most primitive sponges don't pop into existence until long after midnight, at about 2:30 am. Crustaceans begin to crawl about the ocean floors at 3 am, followed soon after by jawless fish. Mammals don't even begin to put in an appearance until the final hour before dawn, and modern humans only show up in the final four seconds. In the following chapter, we're going to look at the specific genetic and environmental changes which triggered these evolutionary events.

SPONTANEOUS ORGANIC ASSEMBLY

In 1938, Soviet biochemist Aleksandr Oparin first demonstrated how organic molecules spontaneously form into membrane-protected droplets called *coacervates* - the precursors to cellular life in Earth's ancient oceans. Later studies at the University of Chicago by Drs. Stanley Miller and Harold Urey showed how organic molecules spontaneously form under early-Earth atmospheric conditions.

For life to emerge, organic elements capable of replication had to be separated from the environment by a constant but adaptable barrier - the cellular lipid membrane. Image: *Coacervates*, NASA, public domain, from *The Origin of Prebiological Systems and of their Molecular Matrices*, S.W. Fox, Academic Press, 1965

Roots of RNA

Biologists believe life developed from RNA strands, which are able to act as their own catalysts to initiate useful chemical reactions. But the problem with this theory is that RNA nucleotide bases can't link up without a polymer backbone. However, researchers say RNA can evolve from simpler, slightly different bases than those found in modern RNA. Adding a small chemical tail to one of these *proto-RNA bases* prompts spontaneous self-assembly into highly-ordered gene-length RNA chains in water.

Georgia Tech Professor Nicholas Hud has triggered spontaneous base-pair assembly into polymers as long as 18,000 bases, and his team is confident they're on the right track. So are the National Science Foundation and NASA, who are backing his research.

Normally RNA expands one nucleic acid base at a time, a linked molecular chain growing in sequence; but ancient Earth RNA had no external enzymes to help catalyze this reaction, so its growth would be too slow to ever achieve more than a few links. However, Italian researchers have recently prompted long chains of RNA to spontaneously emerge from nucleotide subunits in nothing but warm, slightly acidic water.

University of Rome microbiologist Dr. Ernesto Di Mauro has found that under the right conditions – acidic water and temperatures ranging from 40 to 90 degrees Celsius – RNA fragments of 10-24 bases naturally combine into chains of 100 or more bases within little more than half a day. This spontaneous *ligation* (fusing) allows RNA to reach a biologically functional size of about 100 bases, at which point the molecules can start folding into biologically useful three-dimensional shapes.

Like Dr. Hud, Dr. Di Mauro and his team are using proto-RNA bases, in this case *cyclic nucleotides*. These molecules are like conventional DNA-RNA nucleotides, except they form an additional chemical bond, giving them a ring-shaped structure. This extra bond makes cyclic nucleotides more reactive, forming polymers at a faster rate. Cyclic nucleotides themselves easily arise from simple chemicals found in nature such as *formamide*, making them likely candidates for the basis of RNA assembly on ancient Earth.

DNA and RNA promote heredity – the transmission of genetic code, which allows for adaptations over time, and even they themselves evolve through natural selection – survival of the fittest *molecules*. But Dr. John Chaput of Arizona State University's Biodesign Institute says there may have been earlier, simpler precursors – nucleic acids with slightly different chemistry, still able to self-assemble and replicate, which were the chemical stepping-stones to the emergence of life on Earth.

Theories have been advanced that comparatively simpler RNA evolved first, but because even these molecules are relatively complex, some believe more primitive self-replicating organic molecules must have existed first. Because of this, Dr. Chaput and others have been exploring several alternatives to the two primary organic molecules, trying to determine if less complex organic molecules may have first emerged to jumpstart life.

At least four nucleic acid analogs exist – *peptide nucleic acid* (PNA), *locked nucleic acid* (LNA), *glycol nucleic acid* (GNA) and *threose nucleic acid* (TNA), all of which differ from naturally-occurring DNA or RNA in changes to the molecular backbone. The chief contender among these candidates for the ancestor of RNA is TNA.

While TNA's nucleotide base pairs are the same as in DNA, TNA's backbone is comprised of a special sugar called *threose*, instead of ribose or deoxyribose. Threose is much simpler to assemble than ribose, making it a possible precursor to RNA. The sugar backbone is based upon a four-carbon ring, simpler than the five-carbon sugars of DNA and RNA, assembling easily from double-carbon fragments, and able to bind to either DNA or RNA.

Once TNA strands arise, natural selection promotes the survival of the most useful sequences, while less environmentally fit molecules gradually fade out of existence.

There is no solid proof yet that TNA led to RNA, but experiments show that such simpler organic molecules can easily arise, are capable of storing information, undergo natural selection, and fold into useful structures. Chaput firmly believes that eventually proof will emerge of TNA's original role in the evolution of life.

Additional experiments in creating six artificial nucleic acids – *xenonucleic acids* or XNAs – have further strengthened the argument that earlier, simpler forms of nucleic acids may have existed before RNA or DNA. There are at least three environments in which complex organic compounds naturally assemble:

1. Mudflats – Earth's oceans are often bordered by coastal wetlands called "mudflats". Clay mudflats are ideal for incubating complex organic chemistry, forming natural templates whose chemical ions naturally attract amino acids. The nooks and crannies of clays also provide some protection from UV radiation and atmospheric hazards.

90% of the rocks found in the Earth's crust are made up of *silicates*. These minerals are built of repeating chains or sheets of pyramidal molecules, consisting of a silicon atom surrounded by four oxygen atoms. When the central silicon atom is replaced by a smaller aluminium one, it creates an *aluminosilicate*, with surface ions that attract amino acids.

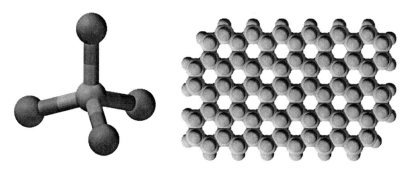

Silicates, Wikipedia, public domain

113

Tide-stacked layers of clay mudflats, rich with layers of aluminosilicate sheets, make a natural template for chaining amino acids drawn from seawater. Amino acid chains hundreds or even thousands of molecules long can continue spontaneously growing virtually indefinitely, given the right ingredients and environments. These ancient polypeptide chains would likely have been more random than modern proteins, crosslinked and contaminated with other organic compounds bound in the chains.

RNA and DNA readily bind to clay particles, and phosphate, common in pool sediments and phosphate-rich rock, is central to the backbone of RNA and DNA, and to ATP energy-extraction, which powers living biochemistry.

2. Condensing Pools – along the Earth's shores, porous rock is full of basins where seawater collects, drying in thick, dense concentrations. This is the equivalent of trillions of small petri dishes of varying sizes, temperatures and mixtures, all randomly connected, making for an ideal organic laboratory, where the tides constantly mix accumulating organic debris.

3. Volcanic vents – both onland and deep in the ocean, volcanic activity releases mineral-rich steam and heated water. Onland, this creates hot springs, mudpots and geysers, and under the sea, black smokers, all rich with minerals vital to organic chemistry. The prevailing theory for decades was that life originated around such undersea hydrothermal vents, which today are found to teem with microbial life that feeds off chemicals dissolved in vent fluids.

Protein synthesis requires a lot of potassium, and the process is inhibited by sodium, so living cells struggle to maintain potassium levels, while actively expelling sodium.

Modern cells have evolved complex protein machinery to actively pump excess sodium out through their membranes, but the first cells would not have possessed such complex molecular machinery. The first primitive cellular membranes would have been highly *permeable* (substances could easily pass through), rendering them at the mercy of the environment, but still needing to maintain a high ratio of potassium to sodium.

Because of this, ocean vents – where the ratio of sodium to potassium is typically 40 to one – are much less hospitable to developing life than land-based volcanic mud pots, like those in Yellowstone National Park, where potassium is much more abundant, and sodium levels low. Such bowls of warm, slimy muck were fed the ingredients for organic molecules over millions of years, and warmed by volcanically-heated steam, creating the perfect "hatcheries" for early life. Modern-day mudpots are full of toxic sulfuric acid, but on ancient Earth, the atmospheric oxygen necessary to create this toxic chemical did not yet exist.

Coacervates

As complex organic chemicals cool in water, the most fascinating phenomenon can be observed: cooling peptide chains and lipids spontaneously form membrane sacs, selectively allowing some chemicals in, and keeping others out – primitive but fully functional cell membranes. These membrane sacs are coacervates, and their spontaneous formation shows the second step in the evolution of life is a natural occurrence.

Coacervates (Latin for *assembly* or *cluster*) are tiny spherical droplets of lipids held together by *hydrophobic* (water-repellent) forces which separate them from surrounding liquid. 1 to 100 micrometers across, they can selectively allow organic molecules to be absorbed through the membrane from the surrounding medium – a primitive sort of metabolism. This is the closest structure to living cells that can be created without the need to engage in complex biochemical life processes.

A Fixation

The early protocells were little more than shaky, unstable chemical systems which survived by cobbling together a handful of carbon-based molecular assemblies.

Carbon is at the center of all organic molecules. That's because it's extraordinarily versatile, with its ability to stabilize by forming four outer bonds. All life on Earth is carbon-based, and living tissues – made of organic molecules such as amino and nucleic acids, proteins, lipids, and carbohydrates – all contain carbon as their central feature.

To synthesize these organic molecules, living organisms use chemical reactions like photosynthesis to harvest carbon from carbon dioxide in the atmosphere. Living organisms use this and a handful of other chemical reaction strategies are classified as *carbon fixing mechanisms*. How these six strategies of carbon fixing first evolved is just now coming to light, with the discovery of a single ancestral form.

By analyzing and comparing these metabolic strategies and the genes which give rise to them, researchers have been able to piece together a complete evolutionary history of carbon fixation. What they've discovered is that earliest life forms seem to have combined multiple carbon-fixing strategies to increase the odds of survival, although it's still not entirely clear if a single organism possessed all the carbon-fixation mechanisms, or whether a community of tightly-coupled organisms regularly exchanged organic components, from which specific lineages would later emerge.

COMMON ORGANIC MOLECULES

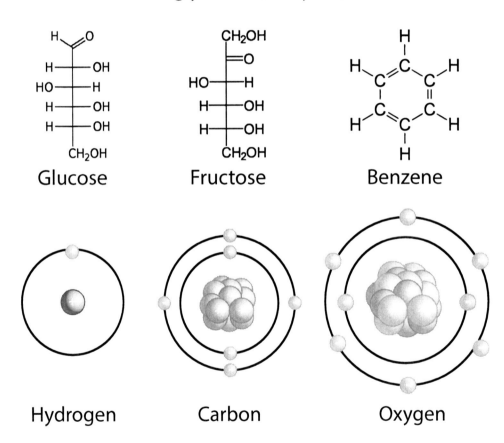

Triglyceride (body fat)

Glucose

Fructose

Benzene

Hydrogen

Carbon

Oxygen

Carbon is Your Friend – Organic chemistry can be said to be the chemistry of carbon, because it's at the heart of all organic molecules. Carbon, with an atomic number of 6, is one of the most abundant elements in the universe and is tremendously versatile in forming a variety of molecules. Each carbon atom has two electrons in its first shell and four electrons in its second.

Because the most stable atomic arrangements are for electrons to exist in pairs, carbon has four electrons available to pair up with other atoms, generally hydrogen, oxygen and nitrogen. By sharing its electrons with other elements, carbon forms strong, stable bonds, potentially up to four per atom. This makes carbon extremely adaptable for constructing chains, rings, tubes, spheres, lattices and other biochemically useful, strong and stable structures.

*When carbon shares its electrons with hydrogen atoms, it forms **hydrocarbons**, the simplest organic compounds. Hydrocarbons are **hydrophobic** (water repellent) oily, fatty or waxy molecules collectively referred to as **lipids**. Their **catenating** (self-bonding) properties mean hydrocarbons bond with themselves to form complex, energy-dense molecules.*

*Hydrocarbons are also the chemical basis of **crude oil**, formed from decomposed, compressed organic tissues. **Petroleum** and **natural gas** are mainly formed by decomposed, prehistoric plankton compressed in the absence of oxygen, under high heat and pressure deep within seabeds and lakebeds. **Coal** and **methane** are generally formed by decomposed prehistoric plants.*

These ancient hydrocarbons are energy-dense molecules, which we purify and burn to push the pistons that drive our gasoline engines. They're currently also the primary source of electric energy and home heating around the world because of the energy they release when burnt.

*Six- through 10-carbon versions of hydrocarbons are used to make gasoline, jet fuel and specialized industrial solvents. Petroleum products are also used in a vast number of plastics, paraffins, waxes, solvents and oils. Unfortunately our heavy reliance upon them contributes to the rise in **greenhouse gases**, which trap heat in the lower regions of the atmosphere, leading to potentially disastrous climate change.*

Hydrocarbons are abundant throughout the solar system, and undoubtedly throughout the Universe. For example, NASA's 2005 Cassini-Huygens Mission to Saturn's largest moon Titan discovered lakes of liquid methane and ethane. They have also been confirmed in distant nebulae.

According to Santa Fe Institute's Dr. Eric Smith, "It seems likely that the earliest cells were rickety assemblies whose parts were constantly malfunctioning and breaking down. How can any metabolism be sustained with such shaky support? The key is concurrent and constant redundancy."

This redundancy – backup metabolic strategies – became the basis of evolutionary splits in the tree of life, the diversification into bacteria such as cyanobacteria (blue-green algae), and archaea, the second major group of early single-celled microorganisms. Each of these early life forms developed ever more finely-tuned biological mechanisms to respond to the environment, such as improved membranes better able to control the flow of materials in and out of the cells, and enzymes better able to control specific reactions. Those that survived multiplied, passing on the genes that expressed their beneficial adaptations.

My Name is LUCA

Modern biologists call the theoretical first ancestor of all life *LUCA*, an acronym for the *Last Universal Common Ancestor*. This theoretically extinct microorganism appears to have lived 3.8 billion years ago.

By comparing the 138,458 proteins generated by the genomes of 66 separate species, it's possible to pinpoint the genetic code they all share – LUCA's genome. This common ancestral DNA shows that LUCA – or possibly a community of various co-existing LUCA types – gave rise to the three *domains* of biological life, Archaea, Bacteria, and Eukaryota. Biologists say that LUCA's genome was RNA-based, capable of advanced protein synthesis, and that it was protected by a fatty acid membrane.

Life Goes On

Animals are *heterotrophs*, meaning they obtain energy and carbon compounds from consuming other organisms, or by absorbing nutrients from them. This makes animals *consumers* in the food chain, and photosynthesizing bacteria, algae and plants the primary *producers*.

The earliest life forms were *autotrophs,* organisms which created their own food, converting energy through photosynthesis – the capture and storage of sunlight energy in organic sugars – or *chemosynthesis*, the capture of energy released by chemical reactions like those in geothermal vents of deep ocean floors.

Volcanic spouts release energy-dense chemicals into Earth's oceans, ponds and streams. Living organisms which feed from such chemosynthesis are found in great numbers even today, thriving around volcanic vents in the depths of the oceans.

Before the Cambrian era, Earth's temperature dropped sharply, and glaciers covered nearly the entire planet. Then the massive supercontinent *Rodinia* fractured and split into separate continents, opening up shallow seas across much of the Earth.

These shallow seas were warmed by plentiful sunlight, providing a hospitable environment with abundant energy for algae and other microorganisms. Surviving creatures naturally migrated to these regions.

Solid evidence of the early emergence of these primitive life forms was found in 2010, in microfossils unearthed from the Makhonjwa Mountains of South Africa, showing a "surprisingly diverse microbial biosphere already existed 3.5 billion years ago."

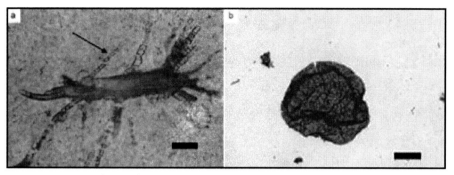

Traces of early life in rocks of the Makhonjwa Mountains in South Africa,
a) Furnes, et al, 2004; b) Javaux, et al, 2010, NASA, public domain

These fossils were dated using both carbon 14 and uranium – elements whose *isotopes* (atoms with extra neutrons) *decay* (neutrons stabilizing into protons) at a very precise, measurable rate. Additional dating techniques have recently been brought to bear, including *electron spin resonance*, which measures electrons absorbed and trapped inside rock or bone, *paleomagnetism*, which compares magnetic particle directions in sediment layers – because the Earth's magnetic field has shifted at known times in history – and the *molecular clock method*, which uses known rates of DNA mutation to compare genetic differences in organisms where DNA can still be sampled.

Other Frontrunners

In 2011 and 2012, Oxford and Caltech paleontologists discovered several apparent microfossils: fossilized *microbial mats* called *stromatolites* and clusters of tubular cells embedded in sandstone on a remote Australian beach called Strelley Pool, the oldest known shoreline on Earth.

The specimens appear to be 3.4 billion-year-old fossilized, anaerobic, sulfur-metabolizing bacteria. They range in size from five to 25 μm (micrometers), and are 10 μm on average, just like modern prokaryotes tend to be, though some outliers are as large as 80 μm. The high degree of sulfur present in the samples is indicative of bacteria which subsisted on sulfur, living at a time when Earth's early atmosphere was thick with methane instead of oxygen, and the oceans were much warmer than in the present day.

Inorganic chemical processes can produce similar shapes, which resemble organic structures, but these specimens appear to have undergone folding, something inorganic shapes don't do. They're also disordered, like most organic matter – inorganic carbon-based molecules are highly-ordered.

Multiple chemical analyses show the apparent cell walls contain isotopes of sulfur, carbon, and nitrogen, all indicative of biological remains, and there are concentrations of heavy carbon chains; only organic activity sifts apart heavier forms of carbon in such a manner.

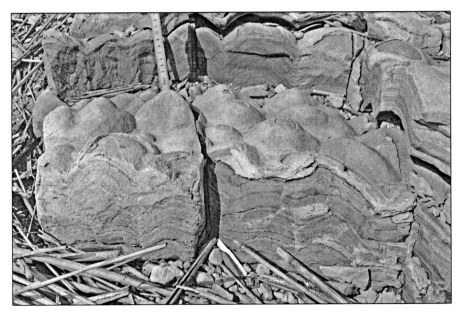

Photo: Stromatolites (Pika Formation, Middle Cambrian) near Helen Lake, Banff National Park, Canada; wikipedia, public domain, 2010

NASA geologist Abigail Allwood also studies stromatolites, dome-like rock formations made from bacterial colonies. These stubby pillars are one form of such colonies, the other being the microbial mat.

Microbial mats are multi-layered sheets of bacteria and archaea, a few centimeters in thickness, which grow on shallow lake floors and seabeds. They're held together by slimy secretions and tangled webs of filaments formed by the microbes. These are some of the earliest forms of life, dating back some 3.45 billion years.

These colonies were responsible for development of the planet's modern atmosphere, and hence its ecosystem. After first evolving, they were dependent upon hydrothermal vents for energy and chemical nutrients, until the evolution of photosynthesis liberated them from these limited environmental niches, providing an abundantly available energy source in the form of sunlight. When the oxygen-producing form of photosynthesis evolved, microbial mats started producing our modern oxygenated atmosphere.

It's still a microbial world; by weight, microbes make up the majority of Earth's biomass, and most genes are derived from microbes or their viruses. They are by far the oldest forms of life, and the most well-adapted, found in virtually every ecological niche on the planet. It's estimated that there may be as many as 5,000 species in the human gut, and a single teaspoonful of soil can contain as many as 10,000 bacterial species. Microbes live on, in and everywhere around us.

Breathe

One single, microscopic change in the structure of early DNA opened the door for complex life to evolve: a slight adaptation in the genetic code of a tiny *cyanobacterium* (blue-green algae) allowed it to split a water molecule, harvesting its energy for the first time. This microbe had perfected *photosynthesis*, and by freeing oxygen from water molecules, it simultaneously unleashed a poison which would lead to the greatest global extinction in our planet's history, and allow plant and animal life to be born.

A breakthrough study in 2013 by evolutionary biologists at the Universities of Zurich and Gothenburg showed that this *Great Oxidation Event* was triggered by multicellular cyanobacteria 2.4 billion years ago, who probably evolved *aerobic respiration* (oxygen-breathing) through *horizontal gene transfer*, the routine exchange of genetic material among bacteria. Oxygen breathing was tremendously beneficial, yielding four times the energy of anaerobic respiration.

Cyanobacteria had developed multicellularity about a billion years earlier than eukaryotes, and coinciding with that appearance, oxygenation began in the oceans and in Earth's atmosphere. This played a significant role in the development of life on Earth. By comparing modern cyanobacteria phylogenies with fossil record data, Dr. Bettina Schirrmeister showed how multicellular cyanobacteria emerged much earlier than previously believed. According to her findings, multicellularity emerged shortly before the rise of free oxygen levels in the oceans and atmosphere referred to as the Great Oxidation Event, the most significant evolutionary event in Earth's history.

"Morphological changes in microorganisms such as bacteria were able to impact the environment fundamentally and to an extent scarcely imaginable," says Dr. Schirrmeister. The oxygen they produced radically transformed Earth's atmosphere forever.

The increase in oxygen knocked the early Earth atmosphere out of balance. Oxygen was poisonous for huge populations of anaerobic creatures, which went extinct, freeing up ecological niches. Many new types of multicellular cyanobacteria also arose immediately after the climatic event to occupy the newly developed habitats.

Photosynthesis harvests sunlight and electrons to create energy necessary for life processes. In the modern form of photosynthesis, water is an electron source, and oxygen is expelled as a waste product. Although photosynthesis had first evolved nearly a billion years earlier (3.4 billion years ago), geological evidence shows no significant atmospheric oxygen at the time, so early photosynthesis instead involved splitting molecules like hydrogen sulphide to scavenge electrons for life-sustaining chemical energy. Combining oxygen and water with minerals like iron weakens rock, changing its color, creating *rust*.

Discoveries of oxidized mineral deposits show that oxygen first began to accumulate in the Earth atmosphere about 2.4 billion years ago. That new oxygen-rich atmosphere formed an *ozone layer*, blocking harmful ultraviolet radiation, paving the way for future life to inhabit shallower waters and eventually land. At that time, the Moon was much closer to Earth, driving 1,000-foot tidal waves, and the Earth was continually beaten by hurricane-force winds. Both conditions, however, are thought to have assisted evolutionary processes, forcing organisms to adapt or perish.

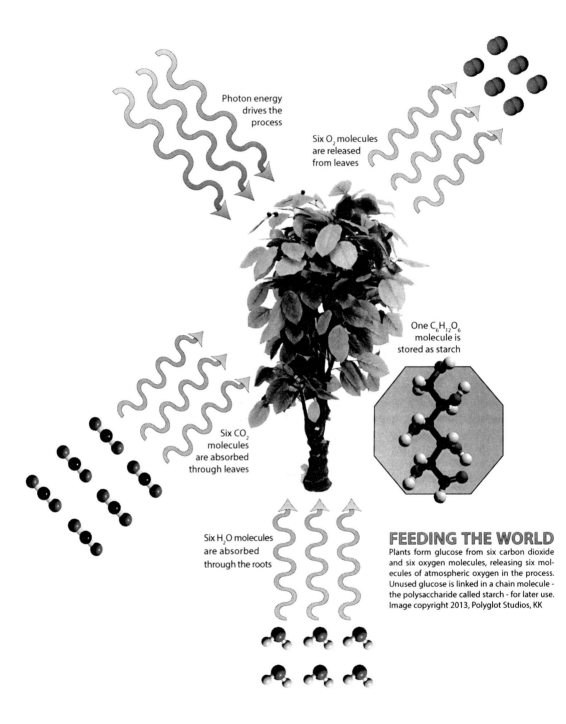

Photon energy
drives the
process

Six O_2 molecules
are released
from leaves

One $C_6H_{12}O_6$
molecule is
stored as starch

Six CO_2
molecules
are absorbed
through leaves

Six H_2O molecules
are absorbed
through the roots

FEEDING THE WORLD

Plants form glucose from six carbon dioxide
and six oxygen molecules, releasing six molecules of atmospheric oxygen in the process.
Unused glucose is linked in a chain molecule -
the polysaccharide called starch - for later use.
Image copyright 2013, Polyglot Studios, KK

122

Splitting

Earth's newly oxygen-rich atmosphere was toxic to early life. Three different metabolic strategies evolved in response, leading to the first evolutionary split in the tree of life. As a result, three distinct forms of life emerged: the archaea, bacteria and eukaryotes LUCA's first offspring were heat-flourishing *thermophilic* archaea. One lineage of archaea shed some of its redundant DNA – the process called reductive evolution – developing into the first bacteria. Both early forms of life were originally little more than membrane-bound, self-replicating sacs of DNA.

Then about 1.2 billion years ago, these two life forms merged through *endosymbiosis*, one living creature absorbing and hosting another to mutual benefit. Astonishingly, DNA analysis shows this began with the infection of an archaean cell by a primitive aerobic bacterium; that bacterium's closest living relative is *Rickettsia prowazekii*, the cell-invading parasite which causes the epidemic typhus, also known as *jail fever, ship fever*, and *famine fever*, so-called because it causes epidemics in the wake of wars and natural disasters, and is transmitted by human body lice. But this arrangement turned out to be mutually beneficial, with the host organism providing shelter and protection, and the symbiont producing chemical ATP energy.

In the world of microbes, temporary engulfment of prokaryotic cells by larger hosts is not unusual, but in this case, the relationship became permanent, when the bacterial cell shed some of its DNA, and became incapable of independent living, while its host cell grew dependent upon its tenant's energy generation. Thus, through reductive evolution, the membrane-enclosed bacteria eventually evolved into *mitochondria* or *chloroplasts*, the energy-production factories of animals and plants. The host archaea resembled those found today in the hot springs of Iceland. In swallowing a bacterial cell, the host became able to delegate energy production to its inner passenger, the symbiont bacterium, giving the host an ability to increase its size, and the complexity of its genome.

---

*Plants, animals, fungi and other eukaryotic cells contain between one and several thousand tiny energy factories called **mitochondria**. These organelles seem like separate cells within cells, and for a good reason – they used to be. Mitochondria are surrounded by their own membranes, carry their own separate DNA and replicate it when they divide. Geneticists have found this mitochondrial DNA uniquely matches bacterial DNA.*

Because of this, biologists know these organelles used to be free-living bacteria, which were engulfed by a single-celled creature billions of years ago, providing survival benefits to the host. These oxygen-consuming bacteria infected early eukaryotes, providing a mutually beneficial arrangement that evolved. The "host cells" abandoned their inferior energy-extracting proteins, taking advantage of the energy provided by the bacterial organelles they now hosted, while the mitochondrial bacteria shed unnecessary genes.

Similarly, the earliest plants evolved from predator species which engulfed photosynthesizing microorganisms, in a mutually beneficially arrangement.

This symbiotic partnership was the emergence of the third domain of life – the world's first eukaryote, an organism with its multi-strand DNA enclosed within a nuclear membrane instead of free-floating within its cell cytoplasm, and equipped with specialized cellular subunit organelles generating energy and performing control and data transmission functions. Over the next 1.3 billion years, electron transport systems, light-trapping pigments like chlorophyll, and other metabolic systems evolved in this lineage.

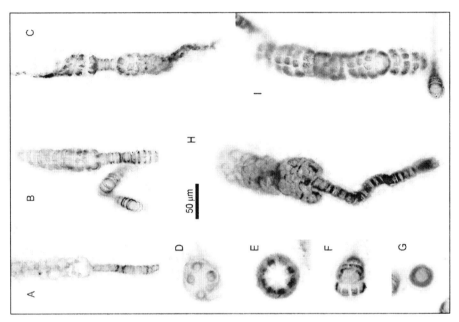

*The oldest known eukaryote, **bangiacean red algae**, ca. 1.2 billion years old, discovered in Arctic Canada in the year 2000. Gamete formation shows B. pubescens reproduced sexually, the oldest occurrence in the fossil record. This is also the oldest evidence of complex multicellularity in the fossil record. Image: Professor Nicholas J. Butterfield, 2000. Used with permission.*

Holding Back

After our atmosphere first formed out of gasses and water vapor from cooling rocks, life first began to appear, some 3.8 billion years ago, probably due to bombardment by meteorites studded with organic molecules. But for more complex life to evolve, a threshold level of atmospheric oxygen was needed, estimated at one to ten percent of current levels. We now know that oxygen first began to appear 2.4 billion years ago.

So why did it take nearly another two billion years for single-celled microorganisms to develop any further? For decades, this "late start" puzzled scientists, until now.

In studying ancient marine sediments, UCal Biogeochemistry Professor Timothy Lyons and his colleagues discovered a significant lack of an essential trace element – the metal *molybdenum*. According to Dr. Lyons, the shortage of this trace metal likely delayed the development of complex life for almost two billion years:

Bacteria use molybdenum to harvest atmospheric nitrogen in a biologically useful form, a process known as *nitrogen fixation*. Without molybdenum, bacteria cannot fix nitrogen, and without nitrogen, eukaryotes (plants, animals, fungi and more) could not develop.

According to Dr. Lyons, this is why life was limited to the simplest life forms until only about 600 million years ago: "The amount of molybdenum in the ocean probably played a major role in the development of early life. As in the case of iron today, molybdenum can be thought of as a life-affirming micronutrient that regulates the biological cycling of nitrogen in the ocean."

Initial low levels of molybdenum match low levels of oxygen in deep early ocean seawater, which hampered life's evolution. Oxygenation of the atmosphere occurred twice: first, around 2.4 billion years ago, as the ocean surface was oxygenated by photosynthesizing algae; and second, around 600 million years ago, when the entire ocean became fully oxygenated. Says Dr. Lyons, "These steps in oxygenation are what gave rise ultimately to the first animals almost 600 million years ago – just the last tenth or so of Earth history."

Before bacteria evolved to fix nitrogen, Earth's early oceans were full of toxic hydrogen-sulphide, further hampering the spread of complex life. These oxygen-deprived conditions were eventually altered by the rise in nitrogen, somewhere around 600 million years ago. Geological data shows that early Earth's deep oceans cycled between two oxygen-free states – one rich in iron, and the other in toxic hydrogen-sulphide, an ocean environment created by early anaerobic bacteria, which survived using little nitrogen.

When bacteria evolved to use *nitrates*, they displaced the less energy-efficient bacteria, which had been producing the toxic ocean sulphides, and rising nitrate levels in the seas permanently blocked a return to the toxic states.

Researchers at the Universities of Exeter, Leeds, Southern Denmark and University College London, say modern organisms use nitrate both in respiration and as a nutrient. In our modern era, nitrate is abundant in highly-oxygenated oceans, preventing a reversion to the toxic environment which blocked the formation of early life.

Flagellation

Just below the base of the animal tree are *choanoflagellates* (Latin for *collared* and *whipping*), unicellular, filter feeding microbes capable of colonizing. These are the closest living ancestors of animals, among the group of organisms called *protists*, which means "the very first".

Choanoflagellates are *sessile* (living attached to a surface), with microscopic tendrils called flagella they use to beat the water, creating currents that draw in microorganisms and organic debris to be devoured. They reproduce through simple cell division and are too primitive to possess nerves, being single-celled.

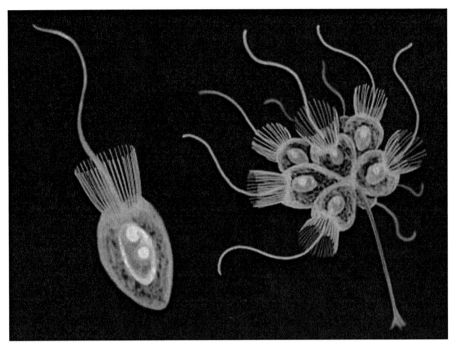

Choanoflagellates, Wikipedia, public domain.

Sexy

Instead of chromosome strands packed into a cell nucleus, bacterial DNA is free-floating, and bacteria multiply by dividing and making copies of themselves. Some bacteria also have the ability to insert tube-like appendages into neighboring bacteria, directly transferring DNA. This *horizontal gene transfer* allows bacteria to evolve tremendously quickly.

But 1.2 billion years ago, multi-celled algae evolved a powerful new trait – sexual reproduction. This method of DNA mingling would allow natural selection to proceed at a comparatively breakneck pace. For two billion years – half of its entire history – life had been confined to primitive single-celled microorganisms. But with a new means of evolving ever more complex DNA, eukaryote life began to diversify much more quickly.

Sexual reproduction was vital to the eventual survival of eukaryotes, as was complex multicellularity, which offered many survival advantages. Together, over the course of a billion years, these two powerful evolutionary tools would lead to the astounding variety of eukaryote species populating the world today.

Simple bacteria link together into chains and mats, but true multicellular organisms require different, specialized cell types. The modern algae *Volvox* is considered something of a living fossil, the simplest example of such multicellularity; it has only two types of cells – reproductive cells, and mobile cells equipped with flagella for swimming and for sensing chemicals and temperature.

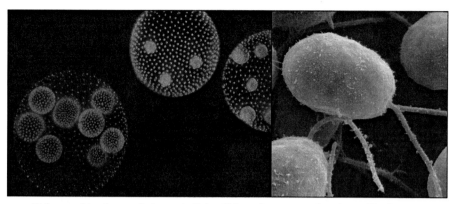

Volvox and its closest relative, unicellular Chlamydomonas, Wikipedia, public domain.

Volvox's close relative is the unicellular *Chlamydomonas*, which has remained largely unchanged genetically since its first emergence a billion years ago. While Chlamydomonas cells divide to produce asexual daughter cells, Volvox has two cell types – one for swimming and perception, and the other for sexual reproduction. Comparing the genomes of these related species lets researchers determine which genes are unique to each, and which proteins these genes produce.

Twelve traits evolved in Volvox that Chlamydomonas does not possess, expressed by very minor modifications to the existing unicellular blueprint: duplications and slight mutations to genes for cell division and other simple functions. The end result was cells capable of differentiating; in the case of Volvox, these genes can be switched on or off to express reproductive cells or non-reproductive *somatic* (sensing and moving) cells. Reproductive cells lose their flagella and the ability to swim, while somatic cells lose the ability to reproduce. This cooperative division of labor was the beginning of complex multicellularity, the cell specialization that is a key to modern evolution.

Enter the Matrix

Berkeley researchers discovered choanoflagellate genes which encode the amino acids used in adhering cells to one another. It's believed that these genes led to multicellularity further down the evolutionary tree. Multicellularity was a critical step in the development of complex life, allowing cells to become specialized for different specific tasks.

The transition from single cells into multicellular organisms was largely made possible by the evolution of an *extracellular matrix*, as cells began to secrete a kind of protein-polysaccharide "glue" to stick together.

The earliest forms were *collagen* proteins and *integrin* receptors, which would evolve into an extracellular matrix, the meshlike supportive network which holds cells together as living tissue. Much of living tissue is comprised of the space between cells, filled with this network of proteins and polysaccharides secreted by cells into the space between them.

PROKARYOTES AND EUKARYOTES

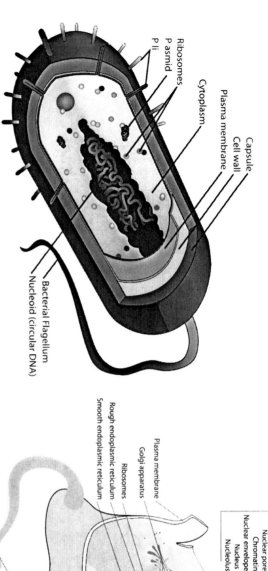

Capsule
Cell wall
Plasma membrane

Ribosomes
Plasmid
Pili

Cytoplasm

Ribosomes

Bacterial Flagellum
Nucleoid (circular DNA)

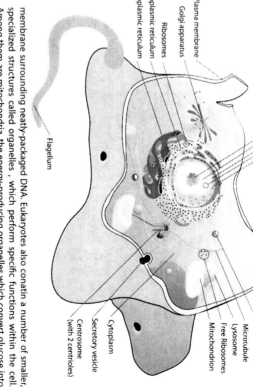

Nucleus
Nuclear pore
Chromatin
Nuclear envelope
Nucleus
Nucleolus

Plasma membrane
Golgi apparatus
Ribosomes
Rough endoplasmic reticulum
Smooth endoplasmic reticulum

Flagellum

Peroxisome
Microtubule
Lysosome
Free Ribosomes
Mitochondrion

Cytoplasm
Secretory vesicle
Centrosome
(with 2 centrioles)

Prokaryotes were the earliest forms of life - bacteria and archaea. Archaea were officially recognized as distinct life forms in 1990, because of major structural and genetic distinctions from bacteria. Most prokaryotes are unicellular, though some species - such as *cyanobacteria* - cluster into large colonies. In prokaryote cells (pictured above left), all proteins, DNA, ribosomes and smaller organic molecules are enclosed within the same outer membrane. These cells contain no central nucleus or membrane-bound organelles. The *nucleoid* is a free-floating DNA/protein complex which contains the prokaryote genome, a single, double-stranded loop of chromosomal DNA, differing markedly from the compact linear chromosomes of *eukaryotic* cells. Additional genes may be stored in separate DNA loops called plasmids. Because of their smaller size, prokaryotes tend to have a much higher metabolic rate, growing and evolving much more quickly than Eukaryotes.

Eukaryotes span four of the six kingdoms of life: Animalia, Fungi, Plantae, and Protista, a range of organisms from single-celled yeasts to blue whales. All visible creatures are eukaryotes, including plants, animals, and fungi, while tinier eukaryotes include yeasts, which can only be seen when gathered into colonies. Eukaryotes share the common trait of a nuclear membrane enclosing their genetic material. Eukaryotic cells (pictured above right) are enveloped by a *plasma membrane*, which forms a protective barrier between the outside world and the cell's interior *cytoplasm* in which internal organelles are suspended. Eukaryotic cells are generally much larger than prokaryotic cells, and while prokaryotic cells contain DNA floating freely within the inner cell fluid, eukaryotic cells are more complex, with a nuclear

membrane surrounding neatly-packaged DNA. Eukaryotes also conatin a number of smaller, specialized structures called organelles , which perform specific functions within the cell. Among them are mitochondria, the energy-producing organelles which convert glucose into ATP to fuel various life processes, such as muscle contraction.

Within the nucleus, DNA is transcribed into RNA to guide protein synthesis. Here too, at the center of the nucleus is the nucleolus, a sphere of proteins and nucleic acids which transcribes ribosomal RNA (rRNA) and assembles it into organelles called ribosomes. Ribosomes in turn assemble proteins within a network called the endoplasmic reticulum, which transports these proteins within and out of the cell. The Golgi apparatus packages materials into fluid pockets called vesicles, which migrate to the membrane, and fuse with it, delivering their contents outside the cell, or transporting materials inside of it. Lysosymes break down unused organic matter, including non-functioning organelles.

Centrioles are tiny cylinder-shaped organelles used in organizing the cell's inner structure and in cell division. Vacuoles are tiny storage units, found in greater abundance within plant and fungal cells. Plants and fungi also have rigid cell walls which contain these cellular contents, including organelles called chloroplasts, which use sunlight to convert carbon dioxide and water into sugars. *Images: Mariana Ruiz Villarreal, 2007-2008, Wikipedia, public domain.*

Collagens are long, stiff, ropelike, triple-helix amino acid chains that form tough fibers used in skin, tendons, ligaments, cartilage and bone. Today, they are the most abundant protein in mammals, making up 25% of their total proteins. But far earlier, cyanobacteria evolved collagen to adhere to one another in colonies, and sponges use a short-chain version of collagen called *spongin* as a cement to attach to seabed rocks. Similar ECM proteins have also been discovered in choanoflagellates.

Integrin receptors are found in all living animals today, from sponges to mammals. Adhesive proteins bind with these receptors to provide cell-to-cell and cell-to-matrix interaction and communication.

Gene shuffling, mutations and duplications have since given rise to the more complex ECM components found in the connective tissues of modern animals. So far, about 25 different collagen chains have been discovered, which combine into thousands of different types of collagen proteins.

Join Together

The organization of single-celled organisms into multicellular clusters was an evolutionary leap forward, allowing much more sophisticated, higher-level functioning through cellular cooperation. This cooperation enabled greater adaptability, ultimately allowing complex creatures like plants and animals to evolve.

Multicellularity has evolved independently at least 25 times, among different groups of living organisms, but just how it occurred was a long-standing mystery among biologists. But the process was demonstrated in January 2012 at the University of Minnesota, using single-celled *Brewer's yeast*. Surprisingly, the process is both rapid and easy: in a single 60-day experiment, the team of four evolutionary biologists used a culture medium and centrifuge to "evolve" the yeast into multicellular snowflake-shaped clusters, which reproduced, adapted to the environment, and worked together in a cooperative division of labor – features central to complex Earth life.

"The finding that the division-of-labor evolves so quickly and repeatedly in these 'snowflake' clusters is a big surprise. The first step toward multicellular complexity seems to be less of an evolutionary hurdle than theory would suggest", said Dr. Ratcliff, who led the experiment.

Brewer's yeast (Saccharomyces cerevisiae), is a species used since prehistory for making bread rise and beer ferment. It's abundant in nature and easy to cultivate. The team grew the yeast in test tubes filled with a nutrient-rich liquid, allowing the cells to grow for one day, then spinning them in a centrifuge to collect heavier cell clusters.

The process was repeated for sixty cycles, and spherical clusters of hundreds of cells emerged. These clusters weren't merely random cells which had stuck together, but were genetically-related cells, showing they had remained attached after the cells had divided.

Simple cell clusters aren't multicellular, but when they cooperate, adapt to change, and sacrifice themselves for the common good in *apoptosis* (programmed cell death), it's an evolutionary transition into multicellularity. Because of this experiment, we know that multicellularity first arose when recently-divided cells simply remained attached.

Vive la difference!

The emergence of cellular differentiation, in which a cellular lineage becomes permanently specialized in response to chemical signals, played a central role in early evolution. Multicellular creatures are made up of a variety of cells, each specialized for a specific function. For example, in humans, blood, muscle and nerve cells all have different structures, functions, enzymes and other proteins. But identical DNA is used to create all of these different cell types, by switching a different pattern of genes on and off with transcription factors and *microRNAs*.

In any one creature, every cell nucleus contains identical, complete DNA derived from the zygote, and even though cells have differentiated, their DNA is identical. Unused genes in these cells are neither destroyed nor mutated, but still retain the potential to be expressed, though only a small percentage of each will actually be expressed.

MicroRNAs can bind to messenger RNA, sealing up and thus silencing genes which would normally express proteins. In this way, miRNAs can act as on/off switches in response to environmental changes. Transcription factor proteins can also turn specific genes on and off and accelerate or decelerate transcription. This controls which messenger RNA are transcribed to synthesize proteins, accounting for different structures and functions specific to each cell type.

Differentiation allows cellular roles to be fixed while an embryo develops. Such fixed cellular roles enabled more elaborate, adaptive organisms to emerge, giving rise to complex organs and sophisticated, stable biological networks such as nervous systems.

It's important to note that no single gene is responsible for expressing a complex trait like a finger or hooves. In fact, a single gene often performs multiple duties, expressing different proteins, depending upon the region of the body. Such genetic multitasking is called *pleiotropy*. Thus, a one-to-one link between a specific gene and a trait is very rare. Because of this, scientists usually exercise caution, saying generally, "Gene X has a very strong association with trait X".

Winter

From about 850 to 630 million years ago, glaciers covered the Earth. During this period, in a tenth of the time it took the first eukaryotes to arrive, a kaleidoscope of diverse tiny microplankton with acid-resistant cell walls evolved. These are the mysterious *acritarchs*, whose fossils are found in abundance around the globe. Over 2000 species are known to have arisen by 800 million BC.

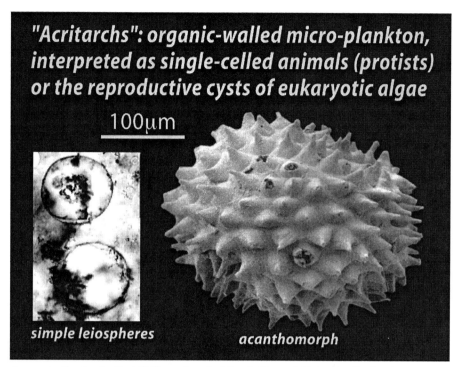

"Acritarchs": organic-walled micro-plankton, interpreted as single-celled animals (protists) or the reproductive cysts of eukaryotic algae

100μm

simple leiospheres

acanthomorph

Image: Acritarchs, Dr. Paul Hoffman, Snowball Earth, Harvard University. Used with permission

As the glaciers slowly retreated – 635 to 541 million years ago – *acritarchs* evolved from the tiny forms pictured on the left into the much larger, more diverse creatures such as the South Chinese specimen seen on the right. These life forms eventually gave way to the first true animals, which evolved into diverse shapes resembling discs, tubes, mud-filled bags and quilted mattresses. These were the soft-bodied forebears of modern sponges, marine worms, jellyfish, corals and anemones.

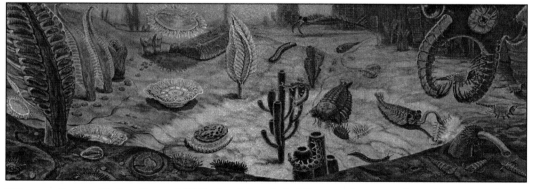

Ediacaran/Burgess Shale – Pre- to Middle Cambrian. Left: Ediacaran fauna, mostly sessile and filter feeding. Right: Mid-Cambrian life forms, like Anomalocaris, Hallucigenia, and Pikaia, with their novel body plans, armor and anatomical inventions enabling predation. Image: D.W. Miller, used with permission of the artist.

131

During the *Ediacaran*, about 635 million years ago, multicellular life was a variety of strange tubular, cylindrical and frond-shaped organisms, primarily *sessile* (fixed in place). The weird creatures populating this unique ecosystem completely vanished, however, leaving trace fossils around the world, but no apparent ancestors, during the period of rapid diversification known as the *Cambrian era*, ca. 542 million years ago.

It's believed that predation and competing species led to the extinction of the Ediacaran ecosystem. The first signs of such predators are tiny holes bored into the sides of ancient Ediacaran organisms.

Ediacaran creatures have proven difficult to classify. In fact, they may not have been animals at all, but instead some long-extinct form of lichens, algae, fungi or microbial colonies, or perhaps some hypothetical precursor which lay between plants and animals on the tree of life. While it's possible they were related to sponges or jellyfish, the difficulty in classifying these creatures has led some scientists to propose they were unique lineages which went completely extinct, a sort of failed attempt at animal life, and that modern life arose again completely anew from single-celled organisms.

Mother Sponge

The oldest true animals yet discovered are prehistoric sponges. 635 million-year-old chemical traces were discovered in an Arabian Peninsula oil field in 2008, by UCal geochemist Gordon Love.

There is a fatty compound called *24-isopropylcholestane,* found only in the protein-silica "skeletons" of *demosponges*, the most common sponge family. Dr. Love's team found the telltale traces of this organic molecule in sedimentary deposits mined by Oman's national oil company.

The deposits formed during the final stages of the *Cryogenian period*, a global ice age that researchers informally call Snowball Earth. The discovery shows that animals existed much earlier than previously believed, allowing primitive sponges at least 100 million years to evolve into the kaleidoscope of life forms which bloomed during the later Cambrian period.

In 2010, Princeton geologist Adam Maloof also unearthed a 645-million-year-old fossil in South Australia's Flinders Ranges that appears to be of sponges, though the classification is a little less certain. Dr. Maloof's team created a precise three-dimensional map of the fossil by grinding down a baseball-sized rock 50 micrometers at a time, shooting an image at each step. The fossil revealed sponge fragments interspersed with a microbial mat. It's still possible the microscopic structures were giant single-celled organisms or slime molds, so studies are ongoing.

While fossil evidence indicates that sponges were the first animal life forms, DNA evidence suggests a forebear of *placozoa* – an amoeba-like creature whose genome was sequenced in 2008 – may have been an even earlier arrival.

Sponges are extremely simple multicellular animals, well adapted to life on Earth. There are as many as 10,000 modern species, largely unchanged since they first evolved. Their bodies are porous, with channels that allow water to circulate throughout, providing oxygen, food particles, and removing waste.

Sponges are the only animals where cells don't form tissues. They have several distinct types of cells, but these aren't organized into tightly-knit, functional structures called tissues. They also lack organs, nervous, digestive or circulatory systems, and are sessile; but like other animals, they're multicellular, *heterotrophic* (eat other life forms), lack cell walls and produce sperm cells. Their bodies are made of undifferentiated, unspecialized cells which can transform into other types as needed, and migrate through the jelly-like *mesohyl* extracellular matrix between thin inner and outer layers of cells.

Interestingly, sponge feeding cells, called *choanocytes* (collared cells), share the structure of choanoflagellates – a single flagellum and collar of food-trapping filaments. These collared cells are the first type of cell to develop in embryonic sponges, and collared cells also appear in other animal groups, such as the ribbon worms, making it easy to recognize the evolutionary progression. Compare the following picture with that from page 128:

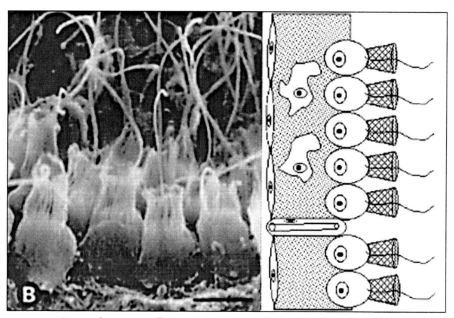

Sponge choanocyte cells. Image Animal Evolution: Interrelationships of the Living Phyla, Oxford University Press, 1995, used with permission

The Nerve!

Sponges are the most primitive animals alive, with only four different cell types in a very simple body. However, at least one species, *Amphimedon queenslandica*, synthesizes an almost complete set of proteins central to neural communication – even though, like all sponges, it lacks any neurons. Sponge larvae apparently use these proteins to sense chemical cues in their environment.

Neurons are cells specialized for communicating with one another, via a *synapse*, the tiny gap between adjacent cells. In order for this signalling to work, on either side of the synapse, just beneath the membranes, signalling components are organized upon a *protein scaffold*.

In 2007, researchers at the University of California Santa Barbara discovered 36 gene clusters in the Amphimedon genome which encode these scaffold proteins. One of them, called *dlg*, expresses a protein which binds all post-synaptic scaffold proteins together – and the Amphimedon gene is identical to that found in human DNA. In fact, Amphimedon possesses nearly all the components for a neural scaffold; all it lacks are human genes which encode ion channel receptors.

However, in 2012, researchers at the University of Texas discovered these genes at the heart of neural communication existed in choanoflagellates. These genes express *sodium channels*, protein receptors embedded in cell membranes which act as tunnels conducting the flow of the positively-charged *sodium ions* which generate the electrical impulses of nerve signals.

Channeling

In a sense, eukaryote cells operate like storage batteries. Usually, negative ionic charges are built up inside their membranes and positive charges on the outside. This difference between inner and outer charges, called a *membrane potential*, is used to power life processes or transmit signals like neural impulses.

Such neural communication uses controlled movement of charged sodium, calcium and potassium ions in and out of cells through ion channels. Ion channels are protein tunnels embedded in the cell membrane, which open and close, allowing ions to flow in and out, building the charges needed for the electrical signalling in nervous systems. Every thought you have, and every move you make is the result of the incredibly precise opening and closing of these ion channels.

Opening these channels lets ions flow into the cell, attracted by the opposite charges within. After a neuron has fired, protein pumps use ATP energy to actively push these ions back out across the membrane and restore the difference in charges between both sides of the membrane.

Interestingly, 2012 studies of cell membrane bioenergetics by Drs. Nick Lane of UCL, Bill Martin of the University of Dusseldorf show that, given conditions like those of underwater hydrothermal vents, these potentials arise naturally in inorganic matter – simple water, rocks, and carbon dioxide. This leads in a direct path to the property's emergence in living cells.

Do the Locomotion

While many animals are *sessile* (unmoving) during part or all of their lives, and others are *sit-and-wait predators*, the huge majority move under their own power at some point in their lifetimes. For example, sea anemones spend their adult lives attached to undersea rocks, but they give birth to larvae which disperse under their own power, acting like plant seeds by migrating to new habitats where they don't compete with their parents for space or resources.

Among animal species which move throughout life however, motion serves three purposes: finding food, finding mates, or escaping predators. The method of accomplishing this goal varies tremendously, including various means of burrowing, swimming, slithering, jumping, bounding, gliding, flying, crawling, climbing, waking and running. But while the means may vary, the power behind the movement is generally provided by four possible structures: *cilia*, flagella, *muscles* pulling upon hard *skeleton*, or muscles compressing a fluid-filled cavity – a *hydrostatic skeleton*.

Cilia (Latin for *eyelash*) are the oldest means of locomotion, hair-like extensions from the body used for both motion and primitive sensory organs. Flagella are long, whip-like structures used to propel creatures through water, and hydrostatic skeletons use a fluid-filled cavity called a *coelum*, which can be squeezed by surrounding muscles to alter a creature's shape and produce movement, such as burrowing or swimming.

This form of movement is used by many cold-blooded and soft-bodied life forms, including earthworms, starfish and sea urchins, jellyfish and other invertebrates. (Interestingly, Dr. Diane Kelly of the University of Massachusetts says the hydrostatic skeleton is the functional basis of the mammalian penis.)

Cilia and flagella are both built of *protein microtubules* – threaded protein filaments which provide structural stability, and *motor proteins* – molecules that convert chemical energy into mechanical work by forcibly flexing.

It's believed that these primitive forms of movement first evolved from transport systems used to move particles within cell cytoplasm, because the proteins and microtubules central to both flagella and to sensory receptors have been found in such primitive life forms as cyanobacteria, showing the molecular components had been in place long before flagella ever evolved.

Muscles contract to provide the basis of movement, and the squeezing or pumping activity of internal organs like the intestine and heart. In general, they operate through the interaction of two filament motor proteins, *actin* and *myosin*, powered by ATP to pull across one another, like dragging a rope inwards, thereby tightening muscle tissue and pulling on connective tendons and bones.

Actin and myosin are very ancient biomolecules, with earlier forms of actin found even in bacteria. Several myosin genes also exist in primitive yeasts and slime molds. Together, actin and myosin appear to have originated as a means of transporting components about within cells, before developing into an intercellular system, such as that which allows multicellular algae like Volvox to migrate into colonies.

Early animal ancestors adapted these proteins into actin *cytoskeletons*, the interior cellular scaffolding that maintains the shape of all living cells. Together with myosin, they evolved motor-protein systems that eventually gave rise to contracting units – the *sarcomeres* found in muscles. Actin and myosin appear in sponges, and *cnidarians* (jellyfishes and related species), allowing tentacle movement, body contraction and swimming.

The transition from cytoskeleton components into fiber muscle cells progressed as actin-myosin filaments were compartmentalized into sarcomere units, the basis of muscle tissue. A buildup of muscle cells organized in this fashion gives a tremendous increase in power over cilia, the ancient hairlike "legs" used to power simpler organisms. Muscles allow contraction over a greater distance, and with much stronger force, enabling movement of large-bodied animals.

The Ancient Ones

Cnidarians – jellyfish, corals, sea anemones, hydras and sea fans – are the most ancient forms of animal life with unified cell structures called tissues. This ancient lineage split from the rest of the animals more than 600 million years ago, before the great diversification known as the Cambrian Age. There are over 11,000 of these predatorial species, living primarily in the oceans.

Their tissues include sensory cells which respond to environmental stimuli with electrical signals; nerves which process and transmit those signals, and muscle cells which contract in response to those signals, allowing coordinated swimming.

Jellyfish and related species contract muscles in a ring around their bells, creating *jet propulsion* (forcible water flow) which pushes them rapidly through water. Their young (called *polyps*) and their adults (called *medusae*) may reproduce asexually or sexually. Also among cnidarians are *corals*, which secrete the *calcium carbonate* that grows into *coral reefs*.

In cnidarians, synapses are *bidirectional*, transmitting in both directions, though synapses which only conduct signals in one direction are also found in sea anemones, functioning like those of more complex animals, including humans. Sea anemones and jellyfish also possess sodium-specific ion channels, more specialized than ancient non-selective ion channels, which also transmitted calcium.

Cnidarian bodies have *radial symmetry*, with a single opening for both feeding and eliminating waste. They feed using specialized *cnidocyte cells* to capture prey: if a creature brushes up against a cnidocyte, the cell ejects a poison-coated barb into the victim's flesh. Some of these toxins can paralyze prey, allowing a cnidarian to bring prey to its mouth.

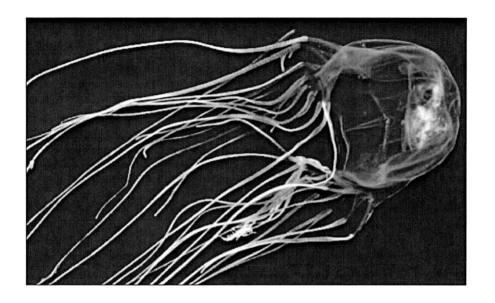

World's Deadliest Venom - *The coastal waters of Northern Australia and the Indo-Pacific Oceans are home to a rather fearsome creature – the world's most poisonous animal, the* **box jellyfish**. *Box jellyfish aggressively hunt, injecting a paralytic toxin into their victims. This jolts the prey into shock, often killing it outright, so it never struggles to escape or damage the jellyfish's delicate tentacles.*

Box jellyfish venom causes cellular leakage, leading to cardiovascular collapse and death within as little as 120 seconds. The toxin is said to be so overwhelmingly painful that humans are likely to go into shock and drown or die of heart failure before being able to swim to shore, and survivors can expect agonizing pain for weeks, followed by lifelong, significant scarring.

For all their deadliness, box jellyfish are strikingly beautiful, pale blue-white and transparent, with a cube-like bell and some four dozen 10-foot-long tentacles. Each of those tentacles, however, contains about 5,000 stinging cells. These animals are highly advanced jellyfish, capable of active movement instead of simple drifting, rocketing through the water at nearly two meters a second – roughly as fast as a human running on land. They also have clusters of six eyes on each of the four faces of their cube-shaped bells. These eyes are quite sophisticated, with a lens, retina, iris and cornea.

Interestingly, some experts estimate as many as one to two hundred unreported victims die annually from box jellyfish stings, twice as many as from shark attacks in Southeast Asia and Australia. But sea turtles are completely unaffected by the toxin, and regularly snack upon box jellyfish. Image: The 10 Most Known. com, public domain

The Very Nerve!

Recently, many genes once thought to be specific for the human nervous system have been found in the most ancient eukaryotes. Thus, the components for neurons have existed long before their use in nerve cells. But the first *nervous systems* evolved among jellyfish, anemones and other cnidarians about 600 million years ago – decentralized, netlike systems that would eventually evolve into centralized brains and nerves.

Chemical signalling is used within a number of biological systems, such as hormones circulating in the bloodstream; but hormones slowly circulate, acting like a molecular broadcast. Nervous systems are specialized for faster, targeted information transmission. Structurally, nerve cells aren't much different from other cells, and the basic chemical units which combine into neurotransmitters are found in many species.

This electrical signalling isn't unique to animals, however; it also occurs in plants. For example, when caterpillars feed on tomato leaves, it creates action potentials which are transmitted to neighboring leaves, triggering the synthesis of toxins.

Animals use many different neurotransmitters to signal between synapses, allowing for diverse signals. Additionally, several different receptors can exist for each neurotransmitter, allowing a variety of responses to the same transmitter, and adding to range of available incoming signals.

A major requirement for neurotransmitters like dopamine, adrenaline, noradrenaline and serotonin, however, is that they be easily synthesized from readily available substances. These neurotransmitters are closely related to substances used for metabolic signalling, so they're even found in unicellular organisms which have no synapses.

Getting in Touch

Although it is the first and most basic sense to have evolved, touch is currently the least understood of the five senses. But the tactile sense is ubiquitous; virtually no creature alive today fails to respond in some way when physically touched. Even simple one-celled organisms feel something brushing up against them, responding by nudging closer or pulling away. Touch is the first sense aroused in a developing baby, and last to fade at the end of life. Even patients in comas show skin responses to touch.

Mechanical senses first originated in unicellular organisms, and the first to evolve was *osmosensation*, in which protein *osmoreceptors* detect the concentrations of chemicals in fluids outside the membrane, allowing cells to adjust their inner chemistry in response. These channels are found in E. coli bacteria, acting as release valves to expel excess water or other substances as needed to maintain stable inner cellular chemistry. Equivalents are found in archaea.

Because it's central to survival, these receptors evolved in animals into force-detecting, mechanosensory cells which change shape in response to physical stimuli such as vibration, stretch, pressure, temperature or injury. Living cells meet with a constant barrage of forces – pressure, stretch, flow, and sound waves. This has all led to the evolution of extraordinarily fast, sensitive, selective, diverse and specialized mechanosensory cells.

The tactile sense is vital to myriad behaviors ranging from avoiding bodily harm to social interaction – from the simplest worm to the most complex mammal, species *propagation* (population increase) depends upon touch-reliant mating behaviors. In mammals, touch is critical to raising young; infants deprived of touch have significantly impaired cognitive and physical development, often unable to survive infancy.

Haptic communication – communication by touch – is a type of nonverbal communication used by humans and other animals. This form of communication is extremely important for social interactions, particularly in conveying physical intimacy, but also in establishing social hierarchies.

A variety of *somatosensory* neurons populate your skin to report sensations of touch, texture, vibration, temperature and pain. But the basic forms of these nerves exist in a wide range of creatures, from the tine roundworm C. elegans to the fruit fly Drosophila, all having evolved from unicellular cilia and flagella. Ion channels are at the heart of all of these systems, which convert mechanical stimuli into neural impulses that the brain then organizes into sensations.

Rise of the Hunters

Kimberella was an early marine organism whose fossils have been found in Ediacaran-era rocks. The creature appears to have been soft-bodied like a slug, and fed upon the microbial mats of the ancient ocean floors some 550 million years ago. Kimberella indicates that species diversification had already progressed significantly by the time of the so-called Cambrian explosion. Image: Wikipedia, public domain

600 million years ago, the Ediacaran seas teemed with *benthic* life – creatures living in or on the ocean floor. Primitive animals shaped like fronds, bags and sponges fed upon microbial mats scattered across the mud and sand. The rise in ocean oxygenation and retreat of global glaciers further opened the door for ever greater adaptations to take hold. Then something wonderful happened.

Quite rapidly, and quite beautifully, there was an explosion in the diversity of life. Zygotes from prehistoric creatures started following different patterning trajectories, and new genetic patterning templates controlling embryonic development gave rise to innovative new forms.

From a common ancestor, these organisms all began with the same genes to guide the formation of three-dimensional animals. But relatively minor DNA transpositions, mutations and sexual reproduction are thought to have had a major impact, radically altering genomes and embryonic development.

In 2012, Dartmouth College palaeobiologist Dr. Kevin Peterson compared microRNA sequences of several species, and found a huge burst of new miRNAs appeared between 550 million and 505 million years ago – more than at any other time in evolutionary history. This is the period in which complex vertebrate features like the head, gills, kidneys and thymus evolved. Says Dr. Peterson, the acquisition of these miRNAs seems to have allowed cells to develop more complex regulatory systems and new and diverse cell functions: "It's those miRNAs that I would argue allow you to get novel cell types," he says.

This was the era of the so-called *Cambrian Explosion*, evolution's "Big Bang", in which up to 80 percent of modern animal phyla first appeared. Over the course of roughly 100 million years, these new branches of life developed down divergent paths. At this ancient crossroads, animals branched out into distinct new groups, and a stunning variety of creatures encased in armored plates, shells and spines began to emerge.

A 2005 Stanford University experiment shows this trait is controlled by protein signalling molecules like *ectodermal dysplasin* (EDA) – switching on a single EDA gene in the lab triggers the growth of bony plate armor on fish. When Professor David M. Kingsley inserted the gene into fish which had lost their armor plates after evolving in freshwater, the plates re-emerged.

The gene is still present in mammals, where it guides embryonic development of *ectodermal* tissue, instructing progenitor cells to form teeth, hair and sweat glands. It also appears to guide the shape of nose and forehead bones, one of countless examples of nature recruiting previously-existing genes for novel traits in later species.

The Cambrian Explosion perplexed biologists for over a century. It seemed to begin roughly 545 million years ago, with an "explosion" of new life, then to have ended with a mass extinction 52 million years later. It was an era in which more diverse life seemed to evolve than at any time before or since.

The Cambrian seemed relatively overnight, a huge growth in complexity among living organisms within just five to ten million years – an evolutionary eyeblink. Prior to this, life seems to have existed in the form of soft-bodied invertebrates; then creatures with hardened skeletons suddenly sprang up and diversified at an astonishing speed. Scientists long puzzled over this comparatively overnight explosion of diversification.

However, in 2012, researchers at the University of Alberta discovered tiny shallow-water burrows in Uruguay at least 585 million years old, showing tiny worms, comparatively sophisticated creatures, had emerged much earlier. This suggests the Cambrian's "explosion" was only a stage of rapid development, likely triggered by genetic transpositions that created the first *genetic tool kit* which governs body patterning.

The process was undoubtedly hastened by predation, climate change, and the rise in ocean oxygenation, all of which occurred about 550 million years ago. Thus, the one-two-three punch of the genetic tool kit, the global rise in temperature and oxygenation 550 million years ago lit the Cambrian fuse, so to speak.

Mass extinctions at the end of the Ediacaran likely led to major changes in the ecosystem, and climate change in particular opened a variety of unique new environmental niches, for which creatures adapted specialized survival traits.

Waste Not, Want Not – Evolution is driven less by the emergence of new genetic mutations which express novel traits than by the "right" habitat which encourages particularly advantageous traits, often from existing genes.

Exaptation – the repurposing of existing structures – is common in evolution. One example is seen in feathers, which initially evolved to provide insulation, but were later adapted for flight and for courtship display. Recently, it became apparent that exaptation also takes place at a genetic level. In genetic exaptation, dormant DNA can also sometimes acquire new functions.

When twin copies of a gene exist in a creature's genome, often one of the pair retains its normal function, while the second is either lost or repurposed to express an entirely new trait.

In the Box

Hox genes are billion-year-old clusters of DNA which control animal limb and *longitudinal* (head-to-tail) axis development. These genes direct the organization and development of anatomical regions, organs, and tissues, and have been crucial in controlling major evolutionary transitions in animal anatomy.

To gauge the importance of Hox genes for life on Earth, consider: most genes have gradually changed over time, chromosomes snipped and spliced, copying errors and advantageous mutations giving rise to a dazzling diversity of life; but while whole continents drifted about the planet, asteroids slammed into the earth, and glaciers advanced and retreated, this fundamental set of genes remained intact for over a billion years, predating even the evolutionary split between animals, plants, and fungi.

Hox (short for *Homeobox*) genes express transcription factors, the regulatory proteins which activate or repress other genes by binding to DNA enhancer regions – in this case, regions which control embryonic tissue production. Transcription factors are thus critical for making the right proteins in the right places at the right times, and, in this case, for guiding anatomical development. The word Homeobox is derived from the word *homeotic*, which means "responsible for a shift in structural development".

Hox genes express protein transcription factors which act as *ligands*, chemicals which act as keys fitting into protein receptor locks in cell nuclei, triggering chemical reactions. This creates a chemical cascade, turning on specific genes that direct uncommitted embryonic cells to differentiate, grow and multiply, to produce cartilage, bone, nerves, muscle, hindbrain, etc.

The proteins which Hox genes express control how an embryo's body develops along its head-to-tail axis, in a progression of segments from the head down, guiding the formation of, for example, legs, ribs and a tail for an alligator, or legs, wings, and antennae for a butterfly. The sequence of each Hox gene matches the sequence of development along the animal's length.

The Hox gene family is divided into 13 groups of highly-related genes, each group called a *paralogue*. These paralogues are found in the same position in each complex.

Mammals have four Hox gene complexes, derived from duplications of the original single complex – found in ancient ancestor species as far back as the *lancelet Amphioxus (see below)*, which has survived relatively unchanged since the Cambrian era.

Hox genes control cell differentiation and thus embryonic tissue expression in a linear sequence, from the anterior to the posterior, and the entire animal kingdom makes use of Hox genes to organize segmented body development starting with the *bilaterians* (animals with *bilateral symmetry* – two-sided evenness, with a front and rear end, as well as an upside and downside).

Hox genes govern development of segmented body parts in vertebrates as they form in the embryo, including the vertebrae of the spine, and the limb and digit bones, as well as the hindbrain and reproductive organs.

Hox genes are one type of *genetic toolkit* which evolved to shape embryonic development. They've been duplicated and extended several times in evolutionary history, leading to progressively more complex organisms. Such gene duplications occasionally occur on the scale of an entire genome, resulting in major alterations to physical traits among animals. This is one of the major drivers of evolution, giving rise to novel features in species, or even entirely new species. (The dividing line for a *species* is generally when a pair of animals can no longer successfully mate.

Researchers have been using mouse, fruit fly, chick and zebrafish for Hox gene experiments, altering individual Hox gene expression to see how it affects morphological development:

Retinoic acid – the biologically active portion of vitamin A – activates Hox genes. By injecting mouse, zebrafish, or chick embryos with retinoic acid, specific sites can be prompted to overexpress Hox genes, developing into new vertebrae or limbs.

Custom miRNAs can also be inserted into viral shells and injected into nuclei to bind to and silence specific genes, allowing researchers to study the effects upon embryonic development. The injection site and timing during fetal development determines what will develop, starting from the posterior end, and working forward.

Because of these experiments, the specific functions of Hox genes are starting to become fairly well mapped out.

This *genetic toolkit* was a major leap forward in animal evolution, enabling the transition from cnidarians to more complex bilaterian animals: the Hox gene toolkit readily allows natural evolutionary alterations to body plans, through transcription factors, microRNA gene silencing, mutations, transpositions, deletions and/or duplications of clusters or individual genes.

Changing the timing, location and level of Hox gene expression radically alters body patterning. Duplicating these regulatory genes allows increased structural complexity.

In humans, there are an estimated 235 functional homeobox genes and 65 *pseudogenes*, which are structurally similar but don't express proteins. Homeobox genes are found in every human chromosome, often appearing in clusters. Among the supercluster are the Hox group, which guides skeletal, limb, hindbrain and organ development, the *PAX genes*, which guide neuron and sensory organ development, and *MSX genes*, which guide head, face, and tooth development.

Since the Cambrian explosion seems to have occurred within a very brief span of perhaps 20 to 50 million years, such tremendous species diversification couldn't have arisen from typical genetic mutations alone. Given a steady rate of 1 mutation per year, it would require 10 million years for even a 1% change to a billion-base-pair genome. Because of this, Dr. Susumu Ohno of the Beckman Research Institute suggests that Hox genes were part of a larger, nearly identical *pananimalia genome* shared by all Cambrian-era animals, who diversified through novel ways of regulating this universal animal-building template.

Thus, approximately 560 million years ago, a common bilaterian ancestor evolved regulatory pathways which modified the universal patterning template, resulting in major morphogical innovations. In addition to Hox genes for anterior-posterior body development, Dr. Ohno proposes that the universal genetic template included a gene for the enzyme *lysyloxidase*, used to form ligaments and tendons; the *Pax-6* gene, which guides eye development in creatures from ribbon worms to humans, and other sensory systems in eyeless animals; and *skeletal patterning genes* inherited from algae.

143

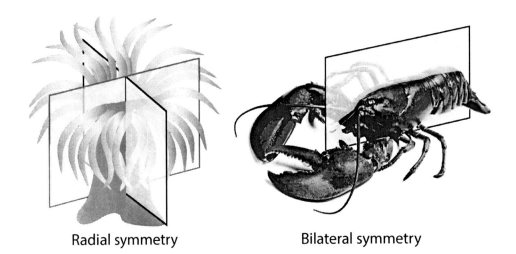

Radial symmetry   Bilateral symmetry

The Shape I'm in

Before the advent of modern genetics research, biologists built phylogenetic trees based upon anatomical similarity, in both the developmental and adult stages. In terms of anatomy, animals are grouped according to four criteria: *1) body symmetry, 2) embryonic tissues, 3) body cavity*, and *4) developmental stages*.

Multicellular animals can either be *symmetrical* – having matching sides – or *asymmetrical* – randomly-shaped like a sponge; and symmetry can be two-, four-, five-sided or even more.

The first major change in body structures was the emergence of *radial symmetry* – the body plan of cnidarians like sea anemones and jellyfish. Next came the evolution of *flatworms*, with the simplest bilateral symmetry along two body axes – *anteroposterior* (head to tail) and *dorsoventral* (back to belly).

Bilateral symmetry is ideal for hunting and foraging; bilateral animals face the environment in one direction. Their body plan is tube-like, running *anterior* (front) to *posterior* (back). The emergence of this organization was a major step in evolution, giving rise to *cephalization*, the development of an anterior head, where structures for feeding, perception and information processing could be concentrated. Meanwhile, the posterior evolved for forward locomotion.

Bilateral symmetry is widespread throughout the animal kingdom, because the structure is very efficient for hunting: quick movement can be directed by the head, and powered by a long posterior region. Organisms organized along this anteroposterior axis take advantage of *pair-rule genes* to build up a muscular grid of fibers, a pattern first seen in ancient flatworms and leeches.

Animals are also classified according to the number of *embryonic tissue layers* which develop. Animals of greater complexity than sponges develop from either two or three primitive collections of cells, called *germ layers,* are used to form tissues, organs and organ systems. Simpler animals – jellyfish, anemones, sea pens, hydra, comb jellies and corals – have two embryonic tissue layers, while more complex *triploblastic* animals have three: the *ectoderm, mesoderm* and *endoderm* (Greek for *outer-, middle-* and *inner skin*).

In humans and other vertebrates, ectoderm tissues develop into the skin and nervous system, mesoderm into bones, organs, circulatory system and muscles, and endoderm into the lining of the *alimentary canal* – the digestive tract.

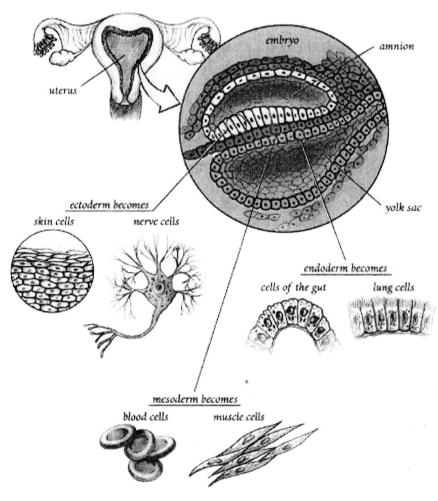

Image: Stem Cell Now, Christopher Thomas Scott,
Plume Books, 2006, used with permission.

145

It's believed that the *epidermis* – skin – was the first organ system that evolved in animals. This tissue layer intervenes between the body's external and internal environments, and has a number of functions – holding an organism together, controlling the flow of substances in and out, and offering protection from dehydration, extreme temperatures, and parasite, bacterial and viral infections.

University of Minnesota Professor PZ Myers teaches evolutionary developmental biology. Says Dr. Myers, at one time Hox genes and related *ParaHox* and *NK gene clusters* were all linked in a "megacluster" of homeobox genes central to body-plan evolution.

Early in animal evolution, he says, before sponges evolved further, this megacluster split it into three blocks – the ParaHox, Hox, and NK regions. He contends that these three banks of patterning genes correspond to the primitive germ layers in triploblastic animals – Hox genes associated with ectodermal development, ParaHox genes with the endoderm, and NK genes with the mesoderm.

From the Humblest Beginnings

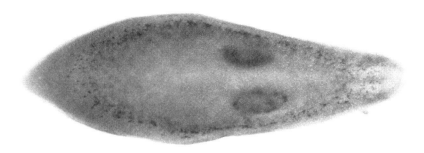

Acoel flatworm Neochildia fusca, Egger, B., Steinke, D., Tarui, H., et al, 2011 Creative Commons Attribution 2.5 Generic License

Acoela are tiny worm-shaped organisms, about 2 millimeters long. These soft-bodied marine animals are only slightly more developed than jellyfish and anemones, swimming as plankton, crawling between sediment grains, or living on algae. Although they look like flatworms, they are much closer to sponges, lacking a *coelom* (inner cavity), without a gut, circulatory or respiratory system. Like sponges, they digest food with a special type of multi-nuclear cell called a *syncytium*, which surrounds and engulfs food.

The ectoderm was coaxed into expressing a primitive neural network by genes like the *sog* and *chd* genes, giving Acoela a simple network of nerves just under the skin, connected to surface cilia. These nerves are slightly more concentrated towards the front, where two sensory organs are located.

Being upside-down exposes this creature's belly to predators. To prevent this, like modern jellyfish, snails and other related creatures, acoela evolved *statocysts*, balance-sensing organs similar to those in human inner ears.

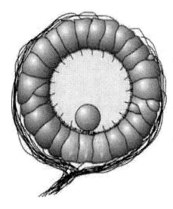

*A **statocyst** is a hollow sac with sensory hairs lining the inner walls, and tiny calcium carbonate particles within. When the acoela is upside-down, the particles shift about, disturbing the sensory hairs and triggering a neural impulse, and the animal reflexively rights itself. Image: Statocyst, Davis, W. J., 1968, public domain.*

The aceola's second sensory organ is a pair of spots, capable of detecting light. These spots contain special proteins called opsins, which change their molecular structure when struck by energy-transferring photons, triggering nerve impulses. They are hermaphrodites, each creating its own young independently. The *Urbilateria*, common ancestor to all modern bilaterians, was something very much like this humble creature.

Tubular

Another major defining feature among animals is the presence or absence of an internal cavity called a *coelom*. Worms were the first to develop a primitive proto-coelom, which eventually evolved into a mesoderm-lined hollow space, lined by muscles and blood vessels. The coelom acts as a container for circulating nutrients and oxygen, and as a space for internal organs.

This ubiquitous design – a tube within a tube – renders tremendously efficient moving, eating machines: broadly speaking, the inner tube comprises an organism's gut, while the outer tube is its outer skin. Sandwiched between, the mesoderm forms its muscles and inner organs. Worms are the starting point for this template, but mounting the design on legs produces everything from komodo dragons, to army ants, lobsters, and even African elephants.

Nearly all animal species alive today follow this body plan: *bilaterally symmetric triploblasts* with a central cavity lined by protective mesoderm. *Segmentation*, the repetition of identical anatomical units along the anteroposterior axis, is a fundamental structure found in many species. Obvious examples include centipedes and millipedes, which have a segment repeating dozens of times over. The genes controlling segmentation have been conserved across species, indicating they originated within a single common ancestor some 600 million years ago, an ancestor who survived due to this segmentation.

Three of the most basic animal groups, the *arthropods* (insects, arachnids, and crustaceans), *vertebrates* (animals with backbones), and *annelid worms* all make extensive use of segmentation, although they've very distantly related.

147

In essence, all vertebrates are modified versions of segmented worms, their bodies comprised of sequentially repeated units – such as vertebral columns and ribs. Arthropods – crabs, lobsters, insects and the like – are also modified segmented worms, made up of stacked rings.

So animals share a fundamentally tube-like, segmented body, with an internal gut running from mouth to anus, and a body cavity filled with muscles and organs. The vast diversity of animal species is derived from the evolution of specialized structures for feeding, perceiving the environment and locomotion – wings and legs are simply more efficient ways of transporting the living tube around its environment.

Eating machines

Morphology deals with the structures of living creatures – external features such as shape, structure, color, and patterns, as well as internal ones, such as bones and organs. In animals, these structures evolved primarily as ever-more efficient means of engaging in the "three F's": feeding, fleeing and reproduction.

After the sponges, animals all developed the following shared traits:

- *multicellularity and tissues*
- *heterotrophy (eating other organisms)*
- *energy storage – long term as fat and short term as **glycogen***
- *no external cell walls*
- *a nervous and muscle system*
- *sexual reproduction*
- *embryonic development in which a zygote undergoes multiple cell divisions*

There are five strategies animals use to eat, although some switch between these strategies over the course of their lifetimes:

1. *Suspension feeders* (filter feeders) capture food particles by filtering air or water. This is how clams eat, burrowing under the ocean floor, and extending siphons out. One siphon draws water in, gills trap microorganisms for the clam to digest, then pump water out the other siphon.

   Tiny, lobster-like krill swim about the ocean, minute cilia (hair-like) projections on their legs capturing plankton and bringing it to their mouths to feed. These krill are, in turn, eaten by baleen whales, giant suspension feeders which gulp great mouthfuls of water, then squeeze it out through a series of long mouth plates called *baleens*, thus trapping the krill inside. Because such creatures belong to very different animal lineages, we know that filter feeding evolved independently several times in Earth's history.

2. *Deposit feeders* eat their way through substances. Earthworms, for example, tunnel through dirt, swallowing as they go and digesting organic matter like bacteria,

archaea, fungi, and dead and partially decomposed remains of leaves, insects and other life forms. Many insects also bore through plant leaves and stems, through animal waste, or through animal carcasses or dead plants. Deposit feeding animals are also diverse, including worms, insect larvae, and hagfish. However, their body structures are always wormlike, and their mouths simple.

3. *Herbivores* consume photosynthesizing organisms – either algae or plant life. Unlike deposit feeders, herbivores have a very wide range of mouth shapes, ranging from the scraping, file-shaped radula of snails, to the curled, extendable sucking proboscis of moths, to the chewing mandibles of grasshoppers and the grinding molars of horses. All these mouth shapes evolved to process plant matter or algae.

4. *Predators* capture and eat other animals, by either lying in wait or actively hunting their prey. Frogs are sit-and-wait predators, which wait for insects or worms to approach, then shoot out their sticky tongues to capture their prey. Of the active hunters, some species travel in packs and others are solitary hunters. Wolves and other members of the dog group run down prey after extended, long-distance chases in family groups called packs. Conversely, mountain lions, like nearly all cats, hunt alone, slowly stalking their prey, then pouncing upon it, or running it down in a short burst of speed.

5. *Parasites* tend to be much smaller than the animals upon which they feed, and usually harvest nutrients without killing their victims. There are two types – endoparasites, which live inside their hosts, and ectoparasites, which live outside them. Tapeworms are endoparasites with hooks in place of a mouth, and they latch onto the intestinal walls of hosts, then absorb surrounding nutrients. Ectoparasites like lice, ticks and mites have limbs and mouths which allow them to latch onto the host, pierce its skin, and suck up nutrient-dense fluids.

Meet Grandpa

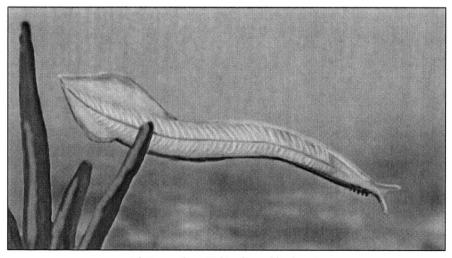

Pikaia gracilens, Wikipedia, public domain.

149

DNA and fossil evidence show that our earliest ancestor was a tiny worm swimming the oceans half a billion years ago. Less than two inches long, *Pikaia gracilens* was one such flat, leaf-shaped creature, which propelled itself over the sea floor by undulating through the water like an eel. Pikaia's fossilized remains were discovered a century earlier in the mountains of British Columbia, Canada, but their significance had long remained unknown, until the creature was re-examined in 2012.

Pikaia is at the base of the branch of life which includes everything from sea cucumbers to humans – the *Deuterostomes*. The name is Latin for *mouth second* because in deuterostomes, an embryonic anus develops before a mouth. Pikaia was one of the first to evolve remarkable new features: its body was bilateral, with lined pairs of segmented muscle fanning out from a flexible central rod – the *notochord*, precursor to the backbone.

All *chordate* embryos develop a notochord, which usually matures into the vertebrate backbone. Pikaia's notochord ran from the tip of its tail to the tip of its very primitive head – the earliest form of *cephalization* (head development). Its head, however, consisted solely of a mouth, the creature's first point of contact with the environment it swam through, feeding on organic particles. Pikaia possessed no true sensory organs, but its quest for food required continuous testing of what lay ahead in the water. It's believed this triggered the evolution of specialized sensory organs for sight, touch and smell, all evolving around the mouth.

Meanwhile, *hypertrophy* and *hyperplasia*, a swelling and proliferation of cells in the central nerve cord eventually evolved into a brain, necessary for processing data gathered by developing sensory organs. Together, these features were the prerequisites for the first vertebrates. However, developmental genetics shows that brains evolved independently at least four times among different bilaterian animal groups – driven by genes such as *sog* and *chd*, which push ectodermal tissue to differentiate into neural networks.

Striking the Right Chord

University of Cambridge Professor Simon Conway Morris says *myomeres* (strips of skeletal muscle tissue) constitute a "smoking gun" that clearly shows Pikaia was Earth's most primitive chordate. This means it's an ancestor to all vertebrates, including fish, amphibians, reptiles, birds, and mammals.

The chordates are uniquely-adapted animals which evolved four shared features. Interestingly, all chordates, including fish, amphibians, reptiles, and mammals, show these features at some point during embryonic development:

1. *pharyngeal clefts* – Embryonic openings connecting the inside of the throat to the outside of the "neck" which develop into structures which vary by species, such as *gills*, for oxygen filtration from water;

2. *dorsal nerve cord* – a bundle of nerve fibers running down the creature's dorsal region (back), connecting the brain to muscles and organs;

3. *notochord* – a stiff but flexible supportive rod from which the chordates get their name;

4. *tails* – a muscle-containing structure that extends past the anus.

BILATERIAN DIVERGENCE

Genetic analyses indicate a hypothetical *Urbilaterian* diverged into two branches of bilaterian animals, perhaps even before the Cambrian era. This urbilaterian must have been a segmented *benthic* (sea bottom-dwelling) animal.

The two bilaterian animal branches are the *protostomes* (proto + stomo = *first mouth*, because the mouth develops first in the embryo) and the *deuterostomes* (deutero meaning second, because the mouth develops after the anus). Both animal groups use *homologous patterning genes* to build their body structures.

Invertebrates such as insects evolved with their spinal cords running along the *ventral* side (belly), and digestive system along the *dorsal* side (back). Vertebrates evolved with their spinal cords running along the dorsal side (back), and gut along the ventral side (belly).

The *central nervous system* is marked blue and the *endoderm* - the innermost embryonic tissue layer - is red. Openings in the endoderm are yellow. The endoderm forms inner linings for the gastrointestinal tract, the respiratory tract, the *endocrine* (hormone-excreting) glands and organs, the auditory and urinary systems.

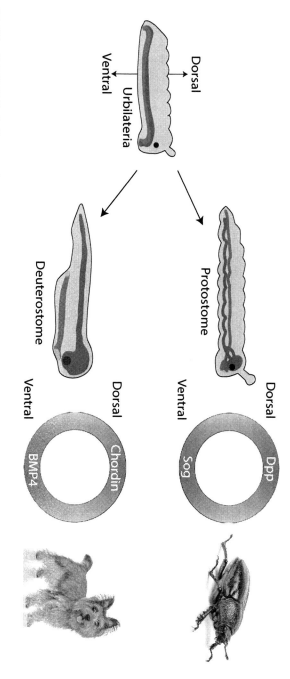

151

The chordate body plan proved enormously efficient and versatile. Today, over 60,000 chordate species exist, half of them bony fish. The family also includes the world's largest and fastest animals, the blue whale, and the peregrine falcon. It also includes the *primates* (of which humans are one species).

Alongside the chordates, the arthropods continued to evolve along separate lines –insects, spiders, and crustaceans would flourish and become the most diverse group, eventually constituting over 90% of all surviving animal species, adapting to nearly every ecosystem on the planet.

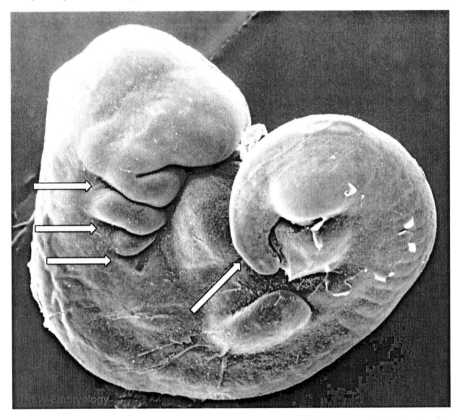

*In vertebrate embryos, **pharyngeal arches** develop into a variety of structures. In fish, they develop into **brachial arches** which support **gills**, while in human embryos, the **Hox, Dlx, Gcm-2,** and **Foxn1** genes transform them into parts of the jaw, upper respiratory tract, middle ear, parathyroid and thymus glands. The pharyngeal clefts are indicated by three left-hand arrows, and the post-anal **vestigial tail** by the right-hand arrow. Images: Human Embryo, Carnegie Stage 13, (26-30 days) and 14 (31- 35 days), Dr. Kohei Shiota, used with permission.*

Innovations

Amphioxus is a tiny, ancient marine animal which has remained essentially unchanged for half a billion years. It's a filter-feeder, more commonly called a *lancelet*, and it burrows in sandy sea floors, primarily in shallow waters of temperate and tropical shorelines. There are about 35 known species, ranging in size from two to four inches long. Superficially, Amphioxus resembles a fish, with a dorsal fin running nearly the length of its body, and a short ventral fin near its tail. Its sharp-edged body earned this creature the name amphioxus, which means *double edged*, while the name lancelet is derived from its lance-shaped tail.

Amphioxus is a *transitional form* between invertebrates (animals without backbones) and vertebrates (animals with backbones). In place of a backbone, amphioxus possesses a stiff, flexible cartilage-like rod called a *notochord*, which extends the length of its body. Running above and parallel to the notochord is a nerve cord, but it has no centralized cluster that could be classified as a brain.

Amphioxus is able to swim, but mainly spends its life buried tail-down in coarse sand or gravel in shallow coastal waters, feeding upon microorganisms which it filters out of seawater via its gill slits. DNA analysis reveals it's at the base of the chordate lineage, and therefore one of the first. The adult is similar to a vertebrate, but simpler, lacking features such as paired sensory organs (eyes or ears), a mineralized skeleton, and paired limbs. Its embryo also lacks *neural crest cells* – cell clusters which are the source of vertebrate features like sensory ganglia, and a bone-encased head and spine. These features would develop later, becoming central to vertebrate evolution and allowing a predatory lifestyle.

Experiments with amphioxus allow biologists to study the specific genes which led to the chordate transition from invertebrates to vertebrates. They've discovered the amphioxus genome contains a single Hox cluster, and this entire genome underwent two duplications en route to vertebrate evolution. These duplications gave rise to a mineralization-controlling gene (*Scpp* – *secretory calcium-binding phosphoprotein*), and gene transpositions gave rise to a vertebrate cartilage matrix gene (*aggrecan*).

Researchers have catalogued other specific transcription factors which govern cartilage and bone formation (*SPARC*, *SoxE*, *Runx* and *collagen* genes). These further evolved in vertebrates, while several non-coding elements remained essentially unchanged for half a billion years, living on in modern mammals.

Placodes are thickening regions of ectoderm setting the site of future embryonic development of sense organs and other structures, including hair, eye lenses, teeth, and structures central to sight, hearing, and olfaction. In fish, they also map out a sensory system called the *lateral line*, used to detect movement and vibration in the water.

Pax, *Six* and *Eya* family genes, central to vertebrate sensory development, as well as specific sex-determining genes, were already present in amphioxus, and would come to be used by vertebrates for placode development. *T-box* genes, which assist in vertebrate limb formation, are also present in amphioxus. Amphioxus' single Hox cluster would be duplicated three times during the course of mammalian evolution.

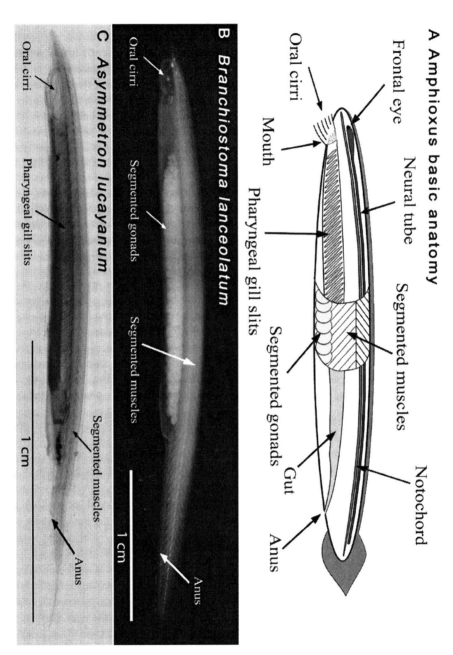

Image: **Amphioxus**, dubbed the "faceless and brainless fish", is a living ancestor of the first vertebrates, and has survived essentially unchanged over half a billion years. This creature has no specific brain or face, but a nerve cord, the precursor to a vertebrate spine, runs down its back. A) Amphioxus shares all the features common to chordates, including a dorsal hollow neural tube (blue), dorsal notochord (red), ventral gut (green) and segmented gonads (yellow). (B) An adult lancelet, with oral cirri, segmented gonads and muscles, and anus labelled. (C) An adult with oral cirri, pharyngeal gill slits, segmented muscles and anus labelled. Image: Dr. Hector Escriva, reproduced with permission, Development Magazine, 2011.

154

Getting Ahead

While Hox genes guide body patterning, 1999 genetics experiments show that *Cerberus* proteins (expressed by the *CER1 gene* in humans) are central to head development. Heads evolved in complexity from a simple bud of sensory and motor *ganglia* – neural clusters – in the anterior end of the body.

In 2013, researchers at the Universities of Bergen and Vienna announced a separate set of three genes which guide bilaterian head development, including the forebrain. These patterning genes – *six3/6*, *foxQ2*, and *irx* – arose in a common animal ancestor before the split between bilaterians and *cnidarians*, some 600 to 750 million years ago.

The cnidarians – jellyfish, corals, and sea anemones – are a sister group to bilaterians. They have nerve networks, but no centrally-organized brain, and their primary sensory organ is at their *aboral end* (opposite the mouth). The genes used to form this sensory region were conserved in bilaterians, where they organize head and forebrain development. In humans, *six3* also regulates eye development.

Braaaaaaaains!

The earliest, most primitive benthic animals led quiet, relatively peaceful lives upon the dark ocean floors, but the rise of *predation* created an evolutionary pressure to adapt, with a system allowing fast responses for hunting or escaping.

Brains began as a series of neural clusters, swellings at the top of the spinal ganglia. The oldest fossil evidence of such a structure was found in 530-million-year-old *Haikouichthys*, a benthic, eel-like *craniate* – a creature with a backbone and head.

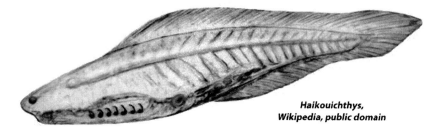

Haikouichthys,
Wikipedia, public domain

Named after the region in China where it was discovered, it had a distinct head, tail, primitive cartilage skull, and what seems to be a segmented, cartilage backbone housing a spinal cord, making it one of the earliest vertebrates. At the front of the creature's body are a pair of eyespots and a cavity which may have housed a primitive olfactory organ. Within the same formation, archeologists also discovered 524-million-year-old *Myllokunmingia*, with a notochord, a pharynx and digestive tract. Both species closely resemble modern lancelets.

The brain evolved as the primary controlling unit for the *central nervous system*, protected by a bony frontal skull and growing near the sensory organs, to efficiently process data. As animals move forward, sensory organs gather information about the environment, relaying it in a direct path to the brain.

The brain also controls the body's organs, either contracting muscles or triggering the secretion of signalling molecules like hormones and neurotransmitters. In addition to a centralized brain which directs complex behaviors, vertebrates evolved a sophisticated spinal cord which provides automatic *reflex responses*, such as flinching away from a source of pain or tissue damage.

The Cognitive Big Bang

Near the early Cambrian, gene duplications and expansions in creatures such as Pikaia triggered a second evolutionary "Big Bang". These gene alterations resulted in the rapid growth of several new signalling molecules. The increased diversity in cell signalling opened the doorway to greater intelligence, allowing for more nuanced and sophisticated responses to the environment.

The emergence of the vertebrate brain would transform the first tiny, frail chordates into formidable predators, enabling *association-* and *reward-based learning*; the formation of new synapses and strengthening of existing ones, creating memories from linking perceptions, for example, a specific shape with a predator, the feeling of pain with fighting, a smell with a food source.

This allowed animals to modify their behavior "on the fly", generating sophisticated responses to the environment which would confer huge survival advantages. The system would slowly evolve to include paired sense organs – eyes, ears, and noses – along with related ganglia.

Key innovations emerged in the chordate embryo, where ectoderm tissue can transform into specific developmental regions. One of these regions, the *neural plate*, generates the vertebrate nervous system. Here, *neural crest cells* migrate and differentiate into neurons, *glial* (brain support) cells, cartilage, bone, and muscle. The process is guided by a network of regulatory genes, activated by three protein signalling molecules – *FGF*, *BMP* and *WNT* – which initiate cell differentiation.

Guided by genes such as *Six* and *Eya*, temporary neural plate regions called *sensory placodes* differentiate into cells which form sensory neurons and ganglia, lens fiber cells, and receptor cells for hearing, balance, olfaction and vision. This system eventually evolved into the system of paired vertebrate sensory organs, pivotal in enabling the emergence of an advanced predatory lifestyle.

The transition also involved the evolution of *monoamine neurotransmitters*, so-called because of their single amino acid chemical structures: *serotonin, dopamine, adrenaline (epinephrine), noradrenaline (norepinephrine), melatonin* and *histamine*. Related systems included enzymes for the synthesis and breakdown of neurotransmitters, and membrane receptor and transport proteins.

Genetic analyses show these monoamine systems evolved with the emergence of the chordates, though serotonin-related genes had existed much earlier. Serotonin receptors exist in all animals, who use it to govern behaviors as diverse as swimming, sleeping, feeding, social interaction, and as a fetal brain growth factor. The roots of the serotonin neural modulating system may extend as far back as photosynthesizing bacteria, who used the serotonin-synthesizing enzyme *tryptophan hydroxylase* for a simpler purpose – to shed excess oxygen waste from photosynthesis.

In vertebrates, serotonin is secreted from neural clusters called the *raphe nuclei* in the *brainstem,* where the spinal cord connects to the base of the brain. Serotonin often doesn't act directly upon other neurons, but instead modulates the transmission of other neurotransmitters, exerting a profound influence: a single serotonin neuron can affect as many as 500,000 target neurons, acting as a *neuromodulator* which regulates signal flow. Due to its widespread influence throughout the nervous system, it's unsurprising that serotonin is linked to many kinds of behavior.

Like serotonin, norepinephrine, and acetylcholine, dopamine (shortened to DA) is also a neuromodulator, acting as a sort of chemical valve for mental activity, helping control signal flow throughout the brain and central nervous system. As such, it helps regulate sensory perception, and such things as body temperature, food intake, and blood chemistry. It's also an extremely versatile neurotransmitter, central to a wide variety of functions, including motivation, motor control and motor learning, memory, emotions and endocrine regulation.

High levels of dopamine have been associated with greater competitiveness and aggression, and, conversely, impulse control – a useful combination of survival traits. But dopamine is most famous for its role in *reward-driven learning*, and it lies at the heart of motivation – without dopamine, fruit flies will not move to feed themselves, even at the point of starvation. Oddly enough, these mutant fruit flies also learn not to avoid painful shocks, but to seek them out.

Dopamine first evolved among the diploblasts (jellyfish, corals, sea pens, anemones, and comb jellies). Chordates capitalized and expanded upon the system's flexibility through gene duplications, spreading the DA system to other regions of the nervous system.

DA neuronal systems began as dopamine-synthesizing cells clustered around photoreceptors connected to anterior neural tubes in ancestral chordates like amphioxus. This arrangement – DA cells in close proximity to photoreceptor cells – was useful in modulating motor responses to light. Eventually, the DA system came to be expressed in the *hypothalamus,* the brain's "thermostat", which reads and regulates body states through blood chemistry. This spreading of the dopamine system was part of larger genome duplications which occurred early in craniate evolution.

Gene duplications, together with the flexibility of the DA system, made it useful for a number of functions, and with evolutionary changes in the organization of the central nervous system, DA systems eventually evolved to modulate sensory information from the retina, olfactory bulb, and hypothalamus, as well as to control motor programming, emotions, motivation, and memory. This expansion of the system into different brain regions significantly improved sensory perception and motor functions, refining their use for environmental adaptation.

Like serotonin, dopamine is synthesized from food, and is a precursor used to synthesize the neurotransmitters *norepinephrine* (noradrenaline) and *epinephrine* (adrenaline), which together control such functions as heart rate, attention and arousal.

In the bloodstream, *norepinephrine* is a *stress hormone.* evolved from the invertebrate signalling molecule *octopamine*. Norepinephrine acts upon brain regions where attention and responses are controlled, and, together with *epinephrine*, underlies the fight-or-flight response. Its release speeds up the heart's contractions, initiates the release of blood sugar stores for quick energy, and increases the flow of blood to muscles in the body, and oxygen to the brain.

Many key enzymes in the monoamine system used for transport, reception and synthesis are derived from the same gene-protein family. Genes which express the enzyme *Tyrosine hydroxylase* (TH) emerged early, as far back as the lampreys, and were duplicated in early vertebrates. In all probability, a single ancestral chromosome bearing at least three key genes was duplicated, perhaps as part of the whole genome duplications thought to have occurred close to the emergence of the earliest vertebrates.

The *acetylcholine* system is found in the entire bilateria family, from nematode worms to humans. Neurons use acetylcholine to trigger muscle contractions, and to enhance *long-term potentiation*, the synapse-strengthening basis of memory formation. The system is an ancient one, and through multiple exon duplications, at least eight gene families responsible for the acetylcholine system emerged, as the chordate nervous system grew in complexity.

Glutamate, central to memory formation, had long been in use as the primary *excitatory neurotransmitter*, meaning that when it binds to a receptor, it increases that neuron's probably of firing. Glutamate is derived from the dietary amino acid *glutamine*, and a precursor to *GABA*, the primary *inhibitory* neurotransmitter. Together, these neurotransmitters work in tandem to excite and inhibit neural activity.

Glutamate may have been the first neurotransmitter, likely used in primitive cell-to-cell signalling before the evolutionary split between plants and animals – there are at least four glutamate receptor gene families, thought to have spread from prokaryotes to eukaryotes through lateral gene transfer.

An active predatory-prey lifestyle is thought to have driven the evolution from flatworm-like ancestors toward more complex vertebrates, resulting in the emergence of many new structures, including complex heads, brains, image-forming paired eyes, and bony skeletons.

What began as simple, bulging neural clusters in the ancestors of chordates gradually evolved into a functionally distinctive tri-part *forebrain*, *midbrain* and *hindbrain*. This progression quite logically arose from increasing selective pressures for better perception and locomotion, leading to increased sophistication, initially in only the midbrain and hindbrain.

Natural selection also led to the evolution of *myelin*, a fatty-protein insulating sheath which forms an insulating coating around long, signal-conducting neural *axons*. Genetic comparisons show *Proteolipid protein (PLP)*, the primary component of myelin, evolved independently among both deuterostomes and protostomes near the start of Cambrian era, likely driven by the first evolutionary pressures of predation.

Myelin greatly increases the potential distance and speed of signals processing sensory data and activating muscles. Its development allowed for much faster and more sophisticated sensory processing and motor systems, resulting in faster reactions to the sight of predators or of prey, and increasing the odds of survival for both.

Grow Some Spine

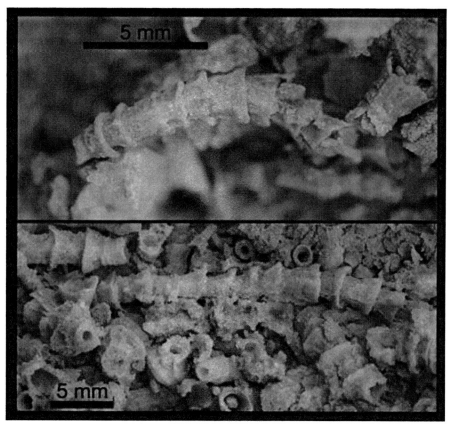

*Fossils of **cloudina carinata**, a newly-discovered pre-Cambrian species found in 2010 in Spain. Cloudina was one of the first organisms to evolve a special new defense – a hardened, calcium exterior – better known as an exoskeleton. This is evidence that protection from predators was needed as a result of the evolution of mouths. The first interspecies "arms race" had begun. Prey would develop ever-more elaborate strategies to elude predators, and predator would respond by becoming better equipped at hunting, a remarkable system of coevolution – the adaptations of one species driving adaptations in another. Image, Iván Cortijo et al., public domain.*

The geological record shows Cambrian ocean volcanic activity created a sudden, massive surge of seawater calcium, which could be exploited to build hardened body parts.

With predators adding selective pressures to evolve defensive strategies, marine organisms took opportunistic advantage of the newly mineral-rich seawater to evolve calcified shells and skeletons. Soft-bodied and sessile organisms, which had become easy targets for sighted predators, developed armor as a defensive response. This is thought to have been the start of first *evolutionary arms race*.

Various adaptations split bilaterians into two distinct groups. Both lineages used crystallized salts – *calcium carbonate* or *calcium phosphate* – as the basis for new structural development. Fortunately, neither molecule dissolves in water, allowing marine bone and shell fossils to be preserved through the eons.

Protostomes (insects, *crustaceans* like crabs and shrimp, and *mollusks* like clams and snails) evolved outer shells and *exoskeletons*; among them, the *arthropods* (insects and crustaceans) began to appear about 530 million years ago, including *eurypterids*, the giant sea scorpions which dominated the seas before fish emerged.

Among the *deuterostomes* (animals ranging from sea stars to humans), early *echinoderms* ("spiny skins" like urchins and starfish) began to leave fossil remains about 540 million years ago, when they first evolved bumpy and spiny skin-covered *endoskeletons*. These endoskeletons are comprised of tiny, hexagonal plates of calcium carbonate armor called *ossicles* buried in the flesh beneath the outer skin, which fit together loosely or tightly, conferring varying degrees of stiffness or flexibility, depending upon the species. This endoskeleton lends rigidity and support to the body.

Meanwhile, the first vertebrates developed skeletons and skulls of *cartilage* – a stiff tissue made of cells in a gel-like matrix of protein fibers and polysaccharides. These same skeletons exist in modern sharks and rays. It would still take nearly 100 million years for the first *bone* endoskeletons to evolve, however. Bone is a tissue made up of cells end blood vessels encased in a calcium/phosphate compound (hydroxyapatite) reinforced by protein fibers.

A vertebrate spinal cord would evolve from the chordate dorsal nerve cord, and cells in the notochord would secrete regulatory proteins that coaxed *somites* – segmented blocks of tissue – to form along the length of the body, developing into cartilage, tendons, vertebrae, ribs, and skeletal muscles.

The cranium emerged, a hard encasing to protect the sensory organs and evolving brain. This brain slowly developed into three distinct regions to process the senses: a forebrain, which originally housed the sense of smell, a midbrain, concerned with vision, and a hindbrain, responsible for balance and hearing. As sensory priorities were molded by each species' habitat and lifestyle, these basic but fundamental concerns of the brain were amplified in some cases, and reduced or overshadowed in others during the course of evolution. It's been suggested that this triple-segmented development pattern arose out of three homeobox gene clusters.

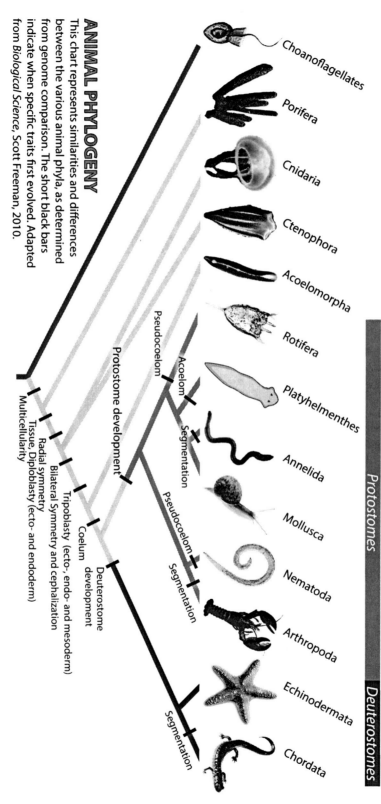

ANIMAL PHYLOGENY

This chart represents similarities and differences between the various animal phyla, as determined from genome comparison. The short black bars indicate when specific traits first evolved. Adapted from *Biological Science*, Scott Freeman, 2010.

Choanoflagellates

Porifera

Cnidaria

Ctenophora

Acoelomorpha

Rotifera

Platyhelmenthes

Annelida

Mollusca

Nematoda

Arthropoda

Echinodermata

Chordata

Protostomes

Deuterostomes

Pseudocoelom

Protostome development

Acoelom

Segmentation

Pseudocoelom

Segmentation

Deuterostome development

Segmentation

Coelum

Tripoblasty (ecto-, endo- and mesoderm)

Bilateral Symmetry and cephalization

Radial symmetry

Tissue, Diploblasty (ecto- and endoderm)

Multicellularity

161

Refined

By this time, the *extra-cellular matrix*, the supportive structure to which cells attach, had also been evolving. Substances contributing to the ECM included complex polysaccharides and fibrous proteins like *collagen* and *elastin*, though the composition varies according to the type of tissue in which it's found.

Collagen fibers provide structural support – hence their popularity in anti-wrinkle skin creams. These are the most abundant proteins in mammals, comprising 25% to 35% of the body's protein content. Elastin proteins, on the other hand, lend elasticity to tissues, allowing them to stretch as needed, and then to return to their original state. These properties are useful for blood vessels, lungs, skin, and ligaments.

Substances central to skeletal development are found in this ECM, proteins, polysaccharide chitin, or inorganic salt crystals such as calcium carbonate and calcium phosphate, which can be integrated with collagen fibers to form a hardened support structure *externally* in exoskeletons, or *internally* in endoskeletons.

The modern ECM is highly dynamic, its molecular components constantly undergoing modifications. This allows the ECM to generate special biochemical and mechanical properties for each tissue, such as compressive strength or elasticity. The ECM also allows for the formation of spherical compartments, which isolate internal from external environments, allowing the state of the inner chamber to be controlled and maintained.

When ECM proteins bind to cell receptors, they don't just provide structural support; they can also regulate intercellular communication, and activate signalling pathways to regulate gene transcription, help control cell structure, migration, proliferation, differentiation, homeostasis and *apoptosis* (programmed cell death). The ECM is also essential for processes like growth and wound healing.

A similar supportive and transport-guidance structure found within cells is the *cytoskeleton*. This is a fiber network of *actin* (a motor protein responsible for cellular contraction, crawling and pinching during cell division); *microtubules* (long, hollow protein tubes used in cell division, cell organization and intracellular transport); and *intermediate filaments* like *keratin proteins* (the substance of which your hair is composed), which act as a physical support within the cell's cytoplasm. Most of the cytoskeleton's "struts" can be disassembled and reassembled as needed throughout the cell.

Promiscuous Proteins

Just as existing genes can be adapted to new purposes, so-called *promiscuous proteins* are recruited for additional purposes distinct from their original ones. For example, in the 1930s, researchers discovered that the bacteria *Sphingomonas chlorophenolicum* had evolved the ability to eat the highly toxic biocide *pentachlorophenal* (PCP). Five proteins these bacteria normally used to digest amino acids had been recruited to break down PCP for consumption. The bacteria had evolved within a few short decades to feed off of this deadly poison.

Similarly, a wide range of animals (and possibly plants) long ago evolved special proteins called *defensins*, toxins for destroying viral, bacterial and fungal infections. In snakes, these defensin genes duplicated, but instead of being expressed solely in the body, they came to be produced in the mouth. Mutations to these defensin-expressing genes resulted in *crotamine*, replacing a toxin for killing invading pathogens with one that causes *necrosis (tissue death)* in muscles – snake venom.

Another repurposing of material is the use of the same signalling molecules to trigger both scale and feather growth; Yale university experiments on duck, chick and alligator embryos have shown that *BMP2* (Bone Morphogenetic Protein 2) and *Shh* (Sonic Hedgehog) proteins trigger the development of both scales and feathers from embryonic placode cells. Birds are modern descendants of the dinosaurs, technically considered warm-blooded, feathered reptiles.

The Eyes Have It

In 2011, six pairs of 515-million-year-old fossilized eyes were discovered on Kangaroo Island off the southern coast of Australia. The eyes belonged to *Anomalocaris* (Latin for "abnormal shrimp"), an extinct early predator, thought to be an ancestor of the arthropods. The find showed that sophisticated eyesight had already evolved by the Cambrian age.

Anomalocaris' 3 cm-wide eyes were multi-faceted like an insect's, each with 16,000 lenses able to clearly distinguish many features in the environment, including the identity of other undersea creatures. Anomalocaris was a *superpredator* at the top of the Cambrian-era food chain, and sometimes reached two meters in length. Fecal pellets show the creature dined on hard-shelled trilobites, which were plentiful in the Cambrian seas. Such advanced vision among predators almost certainly accelerated the first predator-prey arms race, which began over half a billion years ago.

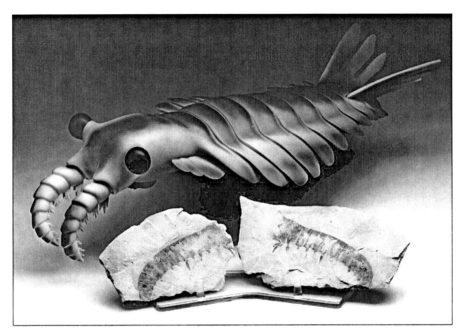

A team of U.S. researchers discovered the fossilized remains of anomalocaris in March, 2011 in Emu Bay Shale fossil beds of Australia's Kangaroo Island. This arthropod possessed the greatest visual acuity of any known organism, with over 32,000 lenses per eye, surpassing even current arthropods (human eyes have only one). Its remarkable vision would have made it a fearsome apex predator of the era. Researchers say that each lens provided a view equivalent to a single pixel, though low light conditions would have hampered its visibility. The recovered specimen was five feet long, and remarkably well-preserved. Image: Saragossa University, public domain.

The evolution of eyes changed predator-prey relationships quickly and dramatically. Prior to sight, hunting and evasion required close-range senses such as touch and vibration, but as predators developed the ability to see from a distance, new defensive strategies became necessary for prey animals. Thus armor, spines, and similar defenses may well have evolved as an adaptive response to vision.

Oxford zoologist Andrew Parker says vision may well have been responsible for the Cambrian explosion. Prior to this, animals only needed simple light sensitivity, but increased pressure to eat or avoid being eaten led to visually-guided navigation. Fossil records show that during this period, eye evolution accelerated rapidly.

Simple light sensitivity is very ancient. A variety of molecules, mostly used in photosynthesis, are photosensitive, and even the most primitive creatures show responses to light, a general *dermal photosensitivity that doesn't require* eyes. This is sensitivity is provided by photoreceptors built of light-sensitive *opsin proteins.*

Opsins are a special class of *G-protein-coupled receptors* (GPCR) which emerged as far back as the yeasts, which originally used them for detecting *pheromones*, chemical communication signals between members of a species. Because they're so versatile,

GPCRs are used widely, in synaptic transmission, hormone function, olfaction and taste. Chemical ligands bind with GPCRs like keys fitting locks, triggering cellular functions. But in opsins, instead of chemical ligands, photons trigger impulses.

Opsins are embedded in the cell membrane, using the vitamin-A derivative *retinal* to trap photons. When photons strike, retinal electrons are excited and switch to higher-energy states, altering the shape of the molecule, and triggering a chemical cascade which leads to a visual nerve impulse. In humans and other animals, the brain reads this signal as a point of light in a visual field.

The earliest light-sensitive forms of opsins may have simply been used to monitor ambient luminance to synchronize *circadian rhythms* – daily sleep-wake and metabolic cycles, to gauge depth control in water, or guide surface emergence for burrowing animals.

Between 755 and 711 million years ago, opsins evolved from the duplication of a single GPCR, in a creature sometime after sponges diverged from other animals, but before the Bilaterian-Cnidarian split. According to Oxford University evolutionary biologist Roberto Feuda, the most primitive creature found to possess them so far is the *placozoan* called *trichoplax*, a tiny, flat, multicellular, benthic scavenger.

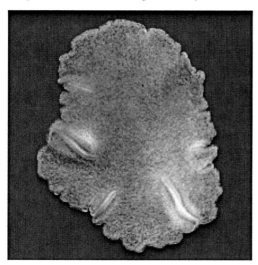

*Trichoplax has the most primitive body and the smallest genome of any known animal, functioning without any internal organs. It's about one millimeter in diameter, built of two layers of cells, using cilia to crawl across the sea floor. It absorbs microbes from its underside, digesting them with simple enzymes. Though it moves in response to light, Trichoplax has opsins which lack the amino acid lysine-296, necessary for **retinal**, the light-binding portion of human opsins. Image: US Joint Genome Institute, public domain.*

In the last common ancestor of Bilateria and Cnidaria, opsins mutated into light-sensing proteins by incorporating retinal with the amino acid lysine-296, and diversifying into the three forms used by humans today.

Human rod photoreceptors use *rod opsins* (*rhodopsins*) for night vision, and cone photoreceptors use *cone opsins* (*photopsins*), for color perception. There are three cone opsins, subdivided according to the wavelength of light they absorb: *long wavelength sensitive cones* respond to red light, *middle wavelength sensitive cones* to green light, and *short wavelength sensitive cones* to blue light.

Rhodopsins in particular are widespread, found in archaea, bacteria, algae and even fungi, and perform a variety of biological functions. For example, they can act as pro-

165

ton- or chloride ion-pumps, or be used to guide *phototaxis* – a movement toward or away from light.

While opsins may have only emerged once and evolved through gene duplication, complex eye structures evolved separately many dozens of times over, using the same genes and proteins in a wide range of organisms. Central to human eye evolution are the *PAX6* (paired box 6) and Six family genes, which express transcription factors guiding embryonic eye, receptor cell, and neural development in all bilaterians, from fruit flies to mice to humans. Because these genes are found in nearly every modern multicellular species, geneticists know they evolved quite early.

The PAX6 gene, located in human chromosome 11, is part of the larger homeobox gene family, and expresses a transcription factor which guides eye development. It's part of a larger family of PAX genes guiding nerve cell, sensory organ and system development.

During human embryogenesis, the PAX6 protein activates genes involved in forming lenses, irises, optic nerves, the brain and central nervous system, as well as the *pancreas*, an organ which regulates blood sugar. In the human brain, PAX6 also helps guide development of specialized cells in the *olfactory bulb* which process smell.

Crystallin proteins are a second part of the eye-evolution puzzle. Human lenses contain a mixture of three types of these transparent proteins, which originally had other functions in the body, acting as enzymes and as *heat-shock proteins*, protecting other proteins from *denaturation* (losing shape and clumping due to heat).

Originally expressed in muscle tissues, a mutation first caused crystallin expression on the surface of eyes, where crystallin transparency bends light and thus magnifies images onto a photosensitive surface – the retina.

The first appearance of complex eyes seems to have been about 540 million years ago during the Cambrian explosion, as there is no fossil evidence of eyes prior to this.

In 1994, Swedish zoologist Dan-Erik Nilsson calculated how long it takes to evolve a modern, fully-functional eye with only a 1% change in shape per generation. His computer simulations show a fully-formed, advanced eye naturally evolves from a simple patch of light-sensitive cells within just 363,992 generations – well under a million years for a short-lived aquatic species.

The evolutionary progression can be clearly traced in species alive even today: Initially, visual receptor cells evolved from the simplest of sensory cilia, which respond to light by either increasing or decreasing sodium flow across the cell membrane. Clusters of photoreceptive proteins result in *eyespots*, found in even the simplest single-celled organisms.

Eyespots can only distinguish light from dark, without being able to discriminate form or direction. This assists organisms in moving toward light to ehance photosynthesis.

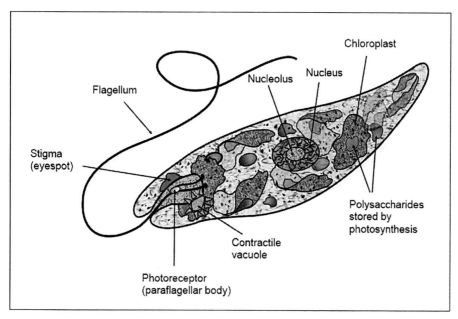

Eyespots are the simplest and most common visual systems found in nature, used by many unicellular micro-organisms such as green algae and the **protist Euglena**. Made only of photoreceptors and pigment, the eyespot senses light direction and intensity, and allows the simplest responses – swimming toward the light (positive phototaxis) or away from it (negative phototaxis). Signals generated by the photoreceptors alter the motion of the whiplike flagella, resulting in the phototactic response. Image: Wikipedia, public domain.

From this, the natural progression is for such a patch to form a simple depression. This very minor change allows light direction to be detected. The cup shape means that incoming light will strike some cells, but not others, depending upon its angle. The deeper the depression in these pigment-cup eyes, the finer the discrimination of light direction becomes. Such primitive eyes still exist in flatworms today – this is in keeping with parsimonious nature of evolution: in the flatworm's environment, there has never been a need for further eye evolution.

The aquatic flatworm *planaria* has such cup eyes, and its ability to rapidly regenerate allows scientists to closely study its eye formation. They've discovered that the genes *sine oculis* and *eyes absent* guide cup eye formation in planaria and other animals, but planaria also use two genes which normally guide limb development in vertebrates and insects – *sp6-9* and *dlx* – to guide organ generation, including eye cup pigment development.

Fast-swimming predators and their prey require more complex vision. The simplest way to achieve a sharper image is through deepening an eyecup depression. Deepening the eyecup and constricting the opening creates a *camera lucida* (pinhole camera) – casting a relatively detailed image onto a surface, in this case a retina of photoreceptors. Such pit eyes are found in the modern-day *chambered nautilus*.

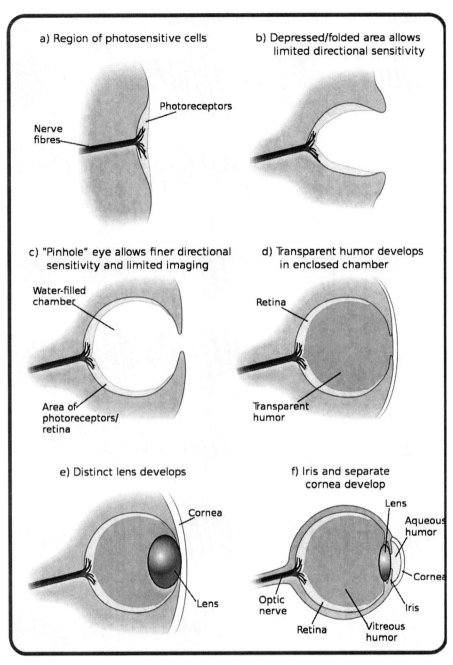

Progressive eye development, Wikipedia, public domain.

At this stage of complexity, eyesight has become rather sophisticated, capable of discerning form, light intensity, direction and movement. But a pinhole opening also decreases the *amount* of light, resulting in a much dimmer image, and pit eyes are open to the flow of sea water, sand and other irritants.

A simple solution is to grow a protective transparent tissue over the open pinhole, similar to the jelly-like film which protects the eyes of modern-day Roman garden snails – *Helix aspersa*.

It's thought that the evolution of a clear lens was a natural progression from this point. *Lobopods*, Cambrian-era deep-sea arthropods which resembled caterpillars, evolved a simple lens early, used to intensify light for deep-sea vision.

Gradually thicken this primitive lens and a progressively sharper, clearer image emerges. Add muscles to stretch or relax the lens, and you have the ability to focus on objects near and far. Such a lens first evolved in cnidarians, and exists in octopi and squid species today. Among the cnidarians, box jellyfish, have 24 eyes, 16 of which are simple pigment cups, but the remaining eight, one pair per side, have quite sophisticated lenses.

For prey animals, eyes on the sides of the head provide a larger field of view, helpful in avoiding predators, while predators have eyes in the fronts of their heads for improved depth perception. Color vision arose as a means of better recognition of predators, food, and potential mates.

Evolution didn't "stop" with the emergence of human eyes however. In fact, as a species, while our eyes are remarkable, they're far from perfect in design. For example, there are at least two "flaws": our photoreceptors are backwards, pointing inward and away from the light; and just off-center of the retina, we have a *blind spot* where the optic nerve connects to the retina. Other species have some distinct visual advantages: birds have evolved eyes which can see in ultraviolet light, some fish have double lenses, allowing them to see both above and below the water simultaneously, and cats have infravision, allowing them to see the heat patterns of living creatures in darkness.

Animal Supersenses

Many animals perceive the world in a completely different way than humans, sensing colors, tastes, sounds and smells beyond the range of human perception. Many have "super senses", able to "see" through sound or touch, or to see heat patterns in darkness, and even to detect electrical or magnetic fields.

Animals have evolved an incredible array of touch-sensitive organs, including whiskers and antennae, which help them navigate, locate food and communicate. Those which live underground in complete darkness have developed extra-sensitive tactile senses to feel their way about.

For example, the star-nosed mole has evolved a "nose" which functions not as an olfactory organ, but as the most touch-sensitive organ known on Earth. With 22 appendages, the star is covered with tens of thousands of tiny, supersensitive bumps called *Eimer's organs*. Though smaller than a human fingertip, a single star has nearly six times the 17,000 touch fibers of a human hand – over 100,000 tactile neurons.

In general, the tactile sense also includes sensitivity to pressure and vibration. Blow flies have an intricate network of vibration sensors along the edges of their wings to sense changes in wind speed and instantly adjust the shape and frequency of wing flapping. Earthworms are eyeless and earless, but so responsive to ground vibrations that they can feel the footfalls of approaching predators like moles.

Sight is also critical, helping creatures navigate, locate food, find mates and avoid predators, whether they're in the ocean's depths or the heights of the sky. Because of this, the vast majority of animals have evolved sight – estimates put it at 95% of all animal species; but only two animal groups evolved hearing – the vertebrates, including mammals, birds and reptiles, and the arthropods, including insects, spiders and crabs.

Insects typically hear via paired *tympanal organs*. Like a tympani, the giant drum used in orchestras, the tympanal organ has a membrane stretched over an air-filled cavity across a frame. The membrane vibrates in response to sound waves in the air.

Grasshoppers, crickets, cicadas, and some moths and butterflies also have a special receptor called a *chordotonal organ*, which senses tympanal vibrations, translating them into nerve impulses. Insects such as mosquitos and fruit flies have a receptor on their antennae called the *Johnston's organ*. The *pedicel*, near the base of the antennae, contains sensory cells which detect vibrations from the segment above.

Some hawkmoths have mouth structures which enable them to perceive ultrasonic sounds, such as bats using echolocation. A tiny hair-like organ called the *labral pilifer* is thought to sense specific sound frequencies. In flight, hawkmoths can avoid pursuing bats by listening for these frequencies.

Animals often have remarkable hearing, attuned to their habitat and life patterns, and can hear sounds beyond the range of human sensitivity. Likewise, our olfactory and gustatory senses are feeble compared with many animal species, who use their keener olfactory sense for hunting or foraging, mate selection, navigation, danger avoidance, and territory recognition.

Dolphins have retained basic vision, hearing, taste and touch, but lost the sense of smell (olfactory regions of the brain), when their nostrils migrated to the top of their heads; olfaction is useless to an air-breathing mammal that spends its life underwater and doesn't sniff at the air. Instead, they have developed senses of echolocation and, evidence indicates, magnetic-field detection.

Tasty

By comparing a wide range of species, researchers have concluded that the sense of taste evolved over half a billion years ago, before the divergence of land and marine vertebrates, when their common ancestor developed a special new type of cell. There are five known basic tastes – sweet, sour, salty, bitter and *umami*, a "meaty" taste with a tongue-coating sensation. To create this taste, the presence of *glutamate*, an ionic form of the amino acid glutamic acid, binds to receptors on the membranes of cells such as those found in taste buds on the tongue.

Dr. Gary Beauchamp, a geneticist at Monell Chemical Senses Center in Philadelphia, says the sense of taste evolved to perform one vital function: to discriminate between good and bad food. Sweet and umami discrimination helps animals detect energy-dense food, while bitter tastes indicate toxins to avoid. As for sour and salt tastes, it's thought that detecting salt helps animals control sodium and other mineral levels, while detecting sour tastes helps them avoid the acids of unripe or spoiled food. All vertebrates share varying degrees of this capacity to locate nutrients and avoid toxins.

Pleasant tastes also act as a powerful reward, and hunger sensations are unpleasant enough that the two complementary states drive animals to seek food. While eating, flavors allow animals to learn and remember which foods are good or bad from taste experiments. If a new potential food makes an animal sick, instinctive taste mechanisms build strong, unpleasant associative memories, and the animal will avoid eating such an item in the future; if a food is dangerous, an instinctive stomach-clearance mechanism is important, which is where the vomiting reflex comes into play. Scientists also recently discovered sweet receptors in the gut which influence insulin levels, as well as bitter receptors in the lungs which clear noxious inhaled substances.

While the combination of taste buds has repeatedly changed with the dietary needs of various species, according to Dr. Thomas Finger of the University of Colorado's Rocky Mountain Taste and Smell Center in Aurora, the world's true connoisseurs are goldfish and catfish. Says Dr. Finger, these fish have significantly more taste buds than any other species studied so far. Although their vision is lacking, taste buds, including taste buds on catfish whiskers, may help them navigate toward food in murky waters.

Umami receptors were the first to evolve 400 million years ago, according to University of Michigan evolutionary geneticist Dr. Jianzhi Zhang. In 2008, his team discovered genes in elephant sharks, which express glutamate receptors. However, sharks have no receptors for bitter taste buds, suggesting those genes evolved more recently.

Bitterness is the most complex taste, and its sensitivity appears to be tailored to the diet of each species. The bitter receptor *T2R16*, for example, is common to all primates, but depending upon the individual, humans possess 24 to 25 distinctive types of bitter receptors, each for a unique chemical combination. Because bitterness can be a sign of toxins or important nutrients (like citric acid), a diverse set of receptors is necessary, according to Dr. Beauchamp.

When encountering unfamiliar foods, animals must be able to instinctively choose between those which are beneficial and those which are harmful. They need to maximize food intake while avoiding eating anything harmful. Certain flavors indicate danger – the smell of decaying food or the extreme bitterness of poisonous chemicals – and these need to trigger strong instinctive distaste. Meanwhile, to keep the range of acceptable nutrients as high as possible, instinctive aversions must be minimized.

Creatures therefore need to be attracted to foods which are nutrient-dense. Sweet, fatty foods are calorie dense, making them ideal for environments where meals may be few and far between, or dangerous to obtain.

Animals like our ancient hominid ancestors often had to snatch and gulp down food as quickly as possible, with no way of predicting when they would be able to eat again. Unfortunately for us, this hereditary preference for high-calorie foods makes maintaining a healthy weight challenging, particularly as one ages and the metabolism slows.

Tastes vary among animal species, because some taste sensitivities offer no survival benefit. University of Connecticut evolutionary biologist Dr. Kurt Schwenk says species taste sensitivity differences are due to diet – if a creature doesn't encounter a specific food in its environment, its ability to sense the chemicals in that food will disappear. Genes which don't directly aid a creature in surviving or reproducing are a dangerous risk – increasing the possibility of mutations which tend to be harmful more often than beneficial.

For example, cats are unable to taste sweet substances. This is because they possess a mutation which disables one of two genes which build sweet receptors, and all felines — from domestic cats to lions — share this mutation. Because of this, the sweet-receptor gene seems to have become inactive in a common evolutionary ancestor.

Dr. Beauchamp believes this is due to switching to a protein-rich meat diet. With no need to consume plant sugars, there was no need for a sweet receptor. This inability to taste sweetness is widespread among carnivores, including sea-lions, otters and hyenas. In fact, the ability to taste sweetness seems to have been gained and lost repeatedly over the course of evolution.

Dolphins, on the other hand, lack the ability to grow umami and bitter taste receptors, while pandas, a vegetarian species, lack umami receptors. Living on bamboo creates little need for detecting glutamic acid, according to Dr. Zhang. His team has also found that vampire bats have no sweet receptors, and all bats, including insectivorous species, lack umami receptors. One pattern that's rather puzzling, however, is that horses, several species of birds, and omnivorous pigs lack sweet-receptor genes.

Jaws

443 million years ago, landmass shifts over the South Pole triggered a global ice age. Massive glaciers formed, global temperatures plummeted, water turned to ice, and sea levels lowered worldwide. At least 70% of all species were wiped out, including many corals and other marine species. Survivors were those best able to quickly adapt. This necessity to rapidly change sped up the evolutionary process. Everything that lives today can be traced back to survivors of this era.

Gradually, as the glaciers retreated, the oceans developed into a rather alien place, filled with armored, jawless fish called *ostracoderms* (bony-skinned ones), which flourished in the mild warmth of the ancient *Silurian age*. According to Oxford University's Matt Friedman, these bizarre jawless fish were covered in protective bone plates, had gills and balancing organs, but seem to have eaten by sucking food into their mouths – like modern-day hagfish and lampreys, these ancient vertebrates were *ectoparasites* (parasites which attach to the outer body), or bottom feeders, scavenging animal carcasses, but unable to bite.

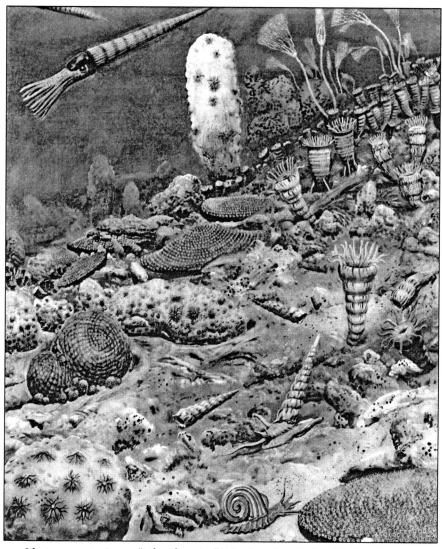

Silurian seascape. Image: "Life Before Man," Zdenek Burian, 1995. Public domain image.

Jawless fish shared the ancient seas with familiar creatures like sea lilies, snails, and corals, but also more bizarre ones like giant sea scorpions (up to two meters long) and shelled relatives of squid and octopus, from which the chambered nautilus has descended. Ostracoderms dominated for the better part of 100 million years, much longer than the current 65-million-year dominance of land mammals.

Eventually, these bottom-feeding mud-grubbers evolved jaws from bony arches supporting their gills. Evidence for this evolutionary process can be seen in all vertebrate embryos, which grow *pharyngeal arches*, nubs of tissue that eventually morph into the jaw in mammals, and into gill-supporting arches in fish. In humans, these arches grow from neural crest cells during an embryo's fourth week, gradually morphing into jaws.

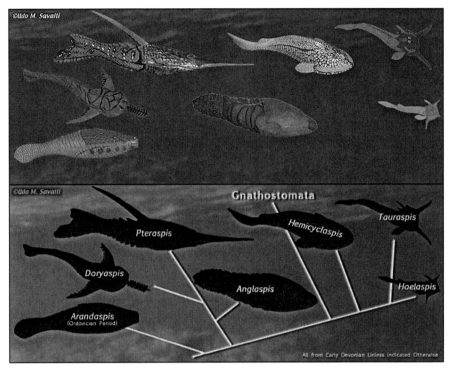

Images: Devonian-era jawless fish, Dr. Udo Savalli. Used with permission.

Fossils unearthed in 2011 in Southern show how jaws first emerged: Dr Zhikun Gai of the Beijing Institute of Palaeontology and Palaeoanthropology says the process began when a 420-million-year-old family of jawless fish called the *galeapsids* (Latin for *helmet shield*) evolved a paired nasal organ. The adaptation arose from an enhanced sense of smell, solving a critical anatomical problem: in earlier jawless fish, the nasal organ sat in the middle of the face, blocking embryonic cells from migrating to new sites. Moving the nose to either side of the face allowed the first jaws to evolve.

Originally, jaws improved suction and helped regulate water flow through the mouth and throat, but over time, the components were adapted and modified for new functions, like crushing shells and biting flesh. Jaws and teeth are thought to be key evolutionary innovations which led to the success of the vertebrate lineage.

The first jawed fish were *placoderms*, from the Greek words for "plate" and "skin". Because placoderms were aggressive predators, they were more powerful, active swimmers than their jawless predecessors.

They would eventually come to dominate, while their jawless competitors almost completely died out, with the sole exceptions of hagfish and lampreys, "living fossils" from the very base of the vertebrate tree which still survive, relatively unchanged for over half a billion years.

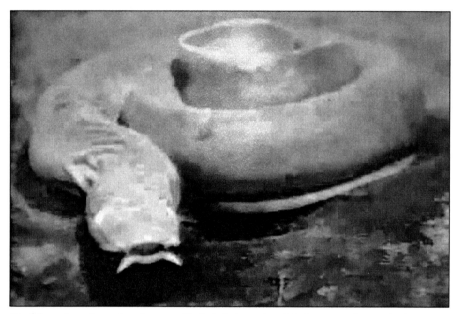

Hagfish are the only creatures known with skulls but no spines. Like lampreys, they are jawless, essentially unchanged since they first evolved 300 million years ago. When agitated, the hagfish excretes as much as five gallons of gelatinous, sticky goo which expands in water. If captured, it will tie itself into a knot, working from head to tail, scraping off slime, to free itself from its captor and its own slime. It's thought this slime clogs the gills of would-be attackers, so hagfish are seldom preyed upon by other fish. Image: National Oceanic and Atmospheric Administration, public domain.

Scientists believe they've discovered the gene responsible for jaw evolution in *BMP4*, which expresses the growth factor *Bone Morphogenetic Protein*. BMP signals cells to begin producing the bone for embryonic jaws, and the more BMP4 protein produced, the thicker the jaw. Thus, differences in jaws among fish species appear to come from different patterns of bmp4 expression in the embryo.

In experiments with zebrafish, manipulating the location, timing or amount of bmp4 expression changes jaw development in ways which parallel natural jaw variation among species. Similar experiments with Galapagos finches have shown that Bmp4 and a second gene, *CAM1*, also govern differing beak development among birds. These genes appear to play a central role in the jaw morphology of many species, including lizards, rabbits, mice and humans.

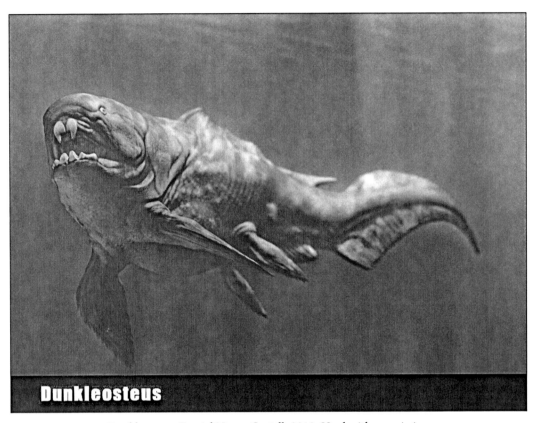

Dunkleosteus, Daniel Navas Castell, 2010. Used with permission.

Some Devonian-era placoderms grew massively – up to 33 feet, weighing as much as two modern elephants. Within twenty million years, they ruled the seas. One such tremendous, rather terrifying sea monster dominated the marine world 380 million years ago.

Dunkleosteus (named after its discoverer David Dunkle, and *osteus,* the Greek word for bone) was a fearsome *hypercarnivorous predator* measuring up to 10 meters (33 ft.) in length and weighing about 4 tons. Although it was originally believed that their plated jaws held no teeth, Drs. Martin Rücklin and Phil Donoghue of the University of Bristol announced findings in 2011 that Dunkleosteus did have teeth, making it one of the earliest known creatures to have evolved them.

Such teeth first emerged as mutated scales; in 2011, University of Alberta paleontologists discovered several bizarre fossils of ancient fish with tooth-like jagged scales jutting from their lips and cheeks.

According to Dr. Mark Wilson, "The first smile would probably have been a prickly one, with many tiny teeth that looked like pointy cheek scales, and other small tooth-like scales wrapping around the lips onto the outside of the head".

400-million-year-old *ischnacanthid acanthodians* sported one such prickly smile. It resembled a modern shark, though its odd lip and cheek scales were transitioning from scales into teeth, evolving in sets which mirrored scale patterns.

We know this progression isn't conjecture, because modern sharks and rays still have tough *placoid scales* covering their outer skin. Just like human teeth, these *dermal denticles* (Latin for *skin teeth*) have an inner pulp core with connective tissues, blood vessels, and nerves, covered by a layer of *dentine* (hard calcium carbonate) and an enamel-like outer coating called *vitrodentine*. Densely packed together, these scales grow with the tips facing backwards, providing protection from predators. In stingrays, placoid scales evolved further into the creature's trademark poisonous tail spines.

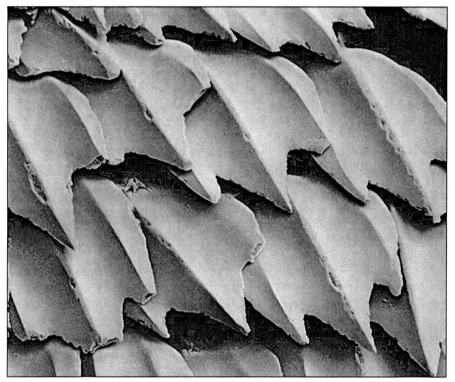

Scanning electron micrograph of the overlapping placoid scales of a White Shark, Australian Museum. Used with permission.

Project leader Stephanie Blais says the evolution of teeth "conferred a major advantage in terms of food acquisition. Pointed scales near the margins of their mouths would have helped them grasp prey and hang onto it until they could swallow it whole."

Jaws and teeth "allowed fishes to change from a filter-feeding or mud-grubbing, more passive, lifestyle to one of active predation. Interactions between predators and prey through time only increased their (teeth's) importance, leading to highly specialized teeth, such as those in mammals," according to Dr. Blais.

Snowballed

In 2001, Oxford University, Exeter University and Penn State researchers came to an astonishing conclusion. They'd just conducted the largest genetic study ever, to determine when Earth's first land plants and fungi emerged. Their findings may well turn decades of evolutionary thought on its head.

According to Dr. Blair Hedges, fungi first appeared about *1.3 billion years ago*, followed by land plants about *700 million years ago*, making both far more ancient than had been previously believed. Theiries of plant colonization have long been based upon 480-million-year-old fossil findings; as of yet, no earlier, indisputable plant fossils have been found, possibly because the first primitive plants were too soft to fossilize.

Says Dr. Hedges, however, the genetic findings easily explain the sudden, dramatic temperature drop and glaciations of the *Snowball Earth* era; plant growth had severely decreased the planet-warming greenhouse gas carbon dioxide, then, by increasing Earth's atmospheric oxygen, eventually triggered the Cambrian Explosion.

The Snowball Earth phase has long been a mystery, as was the sudden emergence of diverse life during the Cambrian Explosion about 530 million years ago. According to this research, plants spread across the continents, drawing in atmospheric carbon, and triggering marked drops in temperature. The geological record shows glaciers advanced across the planet during the *Ordovician period*, as Earth's continents clustered over the south pole, stretching north to the equator.

Oxford University botanist Dr. Liam Dolan agrees that the colonization of land by plants brought about huge climate changes: "...plants have a central regulatory role in the control of climate: they did yesterday, they do today, and they certainly will in the future."

By studying thousands of amino-acid-expressing genes from living plants and fungi, his team discovered a core sequence of 119 genes common to all living plants, fungi, and animals, a sequence which could be used as a molecular clock, steadily accumulating mutations at a constant rate. Since mutations occur at regular intervals, they can be used to determine the emergence of species. These mutation rates were carefully measured against well-known evolutionary events backed by fossil studies.

Exeter University's Dr. Timothy Lenton incubates rocks covered with moss to mimic ancient plant growth and activity. Says Dr. Lenton, Ordovician plants dissolved rocks such as granite, releasing calcium and magnesium ions. These combined with atmospheric carbon, to wash into the oceans. This process alone is thought to have accounted for a temperature drop of five degrees Celsius.

Plants also extracted phosphorus and iron from the rocks, and when they died, these elements washed into the seas, providing nutrients to fuel plankton growth, further locking carbon into ocean floor rocks. According to Dr. Lenton, about 15% of Ordovician Earth's land was covered with early plants, though even a 5% coverage would have created a major cooling. Plants today still cool the Earth, but cannot keep up with the rate of human releases of carbon into the atmosphere.

Drift Away

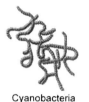

Cyanobacteria　　Diatom　　Dinoflagellate　　Green Algae　　Coccolithophore

Image: NASA, public domain.

Phytoplankton (Greek for *plant which drifts*) are microscopic plant-like organisms at the base of the marine food chain. Like land-based plants, they play a major role in removing carbon dioxide from the atmosphere.

Phytoplankton inhabit both salt- and freshwater habitats. Most are single-celled plants or bacteria, though some are also *protists*, commonly called algae. The most common phytoplankton are photosynthesizing *cyanobacteria*, silica-encased *diatoms, dinoflagellates*, green algae, and chalk-encrusted *coccolithophores*.

All phytoplankton use chlorophyll to trap sunlight energy, converting it into chemical energy during photosynthesis, just like land plants. In the process, they also consume carbon dioxide and release oxygen. Some species also consume other organisms for additional energy. Under ideal conditions, phytoplankton colonies can grow explosively, in a *bloom* covering hundreds of square kilometers, and lasting for weeks.

Brown algae, red algae, and a number of green algae species are multicellular, and the largest forms are known as *seaweeds*. It's from this group that land plants evolved, from freshwater green algae called *charophytes*, which resemble the earliest land plants, in both the structure of their photosynthesizing chloroplasts and sperm cells, and how their cells divide during mitosis.

Octopus's Garden

In 2011, paleontologists under the direction of Virginia Tech's Dr. Shuhai Xiao discovered over 3,000 seaweed and kelp fossils preserved in 150 meter-thick layers of rock in southern China's Lantian formation, long famed for the oldest algae fossils known. These specimens range from 635 to 580 million years old in the *Ediacaran Era*, when Earth began to thaw from one of its most severe periods of glaciation. Freed from the ice, diverse life was finally able to evolve in the Cambrian. Prior to this, says Dr. Xiao, the fossil record is comprised of only algae and bacteria.

Dr. Xiao's rust-colored fossils have the splayed branches, sweeping fans and conical blooms of modern kelps, with a small group of symmetrical tubes and ribbons which could possibly indicate bilaterian animals. Dr. Xiao believes these don't fit into modern classifications, and were possibly early life forms which died out. Together, these early life forms may have helped drive the oxygenation of the oceans prior to the Cambrian explosion.

In the gradual colonization of Earth's landmasses, lichens appear to have been the first fungi to cooperate with photosynthesizing organisms. Because they can survive without rain for months at a time, they provide plants with some protection. They also produce rock-dissolving acids, and together with plants, help fix atmospheric carbon.

Changes

About 416 million years ago, another extinction event at the end of the Silurian destroyed many plants and animals, opening many ecological niches at the start of one of the most important ages in Earth's living history – the *Devonian period*, nicknamed both the *Age of Fishes* and the *Greenhouse* era. Here, the first trees, ferns, seed plants, and many new fish evolved. Named after Devon, England – where most Devonian rocks and fossils were first found – the Devonian lasted from 416 to 359 million years ago.

The planet underwent violent geological upheavals during the Devonian, which radically altered its face forever. Two massive supercontinents, *Gondwana* and *Euramerica*, lay relatively near one another, while the rest of the planet was covered in ocean. A major collision would eventually unite both supercontinents into the single world-continent *Pangaea*.

By this time, oxygen levels had more than doubled, from 10% to 21%, as plants spread across the continents, turning the Devonian into Earth's greenhouse period; at the era's start, plants were only about a meter on average, but the evolution of strong wood stems supported weightier trunks, branches and leaves, and the first ancient forests grew, with trees as high as 100 feet tall.

North America and Europe collided, thrusting the Appalachian Mountains high into the air in eastern North America, and vigorous erosion deposited a torrent of sediment into neighboring valleys and shallow seas. Meanwhile, mountainous reef complexes arose in the depths of the ocean, as corals and now-extinct spongelike *stromatoporoid* populations exploded. Earth's landmass was undergoing its own evolution, a process that is still underway, albeit more gently in modern times.

Fortunately, this affords scientists with the opportunity to watch land colonization, in regions like the volcanic island Surtsey, which formed off the coast of Iceland in the 1960s. Because of this, we know that vegetation colonizes land in stages, not all at once. Each stage depends upon the previous one for food, building upon and adding to the ecosystem until a stable, mature ecosystem emerges, with a wide variety of species, recycling nutrients among organisms which interact to mutual benefit.

Each type of organism originates independently from areas beyond the region being colonised. Usually, the first to colonize fresh land are communities of bacteria, fungi and algae, able to reproduce with spores. These microorganisms release chemicals which help break apart rock, creating smaller grains, along with natural processes such as the fracturing and faulting of earthquakes, and erosion from sunlight, wind, rain, rivers and oceans. These processes allow water to reach deeper soil, working with atmospheric carbon to form clays, as bacteria fix atmospheric nitrogen into biologically useful compounds.

Next come lichens and mosses, and, if the climate is favorable, herbaceous plants, followed by shrubs and trees, with roots and acids to further break up the soil. Burrowing insects such as earthworms and ants also arrive, and gradually, ever-deeper rock is turned into fertile soil.

On Surtsey Island, mosses and nitrogen-fixing cyanobacteria began growing within just three years, around holes and cracks dampened by volcanic steam. A decade later, mosses and lichens had fully colonized the bare rock surface. Insects, mites and arthropods such as spiders and scorpions, swept up by winds and carried hundreds of miles, gradually appeared, as did watertight springtails, shown in experiments to be able to survive floating in seawater for weeks. Other creatures adapting from a marine to a terrestrial environment included *annelids* (earthworms), *onychophorans* (velvet worms), and *molluscs* (slugs and snails). Heavier animals typically arrived on foot or by swimming.

Early Earth's land was much more challenging to colonize, however. Earthquakes and flash flooding were constantly destabilizing the surface, burying it in ever-thickening sand and mud beds, making it difficult for plants to gain a foothold. In the modern world, birds and other animals transport plant seeds, but there were no such helpful species in the ancient world, to help rebuild colonies destroyed by harsher natural processes. This meant that ecosystems had to continually restart the process, in an ongoing, uphill struggle where recovery attempts were under constant disruption.

Fossilized spores from primitive herb-like land plants began to appear in the fossil record from about 470 million years ago. These first plants, classified as *bryophytes*, resembled modern liverworts. Because they can withstand great fluctuations of moisture and temperature, plants like bryophytes, mosses and liverworts are able to survive in comparatively harsh conditions. Well-adapted to Earth's ecology, they have had little need to further evolve, and have thus remained largely unchanged over half a billion years.

FROM SEA TO LAND

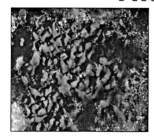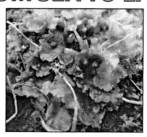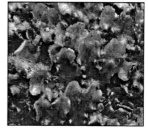

About 2.7 billion years ago, a single-celled eukaryote engulfed a photosynthesizing prokaryote, which stably integrated and evolved into a membrane-bound chloroplast as demonstrated by 2013 green algae feeding experiments by Korean biologist Dr. Eunsoo Kim.

*This evolutionary step marked the origin of oxygenic photosynthesis in eukaryotes, including seaweeds (left). One lineage, the **charophytes**, evolved into freshwater green algae and the first land plants, **bryophytes** such as mosses, hornworts (middle) and liverworts (right).*

Like modern bryophytes, these early species lacked cells for transporting nutrients and water, and required a constantly moist environment for survival and reproduction. Since these primitive plants lack roots, stems, woody tissue and inner transport systems, their growth is limited to tiny "herb-sized" plants. They absorb moisture and minerals through their cell walls, and water moves through their system by diffusion. Water is also needed to transport sperm from male to female forms of bryophyte plants. This limits their range to wet habitats.

These early species migrated first from freshwater onto waterbanks, eventually developing from simple bryophytes into more sophisticated *vascular plants*. This involved the evolution of *roots*, to draw water and minerals and store food; *stems*, to transport fluids, store food, and support branches and leaves; and *leaves*, which generate glucose through photosynthesis. *Cellulose* and *lignin* evolved to provide structural support, allowing the growth of trees, and protecting plant tissue from bacteria, fungus and insects.

Vascular plants have conducting tissues to transport nutrients and water from one part of a plant to another, within the roots, stems, and leaves. This ability allows vascular plants to spread and grow tremendously larger than bryophytes, to stockpile food within, and to further evolve traits which boost their hardiness and allow farther and faster proliferation.

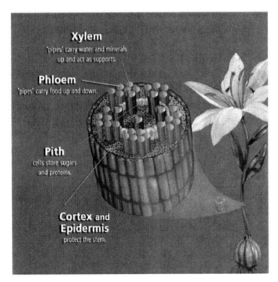

*Vascular plants evolved two specialized tissues to accomplish nutrient distribution: **xylem** tubes, to draw minerals and water from roots to leaves, and **phloem**, to distribute sugar from leaves to roots and areas of the body requiring energy for growth. Xylem, along with lignin, also adds rigidity to stems, allowing plants to grow taller. In contrast with the primarily dead cells of xylem, phloem is made up of living cells which transport sugar-rich, watery sap from the photosynthesizing leaves to non-photosynthesizing regions like the roots, or into storage structures like tubers and bulbs. Image: Boise State University, used with permission.*

In vascular plants, two tube networks, the *xylem* and *phloem*, circulate water and nutrients. The xylem brings up water and minerals from the roots to circulate throughout the plant's body, and the phloem circulates food, nutrients, and photosynthetic material throughout the plant, ensuring its health and growth. When the phloem is loaded with glucose, water is added to create the sugary *sap* which can be transported to growing plant regions, or to roots for storage while a plant is dormant in winter.

Vascular plants also have sturdy cell walls of lignin and cellulose, macromolecules which incorporate carbon into multiple strong chemical bonds, which prevents these macromolecules from easily decomposing after a plant's death. This keeps carbon locked in soil, rather than returning it to the atmosphere. This soil-bound carbon is the basis of fossil fuels like coal and oil, buried in swamps hundreds of millions of years ago. It's the burning of these *fossil fuels* which is re-releasing these carbon compounds into the atmosphere, triggering global warming.

Lignin isn't actually a single compound, but several, which vary by species, and even from cell-to-cell within the same plant. In plants, it regulates liquid flow and reinforces cell walls, allowing trees to grow taller and to compete for sunlight. Lignin and cellulose work in tandem, providing structure to plants.

Lignin is a macromolecule which binds cells, fibers and vessels, resulting in sturdy wood and straw. It's the binding agent coating cellulose fibers, just as resin is the binding agent coating fiberglass, forming the hard, waterproof outer surface of modern boats. Fibrous cellulose is the primary load-bearing element, while lignin forms an extracellular matrix providing stiffness and rigidity.

Photosynthesizing plants absorb carbon dioxide and emit oxygen through their pores, but the chemical reactions require large amounts of water. Because of this, plants need special tissues to draw water up from the ground: water evaporating from leaf surfaces has ionic attraction between its molecules, pulling upon the molecules below, drawing them upward through the plant stem and into the leaves.

Vascular plants left spores as far back as the Cambrian, though the earliest full plant fossils of Cooksonia appeared from the Silurian, when erosion and deposition seem to have been less destructive. Cooksonia was about four inches (10 cm) high, and five species had spread across the globe by the close of the Silurian Era. This was soon followed by a variety of branched, leafy vascular plants, such as the taller, more complex *Baragwanathia*, which reached two to three meters in height.

Most of these early plant forms went extinct, replaced by ferns and horsetails, mosses and liverworts, able to reproduce through spores that could be transported by water and wind. Plant spores have tough walls to protect against damage from microbes, drying out, or injuries suffered in transit. Because of this hardiness, they're the first land fossils to appear in the Ordovician, and possibly as far back as the Cambrian.

Fungi arrived early in the form of *glomerales*, organisms which form a symbiosis with plants, helping them capture micronutrients like phosphorus, sulfur, and nitrogen from the soil. This symbiosis is thought to have played a critical role in land colonization by the first terrestrial plants, and in the evolution of vascular plants. DNA and fossil evidence suggest roots may have evolved specifically to offer a more hospitable habitat for fungi, as well as to provide a means for plants to draw water and nutrients from the soil.

Fungi are multicellular organisms in a kingdom separate from plants. They feed upon decomposing organic matter, recycling it into the ecosystem in forms which other organisms can digest. Fungi usually grow in symbiosis with plants, helping plant roots absorb water and minerals, and receiving carbohydrates in return.

Fungi filaments and spores in the fossil record date back to the Ordovician, and are similar in form to those of modern species. Soils with traces of lichens also began to develop around the same era. Slowly, fungi and land plants rolled out the red carpet for land animals to evolve, plant carbon fixing reducing atmospheric carbon dioxide by 90%, while photosynthesis doubled atmospheric oxygen.

Land colonization by the first plants and fungi created revolutionary ecological changes, allowing the transition of tetrapods from water to land. It was one of the greatest biological revolutions in Earth's entire history, allowing life to thrive and spread across the planet. Plants have become far Earth's oldest living organisms – a patch of 200,000-year-old *Posidonia oceanica* (Neptune Grass) spanning 2000 square miles lies at the bottom of the Mediterranean Sea; they are also its largest – a 380-foot-tall Coast Redwood named *Hyperion* grows in California's Redwood National Park.

The most critical part of Earth's food chain had been colonizing the planet's land-masses for millions of years, initially evolving from green algae, with mosses, liverworts and finally Cooksonia leading the charge, followed soon after by seedless ferns and horsetails. By 428 million years ago, the first fully terrestrial land plants – Cooksonia – had evolved. Cooksonia were a few centimeters tall, without leaves, flowers or roots, simple stalks that branched out, ending in rounded, spore-bearing pods. Over time, more complex plants gradually evolved on land, and began to flourish farther from the coastlines, lakes and streams.

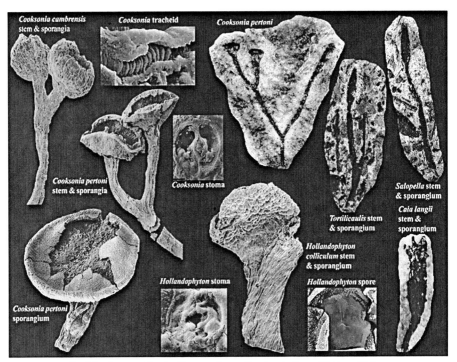

Fossils of Cooksonia, Hostinella, etc, the earliest land plants. National Museums and Galleries of Wales, 2011, used with permission.

By the end of the Devonian, Earth's landmasses were covered with giant super rivers, rainforests, and shallow marshes. Ferns, horsetails and seed plants had emerged to produce the first trees and forests. *Conifers* (named after their seed-bearing cones) were the first seed plants to evolve about 360 million years ago during the *Carboniferous period*, while deciduous (seasonal) and flowering plants would arrive 130 million years ago, during the *Cretaceous*.

Hox genes are at the heart of animal complexity and diversity, while *MADS* genes perform the equivalent function in the plant kingdom, giving rise to, for example, the first flowers. Evolution used essentially the same strategy in two completely different kingdoms of life.

MADS genes express transcription factors in much the same way as Hox genes, thus determining the general structure of parts in plants – what develops when, where and how: stems, petals, reproductive parts, etc. And just as Hox duplications increased in the Cambrian age, an explosion in the number of MADS box genes occurred around the time when flowering plants first evolved, about 140 million years ago.

Creepy Crawlies

The first land animals in the fossil record were insects such as millipedes, which emerged by at least the mid-Silurian, although millipede tracks going even further back have been found in England. Intriguingly, their anatomy suggests they evolved entirely on land, rather than having emerged from the sea. An extinct species of spider-like *trigonotarbids* also appeared, though the first true spiders emerged later, during the early Devonian.

In the Devonian many other arthropods appeared, including mites and *pseudoscorpions*, which lacked tails. The monstrous 8.5-foot ancestral millipede *Arthropleura* appeared, to briefly dine upon rotten tree trunks of Scotland and North America, before vanishing from history. A host of other land-dwelling insects would soon arrive to bring the ancient forests to life, including mayflies, dragonflies, cockroaches, crickets, and many now-extinct creatures, all quickly spreading and diversifying.

As plant growth slowly stabilized the climate and land surfaces, harsh weather patterns, calmed, oxygen levels rose, and plentiful new ecological niches emerged. Swamps, marshes, river plains and deltas formed inviting new habitats, with plant canopies offering shelter, humidity and abundant food for the first tetrapods to exploit.

These early transitional creatures swam instead of walking, gradually encroaching upon brackish and freshwater margins in pursuit of the prey which preceded them onland. These tetrapod predators spread from what would become Australia to North America, attracted by arthropods which had been the first to colonize land.

The Devonian age ended with another major extinction event that wiped out about 70 percent of marine species, though many of the land animals survived. Although it's still unclear why, the latest research suggests there were actually three and possibly seven separate extinction phases over the course of a few million years.

Geological evidence shows another major cooling as well as significant increases in atmospheric carbon dioxide, and some scientists believe a major asteroid impact may have changed the atmosphere as well.

By this time, however, plants and insects had fully colonized Earth's landmasses, and massive coral reefs carpeted the ocean floors, as the supercontinents Euramerica and Gondwana eventually converged into the single supercontinent of Pangaea.

The armored *placodermi* fish didn't survive the Devonian, nor did most jawless vertebrates – today the only survivors are lampreys and hagfishes. Also among the survivors, however, were cartilaginous ancestors of sharks and rays, and the bony fish which would become ancestors of most modern living fish species.

Walking in the Sand

In the oceans, many fish species came and went during the Devonian, from the diverse benthic, armored, jawless fish of the Lower Devonian to the first jawed placoderms and the lobe-finned fish which would eventually evolve into the first tetrapods by the end of the Devonian.

Two major lineages had developed – the ray-finned *actinopterigians*, which produced nearly every fish alive today, and the lobe-finned **sarcopterygians**, which gave rise to tetrapods, including humans.

Three major continental masses had formed. In the north was part of modern Siberia, while in the south, lay a merged supercontinent constituting Africa, Antarctica, Australia, and South America. North America and Europe clustered near the equator, primarily covered by shallow seas.

Paradoxically, events on land seem to have determined the fate of ancient fish, particularly the appearance of Devonian-age forests. Insects and spiders began to flourish among the Earth's first forests, providing a rich new ecosystem to exploit. Early transitional fish began exploring the shorelines, and to make the transition to life on land.

To marine animals, the water's edges offered rich pockets of oxygen, shade, a potential retreat from predators and an abundance of food. The spread of vascular plants at the water's edge in the Middle and Late Devonian allowed large quantities of dead plant material to accumulate in these semiterrestrial ecosystems, offering fertile, nitrate- and phosphate-rich soil and detritus for plant, insect, fungal and bacterial organisms to feed upon in the shallows.

Ever more complex food webs evolved, as greater numbers of marine organisms arrived to exploit these fecund new habitats. Wide, gently sloping mud deposits formed gentle gradients from water to land, offering an array of ecological niches from fully aquatic to fully terrestrial. These came to be colonized by an increasingly diverse range of aquatic vertebrates, as reflected by a striking increase in diversity and number of freshwater animal fossils.

Breathe in the Air

Early aerobic microbes absorbed oxygen from the water in which they swam, using it for *cellular respiration*, the extraction of energy from nutrients they engulfed using oxygen. But while unicellular microbes absorb oxygen across the entire surface of their bodies, larger, active multicellular organisms typically require other means of acquiring oxygen.

In the earliest multicellular organisms, flagella assisted in filter-feeding and in breathing, drawing in water to strain out microbes and oxygen. This is still how modern sponges breathe, using *osmosis*; the sponge's pores draw water into its body, where choanocyte cells use flagella to push it through channels. There, cells absorb food and oxygen, and expel waste and carbon dioxide.

Oxygen and carbon dioxide cross the sponge's cell membranes by simple *diffusion* – the natural movement of a gas from the area of highest concentration to the area of lowest concentration. These expended water and gases are finally pumped out sponge's single main opening, the *osculum*.

From these filter-feeding mechanisms *gills* evolved, filtration systems used to capture dissolved oxygen from water. Gills enable fish to absorb tiny amounts of oxygen dissolved in water. They're functionally similar to lungs, but able to extract much smaller oxygen concentrations. Water molecules trap dissolved oxygen, and fish use their gills to strain the water as they swim, capturing this dissolved oxygen.

Air is about 21% oxygen – 210,000 parts per million – but water typically contains only about 4-8 parts per million. However, fish have lower oxygen needs than warm-blooded land animals, because their metabolic rate is much lower, and they don't shed excess energy as body heat.

Slits on each side of a fish's head are covered by a flap called the *operculum*. Beneath this flap are bone arches, from which tightly-packed, thread-like *filaments* fan out. Fish breathe by gulping in water, and pumping it across the filament of these gills. Please refer to the illustration on the following page.

Bony *gill rakers* act as filters, trapping large particles to prevent clogging, as water passes over the gills. The gill filaments absorb dissolved oxygen, replacing it with waste carbon dioxide, and the oxygen-depleted water is expelled by closing the mouth and opening the operculum flap. On each filament are tiny disk-like protrusions called *lamellae* – membrane-covered collections of blood vessels which separate blood and water, and allow dissolved O_2 and CO_2 to naturally diffuse from one liquid into the other, depending upon which has the highest concentration of either gas.

Particles such as gases seek to equalize, naturally moving from areas of high concentration to areas of low concentration, and in gills, they diffuse across the thin membranes of the lamellae, into and out of the fish's bloodstream. Oxygen can then be pumped by the heart to cells throughout the body.

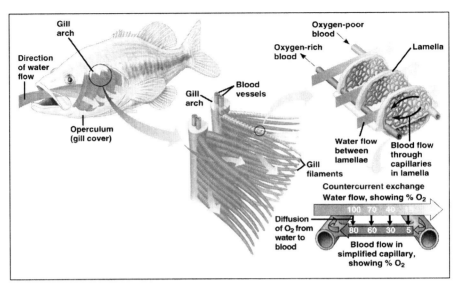

National Ocean and Atmospheric Association, Teacher at Sea Program, public domain.

In the fish's body, this oxygen passes through each cell membrane, where it can be used by mitochondria to generate energy from nutrients. Waste carbon dioxide generated by the process is expelled into the blood, where the heart can pump it to the gills for exhalation. Blood flows in the opposite direction from the water entering the gills, further maximizing oxygen concentration, increasing the system's efficiency 500%.

Gills are tremendously efficient, with a tightly folded surface area to maximize oxygen absorption. Unlike lungs, gills waste no time or energy in expelling gases; the continuous flow of water across the gill surface drives the process.

The Late Devonian marshes offered tremendous survival advantages to any fish living within shallow tropical waters: abundant nutrients, and plentiful shelter from aquatic predators, with few vertebrate competitors. Increased oxygen had thickened the ozone layer, decreasing harmful ultraviolet radiation on land and its potential genetic damage.

However, just as in modern ecosystems, marsh and swamp habitats naturally cycled through *hypoxia*, because of *biological oxygen demand* (BOD) from bacteria and fungi feeding upon decaying plant matter. *Hypoxic waters* contain oxygen at concentrations below 2 ppm – two parts per million. This means that for every million molecules, only two are oxygen, a concentration far too low for most marine animals. Hypoxia and seasonal drought occurred in both marine and freshwater ecosystems on both a daily or seasonal basis, depending upon water flow.

Such environmental pressures rewarded any air-breathing adaptations among aquatic organisms venturing into these ecosystems. Early land plants and insects hadn't evolved defenses against predators, meaning any fish able to survive in the shallows or on land for even brief intervals could easily obtain plenty of food.

To compensate for hypoxic conditions, early vertebrate ancestors used crude air sacs to gulp air from above the stagnant pools in which they lived, supplementing declining oxygen in the water.

These air sacs are derived from the *natatory vesicle,* more commonly called a *swim bladder.* This sac fills with gas, allowing fish to control buoyancy, using the same principle as a submarine: taking in or expelling gas in an enclosed space with a density matching the surrounding water.

The amount of air can be controlled to change depth. Thus, the basic machinery for lungs is derived from the swim bladder – a gas-filled sac which draws in gases from the outside environment, with a network of blood vessels to absorb that gas.

Such environmental pressures rewarded any air-breathing adaptations among aquatic organisms venturing into these ecosystems. Early land plants and insects hadn't evolved defences against predators, meaning any fish able to survive in the shallows or on land for even brief intervals could easily obtain plenty of food.

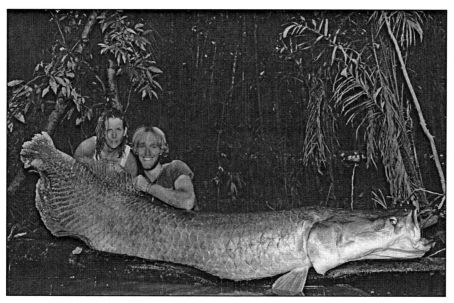

Extreme angler Jakub Vágner with one of the largest freshwater fish ever captured. He released this creature unharmed shortly after the photo was taken. Used with permission.

Just as its ancient ancestors did, *Arapaima,* also known as the *Amazonian Giant,* breathes by using its natatory vesicle like a primitive lung to capture oxygen from the river surface. This enables it to survive in the hypoxic waters of the Amazonian basin. A predatory fish which can grow up to three meters, arapaima has survived since the Jurassic era. It's currently the primary food source of the *Riberinhos,* Brazil's Amazon River Peoples.

189

Similarly, *lungfish* possess both gills and oxygen-breathing lungs, to supplement the oxygen taken in by their gills from the poorly-oxygenated shallows in which they live. When their habitat is stricken by drought, lungfish encase themselves deep in mud. As water evaporates, their skin secretes a mucus which dries and hardens into a watertight cocoon, enveloping the body closely, leaving only a short funnel between the lips and teeth through which they can breathe. In this manner, lungfish can survive up to four years during a dry spell, though rains usually return within six months.

Animals like the lungfish adapted and diversified in this era, colonizing the increasingly fertile freshwater ecosystems, and evolving from marine into freshwater species with their current body plan. Soon after, the first land-living vertebrates would begin to evolve, following the footsteps of terrestrial annelids, gastropods and arthropods – worms, snails, slugs, scorpions, insects and arachnids.

The sarcopterygian lineage gave rise to tetrapods, including humans, while the actinopterygians produced the vast majority of fish alive today, including the fascinating *Mangrove rivulus*, which can live over two months out of water, typically inside fallen logs, breathing air through its skin.

Mudskippers are another species of ray-finned fish which have evolved to become amphibious, able to use their pectoral fins to walk on land and even climb trees in some cases. They range throughout tropical, subtropical and temperate mangroves and mudflats in Africa, Asia, Australia, and the Indies. Like other amphibians, mudskippers employ cutaneous (skin) air breathing. But they also have enlarged *gill chambers*, which close tightly when these creatures emerge onto land, trapping a pocket of air. Periodically, however, mudskippers must return to water to moisten their gills.

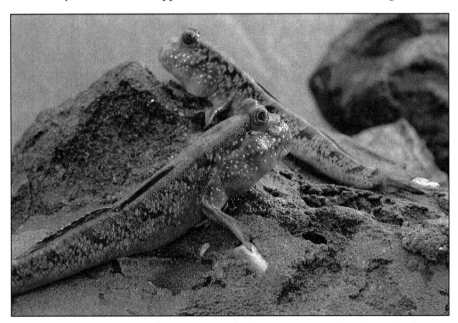

Mudskippers are quite active on land, some even climbing trees. Image: Wikipedia, public domain

Similarly, the *walking catfish* can survive on dry land, using its pectoral fins as stilts to move about in search of water. This animal is indigenous throughout Southeast Asia, where it flourishes in stagnant, often hypoxic waters and frequently lives in muddy ponds, ditches and canals.

Because it is a voracious omnivore, it's a particularly harmful invasive species in Florida, California, Georgia, Nevada and reportedly other more northern states where it has spread since first being imported to Florida from Thailand in the 1960s. Other air-breathing fish which survive to this day include the *Pacific leaping blenny* (rockskipper), the *climbing perch*, and the *oriental weatherloach*.

Air-breathing fish and amphibians like frogs have lungs which expand and draw air by means of a *buccal pump* – a mouth cavity which expands and compresses. They typically have simple balloon-like lungs, and gas exchange is limited to the outer surface area of these primitive lungs. This is sufficient for amphibians, which require comparatively low levels of oxygen, and can supplement their supply by diffusion across their moist outer skin. More active creatures require greater amounts of oxygen, and thus a more efficient system.

True lungs evolved independently several times in different forms over the last 300 million years, as vertebrates diversified, varying considerably in structure between groups. Reptiles may possess only a single right lung, or a significantly smaller vestigial left lung, typically operating by expansion and contraction of the ribs and mouth. The most complex of these lungs have a single *bronchial tube* running through the center, with branches reaching out to comparatively large, simple and sparse individual pockets.

The mammalian breathing apparatus is comparatively remarkable, driven by the *diaphragm*, a dome-shaped bundle of muscle and tendon which separates the chest cavity from the abdominal cavity. During inhalation, the diaphragm contracts, flattening to allow the lungs to expand downward and draw in air. The diaphragm then relaxes, returning to its dome shape, pushing up the bottom of the lungs to produce exhalation.

In mammals, lungs are made up of branching "trees" of tubes. The *trachea* (windpipe) separates into two *bronchi*, which continue to divide into branches called *bronchioles*. The smallest of these, the *terminal bronchioles*, attach to clusters of air sacs called *alveoli*, which look like grapes in a bunch. Human lungs possess about 25 bronchioles and 300 to 700 million of these tiny gas-exchanging alveoli. The system results in a huge surface area for gas exchange – up to 74 square meters in adults.

For all their differences, lungs share a common structure – they're internal, fluid-lined, gas-holding structures which inflate and deflate rhythmically. In the process, fluids (like water) are subject to surface tension because of ionic interactions, making them difficult to pry from surfaces with which they come in contact.

To lessen this potentially deadly stickiness, *surfactants* evolved, which coat the lungs and allow them to freely expand and contract, without adhering to the surfaces of chest cavity walls. In mammals, they also help the alveoli to maintain their shape.

This incredibly complex arrangement greatly increases the surface area across which gases can be exchanged – if an adult human's alveoli were spread out flat, the gas exchange surface area would equal about 74 square meters (800 square feet), over 40 times the total surface area of human skin.

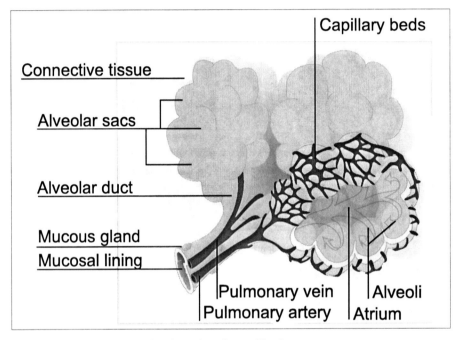

Alveoli, Wikipedia. Public domain.

Alveoli are covered in tiny blood vessels called capillaries, with walls only a single cell thick, and this is where gas exchange occurs. Oxygen diffuses across the alveoli membranes, entering the capillaries where blood is circulating. In the blood, oxygen then diffuses into red blood cells, where it attaches to hemoglobin proteins. The oxygenated red blood cells are then drawn up into the heart.

Chambers in the heart contract, pumping this oxygenated blood throughout the body, where it can diffuse out across capillaries to individual cells, to be used in cellular respiration, the process of nutrient energy extraction.

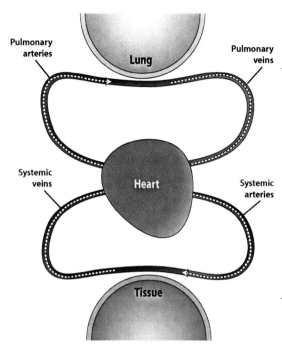

Pulmonary arteries

Lung

Pulmonary veins

Systemic veins

Heart

Systemic arteries

Tissue

After energy extraction, waste carbon dioxide diffuses out from cells into the capillaries, and is pumped from the heart back to the lungs, where it diffuses out from the capillaries into the alveoli and is exhaled. Both gas exchanges – oxygen intake and carbon dioxide disposal – occur simultaneously.

Human lungs have evolved a massive reserve capacity compared to resting oxygen requirements, which is why smokers can continue to destroy their alveoli for decades before contracting emphysema, extreme shortness of breath.

Additional protection comes in the form of cilia which beat upward rhythmically, ejecting dust particles and bacteria caught in the mucous surface of the respiratory passages.

According to the evidence, the mechanism responsible for controlling rhythmic air breathing, which sits atop the vertebrate spinal cord in the brainstem's *medulla,* evolved from ancient fish like the lamprey. Lamprey larvae live in tunnels dug into soft river mud, pumping water through their bodies to breathe and feed. If a lamprey's tube gets clogged, the creature "coughs" to clear the tube using a rhythmic, carbon-dioxide-sensitive system.

Lung structure, on the other hand, was primarily driven by the recruitment of *Fibroblast growth factor receptor 2* (FGFR2), used to guide the growth of limbs and the branching growth of lungs. Meanwhile, *Parathyroid Hormone–related Protein* (PTHrP) triggers the formation of alveoli at the ends of these branches.

As metabolic demands for oxygen increased, PTHrP signalling was central to the evolutionary process. PTHrP is multifunctional however, promoting bone, tooth and mammary development throughout the vertebrate lineage, though it initially guided swim bladder growth. It also plays a role in gas exchange across the alveoli and capillaries, and in producing *surfactants* (lipid-based liquids which prevent surface tension from making lungs cling to surrounding tissue during breathing).

If You Want Blood – You Got It

Hemoglobins are red blood cell proteins which transport oxygen between lungs and tissues of the body. These proteins are found in all kingdoms of living organisms, including prokaryotes, fungi, plants and animals, showing the ancestral genes which produce them are extremely ancient – studies within the last decade show hemoglobin genes existed even before the split between prokaryotes and eukaryotes.

In invertebrates, hemoglobins have diverse functions. In addition to blood oxygen transport, they're also used for oxygen transport within the cells themselves, and as catalysts – enzymes controlling chemical change. They participate, for example, in *redox reactions* (confusingly, **RED**uction means a gain of electrons; and **OX**idation, a loss of electrons), two types of electron transfer which alter chemical compositions.

Hemoglobins are only one of three types of oxygen-transport molecules which evolved independently. These proteins, called *respiratory pigments* because they change color after binding with oxygen, include hemoglobin, *hemerythrin*, and *hemocyanin*. All are structurally different, and there's no indication they share a common ancestry.

Hemoglobins are widespread throughout bacteria, plant, fungi and animal species, while hemerythrin is used by marine invertebrates and at least one species of bacteria. Hemocyanins are respiratory proteins used by molluscs and arthropods, which use copper instead of iron to bind oxygen.

Human hemoglobins evolved through a series of exon shufflings and duplications, and through changes to the regulatory elements controlling their expression. The evolutionary trigger for their modern use is quite logical; hypoxia (low oxygen levels), triggers hemoglobin expression: *Hypoxia-inducible factor* (HIF) is a recently-discovered transcription factor which functions as a master switch in vertebrates, responding to low oxygen levels by triggering hemoglobin production.

Land Ho!

People often picture evolution as a single fish flopping onto land and, with a brave little *Tally Ho!* crawling pluckily forward into history. However, at least 47 distinct species have been discovered that were transitional forms (*tetrapodomorphs*) between lobe-finned fish and tetrapods during the Devonian and Carboniferous Periods.

DEVONIAN AND CARBONIFEROUS TETRAPODS

A comprehensive list of confirmed prehistorical transitional species, adapted from Brian Swartz, Michael I. Coates, Marcello Ruta, Matt Friedman, Davis, M., N. H. Shubin, E. B. Daeschler, Jing Lu, Min Zhu, John A. Long, Wenjin Zhao, Tim J. Senden, Liantao Jia, Tuo Qiao, and Lebedev, O.L.

Tungsenia paradoxa (409 mya)	Eusthenopteron (385 mya)	Ventastega (359 - 372 mya)
Kenichthys (395 mya)	Jarvikina (385 - 359 mya)	Acanthostega (365 mya)
Rhizodontidae (377 - 310 mya)	Cabonnichthys (360 - 370 mya)	Ichthyostega (363 mya)
Marsdenichthys (380 mya)	Obruchevichthys (368 mya)	Hynerpeton (361 mya)
Canowindra (360 mya)	Hynerpeton (360 mya)	Densignathus rowei (361 mya)
Livoniana (374 - 391 mya)	Mandageria (360 mya)	Ymeria (383 - 359)
Koharalepis (374 - 359 mya)	Tulerpeton (363 mya)	Whatcheeria (327 - 342 mya)
Beelarongia (375 - 385 mya)	Eusthenadon (385 mya)	Pederpes (359 - 345 mya)
Gogonasus (380 mya)	Tinirau (365 mya)	Sinostega (355 mya)
Gyroptychius (399 mya)	Platycephalichthys (365 mya)	Eucritta (350 mya)
Osteolepis (398 - 392 mya)	Panderichthys (380 mya)	Colosteidae (342-306 mya)
Medoevia (384 mya)	Tiktaalik (375 mya)	Casineria (340 mya)
Metaxygnathus (358 - 372 mya)	Elpistostege (378 mya)	Greererpeton (330 mya)
Megalichthys (362 mya)	Jakubsonia livnensis (372 mya)	Crassigyrinus (330 mya)
Spodichthys (388 - 382 mya)	Elginerpeton (368 mya)	Baphetidae (326 - 307 mya)
Tristichopterus (385 - 359 mya)	Jakubsonia livnensis	

Jawed fish – *gnathostomata* – are classified into two groups, those with cartilage skeletons, like sharks and rays, and those with bony skeletons. Among the bony fish (*Osteichthyes*) are **ray-finned** (*Actinopterygii*) and *lobe-finned* (*Sarcopterygii*) species. During the Devonian, lobe-fins dominated, morphing into tetrapods over the course of some 120 million years.

Among them are lungfish, which never developed into committed land-dwellers; they're considered living fossils, unchanged for hundreds of millions of years. Three genera exist today, in Africa, South America, and Australia, inhabiting freshwater lakes, rivers and wetlands. In addition to gills they have modified swim bladders that constitute primitive lungs, allowing them to absorb oxygen in gulps of air.

In times of drought, lungfish can bury themselves in mud, remaining in a state of suspended animation for up to four years. This ability required the adaptation of swim-bladders as lungs, changes in circulation, and the ability to slow metabolism to a trickle.

Despite remaining essentially the same since their emergence in the Devonian, lung-fish possess the world's second-largest genome; the African lungfish has an impressive 130 billion DNA base pairs compared to humans with a paltry 3 billion. (Interestingly, certain types of amoebas have the largest genomes yet discovered.)

Today, bony and ray-finned fish dominate the seas. The only surviving lobe-finned fish are lungfish and *coelacanths*, which had been believed extinct for tens of millions of years until a single live specimen was first captured in 1938. Since then, other specimens have been discovered.

> *(Never)* *Mind the Gap* – In 1956, paleontologist Alfred Sherwood Romer noticed a major gap in part of the fossil record, which came to be called Romer's Gap in his honor. This was a stretch of about 30 million years, from the end of the Devonian (363 mya) through the Early Carboniferous (333 mya) Period. Although fundamentalists like to seize upon this as somehow "disproving" evolution, that gap in findings has been fully closed since it first came to light in 1956. Contrary to such Creationist prevarication, the transition from lobe-finned fish to land-walking amphibians has been well traced.

The Devonian Period – also known as the *Age of Fishes* – saw the emergence of Earth's first marshes and swamps. It also saw the transition from fish to *amphibians*, a lineage which would lead to reptiles, birds and mammals. Dr. Jennifer A. Clack, Cambridge paleontologist and author of *Gaining Ground: The Origin and Evolution of Tetrapods*, says this evolution primarily involved three changes: the birth of walking, the birth of limbs with digits, and the birth of terrestriality – life on land.

Walking likely evolved before limbs with digits or life on land, says University of Chicago biologist Dr. Heather King, who studies African lungfish walking along the bottom of test aquariums.

Lungfish share many modern features with the first tetrapods, including four fins with no digits, lungs and the lack of a *sacrum*, a triangular bone joining the hips to the spine, allowing land walking. Dr. King says lungfish are able to push themselves forward because of the buoyancy provided by their swim bladders.

Living organisms adapt from small initial populations in the course of spreading to new habitats, and this was the case during the Devonian Period, when the first amphibians began to appear. Almost all of these transitional species were short-lived – sort of "trial runs" at adapting to the new world. They would only live for short spans and in few numbers, to be quickly outcompeted by their more advanced descendants.

Lobe-finned fish slowly adapted to exploit the new ecosystems with a series of gradual anatomical transformations, over the course of some 120 million years. Each evolutionary "step" seems to have taken about two million years. In the process, all but the lungfish and coelacanths disappeared with the series of extinction events that brought the Devonian to a close and destroyed about 75% of all marine fish from the era.

Among the lobefish, pectoral and pelvic fins slowly morphed into limbs with digits. Their tail fins disappeared, and their skulls separated from their shoulders, forming necks. Their limbs gradually transformed into four fully weight-bearing, jointed appendages, their fins slowly thickening and separating into digits, decreasing in number from eight to five. Their snouts elongated, and curved ribcages grew to protect evolving lungs.

According to the University of Chicago's Neil Shubin, the same genetic toolkit responsible for the formation of shark gills was co-opted for this limb development. The genetic circuitry that builds paired appendages – arms, legs and fins – is the same set of patterning genes governing gill formation in sharks. To test his hypothesis, Dr. Shubin and colleagues injected the gill arches of skate embryos with *retinoic acid* – a vitamin A derivative. The gill arches responded just as paired limbs and fins do, by making mirror image duplicates of budding limb structures while the embryos grew.

DNA analyses show *Dlx* homeobox genes, found in virtually all animal groups, help guide limb development. Dlx genes are highly conserved, existing in nearly all complex animals, including insects. Although this family of regulatory genes is used primarily to grow limbs, it's also involved in forebrain, sensory organ, breathing and feeding system, and craniofacial development. In vertebrates, the present version of this gene family originated from a series of duplications. These Homeobox genes emerged early, appearing as far back as the *annelids* (worms), and duplicating to the point where modern mammals now possess six copies.

Experiments show that Dlx, in tandem with transcription factor *AP2*, is also central to the development of vertebrate neural crest cells, which, like stem cells, are pluripotent, able to differentiate into a number of different cell types, in this case forming skull/facial bones and cartilage, the peripheral nervous system, organ muscles and special *glial* support cells in the brain.

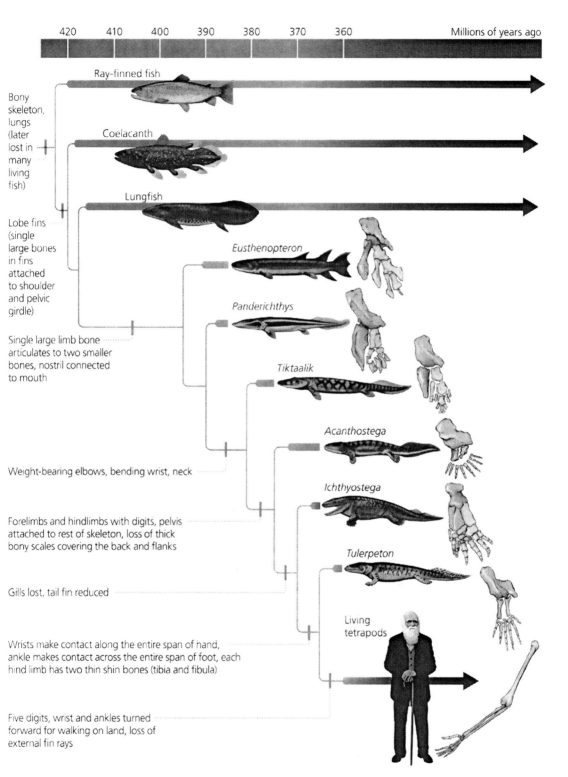

420 410 400 390 380 370 360 Millions of years ago

Ray-finned fish

Bony
skeleton,
lungs
(later
lost in
many
living
fish)

Coelacanth

Lungfish

Lobe fins
(single
large bones
in fins
attached
to shoulder
and pelvic
girdle)

Eusthenopteron

Single large limb bone
articulates to two smaller
bones, nostril connected
to mouth

Panderichthys

Tiktaalik

Weight-bearing elbows, bending wrist, neck

Acanthostega

Ichthyostega

Forelimbs and hindlimbs with digits, pelvis
attached to rest of skeleton, loss of thick
bony scales covering the back and flanks

Tulerpeton

Gills lost, tail fin reduced

Living
tetrapods

Wrists make contact along the entire span of hand,
ankle makes contact across the entire span of foot, each
hind limb has two thin shin bones (tibia and fibula)

Five digits, wrist and ankles turned
forward for walking on land, loss of
external fin rays

Fins to limbs, copyright The Tangled Bank: An Introduction to Evolution,
Carl Zimmer, 2009, Roberts and Co. Publishers, used with permission.

197

Walk This Way

The majority of fish today are ray-finned, and about 25,000 species presently exist, many more than all other vertebrates combined. They get their name from the branching bony rays which radiate out from the base of their fins. The earliest tetrapods, however, evolved from lobe-finned fish, which differ markedly from ray-finned fish, by dint of their fleshy *lobe* fins, the precursors to hands and fingers.

Lobe-finned fish from the Devonian era were already able to breathe air when needed, using *spiracles* in their skulls, and had bottom fins arranged in pairs, supported with internal bones – preconditions necessary for fins to evolve into primitive legs.

Although most lobe-finned fish died out at the end of the Cretaceous period, two lineages still survive – the lungfish and the 400-million-year-old *Coelacanth*, thought to have gone extinct some 65 million years ago, till one was caught live off the South African Coast in 1938. Since then, half a dozen more have been found in the African and South Pacific Oceans. These armor-plated, lunged creatures are just under two meters in length, and are a transition between fish and tetrapods. Within the last decade, fourteen species of *handfish* have also been discovered, which walk along tropic sea bottoms.

Transitional lobe-finned fish date back to the start of the Devonian, but the earliest true tetrapods emerged a little later, some 385 to 380 million years ago. Disputed tetrapod tracks discovered in a Polish limestone quarry in 2010 may have pushed that date back as far as 397 million years, about the same time that *wattieza*, the first trees, appear in the fossil record. The tracks appear to have been made by a creature 2.5 meters (8.2 ft.) long, which seems to have been a scavenger of the tidal flats, living upon washed-up marine animals.

What is certain is that tetrapods evolved several times, in a variety of environments, and they spent most or all of their time in the water, only using their legs and lungs when absolutely necessary.

After the evolution of vertebrae and a central nervous system, the next major event in the development of vertebrates was their transition to life on land. Many of the early tetrapods had limbs with seven or eight digits at each end, which means their lineage died out early, never contributing to the development of modern five-digit vertebrates. The line between advanced lobe-finned fish and primitive tetrapods is somewhat blurred, although *Eusthenopteron*, *Panderichthys* and *Osteolopis* were arguably the earliest tetrapodomorph fish. All three led completely aquatic lives, but had latent tetrapod characteristics.

The evolutionary pressures which drove these lobe-finned fish to evolve into breathing, walking tetrapods aren't entirely certain, but there are at least two possibilities: the shallow habitats of these fish often experienced droughts, and species able to adapt to dryer conditions survived; or predatory threats drove tetrapods out of the water, where dry land offered abundant insect and plant food. Perhaps both were true in different instances or even simultaneously. As lobe-finned fish (sarcopterygians) developed into limbed vertebrates during the Devonian, their lungs, gills, body scales, fin rays, jaw, palate, skulls and ears all evolved, as did mobile necks, weight-bearing limbs, functional wrist joints, and flexible digits. They were adapting to a shallow-water environment, which presumably included forays onto land.

Fish have no necks; their heads are simply a continuation of their bodies. But through Hox gene activations, the vertebral column gradually evolved and extended, as neck vertebrae were added one by one over time in these shallow water dwellers, allowing these creatures to first to move their heads up and down, and then later left and right. This improved the search for potential food or predators.

Meanwhile, limbs and joints evolved into forelimbs and hind limbs with muscular connections, allowing fast locomotion. In the transition to life on land, these creatures also lost their gills, their tail fins shrank, and they shed a special network of vibration-sensing canals in the skull and jaw – the *lateral line system*, which can't function in air.

Possibilities

In 2004, while searching among ancient rock on Canada's Ellesmere Island, high above the Arctic Circle, a team from Harvard, the Academy of Natural Sciences and the University of Chicago discovered the remains of a strange and wonderful creature. Bridging the evolutionary gap between sea and land animals, it was a 375-million-year-old predator with a flattened body and crocodile-like head with a mouth full of sharp teeth.

Tiktaalik, as the creature has been dubbed by the region's Inuit, hunted in shallow streams across its era's wide floodplains, birthplace of the first creatures to emerge on land. During this ancient creature's lifetime, the Canadian Arctic was part of *Pangaea*, a single great subtropical landmass near the equator.

Tiktaalik roseae possessed wrist- and hand-like bones, making it a *fishapod*, the 375-million-year-old nearest ancestor to the first land creatures, a crucial evolutionary development. Fishapods are a cross between fish and amphibians, with four partially formed limbs, each with partially formed digits.

Tiktaalik, discovered by Dr. Neil Shubin and colleagues, provided a missing evolutionary link between fish and tetrapods, and was among the first vertebrates to have walked on land. Tiktaalik sits midway between lobe-finned fishes and true tetrapods, with primitive wrists that may have assisted in propping itself up on stubby front fins, as well as a neck, useful for looking down at the ground for prey.

Tiktaalik was a *transitional form*, a creature which helps shed light on the evolutionary stages leading from one lineage to another, showing characteristics of both the ancestral and the new lineages. It was specialized for a shallow-water habitat, propping itself up on the river and marsh bottoms, and snatching up prey from below with its neck. The adaptations it had made to its ecological niche would later for be co-opted for vertebrates living on dry land.

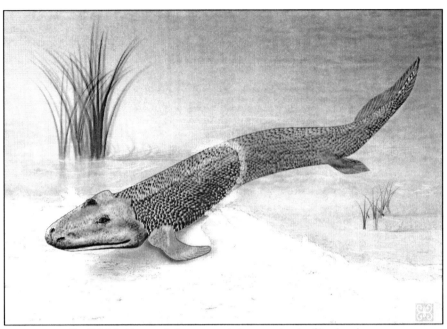

Fossil fish bridges evolutionary gap between animals of land and sea,
National Science Foundation, public domain.

Like most fish, Tiktaalik had fins, scales, and gills, but it also had the neck, thick ribs, sturdy chest, wrist bones and shoulders of a four-legged vertebrate. Its limbs still ended in fin rays, but with smaller bones branching off. These would later evolve into distinct digits in *Acanthostega*.

Tiktaalik's fins had already evolved into flexible appendages, able to extend and splay out on the ground. Although it was definitely not terrestrial, it had muscular, bony limbs and a strong pectoral girdle to prop itself up, perhaps to hold itself partly out of water.

Tiktaalik's discovery proved the predictive abilities of palaeontology, as the expedition that discovered it was specifically in search of an intermediate between the earlier *Panderichthys* and later tetrapods, looking in the most likely environment (rivers) and era (Late Devonian), as indicated by stratified rock layers. Another nine specimens were later retrieved from the same region.

Dr. Shubin followed up his remarkable finding with an even more astounding discovery in the lab: the same genes that guide the growth of limbs and paws in mice not only also exist in fish, but they can be transplanted between fish and mice to trigger normal limb or fin development. This serves as further proof of evolution, according to Dr. Igor Schneider, who conducted the experiments with Dr. Shubin and other colleagues. In other words, we can now conclusively trace the development of limbs back to fish and unequivocally show that the genetic blueprint for legs and digits has existed – in fish – for nearly half a billion years.

Dr. Shubin spliced the *CsB enhancer* for fin development into mouse DNA, and found it triggered normal leg and paw growth. *CsB* guides Hox gene expression, regulating the development of fins in zebrafish and skates, and limbs in chickens, frogs and humans.

Enhancers are short DNA regions to which transcription factors can bind, triggering enhanced gene expression (more proteins). Enhancer regions needn't be close to the genes they act upon, because the complex coiling of DNA strands can bring distant DNA regions into close physical proximity.

By comparing CsB genes in all five species, Dr. Shubin's team discovered identical sequences among them. This means the DNA had been *conserved* – passed down the evolutionary chain unchanged over 400 million years, as prehistoric fish and their ancestors evolved into new animals.

The experiment worked both ways. By swapping genes between the species, the researchers found that mouse CsB genes grew normal fins in zebrafish, and fish CsB genes grew normal paws in mice.

That evolutionary lineage has been confirmed in another lab: 2012 experiments at the University of Andalusia in Seville, Spain further demonstrate the genetic toolkit for limb development existed in fish before tetrapods emerged 395 million years ago.

As in the rest of the bilateral body, Hox genes are central to developing tetrapod limbs, including the *autopod*, the region where digits develop. By switching specific Hox genes on and off, Drs. Renata Freitas, José Luis Gómez-Skarmeta and Fernando Casares narrowed down fin-to-limb evolution to regulation of *hoxd13*. In humans, mutations to hoxd13 result in *syndactyly* (the fusion of fingers and toes) or *polydactyly* (the growth of extra digits).

Dr. Freitas' team engineered a way to overexpress Hoxd13 in zebra fish fins, to see how it affects development. Dr. "PZ" Myers of the University of Minnesota explains:

I work on zebrafish [which] have fins where we tetrapods build legs and arms. Fins are thin membranous folds of ectoderm (our fancy word for skin), infiltrated with thin rods of cartilage called fin rays. Developmentally, they arise from things called fin folds — flaps of ectoderm that flatten to form a double-walled sheet. In development, tetrapods add an extra element to the fin fold: mesoderm, that tissue that forms bone and muscle, expands to fill the fin fold with the raw material of a muscular, bony limb. You can visualize the developing limb as something like a slab of pita pocket bread. Fish are content with just the bread, giving it a little reinforcement, while tetrapods open up that hollow space and stuff it full of filling. That filling represents a field of great potential, which is then organized in reproducible ways to make limb bones and digits and muscle. There are genes... that are more strongly activated in tetrapods than in fish; these genes are associated in space and time with an increase in the volume of mesodermal tissues. The gene of interest here is called Hoxd13.

The Hoxd13 boost resulted in an *autopod* – an embryonic mesoderm bud with the potential to be genetically sculpted into a limb with digits.

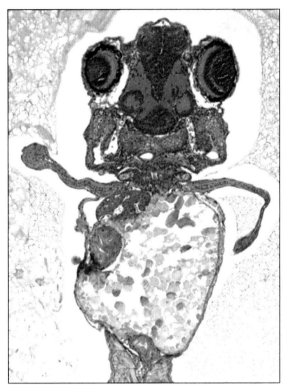

Autopods in place of fins in a zebrafish embryo. Image: Freitas, et al, reprinted from The Conversation, Deakin University, public domain.

Dr. Myers continues:

> *The fish does not build a hand or digits; it lacks the rules to carry out that degree of differentiation. But look at the limbs of fossils from the fish-tetrapod transition. There's a lot of anatomical exploration going on in this series. This fits a model in which tetrapod ancestors carried a genetic variation that expanded the core of mesodermal tissue in their fins, which was then organized by the standard rules of limb mesoderm into bone and muscle. Again, this is opportunity, a new field of potential that in these early stages of evolution hadn't yet been refined into a specific, and now familiar, pattern, although elements of that pattern are foreshadowed here.*
>
> *This morphology fits a simple developmental model. The ancestral change was nothing more than the addition of new regulatory enhancers (and they have a candidate, called CsC, which is found in mouse but not zebrafish) that increased the expression of Hoxd13, which in turn led to an expansion of the raw material of limb mesoderm, which was then shaped by existing developmental rules into a crude bony, muscular strut.*

Subsequent evolution refined that structure into a more specific limb morphology by layering new rules and new patterning elements onto the existing framework of genetic regulators.

So how did fish get legs? By progressive expansion of tissue that was then used autonomously by existing genetic programs to form a coherent structure, and which was then sculpted by chance and selection into the more familiar and more consistent shape of the tetrapod limb. Add raw material first, and the plasticity of developmental rules means that the organism will make sense of it.

Researchers long believed that new traits required new genes; now we know that existing genes are often adapted for entirely new functions. Among them, the genetic keys to limb evolution have long lain dormant in lobe-finned fish, needing just the right regulatory trigger to activate them. These Hox genes had the capacity to build limbs with fingers and toes long ago, but needed the right environmental pressures to exploit that capability.

Says Dr. Shubin, creatures like Tiktaalik developed limbs and fingers with these ancient genes because their shallow-water habitats were entirely new ecosystems, encouraging adaptations through natural selection.

Building a Mystery

It's very simplistic to say that vertebrate limb development in the womb is guided solely by Hox genes. The process is a much, much more complex interplay between signalling molecules, growth factors, enhancers, transcription factors, genes and epigenetic mechanisms. An extremely simplified explanation follows:

In vertebrates, the *mesoderm* (middle embryonic tissue layer) separates into paired blocks of *somites* along the central axis of the notochord. Before forming, these somites have been programmed to differentiate into spinal and rib vertebrae and muscles, growing one-by-one from the head downward. They are programmed to differentiate into muscle, cartilage, tendons, *epithelium* (inner lining of circulatory vessels), and *dermis* (inner skin layer). Their formation into paired blocks will also guide the migration of *neural crest cells*, which will settle and grow into the spinal nerves.

Once mesoderm cells have migrated into place, specific genes are activated in clocklike, oscillating waves of expression. Somites appear to be preprogrammed to switch between "ignoring" and responding to signalling molecules in timed waves.

For the most part, three biochemical control *pathways* govern the process:

- *FGF* (*fibroblast growth factors*, which trigger wound healing and embryonic growth);

- *Wnt* (*wingless type proteins*, cell-to-cell signalling molecules regulating cell fates and cell proliferation);

- *Notch* (receptors regulating cell fates, cell proliferation and cell death).

As the wave of signalling progresses from head to tail, cells in a responsive state undergo transition, and pinch into somite blocks, then reset the process for the next somite down the line. The timing of these gene expression "clock cycles" varies by species.

Give us a Hand

The same system guides limb development in all tetrapods, shaping claws, hooves, fins, paws, hands and feet. Each limb is guided by progressively more hox genes, using a collection of signalling molecules, which set the *axes* (three-dimensional planes of growth) and trigger three development phases, from the *proximal* (closest to the body) to *distal* (farthest from the body): the *stylopod, zeugopod,* and *autopod.*

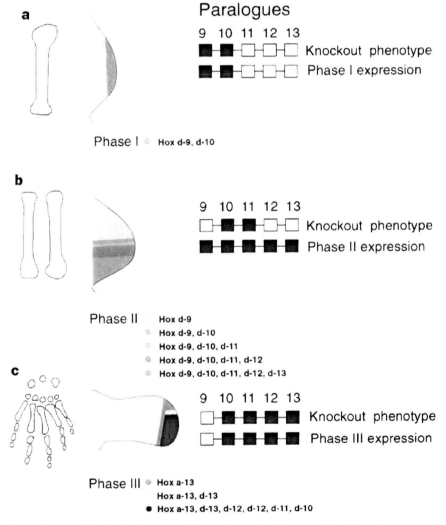

*Three phases of limb development. Pictured on the left are the **stylopod, zeugopod,** and **autopod.** Pictured in the center are the **limb buds,** and pictured on the right are the specific Hox genes activated for each region. Neil Shubin. Used with permission.*

According to Dr. Shubin, these sections evolved progressively over tens of millions of years, starting with the stylopod in the Silurian age, followed by the zeugopod and autopod in the Devonian.

In the womb, at about 28 days, bulges form in specific mesoderm regions called *limb fields*. Depending upon gene expression (signalling molecules), these will differentiate into bone, cartilage, circulatory system and connective tissues. *Retinoic acid* (a vitamin-A derivative) stimulates hox gene expression, guiding the growth and migration of these pluripotent cells.

Each developmental region involves progressively more hox genes, following the same pattern of progression which guides development of the animal's trunk. *T-box* transcription factors determine which limbs will develop: *Tbx4* genes produce hindlimbs, and *Tbx5* genes produce forelimbs (wings in the case of birds and bats).

Signalling molecules sculpt each limb in three dimensions: along the *proximo-distal axis* (the plane extending from the trunk of the body outward) by FGFs; along the *dorsoventral axis* (the line extending from spine to belly) by Wnts, and along the *anteroposterior axis* (the line extending from head to tail) by *Sonic hedgehog* (Shh).

In phase 1, the stylopod develops into a forelimb *humerus* or a hindlimb *femur*. Next, the zeugopod develops into the forelimb *radius* and *ulna,* or the hindlimb *tibia* and *fibula*. Finally, the most distal region, the autopod, emerges. This is where the most marked differences between species appear; among experimental animals, the mouse autopod is most like a human's.

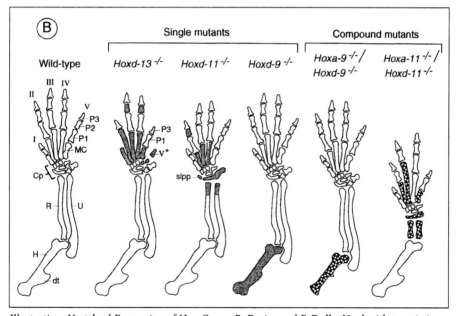

Illustration: Vertebral Expression of Hox Genes, B. Favier and P. Dolle. Used with permission.

Because of ethical considerations, researchers use chicks and mice to study the process. This allows easy modifications to limb development in vivo, to test which signalling molecules and genes affect the process.

In humans, the forelimb autopod will develop into the *carpal, metacarpal* and *phalange* hand regions, as cells proliferate and grow, differentiating according to their relative positions. The hindlimb autopod will differentiate into the *cuboid, navicular, cuneiform, metatarsal, talus, calcaneum* and *phalanges*.

Sonic hedgehog (Shh), determines the number and type of digits produced, and Hox genes d11 through 13 and a13 guide bone and joint formation, targeting transcription factors. Recent experiments indicate Hox genes carve out digits by activating *apoptosis* genes, triggering programmed cell death. BMP signalling triggers either differentiation into cartilage or cell death, sculpting out the joints and digits. Autopods initially form into flat, paddle-like webbed appendages, and apoptosis kills the cells that form webbing between the digits. Examples can be seen in the difference between chicken and duck feet – if cells between the digits are programmed to die, the webbing disappears; if not, the embryo will grow the webbed feet of a duck.

Limb evolution was a revolutionary adaptation, leading to the dominance of modern animals. Limbs grew in complexity from unjointed, sac-like appendages such as the caterpillar's *prolegs,* into the jointed limbs of arthropods and vertebrates. Such jointed limbs allow for extremely fast, precise movement, operating upon the same principles in both cases: muscles attached to either an endo- or exoskeleton contract, pulling upon the supportive skeleton.

Time

The Devonian came to a close about 360 million years ago in two waves of planetwide death. This was one of the five biggest extinction events in Earth history, wiping out about 20% of all animal families and 70-80% of all animal species, mainly among marine organisms. The acritarchs, trilobites, jawless fish, and armored placoderms died out, leaving land plants and freshwater species (including our tetrapod ancestors) relatively unaffected. The reasons are still shrouded in mystery, though major planetary cooling and glaciation may have played a significant factor.

The *Carboniferous (coal-bearing)* period arrived, and would last for about 60 million years, during which amphibians rose to the top of the food chain. The Carboniferous began relatively warm, allowing land-based animals to gain a firm footing, so to speak. Vast, lush forests flourished across the Pangaean supercontinent. Falling trees filled continent-wide swamps and bogs that would eventually form coal beds. The period eventually cooled toward its close, as glaciers once again grew.

Vertebrate fossils from the first 20 million years are scarce. Out of the few archaeologists have recovered, two in particular stand out: *Pederpes*, with a narrow skull and five-toed feet facing forward, features which would later appear in amphibians, reptiles and mammals; and *Whatcheeria*, which appears to have lived primarily in water.

After this brief period, however, a great variety of tetrapods appeared, somewhere around 340 million years ago.

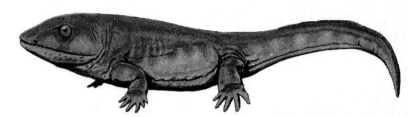

Pederpes lived ca. 350 million years ago, during Romer's gap. D. Bogdanov, used with permission.

As fishapods evolved into *amphibians* (Latin for *living on both sides*), they developed into primarily carnivorous species which fed on land, lay their eggs in water, and breathed through their moist, mucus-covered skin.

These were much closer to true amphibians – tiny *Casineria* with five toes, and *Eucritta melanolimnetes*, which was very like modern salamanders. One special group of amphibians – the *labyrinthodontia* (from the Greek for "maze-toothed") – would evolve into reptiles.

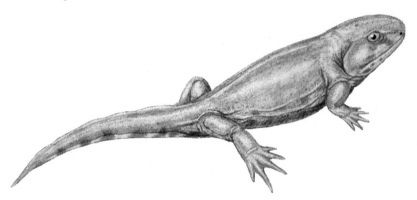

Eucritta, ca. 345 – 328 million years ago. D. Bogdanov, used with permission.

Rise of the Reptiles

During the Carboniferous, tetrapods split into amphibians and *amniotes* – the first reptiles. Amniotes are animals whose embryos grow in a membrane sac called an *amnios* ("bag of waters"). The amnios protects developing embryos from drying out, allowing egg-laying on land rather than in water, and without a larval stage.

Being able to lay eggs on dry land was a tremendous survival advantage, allowing populations to spread further inland. Because of this adaptation, amniotes could spread across the planet and became the dominant land vertebrates.

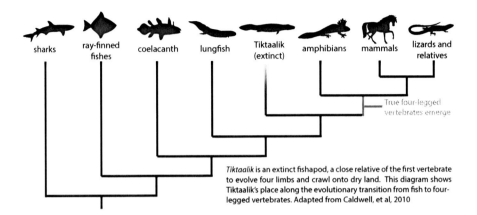

sharks   ray-finned   coelacanth   lungfish   Tiktaalik   amphibians   mammals   lizards and
         fishes   (extinct)   relatives

True four-legged
vertebrates emerge

Tiktaalik is an extinct fishapod, a close relative of the first vertebrate
to evolve four limbs and crawl onto dry land. This diagram shows
Tiktaalik's place along the evolutionary transition from fish to four-
legged vertebrates. Adapted from Caldwell, et al, 2010

Get it On

In a sense, all animals live to reproduce. An animal may be efficient at moving and eating, but if it doesn't reproduce, it will never pass that efficiency on to future generations. Natural selection is an incredibly slow process of trial and error, resulting from individuals with favorable traits reproducing, with more surviving offspring than their competitors with less favorable traits.

As with feeding and locomotion, varying strategies have evolved to allow creatures to reproduce. But whatever the means, there are essentially two paths: asexual or sexual. Asexual reproduction is the result of mitosis, simple cell division; and sexual reproduction is the result of meiosis – the fusing of haploid gametes.

Several species can engage in either form of reproduction, but in the case of sexual reproduction, fertilization will either be internal – with a male inserting a sperm-transferring organ into a female's body – or external – with females generally laying eggs in water, and males ejecting sperm onto them. (Some special cases exist, as with seahorses, where females insert eggs into the male's body for fertilization, and the pregnant male later gives birth.)

Hox genes also played a central evolutionary role in the development of these sexual reproductive strategies, with HoxA and HoxD genes 9 through 13 helping guide the development of both male and female genitalia and the uterus.

Eggs or embryos may be kept in the female's body as they mature, or eggs may be laid outside. Species which lay eggs are said to be *oviparous* (egg-bearing), while those that give birth to live offspring are called *viviparous* (live-bearing). The vast majority of animals are *oviparous* (egg layers), although humans, like nearly all other mammals, and a few fish, lizards and sea stars are viviparous, giving live birth.

Early tetrapod eggs had to be kept in water, or they would dehydrate. This limited the range of habitats the first tetrapods were able to exploit. In contrast, reptiles (including birds), and egg-laying mammals like the platypus produce amniotic eggs, in which the embryos are protected and nourished by a series of membranes, and can be either carried by a female, or laid as eggs.

These membranes include an amniotic sac surrounding the developing fetus. It's primarily these embryonic membranes and the lack of a larval stage which distinguish amniotes from tetrapod amphibians.

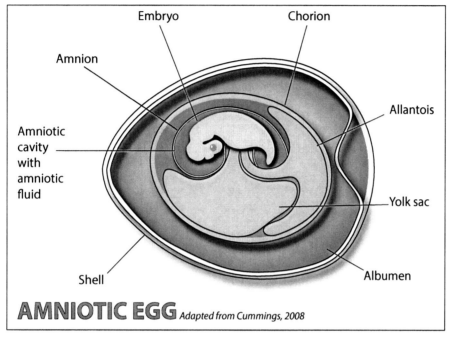

*Image: **Amniotic eggs** are protected against dehydration with shells or watertight membranes, and include a food supply and waste repository. In the egg's outer region, membrane-bound, protein-rich **albumen** supplies a growing embryo with water, while within, the embryo floats in a fluid-filled membrane sac called the amnion. Here, it feeds from the nutrient-dense **yolk sac**, and expels waste into the **allantois sac**. The egg-shell is semi-permeable, allowing gas exchange for breathing. Because their eggs could survive out of water, amniotes were able to branch out into non-aquatic environments.*

Self-sustaining eggs provided a major early survival advantage, allowing creatures to reproduce far from water, even in conditions as dry as deserts. From this point in evolutionary history, amniotes spread across the planet, eventually becoming the dominant land vertebrates.

All reptiles reproduce with amniotic-membrane eggs, including birds, which herpetologists categorize as *avian reptiles*. Some species lay their eggs and some carry them within their bodies until they hatch. Amniotic reproduction is also carried out by all mammals.

Tetrapods were able to breed on land successfully due to three advantages which gradually evolved: 1) the amniotic egg; 2) extended parental care and eventually 3) the *placenta*, among the mammals.

15-cm-long *Casineria* is one of, if not the first amniote, with both primitive amphibian and advanced reptilian features. It lived about 340 million years ago in what is now Scotland, in an era when the climate was warm, humid and highly oxygenated, and amphibians dominated.

Some 20 million years later, adaptations had led to true reptiles such as *Hylonomus lyelli*, a basal species discovered in present-day Nova Scotia, Canada.

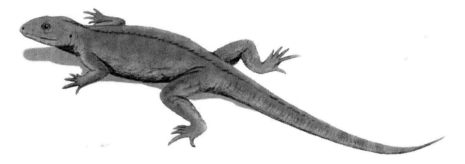

Hylonomus, a basal amniote from the Late Carboniferous, discovered in Nova Scotia, Canada. Pencil drawing, Nobu Tamura. Used with permission.

Have a Heart

For amniotes, the higher energy levels necessary for land-based locomotion created the need for improved oxygen intake. The evolutionary solution was a double-circulatory system, separating *pulmonary* and *systemic* blood flow: with four pumping chambers (two *atria* and two *ventricles*), oxygen-rich blood flowing to the cells of the body is separated from oxygen-depleted blood flowing back to the lungs, an efficient architecture critical for the evolution of warm-blooded animals.

Recent studies indicate the four-chambered heart is shaped by *Tbx5*, the same transcription factor specifying hindlimbs during embryogenesis. Amphibians only possess three-chambered hearts, which means amniotes evolved new regulatory elements that directed Tbx5 to build a tissue wall partitioning the ventricle into two chambers.

Fixing a Hole

Climatic pressures seem to have driven amniotes to diverge into three vertebrate lineages 320 to 315 million years ago. Each used different "approaches" to exploiting life on land. These were the *Anapsids*, *Sauropsids* and the *Synapsids*.

The most easily identifiable differences between the three amniote subgroups is in the *temporal fenestrae* (skull openings) on the sides of their skulls, and the bony arches crowning these openings. These have been used for over a century to classify amniote subgroups:

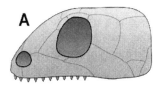 **A) Anapsids** *("no arches"), were a subgroup which, like the first amniotes, had no temporal fenestrae. This group includes modern turtles and their extinct relatives.*

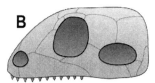 **B) Synapsids** *("fused arch") were a special lineage of* **mammal-like reptiles** *which emerged about 306 million years ago, during the Late Carboniferous.*

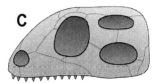 **C) Diapsids** *("two arches") evolved double skull holes/arches approximately 300 mya, and would become modern reptiles – crocodiles, lizards, snakes, tuataras, and birds. Double skull openings above and below each eye allowed for jaw muscles to open widely and provided a more powerful bite.*

Synapsids were among the first amniotes, appearing in the late Carboniferous, around 320 mya. The earliest were lizard-like *pelycosaurs* such as *Archaeothyris*, pictured below. These first fully terrestrial vertebrates would be extremely successful, and their many descendants would eventually include the mammals.

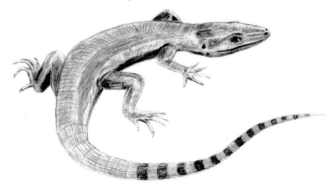

Archaeothyris, discovered in Nova Scotia in 1972, is the earliest undisputed synapsid. Image, Arthur Weasley, public domain.

Soon, however, supercontinent *Gondwana* moved south and glaciated, driving the Earth into a cooler and dryer state, culminating in the *Carboniferous Rainforest Collapse*, an abrupt and dramatic extinction event 305 million years ago.

The mass extinction of continent-wide forests carpeting *Euramerica* flooded the low-lying bogs, marshes, lakes and inland seas with a deluge of dead plant material, which decayed, heated under pressure, and compacted under ever-heavier layers, eventually forming combustible rock – the fossil fuel known as *coal*, humanity's primary energy resource (and the main source of carbon dioxide emissions driving modern global warming, according to the Union of Concerned Scientists).

As Earth's climate and atmosphere slowly restabilized after the rainforest collapse, the surviving pelycosaurs radiated into a number of species, ranging from tiny lizard-like carnivores to giant herbivores over 4 meters long, including the famous fin-backed *Dimetrodon* (*two groups of teeth*), which rose to become a Permian era apex predator.

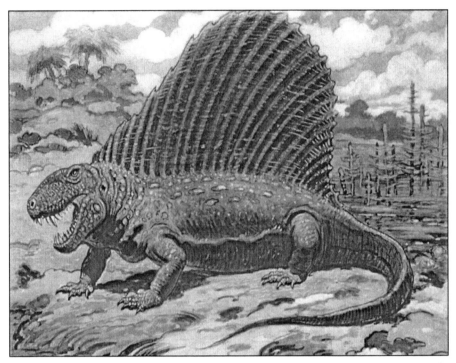

*Pelycosaurs like **Dimetrodon** dominated the early Permian, but declined with rising CO$_2$ levels, heat and aridity, eventually going extinct by the era's close. Dimetrodon's famous fin was a skin-covered, spiky projection of the spinal vertebrae, used for thermoregulation and possibly courting and defensive displays. Image: 1897, Charles R. Knight, public domain.*

These early species were *ectodermic* (cold-blooded), with habitats limited to a narrow range of supercontinent Pangaea's warm, wet equatorial ecosystems. Their back fins appear to have been used for thermoregulation, speeding up warming at dawn, and allowing heat dissipation when the sun was at its apex.

During the Permian, some pelycosaurs grew to be the Earth's first *megafauna*, animals weighing a metric ton or more, both the first *megacarnivores* and the first *megaherbivores*. As they continuing to diversify and grow ever more complex in response to the environment, one special group emerged – the *therapsids*.

Therapsids had developed gradual improvements in their ability to hunt, including three types of differentiated teeth: razor sharp frontal *incisors* for biting, secondary *canines* (fangs) for piercing and ripping away meat, and rear *molars* for grinding food, along with powerful jaw muscles.

Several mammalian traits emerged among the therapsids, such as an erect posture (as opposed to lizard-like crawling upon the belly) and *lactation* (milk production). In place of sprawling reptile legs with feet that splayed out sideways, therapsids developed legs vertically below their bodies, with feet parallel to the directions they faced.

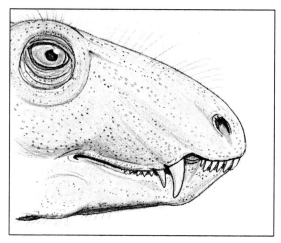

***Raranimus**, the earliest known therapsid. Therapsids first appeared about 270 mya and quickly spread. The earliest known member is Raranimus, an omnivore slightly larger than a house cat, with large, sharp, curved canines. Discovered in 1998 in the Qilian Mountains of Gansu, China, Raranimus fossils show the ancestors of mammals originated in Asia and radiated outward into what would become Africa. Dmitry Bogdanov, used with permission.*

Therapsids also developed more sophisticated joints to accommodate their erect posture, allowing much greater flexibility and a wider range of movement than that of the early synapsids and sauropsids. Together, these traits made therapsids the most successful of the pelycosaurs. They continued to evolve and spread across the supercontinent at the end of the Permian, while more poorly-adapted, non-therapsid pelycosaur competitors died out.

Complex blood chemistry regulation also evolved with the advanced *hypothalamus*, the brain region which reads blood chemistry and directs the *pituitary gland* to release regulatory hormone signalling molecules into the bloodstream. This allowed for better water regulation in dryer times and arid geographical regions – and would come to be at the core of the evolving animal brain's emotion-processing centers.

The more active and adaptable therapsids rose to prominence, better able to regulate their body temperatures and water content than their pelycosaur forebears. Outcompeted, the original pelycosaurs all died out by the end of the Permian, unable to adapt and spread beyond a western belt of *Laurasia*, the northern supercontinent of North America and Europe.

Meanwhile, among the therapsids, a subgroup called *theriodonts* (*beast teeth*) emerged about 265 million years ago in three groups, all thought to have been warm-blooded, among them the direct ancestors of mammals, the *cynodonts*. These reptilian-mammal hybrids would eventually spread worldwide.

The first of the cynodonts is thought to have been the tiny predator *Charassognathus* (*notched jaw*). A fossil of one specimen just under two feet long was excavated in 2007 near Fraserburg, South Africa.

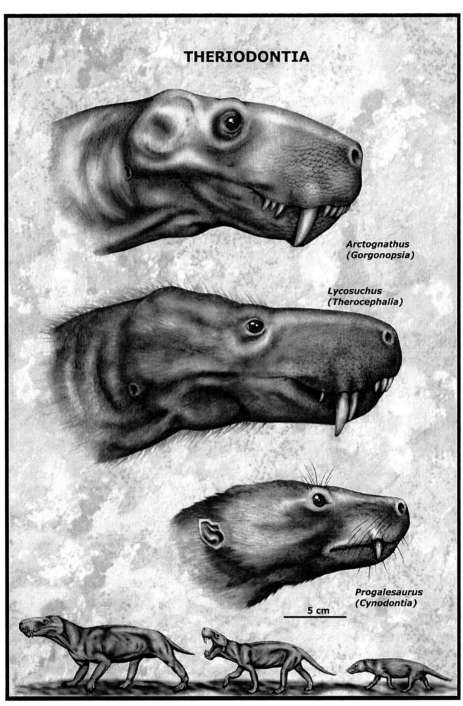

THERIODONTIA

Arctognathus
(Gorgonopsia)

Lycosuchus
(Therocephalia)

Progalesaurus
(Cynodontia)

5 cm

In theriodont fossils, no reptilian scales are evident, but small, regular pitting suggests the presence of whiskers and hair. Image: Mojcaj, Wikipedia. Used with permission.

214

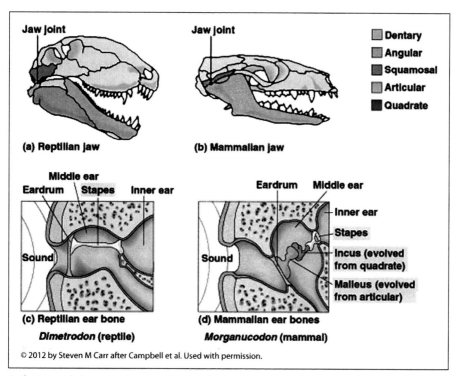

*Left: In amphibians and sauropsids (reptiles), the **hyomandibula** jaw bone slowly shrank to become the **stapes,** a single bony rod connecting the eardrum to the inner ear of modern amphibians, reptiles and birds. Sauropods and the earliest synapsids had 4-part **quadro-articular jaws**, named for the bones in the joint, a configuration still found in modern birds, crocodiles, turtles, snakes, lizards, amphibians, and most fish.*

*Among the synapsids, the quadrate and articular bones slowly shrank and migrated, resulting in the simplified two-part mammalian **dentary-squamosal jaw**. Meanwhile, the quadrate and articular bones came to be used as sound-amplifying bones in the mammalian middle ear – the **incus** and **malleus**, or hammer and anvil. This adaptation significantly improved hearing, and thus, both hunting and evasion.*

On the Hunt

Cynodonts were the transition between reptiles and mammals, with mammalian features like faster, coordinated movement, fur, and the sound-amplifying bones of the middle ear. The quadrate jaw bone shrank to accommodate stronger muscles for greater bite force, thereby allowing expansion of the skull's brain case.

Other adaptations followed over the course of 50 million years, including a *secondary palate*, separating the oral cavity from the nasal cavity, allowing simultaneous eating and breathing – something many modern animals can't accomplish, as their nasal and oral cavities aren't separate. This led to more efficient feeding, and faster food harvesting.

The enhanced ability to quickly harvest food necessitated a faster metabolism to process nutrients, including faster oxygen uptake. These increases in oxygen and food collection in turn provided greater energy for superior hunting skills, allowing sustained muscle activity and improved locomotion, which in turn led to even greater potential increases in food harvesting.

The progressive increase in energy production meant excess energy would be shed as body heat, the basis of *endothermy*. Rather than arising whole cloth however, this feature emerged from a combination of traits, including modern, diaphragm-driven lung breathing, allowing increased oxygen uptake and faster energy extraction.

Endothermic animals need more calories than ectothermic animals, necessitating a faster means of extracting energy. Specialized mammalian teeth evolved to grind food into a more quickly digestible form. Lower jaw bones migrated into the middle ear, providing superior hearing and allowing the creatures to open their mouths wider. Together, these adaptations made cynodonts the most successful synapsids.

Endothermy offered many other distinct advantages – the ability to spread into colder climes, to engage in longer sustained movement, to increase the speed at which offspring grew, boosting their probability of survival, and the ability to be active at night. Cynodonts were almost certainly nocturnal, thus requiring more sensitive hearing and olfaction, as indicated by major expansions in brain regions processing those senses. Nocturnal life also likely caused the evolution of fur, in the final transition from reptiles to mammals.

Apocalypse

A mysterious planetary catastrophe closed the curtain on the Permian 252 million years ago, in what is called *the Great Dying*, or the *Permian–Triassic mass extinction*. This was the worst disaster in history, killing 95% of all life on Earth. Above geographic layers thick with fossils, deep bands of Earth are completely empty of life.

A huge amount of biodiversity was lost, requiring an estimated 100,000 years to recover. The die-off seems to have arisen from a sequence of catastrophes, starting with a *flood basalt eruption* of the *Siberian Traps*. Here the Earth's crust split apart, releasing a continent-wide curtain of lava into the air. This caused a global heat wave, triggering a massive release of frozen methane from ice under the ocean floors, further heating the planet.

Life was nearly destroyed by the Permian-Triassic extinction, and the remaining groups were reduced to a handful of species. Therapsids had come to dominate on land, but the disaster nearly wiped them out, leaving only a line of herbivores and cynodonts to carry on. They inherited an empty world to exploit, and as a result, slowly recovered, eventually spreading across the *Triassic* landscape.

Meanwhile, the *diapsids*, which had also survived the planetary disaster, rose to dominance, with an air-sac respiratory system adapted to the extremely hot, dry and oxygen-poor world of the Triassic. These gigantic creatures would become the direct ancestors of modern crocodiles, lizards, snakes, and birds.

Reptiles are a diverse group of animals which includes turtles, lizards, snakes, crocodiles and alligators, birds, and extinct, air, land, and water-dwelling tetrapods such as the *dinosaurs*. They differ from most mammals in that they lay eggs, have watertight, scaly, keratin-protein skin, and, with the exception of birds, are ectothermic. To regulate their internal body temperature, they bask in sunlight or shelter in water and shade. Their skulls, particularly the jaws, also differ markedly from those of mammals.

Trampled Underfoot

Over the next 35 million years, cynodonts lived in the shadow of dinosaurs, and carnivores like *cynognathus* gradually shrank over the course of the Triassic. At the close of the era, the cynodonts included tiny, shrew-like *trithelodonts*, which eventually died out, but not before giving rise to Earth's first true mammals 225 million years ago, in the *Late Triassic period*.

The earliest of these mammals were small, nocturnal insectivores, eking out their existence by avoiding the great dinosaurs under cover of darkness. They appear to have been egg-layers until the evolution of the placenta 70 million years later.

Alongside the tiny early mammals loomed the stunningly massive *saurupods*, the largest creatures to have ever walked the Earth. These creatures shared the planet with the ancestors of modern birds, *theropods* like *Tyrannosaurus Rex*.

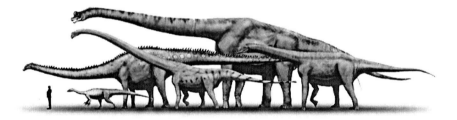

Image: Sauropods, Sergio Pérez, 2012. Used with permission.

The Oldest of the Titans

The evolution of vertebrates can be seen as a progression of steps which began about 540 million years ago: early vertebrates had notochords which developed into cartilaginous skeletons in fish like rays and sharks, then into a bony skeleton and skull with jaws in later fish. Eventually, fins evolved into limbs, and the first salamander-like amphibians began laying amniotic eggs on land.

Reptile evolution followed, and eventually, mammals. It was during the Triassic that many currently-living species first emerged, including turtles, frogs, lizards and mammals. The Triassic is also when dinosaurs first appeared, about 240 million years ago, with the arrival of *Nyasasaurus*. Dinosaurs would rule the planet for 175 million years, until being wiped out by a giant asteroid that smashed into the planet.

The oldest known dinosaur – *Nyasasaurus* – came to light when curators rediscovered an 80-year-old skeleton gathering dust in storage at London's Natural History museum. It turned out to be one of the biggest paleontological finds in history. The fossilized bones had first been unearthed in the 1930s by Cambridge paleontologist Francis Rex Parrington in Tanzania, once a southern region of the supercontinent Pangaea which included Africa, South America, Antarctica and Australia.

According to University of Washington biologist Dr. Sterling Nesbitt, Nyasasaurus is either the earliest dinosaur, or its closest known relative. It was an herbivorous, land-dwelling reptile, about 80 centimeters (three feet) tall and three meters (10 feet) long, with a tail of up to 1.5 meters (five feet), providing evidence that dinosaurs began as relatively small creatures before some species grew larger.

Interestingly, Nyasasaurus is closely related to birds, and shows that dinosaurs evolved at least 10 million years earlier than previously believed. This refutes claims of a puzzling explosion in dinosaur diversification during the Late Triassic, showing that dinosaurs comprised part of a slower, wider diversification of *archosaurs*, the dominant land animals of the Triassic 250 million to 200 million years ago.

Although the age of the dinosaurs ended some 65 million years ago, in a sense, we're still surrounded by them, in the form of modern birds, whose other closest living relatives are, surprisingly, alligators and crocodiles, fellow descendants of the archosaur subgroup.

Birds are direct descendants of small, carnivorous gliding dinosaurs, their feathers derived from the same *beta-keratins* used to form crocodilian scales. A 2006 study confirmed the genes for feather production also exist in American alligators, though these genes are suppressed during alligator embryogenesis, so only scales emerge.

According to a more recent study, birds – the most successful land vertebrates on Earth – emerged as the result of a remarkable adaptation: *progenesis*, a speeding up of sexual maturation. Instead of requiring years to reach sexual maturity like their dinosaur forebears, birds can mature in as little as 12 weeks, enabling them to retain the physical characteristics of juvenile dinosaurs into adulthood.

This, says Harvard's Dr. Arkhat Abzhanov, shows the diversity of evolutionary strategies adapted over millions of years:

> *That you can have such dramatic success simply by changing the relative timing of events in a creature's development is remarkable. We now understand the relationship between birds and dinosaurs that much better, and we can say that, when we look at birds, we are actually looking at juvenile dinosaurs.*

Winds of Change

Dinosaurs dominated the daylit hours of the Jurassic, while our mammalian ancestors scurried about under cover of darkness. However, it would only be a matter of time before fortunes radically changed.

The most significant environmental change in the wake of the Permian-Triassic extinction event was a decline in atmospheric oxygen from 30% down to 10%, conditions which appear to have lasted for at least 20 million years. The sudden drop in oxygen, says a Tokyo research team, awakened dormant genes in therapsids. In response to the emergency brought on by the extreme hypoxia, these genes were repurposed, triggering the beneficial mutations which resulted in mammals.

In addition to the human genome, those of many other chordates have been sequenced within the last decade, including chimpanzees, rats and mice, dogs, horses, chickens, opossums, pufferfish and the platypus. One intriguing finding is the high degree of genetic conservation among chordates; for example, the number of protein-encoding genes is highly consistent among vertebrates – 22,000 in both humans and puffer fish. In fact, astoundingly, this number shows almost no variation among species as diverse as the mustard plant *Arabidopsis thaliana*, the *nematode* (worm) *C. elegans*, and the fruit fly *Drosophila melanogaster*, even though their genomes vary as much as 20 fold in size.

A major source of their biodiversity lies in gene transpositions and whole genome duplications. Among the transpositions are *Conserved Non-coding Elements* (CNEs), which are passed down but lie dormant, until environmental pressures or other factors prompt them to be used for expressing new traits. CNEs comprise about 4% of the vertebrate genome, while the actual protein-encoding regions comprise only 2%.

In 2006, Dr. Hidenori Nishihara of the Tokyo Institute of Technology discovered special classes of CNEs in human DNA which, he says, switched function in synapsids 250 million years ago. This, he believes, gave rise to distinct mammalian traits, such as *auditory ossicles* (bones of the middle ear), a *placenta, diaphragm, mammaries*, and a *neocortex*. There are more than 100 clusters of these non-coding elements in all mammal DNA, suggesting a burst of exaptation occurred, possibly triggered by the Permian-Triassic mass extinction 250 million years ago.

Major changes resulted in a mammalian brain, with a much larger, multi-layered *neocortex* (Latin for *new rind*), a *hindbrain* equipped to process much more complex sensory data, and a sophisticated *cerebellum* to orchestrate coordinated body movement.

Genetic experiments on mice in 2008 show that Dr. Nishihara's CNEs enhance special mammalian signalling molecules – the *FGF8* microRNAs. These give rise to advanced embryonic brain development, upper layers of the mammalian neocortex and other regions of the brain primarily involved with processing sensory data.

These CNEs also influence *SATB2* and *Ctip2* transcription factors, helping direct neural differentiation in the neocortex, spine, and the *corpus callosum*, a sheet of neural tissue joining the brain's twin hemispheres.

The specific CNEs studied by Nishihara's team are of the *AmnSINE1* family, which existed within the genome of a common amniote ancestor over 300 million years ago during the Permian era. These genes remained dormant for tens of millions of years, then – probably triggered by environmental stressors – copied multiple times in great bursts of exaptation during the Permian-Triassic mass extinction 250 million years ago, when 95% of all species perished.

According to Dr. Nishihara, such CNEs are often a source of biodiversity, giving rise to new gene expression. A flurry of duplications of the CNEs in question, *AmnSINE1s,* occurred in the mammalian genome 250 million years ago, probably a response to hypoxia during the Permian-Triassic mass extinction. These duplications, researchers believe, allowed the evolution of mammalian-specific characteristics, including the development of novel brain structures.

Thrinaxodons, the final transition between the cynodonts and mammals, were housecat-sized, burrowing carnivores which managed to survive the Permian/Triassic extinction event. About two dozen adult and juvenile fossils have been discovered in burrows in both South Africa and Antarctica.

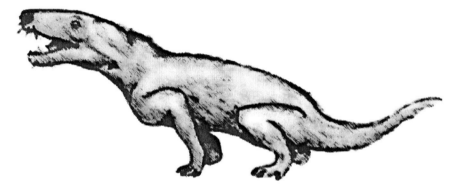

Thrinaxodon, adapted from Dr. Paul Olson, 2005

Thrinaxodon had evolved a diaphragm, significantly improving its oxygen intake, as well as a secondary palate, and small bones inside its nasal passage called *turbinals.* In desert-dwelling mammals like kangaroo rats and camels, turbinals help conserve water, and indicate endothermy in fossilized remains.

Thrinaxodon's snout is peppered with small *foramina* (holes), indicative of *vibrissae,* commonly known as whiskers. This means that thrinaxodon had evolved a *somatosensory* (body sensation) system centered around whiskers, hairs specialized for tactile sensation, which grow around the nostrils, above the lips, and other parts of the mammalian face.

The vibrissal somatosensory system enabled stealthy navigation, scavaging and foraging under the cover of darkness, when the use of other senses is limited.

Dr. Nishihara's CNEs are thought to been exapted to drive development of this sensory-processing system, allowing mammals to adapt to a nocturnal lifestyle after the P-Tr extinction event.

A DEUTEROSTOME PHYLOGENY

Ancestral relationships of the major deuterostome subgroups, showing the development of vertebrates, chordates, tetrapods, reptiles, amphibians, birds and mammals. Adapted from *Biological Science*, Scott Freeman, 2010.

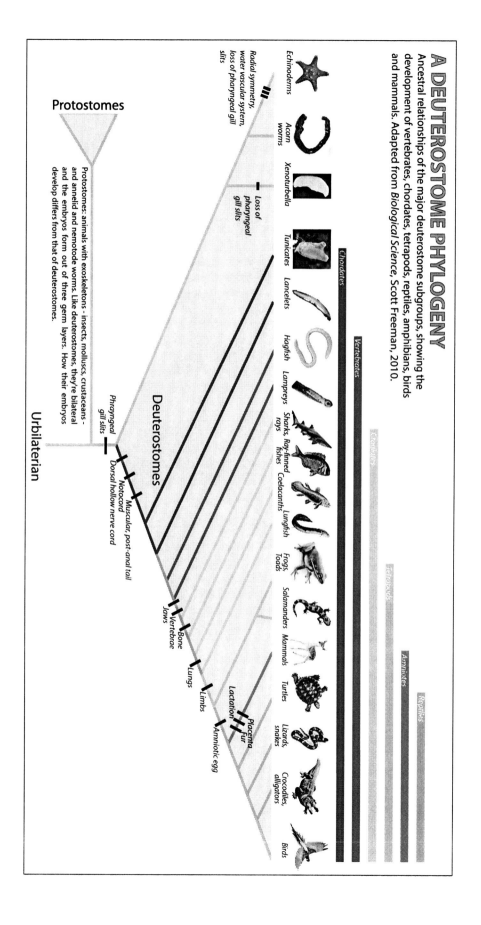

You've Got the Brawn; I've Got the Brain

Over half a billion years, the vertebrate brain has evolved to respond with ever greater sophistication to the environment. In primitive life forms, most or all brain tissue is centered around governing essential life functions or providing *instinctive behaviors*, automatic responses to environmental triggers that *ethologist* (animal behavior specialist) Konrad Lorenz called *Fixed Action Patterns*.

These fixed behavioral sequences are inborn, and appear to be related to anatomical characteristics specific to each species. They run a predictable course, and examples include methods of eating, escape from predators, and social and sexual interactions. Ethologists say these behavioral sequences are genetically programmed into animals at birth.

However, mammals, and particularly *primates* (monkeys, apes, tarsiers, lemurs, bush babies, lorises and humans), evolved a larger outer *cortex* which allows for *learning* to adapt to changes in the environment. Learned behavior involves actions which include *memories*, stored by the physical growth of neural connections in the brain called *synapses*.

Mammals, and humans in particular, have superior mental flexibility, and can predict outcomes based upon learning, and choose between alternatives. Additionally, ethologist Wolfgang Köhler's experiments show that primates have a special mental ability called *insight*, an inspirational ability to find novel solutions to problems.

The evolution of the mammalian brain was driven by the need for keener senses and enhanced alertness in the nocturnal existence of early mammals. But it's built upon a well-conserved foundation. All vertebrate brains are fundamentally *homologous* (anatomically correspondent), having evolved from a common ancestor.

The shared underlying foundation – a distinct set of neuron clusters with specialized functions – is found in lampreys, sharks, amphibians, bony fish, reptiles, birds and mammals. With the exception of hagfish and lampreys, which lack a cerebellum, these species all have brains with the same fundamental architecture.

The shared fundamental vertebrate brain includes major structural regions such as the *medulla oblongata*, which controls involuntary processes such as breathing, heartbeat and digestion; a *cerebellum* governing balance and coordinating multiple discrete muscle contractions into overall movement; a *cerebrum* for sensory integration and controlling voluntary actions; an *optic tectum* for visual processing; and an *olfactory bulb* for processing scent.

Since the Devonian, brain sizes grew in proportion with body weight among fish, amphibians and reptiles, but in mammals and birds, brains began to grow beyond these constraints.

As the vertebrate brain increased in complexity, it allowed for ever more subtle responses to the environment – complex behaviors. Such complex behaviors were made possible by increases in the size and complexity of the *forebrain*, particularly the *neocortex* (Latin for *new rind*), the emotion-generating *limbic system* (Latin for *edge*) and the advanced *cerebellum* (Latin for *tiny brain*), important for orchestrating ever-more complex movements.

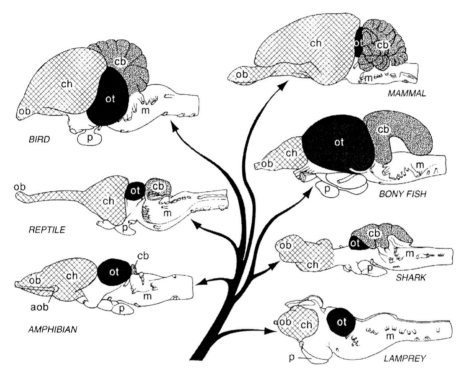

*Brains from several modern vertebrate species (not to same scale). Though there is significant variation in the size of the brain subdivisions and the brains themselves, most vertebrates have brains which can be divided into the same fundamental substructures. Abbreviations: **aob, accessory olfactory bulb** (cross-hatched); **cb, cerebellum** (stippled); **ch, cerebral hemispheres** (cross-hatched); **m, medulla oblongata; ob, olfactory bulb** (cross-hatched); **ot, optic tectum** (black); and **p, pituitary gland**. Image: R. Glenn Northcutt, 2002. Used with permission.*

The cerebellum seems to have evolved with the placoderms, and gradually increased in size among all but the reptiles, though its modern twin-lobed, convoluted form first appeared in birds and mammals. The medulla has changed very little over time; the optic tectum changed to a greater degree, growing in complexity and size, gradually increasing functional layers as vision and complex visual processing evolved.

The cerebrum in particular grew with the transition to land, and in humans, its outermost layer, the *cerebral cortex* (*head's rind*) is the largest region, now constituting

90% of the brain's mass. This region is used for the highest-level mental functions – comparisons, evaluations, predictions, language use, mathematical calculations, and recalling and manipulating memories. It's believed that growth of the cerebrum was spurred by the needs for complex sensory analysis and for social interactions, eventually leading to the use of language.

Just as vertebrates all share homologous brain structures, they also share a dual-network nervous system, the brain and spinal cord comprising a *Central Nervous System* (CNS), and the nerves of the body and its organs comprising a *Peripheral Nervous System* (PNS), which relays information to and from the brain, sensory organs and body. Animal survival depends upon this dual nervous system to continuously monitor and respond to the environment.

Animals, including their brains, adapt to the ecological niches in which they live. For example, the star-nosed mole has little need for eyesight, and so has comparatively little cortical tissue devoted to processing sight. However, a huge amount of its *sensorimotor cortex* is dedicated to processing sensations from the tentacle-like extensions around its mouth. In humans, language use has led to extraordinary tongue and lip sensitivity, and tool use to hand sensitivity –a greater proportion of cortical "real estate" has become devoted to processing signals from these specific regions of the human body.

The late Yale neuroscientist Paul D. MacLean taught that mammalian brains also have a *tripartite* or *triune* brain structure which parallels evolutionary development, and each of the three subsystems plays a part in governing behavior:

1. **The primitive r-complex** or **reptilian brain** contains the oldest structures, which control fundamental functions like muscle contraction, heart rate, breathing, feeding and gag reflexes, body temperature and balance. It includes the same primary structures found in reptilian brains – the brainstem and cerebellum. It also, according to MacLean, incorporates motor control systems called the *basal ganglia*, and governs instinctual behaviors related to aggression, courtship, dominance and territoriality. While reliable, the reptilian brain can be rigid and compulsive. Recent studies show these regions actually evolved much earlier than the first reptiles, having arisen instead in the earliest vertebrates.

2. **The paleomammalian complex** (*old mammal complex*) contains what MacLean called the *limbic system*, the brain's emotional and motivational system, governing feelings and behaviors related to sexual arousal, bonding, nurturing, anger and fear. It includes pleasure-inducing, memory-encoding and alarm structures (the *septum, hippocampus* and *amygdala*), as well as a nervous-system and body chemistry regulator (the *hypothalamus*), and evolved in the first mammals to generate fight-or-flight responses and react to (and learn from) emotion-

ally pleasurable or unpleasant experiences. This system emerged with the earliest mammals, and functions as an instantaneous evaluator, usually unconsciously, exerting a powerful influence upon behavior.

In addition to physical structures, we share core emotions with other mammals: the limbic system's danger-sensing "sentry", the *amygdala*, generates fear responses in all mammals, circuits using the neurotransmitter dopamine generate the anticipatory excitement underlying motivation and addiction; and circuits using the neurotransmitter oxytocin generate feelings of bonding, trust and security, while dampening the fear-inducing effects of the amygdala.

3. ***The neomammalian complex*** (*new mammal complex*) contains the *neocortex*, a structure found only in the brains of mammals. Although we now know that other Great Apes and African Parrots also have both self-awareness and a sense of continuity in experience, the human neocortex gives our species a uniquely powerful flexibility when responding to the environment, and has allowed human culture and technology to develop. It allows for higher-order thinking, and became particularly specialized in primates, culminating in the twin-hemisphered human brain. The neomammalian complex allows abstract thought, reasoning, calculations, language, planning, reflection and consciousness – awareness. The neocortex has a truly staggering capacity. In book two, you will learn how to tap into and use that mind-bendingly vast capacity.

In 2003, Swiss Institute of Biology researchers announced Homeobox genes create this tripartite structure. According to the team, *Otx*, Hox and *Pax2/5/8* genes organize the forebrain, midbrain and hindbrain, respectively. Three homologous gene sets also build a tripartite brain in the fruitfly *Drosophila melanogaster*. This shows, says the team, the genes for tripartite brains evolved even before the urbilaterian ancestor of both protostomes and deuterostomes.

The Genetic Roots of Intelligence

University of Edinburgh researchers spent three years in an historical effort to pin down the physical basis of intelligence, using mice, mutants and schizophrenics as their subjects. Genes to Cognition Director Dr. Seth Grant was conducting a series of experiments that involved knocking out specific genes shared by mice and humans, genes which control synapse formation and signalling.

His team switched off those genes in mice, which were then exposed to seven learning tasks. Their performance was compared with that of human volunteers sharing the same genetic defect, and their genomes compared with those of other species, to determine when genes theoretically empowering those mental abilities first emerged.

According to Dr. Grant, the experiments "unambiguously" point to specific genes which duplicated and mutated to allow complex vertebrate behavior. These genetic changes, he says, "produced a molecular toolbox, which in the case of the brain, produced many, many more proteins that you find in the synapses, the junctions between nerve cells."

Among these genes, he says, the *DLG* (*Discs Large homolog*) genes in particular gave rise to our abilities to analyze, learn and respond flexibly to the environment. DLG genes encode proteins for tuning and balancing chemical signalling in the synapses, the point where two neurons meet and communicate, producing *scaffold proteins* which bind neurotransmitter receptors and enzymes into signalling complexes in *postsynaptic* (signal-receiving) neurons.

Invertebrates such as sea slugs, worms and jellyfish have only one DLG gene, but 550 million years ago, the DNA of a common ancestor of the chordates underwent two rounds of whole genome duplication. In the process, the DLG group duplicated and modified over time, helping confer upon mammals the survival advantage of advanced learning.

Neither intelligence nor any of the specific abilities tested in Dr. Grant's experiments depend solely upon any one protein or gene, but they unquestionably would not be possible without this group of genes. Dr. Grant's experiments demonstrate that DLG proteins directly enhance seven out of 12 measurable mental processes underlying memory, learning, reasoning, problem-solving, language use, focused attention, and decision-making.

Behavioral tests on mice bred with or without each of their natural DLG variations showed the gene family's central role in each of these seven aspects of advanced learning. The case seems airtight: switch on the gene, and an animal can perform specific mental tasks; switch that gene off, and it can't.

All vertebrates, including fish, are capable of selective attention and *association-based learning* – mentally linking a cause with an effect, or an action with a reward or punishment. Memories of these associations then instinctually guide them in modifying their behavior. However, mammals can engage in more complex learning and analysis, including flexible problem-solving, advanced visual recognition and analysis, rapid attention-switching and the ability to inhibit their natural responses deliberately.

These higher-order processes are impaired in sufferers of neurological and psychiatric illnesses like schizophrenia, autism, attention deficit hyperactivity disorder and Alzheimer's disease, all of which are linked to a common mutation in two DLG variants.

When human test subjects with schizophrenia – associated with the DLG mutations – were given the same tests as Dr. Grant's mice, they showed the same learning disabilities as knockout mice bred without the beneficial versions of the genes.

To Dr. Grant, this means "...the very same genes that made us more intelligent and sophisticated are the genes that are damaged in people with learning disabilities, schizophrenia, autism and other brain diseases. If those genes aren't working, then that's when that individual will suffer from some brain disease. That's the price. That's the risk."

This means the evolutionary leap forward in intelligence from these genes came at the price of a greater susceptibility to mental disorders; adding multiple DLG variants to the genome comes with the unfortunate side effect of greater opportunities for harmful mutations to arise.

Humans have four DLG variants. *DLG4* is essential for simple forms of associative learning; *DLG2* and *DLG3* are needed for complex visual discrimination and adaptability to new situations – like learning something in the environment behaves the opposite of how it did previously. DLG2 is critical for processing spatial information such as object locations, and DLG3 for visual discrimination, including the ability to rapidly select the best choice among several alternatives.

Furry, Whiskered Beasts

By comparing *murines* – mice and rats – with their distance marsupial cousins – kangaroos, koalas, possums and the like – University of Sheffield researchers found indications that whiskers played a vital role in the evolution of mammals from reptiles.

Professor Tony Prescott's team analyzed high-speed video recordings of mice and rats moving their whiskers back-and-forth – a means of actively sensing the surrounding environment called *whisking*. Whisking lets murines accurately analyze the shape, texture and position of objects, make rapid and accurate decisions about them, and integrate that information into mental maps of the environment.

If they're running in straight lines, rats and mice wiggle their whiskers back-and-forth equally on both sides, but when they turn, their whisker movements are biased in the direction they're turning. When one side of the head's whiskers encounters an object, whiskers on the opposite side sweep around, gathering additional information. Such tactile sensing strategies greatly assist these creatures in understanding their environments.

Whisking is also found in grey short-tailed opossums, tiny South American marsupials. Opossums are very similar to their 125-million-year-old mammalian ancestors, at the very base of the lineage which would diverge into modern rodents and marsupials. The fact that such evolutionarily ancient mammals whisk like modern mice and rats indicates that moveable whiskers emerged with the first mammals who diverged from reptiles, and their conservation across mammal species shows how important they were to survival.

The first mammals were nocturnal tree dwellers who integrated sight, sound, smell, and touch to successfully hunt and avoid predators in the dark. Facial whiskers were new tactile organs which provided a survival advantage unavailable to reptiles.

According to Dr. Prescott, "This latest research suggests that alongside becoming warm-blooded, giving birth to live young, and having an enlarged brain, the emergence of a new tactile sense based on moveable facial whiskers was an important step along the evolutionary path to modern mammals. Although humans no longer have moveable whiskers, they were a critical feature of our early mammalian ancestors."

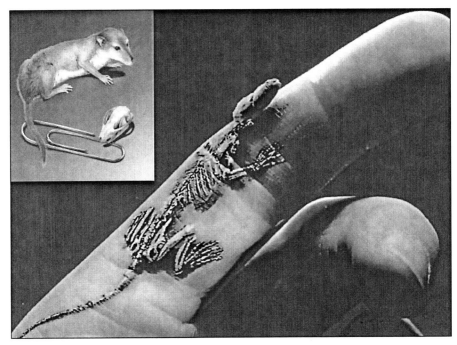

Hadrocodium, Zhe-Xi Luo, PhD, University of Chicago 2011. Used with permission.

Our Tiny Ancestors

In 2001, scientists unveiled the 195-million-year-old remains of a tiny creature from Early Jurassic China. *Hadrocodium wui*, as it was dubbed, was 40 million years older than any mammal previously discovered. It was an insect-eating, nocturnal tree dweller, the size of a bumblebee, which led a life of hiding from the era's massive predatory dinosaurs.

Hadrocodium was one of the first animals to evolve the mandible, middle-ear ossicles and large brain of a mammal. Its discovery pushed back the evolution of these features by some 45 million years earlier.

The usefulness of a heightened sense of smell really kicked mammalian brain development into high gear. University of Texas paleontologist Tim Rowe used X-ray computed tomography on fossilized molds of Hadrocodium skulls in 1985 to show how the early mammalian brain developed in three major phases: improvement of the olfactory sense, followed by refinements of tactile sense through body hair and advanced neuromuscular coordination to take advantage of advanced senses.

Dr. Rowe's 3D images gave a detailed inside view of the brain and nasal cavities, showing how olfactory organs evolved in pre-mammals, alongside special brain regions to process the olfactory information. Distinguishing and analyzing odors to a fine degree gave mammals a distinct survival advantage over other creatures of the era.

The development of body hair also influenced brain size: fur first evolved not for warmth, but to enhance tactile sensitivity and motor coordination. The first body hairs are thought to have served as whisker-like sensors, functioning as *vibrissae* (whiskers which generate tactile information in mammals like cats), allowing Hadrocodium to navigate within small spaces and avoid harm. This heightened tactile sensitivity, in turn, drove formation of the mammalian neocortex, granting complex sensory analysis.

Meanwhile, the cerebellum at the base of the brain, which uses sensory feedback to fine-tune movement, grew so large its surface began to fold into ripples, proving early mammals had begun to evolve superior neuromuscular coordination.

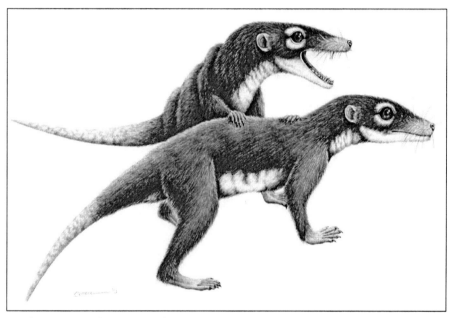

*5-inch **Morganucodon**, named after the region of Wales in which it was first found, predated Hadrocodium by as much as 10 million years, but as it hadn't yet developed the fully-articulated lower jaw of a true mammal, it's instead classified as a mammaliaform. For all its reclusiveness, numerous fossils of Morganucodon have been found throughout Europe, North America and Asia. Image: Cristóbal Aparicio Barragán, used with permission.*

That Smell

Chemosensory receptors are essential for the survival of organisms ranging from bacteria to mammals, but the number of chemosensory receptor genes varies enormously between species, due to adaptation to different environments.

The senses of smell and taste rely upon *odorants* – tiny amounts of *aroma compounds* inhaled through the nose onto the *epithelium* (a 3 cm-square region of specialized tissue inside the nasal cavity) or landing upon the tongue. Odorants act as *ligands* – chemicals which bind to receptors and activate them – in this case, olfactory receptors.

229

Surprisingly, both taste and smell evolved from the most primitive of single-celled bacteria. Since the entire genome of the bacterium E. coli (Escherichia coli) has been sequenced, recent experiments have shed light upon how these senses first emerged.

E. coli is a rod-shaped bacterium found in the digestive tracts of endothermic animals. There, it functions as a symbiont, helping break down nutrients in the large intestine, producing K- and B-complex vitamins and combating harmful *pathogens* – invading disease-causing organisms such as viruses, bacteria, prions or fungi – in return for nutrients such as glucose or amino acids absorbed from the host. Harmful strains of e. coli also exist, which can cause a number of illnesses, including food poisoning, diarrhea and respiratory diseases.

These E. coli strains produce *Shiga toxins*, which disrupt protein synthesis, and can damage blood vessels in the kidney and heart. Since shiga toxins can only attach to and enter cells with specific membrane receptors, species like cattle, pigs, and deer which lack these receptors can carry harmful strains without experiencing any damaging effects. The bacteria is shed in their feces, where it can spread among humans, contaminating food or water, or being transmitted by physical contact.

After E. coli and its nearest bacterial relative *Salmonella* diverged from a common ancestor 100 million years ago, E. coli would become a symbiont hosted in the large intestines of mammals, while salmonella would take up residence in the digestive tracts of birds and reptiles.

E coli survives by moving about in search of nutrients, attracted to areas of high glucose or amino acid concentration. To do this, it uses five different chemosensitive protein receptors (*Trg, Tar, Tsr, Tap,* and *Aer*) to locate nutrients like glucose, and to avoid toxins like chlorine, iodine, alkalis and concentrated alcohols.

On the outer surface of its body, E. coli has up to six randomly-distributed whip-like flagella, used for locomotion. The flagella normally spin counterclockwise in a cooperative bundle, propelling E. coli forward through liquid.

About once per second, a *che-family protein* in the cell binds to the base of a flagellum, switching its rotation to the reverse, clockwise direction. This disrupts the cooperative spinning of the members in the flagellar bundle, and the flagella spread apart. When the flagella bundle spreads, the cell randomly spins in place, pointing in a new direction, a sequence called *tumbling*.

The combination of forward motion and tumbling is the default, random exploratory movement of a bacterium, called a *random walk*, a pattern of movement which changes in response to the concentration of chemicals in the environment.

When a nutrient (or toxin) binds to a receptor, it triggers the suppression of the tumbling sequence, resulting in a straighter swim pattern toward the nutrient (or away from a toxin).

Receptor proteins in the anterior of the bacterial cell – opposite the flagellar bundle – sense chemical concentrations in the environment. When an attractant like glucose binds to these receptors, it inhibits the tumble signal sent to the flagella, so the bacterium tumbles less often as attractant concentration increases. This results in swimming in an increasingly straight trajectory toward an attractant – a *biased random walk*.

When attractants bind to bacterial chemoreceptors, motor proteins propel the organism toward nutrients it will ingest; when repellents bind to these chemoreceptors, it swims away from toxins. This reaction is called *chemotaxis*, movement of an organism either toward or away from a chemical stimulus guided by *chemical gradients* – the concentration of solutes in a solution.

Use the Force – *Living organisms use two fundamental properties to drive vital biological processes:*

Chemical Gradient – *Because of the energy contained within them, atoms and molecules are in constant random motion. As they move about, they collide with one another, causing them to disperse from areas of high concentration to areas of low concentration until a balance has been reached, a state of equilibrium where concentration is equal throughout an area.*

*This is the process called **diffusion**. A chemical gradient, like the gradient of a hill, is a state of imbalance – an area of high concentration separated from an area of low concentration. Like a hill down which objects can roll, a chemical gradient contains potential energy to drive biological processes.*

Electrical Gradient – *When two particles of opposite charge are separated, there is a tension between them; they "want" to come together or move apart due to their charges. Ions – molecules which carry a repellent or attractant electrical charge - are subject to the distributive force called the electrical gradient.*

Protons carry the same positive charge, so when they are close to one another, they exchange bosons, which act like packets of energy pushing them apart. When protons encounter electrons, the boson exchange is an attractive force. Because of this, protons move from positively-charged areas toward negatively-charged areas.

*Since hydrogen atoms seldom contain neutrons, when the single electron leaves the atom, all that's left is a proton. Thus, hydrogen ions (H+ – the source of **acidity**) are usually just called protons.*

Cells can store charged particles such as protons (H+ ions) on one side of a membrane, to build up a strong difference in electrical charges between the inside and outside of that membrane. Releasing these ions carries a force that can be used to drive many biological processes. The "tension" from the differences in charges can also be used to maintain biologically useful states.

231

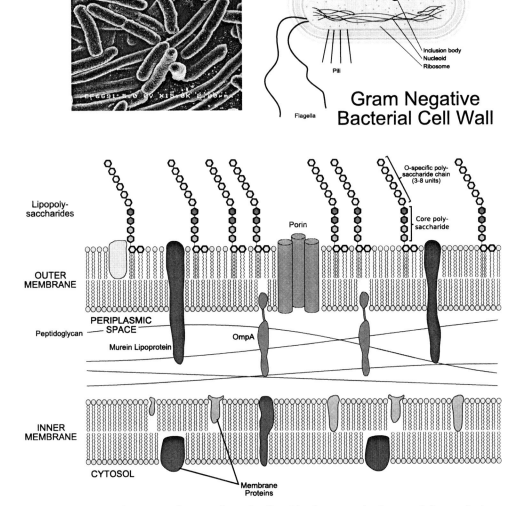

Gram Negative Bacterial Cell Wall

Capsule

Enlarged section

Inclusion body
Nucleoid
Ribosome

Pili

Flagella

Lipopoly-saccharides

O-specific poly-saccharide chain (3-8 units)

Porin

Core poly-saccharide

OUTER MEMBRANE

PERIPLASMIC SPACE

Peptidoglycan

Murein Lipoprotein

OmpA

INNER MEMBRANE

CYTOSOL

Membrane Proteins

*Gram-negative bacteria such as E. coli aren't affected by dyes using the Gram staining method, because they have an outer membrane preventing penetration of the dye. This tough protective surface is like a stiff canvas sack surrounding bacteria, making them resistant to immune-system antibodies and to antibiotics. It forms a barrier to large molecules and provides protection from adverse environmental conditions such as acids in the digestive system of a host. The outer surface is composed mainly of lipopolysaccharides (LPS). These are **endotoxins,** which trigger extreme immune system responses in animals, including fever and shock. Photo: E. coli, US Department of Agriculture, public domain. Illustration: Jeff Dahl, Wikipedia, Creative Commons Attribution-Share Alike 3.0 License, 2013*

Bacterial chemoreceptors would evolve over hundreds of millions of years into much more specialized olfactory receptors (ORs). OR genes seem to have evolved through gene duplication, emerging among the first chordates – these genes are found in the headless amphioxus, the lamprey, and other basal chordates (which lack any olfactory organs), but they are not found in any animals "prior to" the chordates.

See illustration, following page. Flagella are composed of thousands of repeating copies of a protein called ***flagellin***, arranged like a string of pearls spiralling tightly upward into a long helical tube called a filament. At the base of each flagellar filament is a ***reversible rotary motor assembly***, which drives rotation of the flagellum at about 100 Hz (cycles per second). The following is rather complex and completely optional information about the deatils of the process:

Each flagellum has its own reversible motor assembly, a collar of proteins surrounding the base of the rod-shaped filament. The motor has a nonrotating part called the ***stator***, and a rotating part called the ***rotor***. The stator is made up of two proteins, MotA and MotB. These two proteins combine to form an ion channel through the bacterial cell membrane. The rotor is made up of three ringed layers of protein complexes, made of the rotor proteins FliF, FliG, FliM and FliN. Energy driving the flagellum's rotation is supplied by a hydrogen ion flow through this ion channel into the cell, caused by a ***concentration gradient*** - a difference in charges between the inner cell and its ***periplasm*** – a thin layer in the cell where protons can be stored for an energy buildup.

A steady flow of hydrogen ions shifts the molecular shape of **MotA** proteins at the filament's base, and this **conformational change** creates a **power stroke**, spinning the rotor. In E. coli, the flow of protons from the high concentration in the periplasm toward the low concentration within the cytoplasm provides the driving force for the motor. This proton flow causes changes to the molecular shape of MotA proteins encircling the rod. When these proteins change shape, they sweep across the FliG proteins of the rotor collar, generating **torque** – the force driving the rotation of the rod (the flagellar filament). When the energy-supplying proton has been shed, the protein returns to its original shape, resulting in a second power stroke. A sequence of these power strokes rotates the flagellum at high speed. To stop the spinning, a protein block is inserted between the ion power source and the rotor protein which spins the flagellum.

Three proteins (FliG, FliM, and FliN) in the rotor form a controlling "switch complex", used as forward and reverse gears to change the motor's direction. As long as the chemosensing receptors are empty, flagellar rotation will switch about once a second from counter-clockwise to clockwise rotation as directed by the normal, steady flow of the signalling protein CheY. CheY is regularly charged by an ATP phosphoryl group. It then migrates to the flagellum's base, where it binds to the protein assembly switch and changes the direction of the flagellum's rotation. After about a tenth of a second, a ChemZ protein removes the phosphoryl molecule for recycling, causing the CheY protein to detach from the flagellar motor assembly, and this assembly then returns to rotating in a counterclockwise direction.

When a ligand called an ***effector*** (an attractant nutrient or repellant toxin) is encountered, a molecule of that effector binds to the appropriate receptor embedded in the E. coli membrane. This binding alters the receptor's molecule, activating signalling proteins within the cell's cytoplasm.

CheA Protein acts as a master steering mechanism, using phosphoryl groups from the energy molecule ATP. Adding a phosphoryl group to the **CheY** protein triggers a change in flagellar rotation, while phosphorylating the **CheB** protein triggers a return to full sensitivity of a receptor. When a receptor is bound to a repellant **or** an attractant receptor is empty, phosphorylation normally occurs: CheA autophosphorylates, then transfers its phosphoryl group to CheY, which migrates to the base of the flagellar motor to switch rotational direction. CheA's autophosphorylation is **suppressed** when attractant receptors are occupied, thus suppressing the switching sequence, and the tumbling it causes.

The CheY binding sequence which switches flagellar rotation is suppressed by attractant-bound receptors, so the flagellar motor undergoes fewer rotation reversals, and the bacterium tumbles less frequently, spending more time in a **run** (forward motion) toward a favorable direction. In this way, bacteria make a progressively straighter overall movement toward attractants like amino acids and sugars, and away from repellents such as Nickel ions.

Bacterial chemoreceptors are members of a class of transmembrane **methyl-accepting chemotaxis** (MCP) proteins. This means they are embedded in proteins (transmembrane), accept methyl groups which change their molecular shape, and these changes in shape affect the movement (taxis) in response to chemicals (chemo). From within the cell, CheR protein can **methylate** a receptor, **decreasing its sensitivity** to an effector, while CheB can **demethylate** a receptor, **increasing its sensitivity**. When CheA phosphorylates CheB, it increases CheB demethylation activity 15-fold, very strongly heightening the receptor's sensitivity.

Illustration, next page: Tar is the E.coli receptor to which the attractant aspartate binds. The extracellular portion of its protein molecule is called the **periplasmic binding domain**, and the intracellular portion is the **cytoplasmic signalling domain**. The signalling domain communicates with e. coli's flagellar motors using a **phosphorelay sequence** that involves the CheA, CheY, and CheZ proteins. CheA autophosphorylates, then transfers its phosphoryl group to CheY. Phosphorylated CheY binds to the switch proteins of the flagellar motors, augmenting clockwise rotation. Counterclockwise rotation is the default state in the absence of phosphorylated CheY. CheZ helps stop rotor switching by dephosphorylating CheY.

Tar controls phosphate circulation through this circuit by forming a stable chemical complex that binds up phosphoryl molecules, preventing their use by CheA when an attractant has bound to its receptor. This slows the phosphorylation of CheA. The less CheY-P that is made, the less it binds with FliM and FliN, and the motor spends a greater amount of time spinning CCW - the direction that promotes smooth swimming. This propels the cell in a favorable direction.

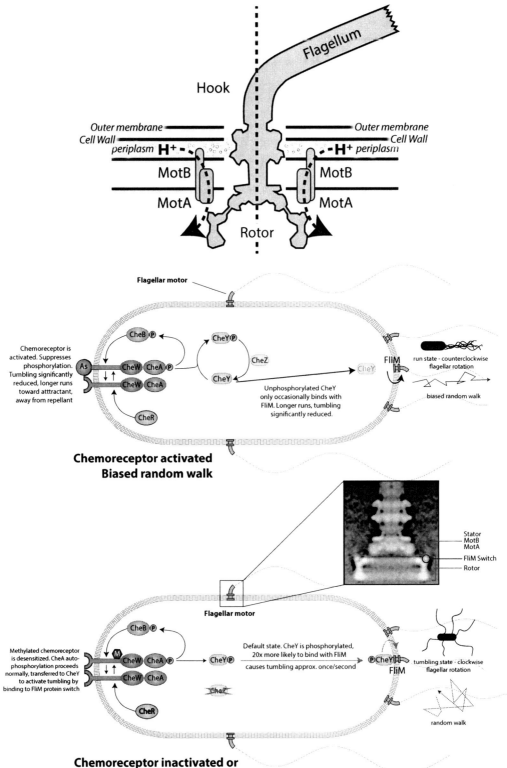

**Chemoreceptor activated
Biased random walk**

**Chemoreceptor inactivated or
desensitized. Normal Random walk**

Studying odorant receptors of humans, mice, catfish, dogs, salamanders and even insects shows how a huge variety of olfactory receptors eventually evolved. Odorant receptor (OR) gene expression changes dynamically depending on each species' living environment; for example, two OR gene groups which detect airborne odorants greatly expanded after tetrapods adapted to land life, while fish retained the same OR genes present in ancestral aquatic species. All vertebrates possess functional OR genes, and they form one of the largest vertebrate gene families. Fish have an average of about 100 OR genes, significantly fewer than mammals, but the number of functional OR genes varies considerably by species, ranging from 1,200 in rats and 388 in humans to 150 in zebrafish and only 15 in pufferfish. The number is generally much smaller in insects – the fruit fly *drosophila melanogaster* has only 62 olfactory receptors, encoded by 60 genes. In every species, however, a significant percentage of these are apparently nonfunctional *pseudogenes*, anywhere from 20 to 50% of the total, having gone dormant over the course of evolution.

Fish can distinguish water-soluble biomolecules such as amino acids and sex steroids, but mammals detect significantly more types of airborne and (some waterborne) odorants. In fact, mammals have approximately 1,000 olfactory genes, comprising the largest known gene family. This huge amount of DNA dedicated to the sense of smell is testament to its importance in animal survival.

Olfaction is particularly vital for mammals, in finding food, mates and offspring, in recognizing territories and avoiding danger, in evaluating the environment, and even in social behavior, although mammals differ in their reliance upon smell, and in their olfactory sensitivity and discrimination. Most mammals possess a special olfactory *vomeronasal organ* (VNO) with special *vomeronasal receptor* (VR) neurons and chemosensory receptors, used to detect *pheromones* – airborne chemical signals which impact the behavior of members of the same species, generally by triggering responses in the hypothalamus.

Run Away! Run Away! Pheromones communicate diverse signals such as alarms, food trails, sexual status and territorial marking. Even plants have been found to use a class of pheromones called **semiochemicals**, used to perfume the air with a variety of volatile compounds for reproduction, defense and internal signalling. These substances have long been used for perfumes, flavoring, pharmaceuticals, and pest protection.

These "plant pheromones" communicate to neighboring organisms warnings about pests. 1983 experiments by Drs. David Rhoades and Gordon Orians at the University of Washington showed that when caterpillars infected a willow tree, other nearby trees excreted toxins as a means of protection. When leaves are damaged by caterpillar infestation, the damaged leaves release **phenols** and **tannins**, which make them unpalatable to caterpillars. Pheromones related to these compounds are released into the air, alerting nearby trees, which then release higher levels of the caterpillar repellant chemicals in response to the warning signal.

235

In primates however, recent studies have shown that there was an evolutionary trade-off. Many primate OR genes lost their functionality, becoming *pseudogenes* with the evolution of *tricolor vision*. It's believed the emergence of color vision decreased primate reliance upon olfaction, explaining this loss of function.

On average, humans can distinguish an estimated 10,000 separate odors, and possess 802 olfactory receptor genes – about three percent of the entire human genome – but only 388 encode working olfactory receptors. The remaining 414 appear to be pseudogenes – those which no longer express proteins or no longer appear to function.

Surrounded by odorant molecules shed by food, soil, trees, flowers, animals, industrial activity, bacterial decomposition, and other people, during inhalation, the nose channels odorant-laden air into the nasal cavity, to a patch of tissue called the *olfactory epithelium*, where odorants bind to neural odorant receptors. Signals from olfactory receptors in the nose travel to the brain's *olfactory bulb*, and are then relayed to the *olfactory cortex*, which connects directly to the brain's main regulator – the hypothalamus.

At the top of the nasal cavity, the olfactory epithelium is made of two membrane patches only a few centimeters square, lying in a horizontal line just below eye level. (see the chapter on senses for diagrams). These patches are embedded with about 5 million olfactory neurons, along with supporting cells and stem cells. Millions of different odorants can be detected by a limited number of receptors by combining multiple ORs that detect a single odorant, or single ORs which can detect multiple odorants.

Olfactory Sense Drove Brain Development

The Triassic period came to a close 190 million years ago, ushering in the Jurassic. Northern and southern Pangaea had split, with North America and Eurasia forming a single northern supercontinent and Africa, South America, and the remaining landmasses forming the southern supercontinent.

Dinosaurs grew even more massive, such as *Seismosaurus* (*Earth-Shaking Lizard*), said to have grown as much as 120 feet long – the equivalent of a 12-story building. Such massive sizes were possible because of the dinosaur's efficient respiration and heat exchange. These titanic herbivores ate most of the time, and moved very little.

Such giants of the Jurassic roamed the supercontinents, perpetually feeding on ferns and palm-like *cycad plants*, and many were in turn preyed upon by smaller, faster carnivorous dinosaurs. At this time, the oceans teemed with fish and squid, though the armored trilobites had gone extinct. The earliest birds emerged, as did tiny, furry, mouse-like creatures the size of paperclips. These were the first mammals.

These tiny creatures began to evolve massive brains, 10 times larger than their relative body size. By using 3D scans of skull cavities, paleontologists such as the University of Texas' Dr. Timothy Rowe have discovered which brain regions were the first to develop. And, according to Dr. Rowe, we owe the current size of our brains to evolutionary leaps in our tactile and olfactory senses. Rowe and his team created brain models for the early mammals Hadrocodium and *Morganuocodon*, and found their skulls had morphed over time to accommodate larger olfactory bulbs, the regions of the brain dedicated to the sense of smell. Their fur, adds Dr. Rowe, originally evolved to enhance their tactile sense, with nerves activated by each hair.

Astonishingly, the brains of Morganuocodon and Hadrocodium were about fifty percent larger than those of their evolutionary predecessors. This rapid growth began with the processing of smell. It's thought that because these proto-mammals were nocturnal to avoid daylight predators, their heightened senses of touch and smell grew to allow them to forage and hunt for insects in darkness. This also allowed them to avoid competing for food resources with the dinosaurs sharing their habitats.

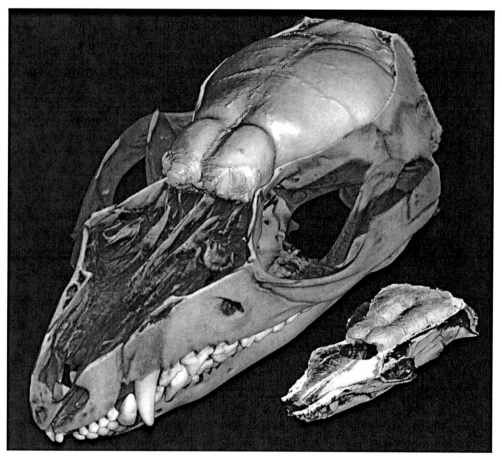

Computed Tomography scans of the skulls of a modern short-tailed opossum (upper left) and Hadrocodium (bottom right). Based upon their brain cases, their brains (pink) have been reconstructed as above. The olfactory bulbs appear at the front of their brains (reddish pink). Image: Matt Colbert, University of Texas, Austin. Used with permission.

Hadrocodium and other Jurassic mammals had already evolved all the key mammalian traits: large brains, limbs positioned under the body instead of being splayed out like a lizard's, milk-producing glands, and four sets of specialized teeth, including incisors, canines, premolars, and molars.

Today, mammals are the only surviving therapsids, their forebears all consigned to extinction when they were supplanted by the first mammals around 100 mya. Their descendants would soon diverge into three lineages: egg-laying *monotremes* like the platypus and spiny anteater; pouch-bearing *marsupials* like kangaroos and possums; and womb-bearing *placentals* like humans, cows and horses.

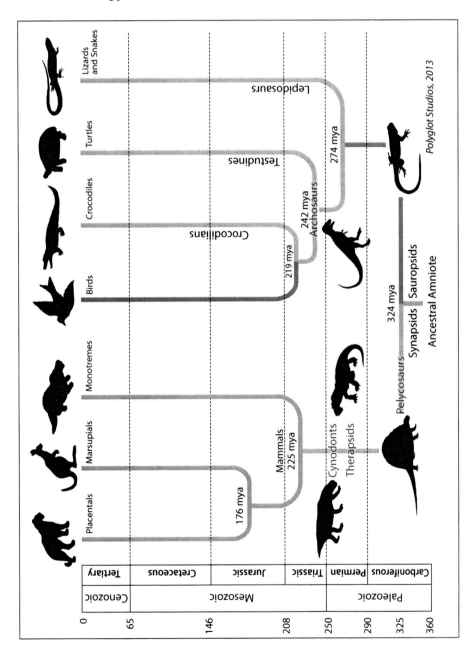

Now Hear This!

Hearing is vital for many living organisms, warning of danger, enabling communication over distance, and in some cases even enabling the reading of surroundings through *echolocation*. Ears receive information from a distance in any direction, without the need for focusing. A secondary function is a means of gauging balance. Given their utility, it's surprising that such useful paired organs were the last to emerge. Complex ears evolved only within about the last 300 million years, as tetrapods made the transition to land.

Although it's also critical for balance, the primary purpose of the ear is to detect sound – fluctuations in pressure travelling through air or water. On land, even the tiniest disturbance in the air causes a compression wave which spreads out in all directions. Sound waves also travel through ground and water, in fact better than through air because of the higher densities of water and rock, making sensitive hearing unnecessary.

Hearing occurs when compressive waves or vibrations trigger *resonance* (sympathetic vibration) in an animal's body. This resonance gets converted into neural impulses which are sent to the brain for interpretation.

The start of what would eventually evolve into the inner ear first emerged during the Devonian Period in the earliest amphibians. The *lateral line system* – sensors used by fish and amphibians to sense pressure changes – may have eventually evolved into the primitive inner ear of amphibians, although some evolutionary biologists suggest the amphibian form developed independently. Whatever the case, fish ears and early amphibian ears have similar principles of operation.

The first amphibian ears were much simpler than modern ones, probably responding to vibrations through the ground and water. The creature's entire body would resonate with these vibrations, especially in the densest parts – the bones. The bone resonated, transferring the vibrations through the body, where these vibrations would eventually reach the *inner ear*, a fluid-filled region encased in dense bone. Inside, tiny hairs converted the vibrations into electrical signals which would be fed to the brain for interpretation.

Thus, the first amphibians, just as with modern salamanders, apparently perceived sound by picking up ground vibrations through their skulls, an arrangement not particularly suited for sounds transmitted through air. The density of water easily transfers sonic energy, vibrating dense bones, but airborne sounds have significantly less energy, and therefore need a more sensitive arrangement.

In response, the auditory sense grew gradually more sophisticated over the evolutionary history of reptiles and mammals. A major adaptation in ear structure came with the evolution of the *basilar papilla*, an organ composed of hair-like sensory cells which multiplied over time, allowing greater sensitivity.

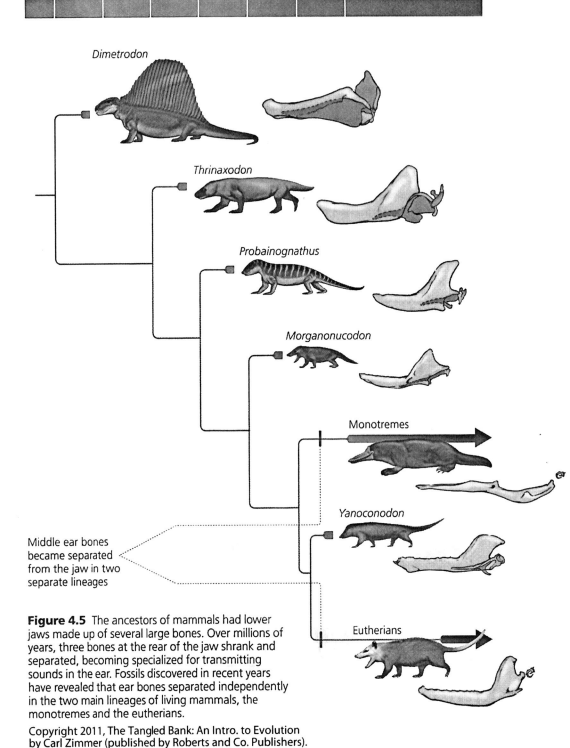

290   270   250   230   210   190   170   Millions of years ago

Dimetrodon

Thrinaxodon

Probainognathus

Morganonucodon

Monotremes

Yanoconodon

Middle ear bones became separated from the jaw in two separate lineages

Eutherians

Figure 4.5 The ancestors of mammals had lower jaws made up of several large bones. Over millions of years, three bones at the rear of the jaw shrank and separated, becoming specialized for transmitting sounds in the ear. Fossils discovered in recent years have revealed that ear bones separated independently in the two main lineages of living mammals, the monotremes and the eutherians.

In the Triassic period, reptiles evolved a *tympanic membrane*, better known as an *ear drum*, separating the middle and inner ears. This allowed for much greater clarity in hearing. Parts of the jaw shrank and receded to become the *ossicles,* three tiny bones in the ear to amplify sound and transfer it to fluid in the snail-shaped, fluid-filled *cochlea,* where vibrations in the inner ear fluid displace hair cells, generating signals for the brain. The three ossicles in the middle ear developed slowly as reptiles evolved into mammals, allowing for a much wider range of detectable frequencies, an adaptation which would become tremendously significant for the evolution of speech.

Meanwhile, during the Cretaceous, the cochlear duct coiled among mammals, allowing for ever greater sensitivity across the auditory spectrum. The outer ear, with its ear canal and protruding *pinna* was last to evolve. The pinna is the outer, protruding portion of the mammalian ear, which collects sound waves and directs them through the ear canal into the middle ear. In addition to collecting sound waves, the pinna helps animals determine the direction from which sounds emanate.

Advanced Senses

In 2012, an international team led by Dr. Stephan Lautenschlager found that smell, hearing and balance were already well developed in a special group of dinosaurs called *Therizinosaurs*, which lived 145 to 66 million years ago. Since therizinosaurs were herbivorous, these exceptionally-developed sensory abilities are surprising, as they would seem more beneficial to predators than to plant-eaters. Close relatives of the famous carnivores Tyrannosaurus rex and Velociraptor, therizinosaurs were instead peaceful herbivores, up to 23 ft. long, with 20-inch claws on their forelimbs, long necks and primitive, downy-soft feathers coating their bodies.

Puzzled by the anomaly, Dr. Lautenschlager's team chose to scan the skull of *Erlikosaurus andrewsi*, a 12-foot therizinosaur species which lived 90 million years ago in ancient Mongolia. The team reconstructed Erlikosaurus' brain structures using high-resolution CT scanning and 3D computer modelling on the skull cavities of fossil specimens, allowing them to deduce the relative development of the creature's sensory and cognitive capabilities.

According to Dr. Lautenschlager, "Our results suggest that therizinosaurs would have used their well-developed sensory repertoire to their advantage which, for herbivorous animals, must have played an important role in foraging, in the evasion of predators or in social complexity. This study sheds a new light on the evolution of dinosaur senses and shows it is more complex than we thought."

N.C. State University co-author Dr. Lindsay Zanno added, "Once you've evolved a good sensory toolkit, it's probably worth hanging onto, whether you're hunting or being hunted."

Therizinosaurs were a subgroup of *theropods*, the lineage from which birds evolved. Special skin cells called placodes can be induced to grow into feathers instead of scales by manipulating the fetal expression of *BMP2* and *Shh* genes. Feathers provide egg and body insulation as well as camouflage, and were also likely used for courtship, and as a means of increasing lift and escape velocity when fleeing from predators.

Wired for Speed

Shifts in only three genetic letters from among billions helped lead directly to the advanced, precise mammalian motor system, laying the groundwork for advanced human coordination, according to 2012 Yale University research.

Among the estimated 22,000 mammalian protein-encoding genes, the critical evolutionary drivers are believed to be *cis-regulatory elements* – non-coding DNA which regulates when, where and how much genes are expressed. *Cis* is Latin for *on the same side*, because these DNA regions are upstream or downstream on the same DNA strand as the genes they regulate.

Cis-regulatory elements are critical to embryonic development in all living organisms. One example is the TATA box, the repeating sequence of Thymine and Adenine nucleotides used as a protein-complex binding site where transcription begins.

The Yale team discovered a very minor change in the mammalian genome which allowed evolution of the *corticospinal tract* – long axons connecting motor control circuits of the brain and spinal cord. This circuitry connects the cerebral cortex – the outer "executive control" portion of the mammalian brain – to the brainstem and spinal cord, allowing precise, delicate motor skills, particularly in the most distal muscles, such as those in the hands, feet, toes and fingers.

The *E4* DNA region controls the *Fezf2 gene*, which directs formation of the corticospinal tract. FezF2 (*Forebrain Embryonic Zinc Finger 2*) is a transcription factor in the *Zinc finger* family, which controls neural differentiation within the forebrain.

FezF2 directs development of motor-sensory circuits joining the cortex and spinal cord. It guides the formation, connection and positioning of brain-to-spine *axons*, the long "tree-trunks" down which neural impulses travel, and *dendrites*, the signal-receiving "branches" of the neuron. Dendrites are the *post-synaptic* side of the *synapse*, the connection point neurons use to send signal-transmitting chemicals.

The E4 enhancer is a cis-regulatory element which ramps up FezF2 expression. Yale University's Nenad Sestan bred mice without the E4 enhancer region and found FezF2 expression dropped significantly, completely preventing formation of the deepest two layers of the cortex and of the corticospinal tract.

Says Dr. Sestan, the modern form of the E4 enhancer first appeared in early amniotes, creating the regulatory mechanism which enabled advanced motor-sensory circuits to evolve in modern mammals and birds. Around the same time, the evolution of gene-patterning programs guided expansion of the vertebrate forebrain into the modern, six-layered upper surface of the cerebrum.

242

Hot-Blooded

Mammals derive their name from *mamma*, the milk-secreting glands females use to provide their young with nourishment, during comparatively prolonged and intensive parental care. Like birds, mammals are endotherms, generating their own body heat by oxidizing large amounts of food. Endothermy is thought to have evolved to allow consistently high activity levels, especially during the night or cold weather. mammals are also unique in having fur or hair, which serves to insulate the heat their bodies generate.

The earliest mammals appear in the fossil record from about 195 million years ago. They began primarily as small creatures thought to have only been active at night, as most share enhanced night vision, three middle ear bones which amplify sound, and an acute sense of smell, with highly developed brain centers to process these senses.

Upon the mass extinction of the dinosaurs, new ecological niches opened, allowing diversification into the 5,488 living mammal species today – small and large herbivores, predators, and marine hunters which dominate Earth's present-day ecosystems.

Among mammals, teeth size and structure vary according to diet. Herbivores have large, flat teeth for crushing plant material, while predators have sharp teeth for biting and tearing flesh. Omnivores like humans have sets of several distinct teeth. Similarly, digestive tracts vary among species, with plant-eating species hosting gut microbes capable of fermenting tough cellulose plant cell walls, allowing nutrients to be extracted.

The majority of mammals are *Eutherians*, named after the Greek word for "good beasts". They're distinguished by the presence of a sac called a placenta, which nourishes young in the womb. There are about 4,000 known eutherian species alive today, classified into 26 lineages called *orders* (though biologists' opinions differ as to how many orders exist). By far the largest order is the *rodents* (mice, rats and squirrels), followed by *chiroptera* (bats), *insectivores* (hedgehogs, moles and shrews), *artiodactyls* (pigs, hippos, whales, deer, sheep and cattle), *carnivores* (dogs, bears, cats, weasels and seals), and *primates* (lemurs, monkeys, and apes, including humans).

Placental mammals give live birth and feed their embryos via the organ from which their name is derived, which is attached to the wall of the mother's uterus. Placental species range from 1.5-gram *bumblebee bats* to 190-ton blue whales.

Eutherian (placental) young are fed milk until they have developed to the point of being able to digest solid foods. But eutherian parental care often extends past the nursing stage; these animals foster their young until they are able to escape predators and find food on their own.

Fossil records show mammals co-existed with the dinosaurs, but didn't diversify or grow in size until their dinosaur competition went extinct and the ecosystems recovered. After that, however, an evolutionary "big bang" similar to that of the Cambrian occurred among mammals, with 10 major placental groups emerging in a span of only 200,000 years, according to genetic analyses by NY paleontologist Maureen O'Leary.

Dr. O'Leary and her colleagues created a massive database of over 4500 phenomic characteristics from 86 living and extinct species of placental mammals. All major groups of placental mammals were represented, varying in size, fur color, and various other physiological aspects. 27 specific genes common to all placental mammals were discovered by the analysis.

Their data defined a tiny, shrewlike insectivore as the first placental, and thus the ancestor of almost all mammals alive today, including humans.

Dr. O'Leary says the creature discovered through her DNA and fossil detective work was a tree-dweller, furry and long-tailed, which gave live birth, and possessed a complex brain with a large olfactory-processing lobe, and a *corpus callosum*, the nerve fiber bundle connecting the brain's left and right hemispheres.

*A **Living Database** – Geneticists have catalogued the human genome – the "standard" genes needed as a baseline to create a human; and since 2010 have been working worldwide to catalogue the **proteome** – all the proteins those genes express – but little attention has been paid to the higher-order product of those constructs – the **phenome**.*

*While the genome and proteome represent all of a creature's genes and proteins, the phenome is the "next step up" in scale – the total of all the traits created by those genes and proteins. In humans, those traits include hair, skin and eye color, height, personality, etc. Thus, a phenome is all the **phenotypes** (possible trait manifestations) expressed by a cell, tissue, organ, organism, or species.*

The phenotype of an organism – all an individual's traits, which can differ from the typical traits of its species – is created from a combination of its species-specific genome, as well as environmental influences, genetic variations and mutations.

The first attempt at cataloguing the human phenome was a collaborative study among three universities in the Netherlands conducted in 2006 to record 5,000 human phenotypes. Though this was the first study of its kind, future additions to this database are likely to yield a wealth of information about human disease.

*Dr. O'Leary has taken this a step further, however: in 2012, with the backing of the National Science Foundation, Dr. O'Leary spearheaded the **Tree of Life** project, including the **MorphoBank** online phenotype database. Its ambitious aim is to allow scientists worldwide to participate in cataloguing and sharing phenomic data for every species on Earth.*

Mother

In 2011, archaeologists had unearthed precisely the creature Dr. O'Leary's analyses had predicted. Dubbed the *Jurassic Mother from China (Juramaia sinensis)*, this tiny, shrew-like animal lived alongside Jurassic-period dinosaurs 160 million years ago. Its discovery pushed back placental evolution at least 35 million years, and provided new information about the earliest mammalian ancestors.

Carnegie Museum paleontologist Zhe-Xi Luo led the team of paleontologists who unearthed Juramaia's nearly complete skeleton from a site in what is now the Liaoning Province in northeastern China. According to Dr. Luo, Juramaia is the earliest known common ancestor of mice and humans, as well as the earliest known Eutherian, animals which evolved a placenta in place of laying eggs.

Placental mammals are a diverse group of almost 4,000 known species, primarily rodents and bats, but also including whales, elephants, shrews, and armadillos. Also among the group are some of mankind's closest domesticated animal allies: dogs and cats, rabbits, goats, sheep, pigs, cattle, horses, and humans.

"Juramaia, from 160 million years ago", said Dr. Luo in a press release, "is either a great-grand-aunt, or a great-grandmother of all placental mammals that are thriving today."

Juramaia weighed only half an ounce (15 grams), making it lighter than a chipmunk. It had forepaws adapted to tree-climbing, and scurried about temperate Jurassic forests, feasting on insects and worms under the cover of darkness. In the trees, it enjoyed a number of ecological advantages unavailable to earthbound animals. "It is their early adaptation to exploit niches on the tree that paved their way toward this success," added Dr. Luo.

Finding Juramaia shows that a major milestone in mammalian evolution – the divergence of eutherians from the earlier *metatherians* (whose descendants would include *marsupials*, which carry their young in pouches like the kangaroo; and the egg-laying *monotremes* like the platypus) – was reached 35 million years earlier than previously thought; it also corroborates DNA evidence of the course of mammalian evolution. The DNA evidence had long indicated the split between ancestral marsupials, monotremes and placentals had occurred about 160 million years ago, much earlier than existing fossils showed.

Secondary physical differences between eutherians and metatherians were adaptive changes to their wrists and teeth. Both ancient lineages began as the tiniest of creatures, which survived by adapting to the forest canopy, out of reach of most predators on the ground. The environmental events which drove the evolutionary split, however, still remain a mystery. As Luo puts it, "We don't know what would be the specific environmental trigger for that."

Just like *oviparous* (egg-laying) animals, placental females produce eggs, but instead of laying them, mothers carry them inside their bodies until the embryos mature, a period known as *gestation*. In place of a nutrient-filled yolk sac, within the mammalian uterus, growing embryos are sustained by a placenta.

The placenta is a specialized organ in the wall of the uterus, which evolved out of membranes like those in the eggs of reptiles, birds, and *monotremes* (the platypus and spiny anteaters), the only mammals which still lay eggs.

Developing embryos inside the womb are nourished by the placenta. This organ is rich in blood vessels, allowing breathing and feeding via the mother's bloodstream. The *umbilical cord* acts as a conduit between the embryo and mother, exchanging oxygenated, nutrient-dense blood and deoxygenated, nutrient-depleted blood back and forth with the placenta.

This evolutionary adaptation allows the pregnant mother to roam in search of food, without risking leaving behind eggs for predators to find. Giving birth to live, relatively mature young also protects them from exposure in harsh environmental conditions.

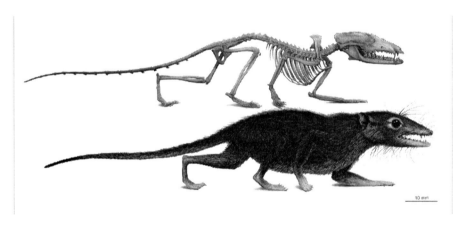

*Skeletal and fur reconstructions of the Jurassic eutherian Juramaia sinensis. Juramaia was a shrew-sized mammal with a skull 22 mm long (just over 3/4 of an inch). It weighed around 15 grams (about half an ounce), fed on insects and worms, and had a great ability to climb. The name of this 160-mya placental comes from **Jura** – the **Jurassic Period**, while maia means **mother** and sinensis means from **China**, so the full name means **Jurassic Mother from China**. Image: Mark Klinger, Carnegie Museum of Natural History. Used with permission.*

A 2011 Yale University study found that *lateral gene transfer* was responsible for this radical change in mammal reproduction. The team, led by Dr. Vincent J. Lynch, pinpointed the precise molecular changes which caused mammals to develop a placenta, and begin carrying embryonic offspring within the womb instead of laying them in nests or carrying them within pouches. Dr. Lynch says transposons functioning as "genetic parasites" had transformed the mammal genome, altering the uterus from producing eggs to providing an inner nurturing environment for embryos.

By comparing the genetic make-up of uterine cells in opossums to those of armadillos and humans, all of which are placental, his team was pieced together the evolutionary history of pregnancy. They discovered over 1500 genes expressed only in the placental uterus and controlled by transposons, "selfish pieces of genetic material" which replicate within a host's genome.

"Transposons grow like parasites that have invaded the body, multiplying and taking up space in the genome," according to Dr. Lynch. But in the case of our species, they also activate or suppress genes which govern pregnancy.

"These transposons are not genes that underwent small changes over long periods of time and eventually grew into their new role during pregnancy," Lynch said. "They are more like prefabricated regulatory units that install themselves into a host genome, which then recycles them to carry out entirely new functions like facilitating maternal-fetal communication."

Said co-author Dr. Gunter Wagner, "We used to believe that changes only took place through small mutations in our DNA that accumulated over time. But in this case we found a huge cut-and-paste operation that altered wide areas of the genome to create large-scale morphological change."

Because of finite energy and the enormous importance of reproduction, females of a species can either produce a large litter of tiny offspring (insects and echinoderms lay thousands to millions of eggs), or a small litter of large offspring, as with mammals. However, nurturing the young inside the body greatly increases the odds that members of a small brood will survive.

Birds and mammals take this energy investment much further, however, investing significant time and energy in parental care, even for years in some cases. Female mammals also lactate, producing nutrient-dense milk to feed their young. This major investment in the protection and care of offspring is thought to be one of the main reasons mammals and birds have been so successful at surviving.

The End of the Dinosaurs

65 million years ago, the reign of the dinosaurs came to an apocalyptic end, as an asteroid fragment the size of Mt. Everest broke off in a collision and slammed into the coast of Mexico. The titanic, lumbering dinosaurs had ruled the continents and seas for over 500 times the length of human existence, but abruptly perished when the 6-mile-wide chunk of space rock struck the Earth 20 times faster than a bullet, with an impact a billion times more powerful than the Hiroshima atomic bomb, blasting hot rock and gas at high velocity into the atmosphere, and triggering a chain of events that led to a global winter and wiped out nearly all life on Earth in a matter of hours.

The initial impact of the *Chicxulub Asteroid* gouged a hole 112 miles wide and 20 miles deep, a crater eight times the width and sixteen times the depth of the Grand Canyon's south rim. The collision vaporized tremendous quantities of rock, blasting sand-grain-sized spheres high above Earth's atmosphere. As the ejecta re-entered, the upper atmosphere reached a searing 2,700 degrees Fahrenheit for two to three hours.

Firestorms raged across the entire planet, roasting every living organism not sheltered in burrows or underwater. The collision generated about 100 million megatons of energy, heat equivalent to "...a 1 megaton bomb exploding every four miles over the entire Earth." – each of these with the same explosive power as 80 Hiroshima-type nuclear bombs.

That the Chicxulub asteroid caused the K-T is no longer in dispute, due to a 2013 study at the University of Colorado Boulder and the National Oceanic and Atmospheric Administration. The team found a layer of soot at the K-T boundary layer which could only have been created by a global firestorm burning every twig, bush and tree on the planet's surface, causing the extinction of 80 percent of all Earth's species. The study backs the findings of experts from 33 worldwide scientific institutions which also concluded the Chicxulub impact triggered the K-T mass extinctions.

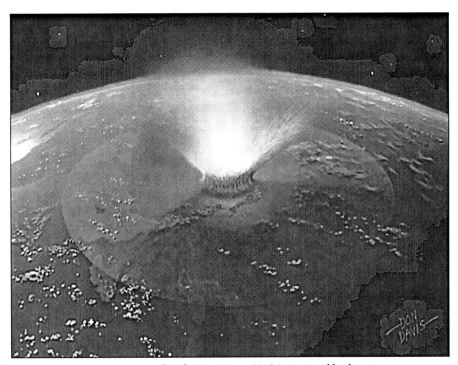

Massive Terrestrial Strike, Don Davis, NASA, 2010, public domain

After instantly cooking the surface of the planet, the impact triggered continent-wide infernos, landslides, skyscraper-sized tsunamis, and earthquakes with a magnitude of over 10 on the Richter scale.

Mass extinctions came from a combination of devastating effects over different time scales; larger dinosaurs were completely exposed and instantly flash-cooked as ejected material fell, heating the atmosphere and triggering massive firestorms. But the deadliest effect was the high-velocity ejection of material into the atmosphere, shrouding the planet in darkness and causing a year-long global winter. This killed many species unable to quickly adapt to the hellish environment.

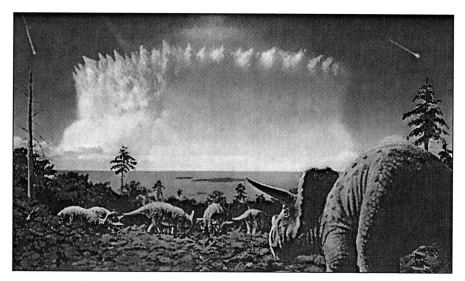

Image: The End, Beyond Genes, 2007, Bravenet Services Inc. Used with permission.

New imaging technology shows Chicxulub struck in coastal waters off the Yucatan Peninsula, ejecting a tremendous volume of vapor into the atmosphere. Sulfur deposits at the impact site reacted with this water vapor, producing global storms of acid rain lasting a decade. Climate change and ocean acidity triggered a complete breakdown in marine ecology, and a slower die-off in the oceans. pH-adaptive marine creatures survived, but more sensitive varieties eventually went extinct.

The global catastrophe spelled the end of the 160-million-year reign of the dinosaurs, but was incredibly fortuitous for the tiny proto-mammals who had previously lived in the shadow of the dinosaurs. In this way, the *Cretaceous–Paleogene extinction* became a pivotal event in Earth's history, ultimately paving the way for humans to rise to planetary domination.

The survivors included many small mammals which were able to burrow underground or immerse themselves in water during the brief but deadly temperature increases. After days of baking heat, Earth's surface temperature returned to habitable levels, and surviving creatures emerged from their burrows into a barren wasteland.

Most surface vegetation had been destroyed, so the herbivorous dinosaurs which had survived were left without food. Their massive bulk had required tremendous amounts of oxygen and high, stable temperatures much different from those of present-day Earth. Global climate change from Chicxulub's impact was too extreme for their bodies to adjust, and they quickly died off.

Small mammals and birds fed upon aquatic plants which had survived the catastrophe, as well as insects, worms, and snails which fed on dead plant and animal matter. Other animals, such as crocodiles, also survived by retreating into the water; on land, mammals benefited most and continued to evolve after the Cretaceous–Paleogene extinction event, which had opened ecological niches for them to diversify and dominate the Earth.

15 million years after the passing of the dinosaurs, the early *Eocene* saw an explosion of growth in mammal populations and diversity. Many of today's mammals appeared, and large land-based herbivores spread widely. During the *Eocene*, atmospheric oxygen had risen slightly above its present-day level.

Mammals and birds, which require three to six times as much oxygen as reptiles, were freed of growth constraints, and began to increase in size, diversity, and geographic distribution. Within a relatively very short span of time, approximately 130 genera of mammals had evolved, with a total of about 4,000 species, including the first rodents, primates, flying and aquatic mammals.

Endothermy in general and placental reproduction in particular require high levels of oxygen, and a large increase in eutherian fossils coincides with these historically high, stable oxygen levels. (Modern eutherians still require high oxygen levels, which is why few mammals live at elevations above 14,800 feet.)

Such rapid diversification into new roles and environmental zones is called *adaptive radiation*. It's occurred repeatedly throughout evolutionary history, on both a large and small scale, usually as a result of the abrupt emptying of previously-occupied environmental niches, allowing other species to take over. The dinosaur mass extinction was one example, in which the dominant competitors died off, while mammals thrived. Surviving mammal species didn't simply jump into the newly-vacant environmental niches, however; they adapted slowly, over millions of years, gradually growing in size and acquiring new beneficial traits through natural selection.

Part of the driving force behind the incredibly rich diversity of mammals is the ongoing breakup of the supercontinents, beginning 200 million years ago, isolating Australia, Eurasia, the poles and North and South America. Marsupials thrived and diversified in the isolated southern continents, while placentals rose to dominance elsewhere.

By this time, the Earth had changed radically. New habitats and food resources had arisen. The end of the Cretaceous saw flowering plants flourishing worldwide, providing fruits, nuts and berries, as well as other nutrients for swarms of new insects, which themselves became a highly-nutritious source of food for mammals.

Forests of emerging species grew and spread, offering novel habitats for creatures which would evolve into the tree-dwelling *primates* (gorillas, shrews, lemurs, monkeys, orangutans, chimpanzees and humans) which first appeared around 50 million years ago. These creatures had evolved with forward-facing, stereo vision, with hands specialized for grasping and climbing, and with superior leaping abilities.

Prime Time

The first primates emerged from the fading smoke of the Cretaceous-Paleogene into the dawn of the *Paleocene* (*early recent*) era. Among the oldest, a squirrel-like tree-dweller called *Purgatorius* lived 65 mya in what is now northeastern Montana, just after the passing of the dinosaurs. Many of its remains have been found scattered right above those of Tyrannosaurus Rex in Cretaceous-era rocks of the Hell Creek Formation.

Purgatorious was the size of a mouse and weighed a little over an ounce. Fossilized ankle bones found in 2012 show this first primate was *arboreal*, with the joints of a tree-climber, providing a wide range of motion to adjust to precarious, uneven branches. Purgatorious had molars specialized for eating fruit, and likely also enjoyed tasty grubs, beetles, worms and termites. It thrived as flowering plants (*Angiosperms*) exploded in diversity, indicating primates and angiosperms probably co-evolved to exploit an entirely new niche. In essence, fruit lured these first primates into the trees, after the need to escape predatory dinosaurs had passed. Bright flowers and fruit likely evolved specifically to recruit animals into spreading pollen and seeds – something modern animals still do. Thus, primates and flowering plants co-evolved in ways benefiting both groups.

According to Chester, plants began to produce something attractive to primates, as a way of spreading their seeds. At the same time, primates were becoming specialized for life in trees, allowing them to climb onto branches and collect fruit. Tree-climbing gave primates an edge over land-dwellers, contributing to their evolutionary success.

The next 10 million years of primate evolution centered around this lifestyle, a remarkably successful survival strategy; nearly all primates today are at least partly arboreal. Humans are a rare exception, our more recent ancestors having abandoned the trees for the grasslands of Africa some 60 million years after the era of Purgatorious. However, according to Dartmouth anthropologist Vivek Venkataraman, 2012 studies show that at least four human hunter-gatherer tribes still climb trees to gather honey, and it's likely our hominin ancestors spent some of their time in trees as well.

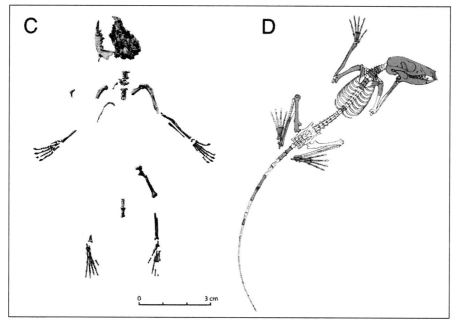

Skeleton and diagram of 55-million-year-old Dryomomys szalayi found in 2007 outside Yellowstone National Park in Wyoming's Bighorn Basin.Bloch, et al; used with permission

Just Like Paradise

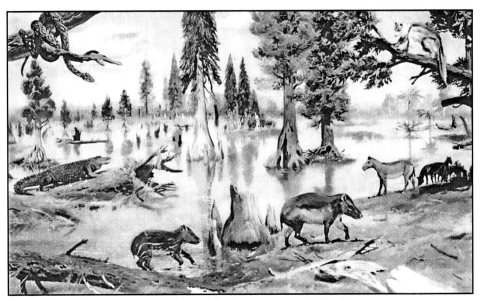

Eocene marsh fauna, Zdenek Burian, 1976. Public domain

During the *Eocene*, Earth was considerably warmer than today, creating a global paradise for primates, which spread and diverged extensively. With little polar ice, the geographic range of primates extended much farther north than in modern times, up to about 60°N latitude – Alaska, Northern Canada, and Siberia. But eventually the planet cooled, and primates all but disappeared from the northern continents. Today, with the exception of humans, primates are restricted to a band of tropical and equatorial climes, from about 40°S latitude to 40°N.

As primates evolved, their eyes moved from the sides to the fronts of their skulls, providing superior depth perception. They lost their claws, which flattened into fingernails, their hands and feet adapted to grasping, and their brains grew substantially, granting the ability to engage in complex social behavior and learn through *insight* – the spontaneous flash of creative problem-solving – instead of being limited to simple trial-and-error problem-solving.

After the earliest primates such as Purgatorious and Dryomomys, a dizzying variety of transitional species would come and go along the evolutionary path to seven primate superfamilies, each physically adapted and specialized for a particular ecological niche.

The radiation began about 56 million years ago, as the earliest primates diverged into two groups. The first were *"wet-nosed"* (*Strepsirrhine*) primates, which would develop into lemurs, lorises and bush babies, all distinguishable by their moist, touch-sensitive and whisker-bearing *rhinarium* – dog-like snout noses. The second group were the *Haplorhines, simple-nosed* tarsiers and *anthropoids.*

252

The *Anthropoids* (*human-like*) would diverge into the *Platyrrhines,* five families of flared-nostril New World monkeys in South and Central America, and the *Catarrhines* of the Old World – Asia and Africa. These latter Catarrhine monkeys and their Great Ape descendants, including humans and extinct ancestral forms, all have downward-pointing nostrils.

Our trichromatic color vision had its genetic origins in the divergence of the Catarrhines into its two superfamilies, Old World monkeys (*Cercopithecoids*) and apes (*Hominoids*). Apes are tailless, larger, and generally ground-dwelling, though the term ape technically refers to the Hominoid superfamily, comprising *Lesser Apes* (gibbons), and *Great Apes,* (orangutans, gorillas, chimpanzees, Homo sapiens, and related extinct species).

As dozens of extinct primate lineages have been discovered, the primate family tree has grown quite complex, but our early primate ancestry is slowly becoming quite well-defined:

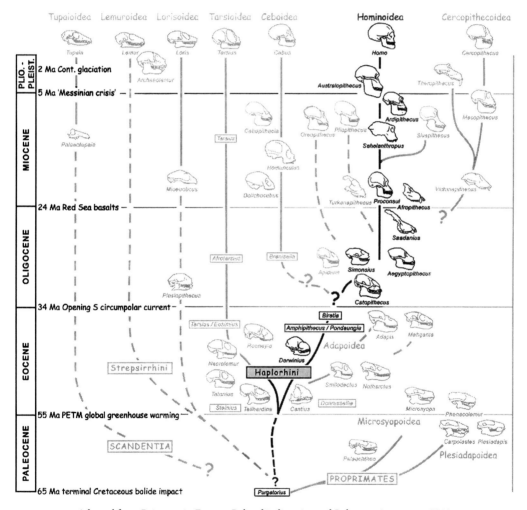

Adapted from Primates in Eocene, Palaeobiodiversity and Palaeoenvironments, 2012,
Philip D. Gingerich, PhD. Used with permission.

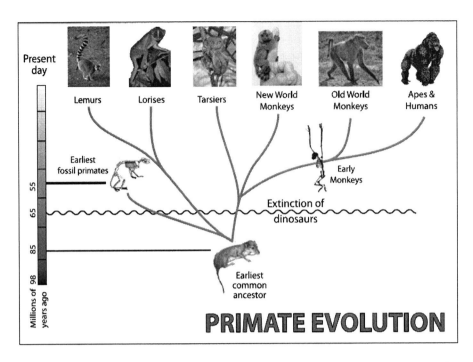

Present day

Lemurs Lorises Tarsiers New World Monkeys Old World Monkeys Apes & Humans

Earliest fossil primates

Early Monkeys

Extinction of dinosaurs

Earliest common ancestor

Millions of years ago
55
65
85
98

PRIMATE EVOLUTION

There are now seven primate superfamilies, with humans belonging to the *Hominoidea* – African, Asian and human apes. From among them, the chimpanzee is our closest ancestor, sharing 96-98% of our DNA.

Like us, chimpanzees are highly social and intelligent, capable of learning rudimentary sign language and, like humans, of experiencing such emotions as anxiety, depression, distress, empathy grief pain, and pleasure. For all their smaller size, however, they can significantly stronger than humans, and deadly when angered.

In 1923, Dr. John Bauman measured chimpanzee pull strength with a device called a dynamometer at the Bronx Zoo, where a female called Suzette pulled 1,260 pounds, and a male called Boma pulled 847 pounds – singlehandedly.

In 1943, Yale University's Dr. Glen Finch conducted similar tests of chimpanzee arm strength, and found the test subjects were stronger than human, but not by a factor of five times. It's been concluded that the reason Dr. Bauman's subjects were so much stronger was that they were enraged at the time, and the adrenaline allowed them to exert far more force than normal.

Chimpanzees are smaller than humans, but their arms are more powerful, due to the muscle structure. Chimpanzee muscle fibers can generate more power, primarily because of changes in the MYH16 and ACTN3 genes, which affect myosin and actin fiber growth. MYH16 has gone dormant in humans, and specific variations of ACTN3 are found among Olympic-level athletes.

Hominids – apes and humans – have the largest bodies and longest limbs, lack tails, and live primarily on land. Their walking styles vary to a degree: orangutans walk with the backs of their fists upon the ground, while chimps and gorillas walk with their knuckles upon the ground, occasionally rising on two legs to display aggression.

Humans are the only great apes which are completely *bipedal* – walking on two legs. It is primarily this bipedalism that distinguishes the *hominins* (humans and our humanoid ancestors) from among the hominids (humans and other great apes).

DNA analysis shows we are most closely related to chimpanzees, and gorillas are our second closest relatives. The chimpanzee and human lineage diverged about seven million years ago from a shared ancestor.

The Journey of a Thousand Miles...

"We are all children of Africa. They say this is where it all began. Africa was our only home for tens of thousands of years, until a small handful of people made their way out of Africa."
– Dr Alice Roberts, "The Incredible Human Journey:
Out of Africa", BBC Two, August 28, 2009

"Those early Europeans were people like you and me, but it is humbling when you see the challenges they faced. People like you and me overcame the Neanderthals; people like you and me made it through the ice age." – Dr Alice Roberts, "The Incredible Human Journey: Europe", BBC Two, May 24, 2009

Just One Look

Approximately 30 million years ago, Old World monkeys and apes diverged from a common ancestor, and some only 200,000 and 250,000 years ago, Homo sapiens emerged, to begin its slow ascent toward planetary dominance. As blogger Robert Lamb so eloquently puts it: *What truly set this particular strain of life apart? Why are we the ones standing on the free side of the cage?*

The story might have begun 30 million years ago, with *Saadanius hijazensis*, a very special tree-dwelling monkey discovered in 2009 near Mecca, Saudi Arabia by University of Michigan Paleontologist Iyad Zalmout. Saadanius was one of the earliest Catarrhines, the larger primates with narrow, downward-facing nostrils instead of rounded, outward-flaring ones. Saadanius seems to have been a tree-dweller before the Arabian Peninsula and African continent separated.

Dietary changes probably led our common ancestor to rely more upon sight than smell. A duplicate opsin gene evolved in the catarrhines which enhances sensitivity to the orange and red range of visible light, matching the colors of ripe fruits indigenous to the region.

Similarly, primates had come to rely upon sight instead of pheromones to process social cues. The genes expressing *TRP2 ion channels* and *V1R pheromone receptors* went dormant in hominoids and Old World monkeys 23 mya, according to University of Michigan Geneticist Dr. Jianzhi Zhang.

TRP2 ion channels and V1R receptors are central components of the *vomeronasal organ*, used for pheromone signal *transduction* – the conversion from sensory stimuli into neural impulses.

Many animals rely heavily upon pheromone signalling, but primates instead evolved specialized facial muscles to convey emotions, and specialized brain regions such as the *fusiform gyrus* and amygdala to interpret those facial expressions. The ability to interpret social cues is vital – in modern primates, social skills are a greater predictor of survival and reproductive success than size or physical prowess.

Crown of Creation

We often forget humans are simply another animal species, and it's the height of arrogance to somehow assume we're superior to other species in importance or evolutionary progression. Far from the pinnacle of evolution, the human body is, for all its truly astounding potential, an imperfect machine.

For example, during primate evolution, we lost the ability to naturally break down *uric acid*, a natural byproduct of digesting the muscle protein *purine*. The gene encoding the enzyme which breaks down uric acid – *urate oxidase*– was switched off in the common ancestor of hominids, leaving us vulnerable to disease.

Human kidneys usually excrete uric acid in urine, but in the case of renal failure – inadequate filtering of waste products from the bloodstream – high levels of uric acid can crystallize as kidney or bladder stones. Uric acid crystals can also form in cartilage, tendons or tissues around the joints, causing swelling, redness, and severe, burning pain – the condition known as *gout*.

Although most people generally believe there's a distinction between apes and humans, humans are actually an ape species. Thus, evolution isn't a progressive march toward humankind from apehood, because there is no distinction between the two – humans are simply one more variety of ape.

Time

When two species diverge from a common ancestor, accumulated mutations create a genomic divergence. If the rate of mutations is known, it's theoretically possible to calculate the time that has passed between a living creature's genome and that of its ancestor. This method was used to determine when our forebears left Africa, some 100,000 years ago.

In examining modern orangutans – which genetic analyses show split from our lineage about 13 mya – researchers used this method to calculate a primate mutation rate of about 75 per generation.

The problem is that such a calculation produces an answer of about 6 million years for the human-chimp divergence at the high end of estimates, while anthropologists say the fossil record clearly shows human ancestors were already far too sophisticated at that point for the divergence to have been so relatively recent.

Fortunately, rather than having to approximate the rate at which the molecular clock works and applying it to rare fossils, we can watch the rate of mutations in humans alive today, comparing the genomes of parents and children.

Augustine Kong of Decode Genetics in Reykjavik, Iceland has scanned and compared the genomes of 78 sets of parents and children, and shown the rate of mutations in humans is actually an average of 36 per generation, half of what had been earlier predicted.

What this means is humans and chimpanzees must have split from their common ancestor much earlier than previous estimates predicted. Based on the average age of chimp reproduction and human reproduction, Kevin Langergraber of Boston University says the split occurred at least 7 million years ago, and perhaps as far back as 13 million years ago.

David Reich and his team at Harvard published a similar study a week later – after analyzing the DNA of over 85,000 Icelanders, focusing on short DNA strands called microsatellites, said to be a more accurate measure of mutation rates. The Harvard team said the mutation rate was not nearly as slow as Kong's team had estimated. Instead, they capped the timing of the split at 7.5 million years – a calculation that nicely predicts the era in which the most primitive hominid ancestor ever found is known to have lived, a creature discovered in 2001 and christened *Toumai*.

It's possible that the rate of hominid mutations has slowed over time, something that has been observed in some modern mammals. Such a deceleration would explain the discrepancy between the two dates.

Planet of the Apes

Some ten million years ago, during the late *Miocene* (Greek for *less recent*), Earth was covered in dense and lush tropical forests, and they were filled with a great variety of apes, which roamed the breadth and width of the planet. They had come to reign supreme, some 100 different species, ranging from the massive Eastern *cevapithecus*, twice the size of a modern human, to tiny *limnopithecus*, scampering about the heights of the forest canopy, feasting upon fruits inaccessible to any other creatures. To an ape, it was paradise. They had literally taken over the planet.

The Miocene ranged from roughly 23 to five million years ago. But after initially warming, the planet slowly began to cool. This radically altered the planet's ecosystems. By the end of the era, nearly all the jungles had vanished, replaced by global grasslands, in which modern grasses and sedges first evolved. In the northern climes, coniferous forests arose, and the seasons became fixed. In the oceans, the first *kelp bed* (brown algae) ecosystems appeared.

It was during this era that most recognizably modern life first emerged. On land, the global spread of tough, fibrous and fire-tolerant grasses drove many herbivores into extinction, but gave rise to new grassland ecosystems, displacing woodlands and jungles. The continents eventually teemed with fleet herds of long-legged, roaming grazers pursued by large predators across broad sweeps of open grasslands.

Among the recognizable mammals that emerged were dogs, raccoons, horses, beaver, deer and camels. In the oceans, the kelp forests gave rise to similar changes, as otters, whales and many modern fish adapted to the new ecosystem. By the era's end, nearly every modern bird family was present, including ducks, owls, crows, plovers and cockatoos, while marine birds reached their highest point of diversity.

Less recognizable species arose and vanished; in the seas were a variety of massive *macro-predators* such as the megatoothed shark *C. megalodon* and the predatory sperm whale *L. melvillei*. On land, a variety of tiny three-toed horses came and went, as well as hornless rhinos, gigantic crocodilians and meter-long piranha.

Planetary cooling and the loss of their jungle habitats doomed most of the Miocene apes, who all but vanished, leaving only a few species to evolve. Among them, however, were the ancestors of today's Great Apes.

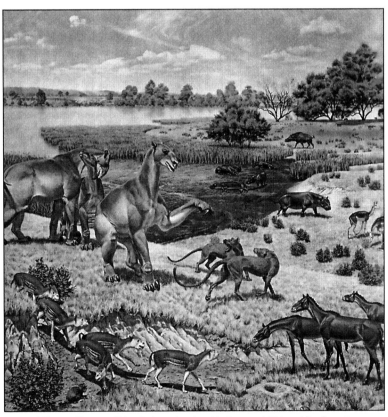

Miocene Fauna of North America, Jay Matternes, 1964, public domain

Apeman

When human and chimp genomes are compared, there are an estimated 15 million base-pair differences, with large sections of deleted or duplicated DNA, and mutations to regulatory DNA. The vast majority of these changes are too minor to affect physical traits or influence gene function. Only a few thousand affect genes sufficiently to alter body development and become eligible to be passed down through natural selection.

Through experimentation with transgenic animals, several genes have been identified which helped drive human evolution, genes central to critical junctures in the process, such as Homo sapiens' rapid brain expansion, the emergence of language production, and the origin of opposable thumbs.

For example, about 15 to 10 million years ago, a mutation in the *RNF213* gene led to improvements in the brain's blood supply, opening the door to the evolution of more sophisticated brains. A different mutation to this same RNF213 gene region results in *Moyamoya disease*, which produces narrowed arteries supplying blood to the brain.

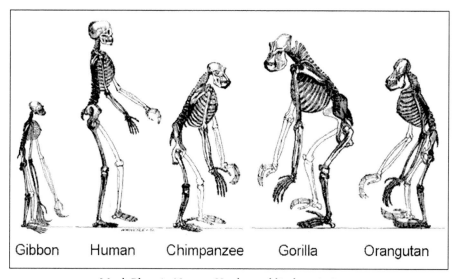

| Gibbon | Human | Chimpanzee | Gorilla | Orangutan |

Man's Place in Nature, Huxley, public domain image

The Final Split

Genetic analyses show that about ten million years ago, the gorillas split from the hominin lineage, followed by the chimpanzees about seven million years ago. The human branch of early hominins differed from both of these apes lineages in that they walked upright and had smaller *canine* teeth (fangs).

As far as we know, humans are the only species of our hominin lineage which survived. Our earlier hominin predecessors spent nearly seven million years of life in Africa, before modern humans ventured out approximately 100,000 years ago, then swept across the entire planet within a span of 40,000 years.

259

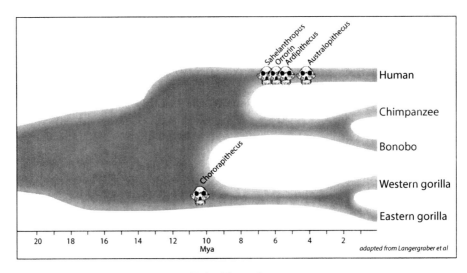

adapted from Langergraber et al

Join Together

En route to becoming human, we "lost" a chromosome. Great Apes – chimps, gorillas and orangutans – have 24 paired chromosomes, while humans have 23. In fact, when humans and chimps diverged, two of our chromosomes fused to form a single longer one, reducing our complement of pairs from 24 to 23. This can be clearly seen in chromosome two, the second longest in the human genome. In the following picture, the human chromosomes (on the left) are stacked next to the corresponding chimpanzee chromosomes (on the right), and all have a great degree of similarity, with the exception of chromosome two.

Human chromosome two is unique in that two smaller ancestral chromosomes are joined end-to-end. Two shorter chromosomes from the chimpanzee genome align nearly perfectly with this single, longer human chromosome two, and these genes between the two species are nearly identical, solidifying the case for evolution. In addition, human chromosome two has remnants of two *centromeres*, the midpoint at which chromosome pairs connect, as well as the remnants of two additional *telomeres*, the "caps" at the ends of chromosomes which protect DNA from unravelling.

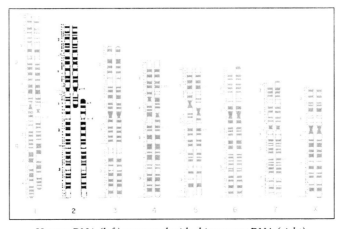

Human DNA (left) compared with chimpanzee DNA (right).

Humans Being

Chimpanzees and humans share somewhere around 98% of the same genes, but their brains differ substantially in volume, organization and complexity. The mechanisms behind that difference are under intense study.

Amino acid differences between chimps and humans are so minimal that they cannot explain most of the differences in traits between us and our nearest living Great Ape cousins. The main differences between chimps and humans is derived from non-coding regulatory DNA – in other words, most of our differences arise from the *regulation* of gene expression rather than differences among the genes themselves.

Only one of every hundred nucleotides differs between chimps and humans. This is substantially fewer than between rats and mice, whose nucleotides differ four times as much – by one in 25. Most of these differences create no effects. Entire gene substitutions between chimps and humans occur at a slightly higher rate than nucleotide substitutions, about 3%. These regions have been duplicated, deleted or inserted.

Gene duplications are particularly important – in fact the primary means by which any species evolves new genes: when a gene is duplicated, it frees up existing copies to perform the original function, while the extra copies can evolve new functions.

A classic example is found in *crystallins*, three transparent proteins found in human lenses, which focus light onto the eye's retina. Crystallins were originally *heat shock proteins*, produced in greater quantities (*upregulated*) in response to environmental stresses.

Crystallins and other heat shock proteins were originally used in muscles to protect critical proteins from *denaturing* – losing shape and clumping under environmental stresses like heat, infections, toxin exposure, starvation, hypoxia, or dehydration. Gene duplication in vertebrates during the Cambrian era half a billion years ago led to crystallins being expressed in the eyes, leading to the formation of lenses.

Win Some, Lose Some

Evolution also comes from differences in gene regulation and from gene "losses". When duplicated, genes usually don't come equipped with the necessary transcription machinery to activate them, so in their new positions they can no longer function, and lie dormant in the genome. They may also get "scrambled", so a stop codon is inserted within the protein-expressing region, causing RNA translation to prematurely end before a protein can be produced.

These are *pseudogenes* – non-functioning relics which lost their protein-coding capacity or transcription-influencing capabilities. This *pseudogenization* is common, and thought to be a major driver of evolutionary change. A total of 19,537 pseudogenes have been catalogued within the human genome, which can be compared with ancestral versions and matched to functions lost during the course of evolution.

After hominins diverged from the chimp-human lineage, 80 genes were inactivated. 36 of these encoded olfactory receptors, and one was for the bitter taste receptor *T2R62P*; others included the *hair keratin gene KRTHAP1*: humans still have nine keratin genes, but loss of KRTHAP1 may have resulted in the thinning out of human body hair 240,000 years ago.

Loss of the *Myosin gene MYH16* may have removed the final physical impediment to brain growth. Losing two base pairs from MYH16 led to smaller *masticatory* (chewing) muscles, allowing for a major increase in cranial capacity in the first true humans – *Homo habilis*.

CASPASE12 is an enzyme used in the mammalian immune system response that was silenced in humans by a premature stop codon. This counterintuitively reduced the deadliness of bacterial infections: bacteria fungi, viruses and some parasites can release complex molecules called *endotoxins*, which sometimes trigger a dramatic response by the body's immune system.

Endotoxins can be released into the blood, urinary tract, lungs, skin, or other tissues, but are particularly dangerous when released in the bloodstream, because they can be widely dispersed throughout the body. When CASPASE12 deactivated in humans, it significantly lowered susceptibility to *severe sepsis*, a potentially deadly immune system reaction to endotoxins which can cause organ failure and death.

Gene Genie

Leading the effort to identify the genes behind human evolution is Dr. Katherine S. Pollard of the University of California. Part of an international team which sequenced the chimpanzee genome in 2005, Dr. Pollard wrote a computer program to compare billions of base pairs which changed during our divergence from a common ancestor.

Her research uncovered 202 DNA regions highly conserved among vertebrates, relatively unchanged for hundreds of millions of years, which suddenly changed dramatically in humans. Five regions in particular changed drastically in humans, with a sevenfold increase in substitution rates among humans, but not other primates. These were mostly non-protein-producing, and near genes for transcription and binding.

Humans and chimps are so different despite nearly identical genes because creating a new species requires very little change; tweaking just a few key sites can have a major impact upon an organism's morphology and functioning. Dr. Pollard has uncovered perhaps the most important among these key sites – the *Human Accelerated Regions* (HARs), a set of genetic regions conserved throughout vertebrate history, but suddenly and markedly changed in the human genome.

These *conserved non-coding element* (CNE) regions experienced a burst of substitutions which led to the evolution of distinctly human traits. Two examples are *HAR1F*, believed to guide neural development in the brain, and *HAR2*, which seems to have played a central role in the development of the *opposable thumb*, enabling precise object grasping and manipulation.

Characteristic	HAR1	HAR2	HAR3	HAR4	HAR5
Location	5' region	Intron	Intron	Intergenic	Intron
Chromosome	Chromosome 20	Chromosome 2	Chromosome 7	Chromosome 16	Chromsome 12
Start[a]	61,203,966	236,556,014	1,979,228	71,686,982	844,471
Length	106 bp	119 bp	106 bp	119 bp	346 bp
Substitutions[b]					
Human	13.93	11.96	5.98	4.98	8.34
Chimp	1.08	0.10	0.05	0.02	0.44
LRT statistic[c]	60.31	35.62	14.40	13.88	10.36

[a]Coordinates from hg17 human genome assembly (build 35).
[b]Expected number of substitutions reported by the phyloP program.
[c]FDR adjusted $p < 4.5e-4$ for all five LRTs.
DOI: 10.1371/journal.pgen.0020168.t001

HARs also include genes expressing proteins central to embryonic neurodevelopment. Each region number is based upon how much it differs between humans and chimpanzees, with *HAR1* signifying the highest degree of human-chimp differences.

HAR1 is a stretch of 106 nucleotide base pairs located on the longer arm of chromosome 20. It contains parts of the RNA-expressing gene *HAR1F*, which participates in human brain development.

Comparing HAR1 between humans and 12 other vertebrates, Dr. Pollard discovered major differences in the human form: Until we emerged, HAR1 had evolved at a crawl – only two out of the 118 base pairs in HAR1 differ between chimps and chickens, vertebrate species separated by 300 million years of evolution.

HAR1's conservation over hundreds of millions of years shows its extreme importance for survival. But in humans, this region changed incredibly rapidly and drastically: 18 novel base pairs sprang into existence since the split from our common chimp-human ancestor eight million years ago – a 900% increase in evolutionary change in one-fortieth the time.

Human HAR1 is expressed mainly in the brain and testes. It's a region encompassing two overlapping genes which encode a special type of RNA – in fact, an entirely new class. Tests show this RNA helps guide embryonic formation of the *cerebral cortex*, the brain's wrinkly outermost layer. HAR1 switches on in fetuses between the seventh and nineteenth weeks, in cells which differentiate and migrate to the cortex.

The main feature distinguishing a human brain from that of a chimp is this hugely expanded cortex, the outermost layer responsible for our most sophisticated cognitive processing – planning, reasoning and language production.

Interestingly, over half the genes clustered near the HAR regions participate in brain development and function, and other human-accelerated regions may also indirectly affect brain development. The majority of these don't encode proteins or RNA, but are regulatory sequences which switch nearby genes on and off, or give rise to regulatory molecules.

Because of this role in regulation, though HARs are only a tiny fraction of the human genome, even minor changes to these regions result in major changes to the evolving human brain, influencing entire networks of other genes.

Human brains more than tripled in volume after our divergence from our common human-chimp ancestor, and a second gene called *ASPM* (abnormal spindle-like microcephaly-associated), which encodes a protein in immature neurons, is a major part of that size increase, in both humans and other animals.

Studies of patients with *microcephaly*, whose brains are 70 percent smaller than average, have shown the key role of ASPM and three related genes (*MCPH1, CDK5RAP2* and *CENPJ*) in controlling brain size, and research at the Universities of Chicago and Michigan has demonstrated that ASPM underwent several evolutionary bursts during primate evolution. One such burst took place specifically among humans, and is likely to have been instrumental in the development of our comparatively large cortices.

In 2012, scientists also discovered that, about 3 million years ago, two duplications of the *SRGAPz* gene emerged. SRGAP2 accelerates the migration of fetal neurons from their development site to their final location, and triggers the formation of more neural spines, allowing for more plentiful neural connections.

The second fastest evolving HAR – *HAR2* – is a 119-base-pair sequence on chromosome two, which includes the gene enhancer *HACNS1*. Enhancers such as HACNS1 can ramp up gene expression, usually protein production.

Out of every 110,000 known human gene enhancers, HACNS1 changed the most since humans diverged from the evolutionary lineage that includes chimpanzees. The human version drives gene expression in the wrist and thumb during fetal development, and likely is at the heart of the anatomical development of the human hand, allowing the crafting and use of tools – thought to be the turning point at which we truly became "human". HACNS1 may also have led to modifications to the ankle and foot which allowed bipedalism.

While such key shifts in physiology helped our ancestors adapt to changing circumstances and migrate to more favorable climes, genetic adaptations also enabled our ancestors to thrive upon a much more diverse diet. To digest foods high in starch, we evolved multiple copies of the *AMY1* gene, which encodes the salivary enzyme *amylase*. Cooking and agriculture would allow us to make use of an even broader range of foods.

Similarly, the *lactase enzyme* gene *LCT* allows us to digest *lactose* – milk sugar. Among most other species, only nursing infants can digest lactose, but about 9,000 years ago, we evolved a version of LCT which allows adults to consume milk. Since the human form of LCT evolved independently among different populations worldwide, lactose tolerance varies by race. The descendants of ancient European and African herders are significantly more likely to tolerate lactose than those from Asia and Latin America.

Right Here, Right Now

Says Dr. Pollard, the chimp genome project discovered 15 genes shifting from earlier primate versions which are beneficial to other mammals, but linked to diseases like Alzheimer's and cancer in humans.

Since many of these diseases only afflict humans or have a much higher prevalence than in other primates, it appears the ancestral versions of these genes became maladaptive in Homo sapiens.

Struggling with infectious diseases results in an ongoing genomic arms race between microbes and their hosts, as animals try to survive long enough to pass along their genes to future generations. Because they're so central to species survival, immunity-related genes are frequently top candidates for evidence of natural selection in humans. Says Dr. Pollard, evolution constantly tinkers with these genes:

> ...in the absence of antibiotics and vaccines, the most likely obstacle to individuals passing along their genes would probably be a life-threatening infection that strikes before the end of their childbearing years. Further accelerating the evolution of the immune system is the constant adaptation of pathogens to our defenses, leading to an evolutionary arms race. Records of these struggles are left in our DNA. This is particularly true for retroviruses, such as HIV, that survive and propagate by inserting their genetic material into our genomes. Human DNA is littered with copies of these short retroviral genomes, many from viruses that caused diseases millions of years ago and that may no longer circulate. Over time the retroviral sequences accumulate random mutations just as any other sequence does, so that the different copies are similar but not identical. By examining the amount of divergence among these copies, researchers can use molecular clock techniques to date the original retroviral infection. The scars of these ancient infections are also visible in the host immune system genes that constantly adapt to fight the ever evolving retroviruses.

Among these relic viruses is *PtERV1*. Genetic analyses show the PtERV1 virus triggered an epidemic about four million years ago among ancient African primates. In response, primates evolved specialized enzymes to destroy the threat. The human version that modified after we inherited it is protein *TRIM5a*, which blocks replication of PtERV1 and other related retroviruses.

To see how different primates respond to this long-dead virus, researchers reconstructed PtERV1, guided by randomly-mutated copies of it which had become incorporated into the chimpanzee genome. They next tested human and ape versions of the enzyme TRIM5a on the resurrected virus and found a single change in human TRIM5a equipped us to fight PtERV1 more effectively than earlier primates.

But while mutations to the TRIM5a gene aided humans against PtERV1, the same shifts, says Dr. Pollard, made it significantly harder for us to fight HIV. Because of this, humans develop AIDS from HIV, while other primates don't.

De Novo

A 2011 study by four Chinese, American and Canadian universities found 60 protein-encoding genes which arose *de novo* in humans. *De novo* is Latin for *anew*, meaning these genes are mutations which didn't exist in an ancestor, as opposed to duplications, transposons or dormant genes exapted for novel functions. In other words, they're mutations which spontaneously arose in one hominin and were passed down, to remain in the human genome over the past eight million years.

These 60 protein-encoding genes are most highly expressed in the cerebral cortex and testes, indicating they produce uniquely human traits, such as improved cognition. Drs. Wu, Irwin, and Zhang said the high expression of these genes in the testes shows their role in human reproduction, while their high expression in the cerebral cortex contributed to the evolution of the human brain and cognitive abilities.

The following year, in 2012, University of Edinburgh researchers announced the discovery of a powerful gene they believe helps explain the evolution of modern human cognition. *miR-941* is unique to humans, and seems to have played a central role in our brain development, particularly in regions critical for tool use, decision-making, advanced coordination, and language.

miR-941 regulates genes during stem cell differentiation and neural formation, as well as neurotransmitter signalling. It's comparatively highly expressed, acting upon the executive control center of the human brain – the prefrontal cortex, as well as, to a lesser degree, the brain's coordination and balance center, the cerebellum. It operates chiefly upon two signalling pathways: hedgehog and insulin signalling:

Hedgehog signalling is central to embryonic development and the maintenance of adult stem cells, and its abnormal activation is associated with some cancers. miR-941 expression is highest in embryonic stem cells and in several cancer-derived human cell lines, where cancer appears to be a form of runaway production.

The *insulin-signalling* pathway plays a central role in lifespan regulation among many species, including humans, and insulin-pathway targets of miR-941 include genes directly involved in lifespan extension in model organisms. One of its targets in particular, the *FOXO1* gene, has been linked to increased human longevity.

Because humans are both longer-lived and have higher rates of cancers than other primates, the authors think miR-941 helped enable a longer human lifespan by maintaining adult stem cells, but simultaneously made humans more susceptible to cancer.

The miR-941 gene is found on human chromosome 20, where it expresses *microRNA 941*, a 24 base-pair segment of microRNA. MicroRNAs silence gene expression by binding to messenger RNA, blocking protein synthesis by the ribosome. The emergence of new miRNAs is comparatively rare, and is generally linked to significant evolutionary changes, as they tend to have a profound influence.

Since they target most of the human genome, miRNAs exercise major regulatory influence; the emergence of a single new miRNA can influence the expression of potentially hundreds of genes at once. miRNA mutations are therefore thought to be a much more powerful evolutionary mechanism than mutations to single protein-encoding genes. The Edinburgh team believes the miR-941 gene thus played a central role in driving human evolution.

DNA analysis of a tooth from an extinct hominin race called the *Denisovans*, which split from humans about one million years ago, shows they possessed at least two miR-941 copies, while contemporary humans have an average of seven, though this varies by geographic region.

Failsafe

As primates evolved, their genomes grew increasingly complex, multiplying the risks of generating "faulty" DNA. Increasing genomic complexity escalates the possibility of problems arising – deleterious transposons, damaged DNA or its faulty repair, all associated with cancer. However, 18 million years ago, two genes fused to protect primates from these growing risks, at a time when the Great Apes were first starting to diverge.

SETMAR (also known as *Metnase*) is a *chimeric gene*, the product of a merging between a 50-million-year-old DNA region that promotes gene-jumping, with one that has controlled vertebrate gene silencing for half a billion years. In its present form, SETMAR appears to repair DNA damage, helping to protect against cancer.

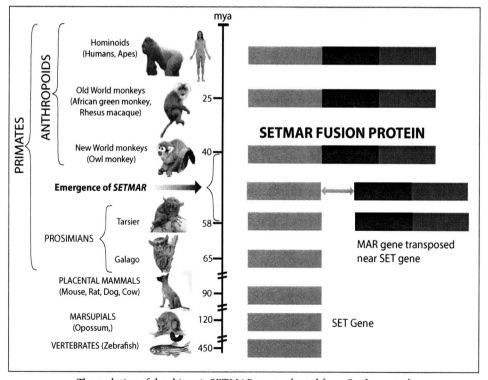

The evolution of the chimeric SETMAR gene, adapted from Cordaux, et al.

The human version of SETMAR is located on chromosome three, and it's widely expressed in the human body, particularly the placenta and ovaries. It's fusion of a transposed enzyme gene – *MARiner*, exclusive to primates – with an ancient epigenetic-control vertebrate gene called *SET*. Together, the two improve genomic stability.

Four American and French geneticists have reconstructed the evolutionary history of this chimeric gene. According to the team, the original SETMAR is now found in all apes, but in humans it has modified via natural selection. The SET portion now matches binding sites which duplicated 1,500 times in humans, pointing to the enzyme's extreme importance. SET is a 450-million-year-old gene which expresses an enzyme that methylates histones, tightening chromatin coils so their DNA cannot be accessed for transcription.

MARiner promotes transposition, but in fusing with SET, the gene switched from promoting migration of DNA fragments to promoting their repair. In other words, by joining to a SET gene, the MARiner enzyme has been "tamed", so instead of causing genome rearrangements which might lead to cancer, it represses such DNA shuffling.

Genetic damage from radiation, toxins, or faulty processing can lead to *double-stranded breaks* (DSBs), one of the major causes of cell death. To repair this, most living cells usually engage in *Non-Homologous End Joining* (NHEJ). The process is *non-homologous* because DNA ends which don't match can be directly sealed using short DNA sequences called *microhomologies*, without the need for more complex, error-prone processes – faulty DNA repair has been linked to leukemia and other cancers, and malfunctions in double-stranded break repair appear to be the main culprit.

SETMAR's enzyme nicks the free ends of DNA so they fuse together efficiently. It increases the rate of Non-Homologous End Joining, repairing faults, and thus reducing the chance DNA fragments can migrate into other nuclear domains (*translocation*). By suppressing chromosomal translocations and faulty DNA repair, SETMAR significantly reduces the possibility of *oncogenicity* – the promotion of tumor formation.

If the incorporation of new DNA is a kind of bug-prone "software upgrade", SETMAR acts as a checksum and patching routine. And since novel genes are a central part of evolution, SETMAR is thought to have played a key role in human development.

Big Brains

Human brains are, on average, 300% the volume of those of chimpanzees, our nearest relative. Dr. John Hawks of the University of Wisconsin-Madison believes that, rather than being due to separate, unrelated mutations, the rapid human brain expansion was due to a cascade of mutations. The first of these mutations initiated beneficial changes which allowed subsequent mutations, further enhancing the brain.

By comparing DNA sequences between humans and other animals, as well as the genomes of people with *microcephaly* – where the brain is abnormally small – and *macrocephaly* – where the brain is abnormally large, Dr. James Sikela believes he may have found what triggered that cascade, concluding in 2012: "...what drove the evolutionary expansion of the human brain may well be a specific unit within a protein – called a *protein domain* – that is far more numerous in humans than other species."

Protein domains are protein regions able to function and evolve independently from the rest of the molecule. Each domain has its own three-dimensional structure, which can act independently of the other domains, folding and functioning as a unit. Many proteins have several such structural domains, and a specific domain may exist among a variety of different proteins.

Protein domains can be used as modular building blocks, and can be recombined in different arrangements, to create proteins with different functions. They vary in length, ranging from 25 to 500 amino acids in length, and are independently stable, allowing domains to be "swapped" between proteins during genetic engineering, to make new combinations known as *chimeric proteins*.

The protein domain on which Dr. Hawks has focussed is *DUF1220*. Modern humans have over 270 copies of it in their genome, far more than any other animal. And the closer a species is on the evolutionary scale to humans, the more copies of DUF1220 it possesses. Chimpanzees possess 125 copies, gorillas 99, marmosets 30, and mice just one. The single overriding theme Dr. Hawks' team repeatedly observed was that the greater the number of DUF1220 copies were in the creature's DNA, the bigger its brain was. DUF1220 has also been linked to brain disorders – a lower number results in microcephaly, while larger numbers were linked to macrocephaly.

In the spring of 2011, a research team from Yale, Cambridge, Harvard, and Northwestern Universities found a single gene involved in cell division called *NDE1* can control this difference in cortical size.

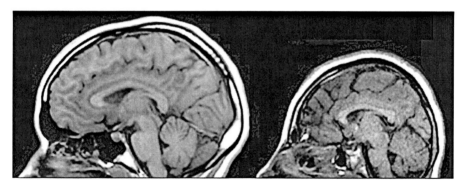

MRI scans of a healthy patient (left), and one with microcephaly. Primary microcephaly is caused by two copies of a mutation in one of the microcephalin genes. Image: PLOS, public domain.

Later that same year, an international research team at Yale and in Turkey was analyzing the unfortunate genetic disorder of a Turkish man with a smooth-surfaced brain, and located the specific gene which produces the deep folds and wrinkles on the surface of the human brain. These wrinkles and folds expand the available surface area of the cerebral cortex tremendously, granting the capacity for abstract and logic thought.

Cortical wrinkling only occurs in the largest-brained mammals – dolphins and apes – but it's most prominent among the human species. The deep grooves – called *sulci* in Latin – greatly expand the brain's surface area within the skull's confines, allowing more neurons to fit within a compact space.

The gene which gives rise to these convolutions is *laminin gamma 3 (LAMC3)*, and the deletion of only two of its base pairs leads to a smooth cortex. LAMC3 is expressed in embryonic development, during the formation of *dendrites,* the rootlike extensions nerves use to connect.

Energy

The human brain uses about 20 percent of the body's total energy intake at rest; as Duke University evolutionary biologist Greg Wray puts it, "It's a very metabolically demanding tissue." In comparison, the brains of other primates only require about eight percent. According to Dr. Wray, a uniquely human adaptation arose to help meet the demands of our ever-more voracious brains: glucose, our main energy source, was diverted from our bodies to our brains.

Glucose is drawn into the cerebral cortex by special glucose-transporter molecules in the bloodstream. Uniquely human genes encoding those transporter molecules (*SLC2A1* and *SLC2A4*) enhance glucose transport to our brains at the expense of our muscles. The human mutations led to more glucose transporters in the brain and fewer in the muscles. In other words, our lucky forebears developed and passed down genes that sacrificed brawn for brains, to our immense adaptive advantage.

Dr. Wray notes other genes are probably involved in a complex web of energy trade-offs between the brain and other tissues, including genes for carbohydrate and lipid digestion – and the shrinking of the human gut also likely played a role.

Hope

In 2001, French and Chad paleontologists were stunned by the discovery of a seven-million-year-old hominin skull in the Djurab desert of Northern Chad. They had just stumbled across remains of one of the first humans ever to walk the Earth. The team named their discovery *Toumai – Hope of Life* in the African Gouran language.

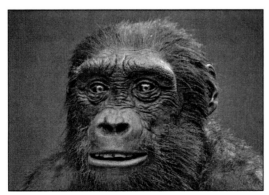

Sahelanthropus tchadensis, *better known by the name of* **Toumai***. Artist John Gurche created this likeness for the Smithsonian's National Museum of Natural History.*

Toumai lived between seven and six million years ago in West-Central Africa (Chad). Used with permission.

Toumai was male and bipedal. Geological analyses show the area had been a wooded lake shore, At the time he was alive. He was given the formal scientific name *Sahelanthropus tchadensis*, and is likely the very first human ancestor.

Like chimpanzees, Toumai's species lived in groups of six or more, headed by a single dominant male, alternating between walking and tree-climbing. About as tall as a modern chimp, Toumai had forward-facing eyes and comparatively nimble hands, and its brain was about a third the size of a modern human's.

Biting Down

Compared to the formidable bone-shearing bite of a chimpanzee, humans have a weak bite. This appears to be due to a single mutation which deactivates the muscle-protein-encoding *MYH16* gene. Human jaw muscles are made from a different version of the protein than those of chimpanzees, and as a result are much less robust.

According to the University of Pennsylvania's Dr. Hansell Stedman, primates with thicker jaw muscles have more supporting bone at the back of their skulls, constraining skull expansion. Our evolution of smaller jaw muscles allowed our brain cases to expand, removing a major evolutionary constraint upon brain development.

The mutation arose sometime between five to two and a half million years ago – right before a major expansion of hominid brain mass. Dr. Stedman believes that this is because our ancestors had stopped relying upon biting attacks in combat at this point.

The Long and Winding Road

Along the path to modern human development, a host of small-brained, bipedal apes came and went, with brains roughly the size of a chimpanzee's. The differences between them were subtle, but they were all bipedal, with large snouts, and generally chimp-sized brains. They were extremely well-adapted to their environments, and so their suite of adaptations and way of life persisted for millions of years.

In fact, for nearly 5 million years, the brains of hominin bipeds barely grew at all, with the group of apelike hominins called the Australopithecines collectively surviving for a little over two million years. Together, the primitive hominins flourished over 25 times the entire length of modern human existence, sometimes living side-by-side.

At least 20 other hominin species have been identified, all but our own line vanishing in the mists of time. More almost certainly existed. Controversy still centers around which of these are our direct ancestors, but one sure sign of our common ancestry is the human *coccyx*, a *vestigial* tail – an ancestral trait which remains in us, even though it's no longer functional. Those species which are generally agreed upon include:

- *Sahelanthropus tchadensis*: Africa, 7 mya

- *Orrorin tugeninsis*: Africa, 6 mya

- *Ardipithecus kadabba*: Africa, 5.8 - 5.2 mya

- *Ardipithecus ramidus*: Africa, 4.4 mya

- *Australopithecus anamensis*: Africa, 4.2 to 3.9 mya

- *Australopithecus afarensis*: Africa, 3.85 to 2.95 mya

- *Kenyanthropus platyops*: Africa, 3.5 mya

- *Australopithecus africanus*: Africa, 3 to 2.4 mya

- *Paranthropus aethiopicus*, Africa, 2.7 to 2.3 mya

- *Australopithecus garhi*: Africa, 2.5 mya

- *Australopithecus sediba*: Africa, 1.95 to 1.78 mya

- *Homo habilis*: Africa, 2.5 to 1.6 mya

- *Paranthropus robustus*: Africa, 1.8 to 1.2 mya

- *Paranthropus boisei*: Africa, 2.3 to 1.2 mya

- *Homo rudolfensis*: Africa, 1.9 to 1.8 mya

- *Homo erectus*: 1.8 mya to 300,000 years ago

- *Homo heidelbergensis*: Europe, Asia, Africa, 700,000 to 200,000 years ago

- *Homo floresiensis (Hobbits)*: Indonesia, 95,000 – 17,000 years ago

- *Homo neanderthalensis*: Europe, Asia, 200,000 - 28,000 years ago

- *Homo sapiens*: Evolved in Africa, now worldwide, 200,000 years ago to present

The first hominins appear to have been scavengers, and several species existed at the same time, and likely had mutual interactions. The 20 hominins most widely agreed upon come from four main groups, sharing the same broad characteristics:

1. ***Ardipithecus (7 to 4.4 mya, incl. Toumai and Orrorin)*** – The oldest group of hominins, several species of *Ardipithecus* (from the Afar language for *ground monkey*) have been unearthed. They are unique among hominins in possessing a big toe with grasping capabilities, indicating they spent at least some of their lives in the trees.

   In these early humans, the hole in the skull where the spinal cord enters and connects to the brain, the *foramen magnum*, is located at the bottom of the skull, showing these creatures were the first primates to walk upright – all other primates have a foramen magnum at the back of the skull.

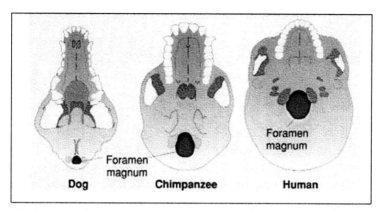

Position of the foramen magnum across three species. Wikipedia, public domain.

Like later hominins, Ardipithecus had smaller canine teeth. They also had relatively small brains – about the same size as a modern chimpanzee's, but much smaller than that of the later australopithecines – approximately 20% the size of a modern human's. Their upper and lower jaws also jutted forward like those of a chimpanzee. Ardipithecus had unspecialized teeth, and appear to have been omnivores, primarily subsisting on fruit.

2. *Australopithecus (4.2 to 1.78 mya)*– Four small species of apes called *gracile australopithecines (graceful southern apes)*, which were bipedal and emerged from South Africa. They ranged from four to five feet tall, with brain sizes from 350 cc to 600 cc. Famous fossils include *Lucy* and the infant *Selam*.

3. *Paranthropus (2.7 to 1.2 mya)* – Three species of *paranthropus (beside humans)* have been discovered. Alternatively referred to as *robust australopithecines*, these creatures were the same height as their namesake brethren, but of a much sturdier build, with broader, stronger skulls. They also stand out for having extremely large cheekbones, jaws and teeth, for a powerful bite, as well as a bony, spinelike ridge atop the skull called a *sagittal crest*. This side branch of hominins went extinct well before the appearance of modern humans.

4. *Homo (1.9 mya to present)* – These are the most modern hominins – humans. There appear to have been a few species, including the famous *hobbits (homo floresiensis* from Indonesia) and *Neanderthals*. The members of the homo group had flatter, narrower faces, smaller jaws and larger braincases, housing larger brains. Hand-crafted prehistoric tools have been retrieved from the sites in which these hominin species lived, generally chipped stone hand choppers, scrapers and knives. There is some evidence, however, that *Australopithecus garhi* may have been the first to create such technology, much earlier, though such findings are in dispute.

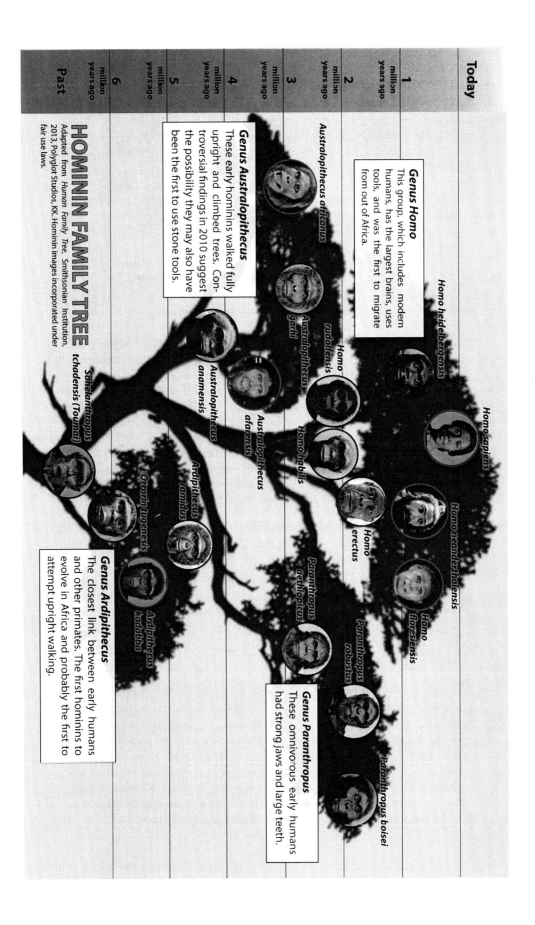

Today	
1 million years ago	
2 million years ago	
3 million years ago	
4 million years ago	
5 million years ago	
6 million years ago	
Past	

HOMININ FAMILY TREE

Adapted from *Human Family Tree*, Smithsonian Institution, 2013, Polyglot Studios, KK. Hominin images incorporated under fair use laws.

Genus Homo

This group, which includes modern humans, has the largest brains, uses tools, and was the first to migrate from out of Africa.

Genus Australopithecus

These early hominins walked fully upright and climbed trees. Controversial findings in 2010 suggest the possibility they may also have been the first to use stone tools.

Genus Ardipithecus

The closest link between early humans and other primates. The first hominins to evolve in Africa and probably the first to attempt upright walking.

Genus Paranthropus

These omnivorous early humans had strong jaws and large teeth.

Homo sapiens

Homo heidelbergensis

Homo neanderthalensis

Homo floresiensis

Homo erectus

Homo rudolfensis

Homo habilis

Australopithecus africanus

Australopithecus garhi

Australopithecus anamensis

Australopithecus afarensis

Sahelanthropus tchadensis (Toumaï)

Orrorin tugenensis

Ardipithecus ramidus

Ardipithecus kadabba

Paranthropus aethiopicus

Paranthropus robustus

Paranthropus boisei

In Europe, *Homo Heidelbergensis* would eventually evolve into the *Neanderthals*, a species we appear to have coexisted with for thousands of years, and, as new DNA evidence indicates, with which we even interbred.

Recent Homo (homo sapiens/cro-magnon 200,000 to present) – Fully modern humans have the flattest faces, smallest teeth, and largest brains of the homo lineage. Like Homo sapiens, however, Neanderthals might have also been painters and artisans, and there is evidence that Heidelbergensis buried their dead in a ceremonial fashion.

Walk

So how did humans evolve from the other primates?

One monumental physical adaptation is believed to have been the defining trait which triggered the emergence of our species about six million years ago: a 4-foot tall creature called *Orrorin tugenensis* began walking upright on the ground.

It's believed this is the single critical act which led to the first humans. Since then, our nearest ape relatives – bonobos and chimpanzees – have evolved very little over the last 7.5 million years, while our line diversified significantly. The first major difference between these lineages was in our ability to walk upright.

Human evolution is highly contentious, however, with major disagreements about which hominids walked bipedally, what they ate, and which can be classified as truly "human".

To determine whether common ancestors of humans and chimps lived in the trees or upon the ground, anthropologists focus on anatomy and behavior. Apes like gibbons and orangutans, more distant from humans than chimpanzees, are mainly *arboreal* (tree-dwelling), while closely-related apes like gorillas and chimps tend to be terrestrial, though they are still skilful tree-climbers.

The first hominins had the opposable big toes and flat feet of arboreal apes. In addition to the *foramen magnum* at the bottom of their skulls, they would develop shorter, flared hips, and larger *femur* (thigh bone) heads. The earliest seem to have retained arboreal and quadrupedal anatomical features even after having evolved bipedalism, suggesting the transition to life on the ground may have been gradual.

The splayed walking stance of chimps would eventually disappear during the progression to human bipedalism – walking with one foot placed in front of the other; this came from anatomical changes to the hip joint, femur, and foot. Early *Australopithecine* footprints are bipedal, but still splayed, when compared to modern humans.*

Bipedalism and an upright stance are not equivalent – animals like T. Rex which lacked vertical backbones were still bipedal, and fossil evidence shows bipedalism was habitual before a modern spine and upright stance emerged.

Charles Darwin proposed that early human ancestors first stood upright to free their hands for tools and weapons, but more recent studies indicate bipedalism evolved for a variety of simpler reasons, including food transport, efficient running, fighting, traversing rugged terrain, and for reaching distant branches while foraging among trees.

Take it Easy

Chimps are, says Harvard's Dr. Daniel E. Lieberman, "energy gluttons", expending four times as much energy walking as humans. Even the smallest anatomical changes result in major energy savings, and when open grasslands began to take over the African landscape, it placed greater energy demands upon our quadrupedal ape ancestors. As the rainforests shrank, they needed to travel progressively farther to find food among shrinking fruit patches.

Orrorin thus probably began walking on two legs simply because it was easier, i.e. more energy efficient; bipedalism requires significantly less food and rest than adding the use of forelimbs for quadrupedal walking.

In 2007, anthropologists at the University of California compared metabolic and kinetic data from chimpanzees and humans using a treadmill. The chimpanzees were trained to walk bipedally on the treadmill in addition to their natural quadrupedal manner. Tests showed that humans on two legs only require 25% of the caloric energy of chimpanzees walking on four legs, and that chimpanzees who were most skilled at bipedal walking used significantly less energy than their peers – getting most of the caloric savings from taking longer strides.

Dr. David Carrier of the University of Utah, however, argues that bipedalism is actually more energy-expensive when it comes to speeding up and slowing down, and that there is an additional loss of agility, suggesting there must have been a different advantage to the adaptation.

Modern great apes and other mammals often stand to fight or threaten rivals over territory and access to mates. In fact, while almost every mammal moves on all fours while running or covering long distances, many stand to use their front limbs in a fight, including anteaters, bears, horses, lions, rabbits, and wolves.

Standing upright, says Dr. Carrier, confers advantages in a fight, perhaps one reason natural selection led to modern-day humans – and why women often prefer tall men. Kinetic measurements show striking downward from an upright, two-legged position delivers more powerful blows than blows delivered upward, sideways or from the front on all fours. Because of this, tall men fight at an advantage.

Using a punching bag with a sensor to compare the kinetic force of punches, Dr. Carrier had boxers and martial artists punch the bag at four different angles: forwards, sideways, up and down. All the volunteers struck from 44 to 64 percent harder while standing, and generated 3.3 times as much force when hitting downward rather than upward.

It's long been assumed that women prefer tall men because height demonstrates superior genetic stock. But Dr. Carrier says this would mean men would also prefer tall women, when in fact men tend to prefer women of average height or less.

In Dr. Carrier's opinion, tall males in human prehistory were at an advantage in fights because they had more force when punching downward, making them better at defending their resources, children and mates. Greater force when striking opponents probably gave tall men a competitive advantage in territorial defense and in mate selection.

This doesn't mean women prefer violent or abusive men, he hastens to add, but that tallness subconsciously demonstrates an ancient evolutionary advantage. Women, he says, "are attracted to men who are powerful, because they can better protect them and their children".

Carry that Weight

Three million years ago, the Earth's axis shifted, causing the planet to point away from the Sun for longer periods of time. The result was an overall planetary cooling, and a locking away of moisture in ice at the North and South Poles.

Temperatures plummeted, and the formerly humid African air became stripped of moisture. The woodlands shrivelled, leaving wide belts of open terrain in their place. The current slight tilt to the Earth's axis of rotation as it orbits the Sun makes the planet point toward the Sun some of the time and away from it at others. This gives rise to seasons. Africa started to dry out, forcing the apes to adapt or perish.

An international research team led by Dr. Brian Richmond of George Washington University says scarcity drove bipedalism: the ability to carry rare, high-quality resources. To understand what ecological conditions could lead apes like our eight-million-year-old ancestors to walk on two legs, Dr. Richmond was among an American, British, Japanese and Portuguese research cooperative which studied the behavior of modern chimpanzees competing for food resources.

Says Dr. Richmond, an item's scarcity makes it difficult to predict when it will be encountered again, and in conditions of scarcity, chimpanzees switch to walking on two limbs rather than four to carry more at once. Over time, intense bursts of such bipedal activity led to physical adaptations, which became the subject of natural selection where competition for food or other resources was most pronounced.

In 2013, however, researchers at the University of York and the Parisian Institut de Physique du Globe concluded that bipedalism was born out of the need to scramble over rugged terrain in East and South Africa, formed during the Pliocene era by tectonic plate and volcanic activity. Rocky outcrops and gorges provided shelter and a superior means of trapping prey, though accessing them required upright scrambling and climbing.

As Dr Isabelle Winder puts it, "The broken, disrupted terrain offered benefits for hominins in terms of security and food, but it also proved a motivation to improve their locomotor skills by climbing, balancing, scrambling and moving swiftly over broken ground -- types of movement encouraging a more upright gait."

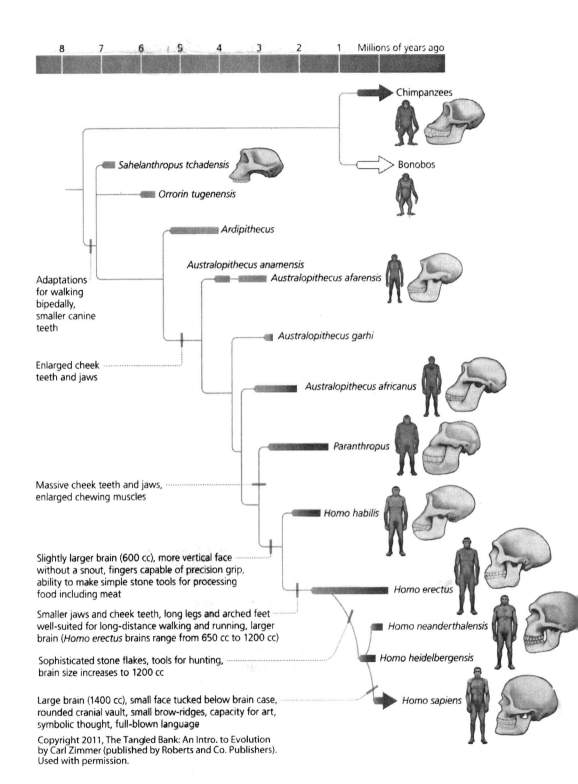

8   7   6   5   4   3   2   1   Millions of years ago

Chimpanzees

Sahelanthropus tchadensis

Bonobos

Orrorin tugenensis

Ardipithecus

Australopithecus anamensis
Australopithecus afarensis

Adaptations
for walking
bipedally,
smaller canine
teeth

Australopithecus garhi

Enlarged cheek
teeth and jaws

Australopithecus africanus

Paranthropus

Massive cheek teeth and jaws,
enlarged chewing muscles

Homo habilis

Slightly larger brain (600 cc), more vertical face
without a snout, fingers capable of precision grip,
ability to make simple stone tools for processing
food including meat

Homo erectus

Smaller jaws and cheek teeth, long legs and arched feet
well-suited for long-distance walking and running, larger
brain (*Homo erectus* brains range from 650 cc to 1200 cc)

Homo neanderthalensis

Sophisticated stone flakes, tools for hunting,
brain size increases to 1200 cc

Homo heidelbergensis

Large brain (1400 cc), small face tucked below brain case,
rounded cranial vault, small brow-ridges, capacity for art,
symbolic thought, full-blown language

Homo sapiens

278

Millennium Man

Orrorin tugenensis (*original man* in a Kenyan dialect) was nicknamed *Millennium Man* because of the 2000 discovery of this group of fossils in four sites of the Tugen Hills in Kenya. The sediments in which they were recovered are between 6 and 5.8 million years old, according to radioisotopic, paleomagnetic and biochronological dating. Orrorin, possibly along with Sahelanthropus tchadensis, was likely the earliest bipedal human ancestor.

20 Orrorin fossils have been recovered from five individuals, including teeth and lower jaw fragments, pieces of the *humerus* (upper arm bone), *femur* (thigh bone), and *phalanx* (finger bone). Orrorin's teeth are a mixture of the apelike and modern hominin varieties. Its femur and phalanx also show it had the ability to walk bipedally or to climb in trees. Its habitats were near lakes and stream, and it seems to have lived primarily in a woodland environment.

Man from the South

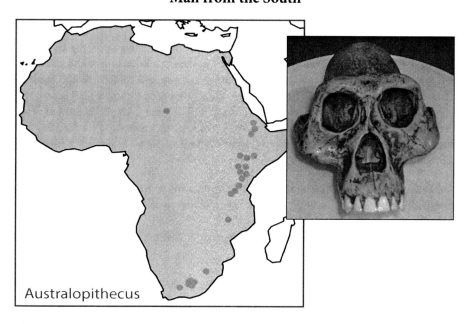

Australopithecus

If it could be said there was truly a "missing link" between humans and chimpanzees, it would be *Australopithecus*, whose name is derived from the Latin and Greek words for *southern* and *ape*. This extinct group of hominins arose in eastern Africa around four million years ago, and spread across the continent over the next two and a half million years, before finally going extinct.

Several species of Australopithecines came and went, including *Australopithecus afarensis, A. africanus, A. anamensis, A. bahrelghazali, A. garhi* and *A. sediba*. Some scholars assign A. robustus and A. boisei to the same genus and call them *robust australopiths*, while others classify them within the *Paranthropus* genus.

279

The Australopithecines were all members of the relatively small-brained, bipedal species which lived in ancient Africa. As they evolved into new species, however, their lower jaws and teeth shrank, brows receded, and brains enlarged, eventually to three times that of a chimpanzee's.

The first australopithecine remains ever discovered were those of the *Taung child* – the 2½-million-year-old fossilized skull of an Australopithecus africanus infant. It was unearthed in 1924 in Taung, South Africa by workers digging at a limestone quarry, but recent sophisticated analytical equipment has yielded further fascinating insight into human evolution from this specimen.

In 2012, Florida State University evolutionary anthropologist Dr. Dean Falk led a team which analyzed the Taung skull and found two striking and telltale features: the first is an unfused seam in the frontal skull bone called a *persistent metopic suture*, a feature which makes baby skulls more pliable during childbirth, as they squeeze through the birth canal. Among great apes such as gorillas, orangutans and chimpanzees, this metopic suture closes shortly after birth, but among humans, this fusion doesn't occur until around age two, thus accommodating rapid infant brain development.

The second feature found by Dr. Falk is the imprint of the brain upon the inner surface of the fossilized skull, allowing his team to analyze the brain's form and structure. By comparing the Taung fossil to huge numbers of ape and human skulls, in addition to corresponding 3D CT (three-dimensional computed tomographic) scans, and considering the fossil record of the past three million years, Dr. Falk and her team concluded that the persistent metopic suture is a specific adaptation for birthing babies with larger brains, allowing rapid development of those brains after birth and allowing the evolutionary expansion of the human cortex.

Dr. Falk adds that the persistent metopic suture seems to have occurred in conjunction with bipedalism: "The ability to walk upright caused an obstetric dilemma. Childbirth became more difficult because the shape of the birth canal became constricted while the size of the brain increased. The persistent metopic suture contributes to an evolutionary solution to this dilemma."

Another major change in hominid evolution has been in the degree of *sexual dimorphism* – the physical differences between sexes; such traits affect social interactions and competition for mates among many animal species. Modern humans have comparatively low sexual dimorphism, but among the other apes, sexual dimorphism tends to be moderate to high.

Among the hominins, *A. afarensis* had a high degree of sexual dimorphism, with significantly larger males than females. The size of males may have played a role in sexual selection, serving to attract females or to intimidate rivals. It may also have been related to different sex roles, with males acting as hunter-gatherers and females as caretakers for the young. This difference was less marked among *A. africanus, Paranthropus*, and the rest of the Homo lineage, however.

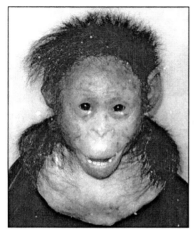

Lucy, christened after the Beatles song Lucy in the Sky with Diamonds, was another famous Australopithecine, discovered in 1974. But only 4 km (2.5 miles) away lay perhaps the most famous Australopithecine discovery of all: the 3.3-million-year-old Australopithecus afarensis girl named **Selam**, *after the Ethiopian word for peace. The nearly complete fossilized skeleton was recovered from the Dikika region of northeastern Ethiopia on December 10, 2000, by a team led by Max Planck Institute's Dr. Zeresenay Alemseged. This is the oldest child yet discovered from humanity's family tree, and one of the most important hominin fossils ever found. Image: Facial reconstruction, National Museum of Addis Ababa, Ethiopia; Wikipedia Creative Commons Attribution 3.0 license*

Dr. Zeresenay Alemseged and his team spent nearly six years extracting Selam's remains from the sandstone in which it was preserved, using dental tools to remove the rock one grain at a time. Because infant remains are so fragile, it is very rare to find a such well-preserved specimen, until the last 100,000 years, when ceremonial burial began.

The entire skull, torso and most of the limbs are present, and leg and foot bones show Selam was already adept at walking upright by the age of three, showing conclusively that A. afarensis was a habitual biped. Her shoulder blades are similar to those of a modern gorilla, while her fingers are long and curved, like those of a chimpanzee. Her inner ear, central to maintaining balance, is also very similar to a chimpanzee's.

Selam's anatomy is a transition point midway between humans and other apes, showing adaptations for both bipedal locomotion and for climbing and swinging from trees. Her species was on the cusp of the hominin transition to a completely bipedal, ground-based existence, one of the most crucial events in the evolution of modern humans.

A. afarensis divided its time walking upright on ground, and climbing trees. Like modern gorillas, females and infants probably spent more time in trees, safe from predators, while more robust males tended to be ground-based. Selam's *hyoid bone*, a structure found just under the tongue, is closer to a modern ape's than a human's, so A. afarensis was incapable of complex language (the hyoid influences the voice box and is critical to human speech).

The discovery of Selam illuminated a major difference between humans and other apes – the length of our childhoods. Baby chimp brains have an early growth spurt and are almost fully formed by the age of three, while human babies undergo a much slower growth spurt, and it takes nearly twenty years for human brains to fully mature.

X-rays of Selam's skull show she had both milk teeth and adult teeth, at the formative stages of a three-year-old. A cast of her skull also gives clues about her brain, so it's possible to measure how much her brain had developed by three years of age. This development can be compared with other fossils, which show how large Australopithecine brains become by adulthood.

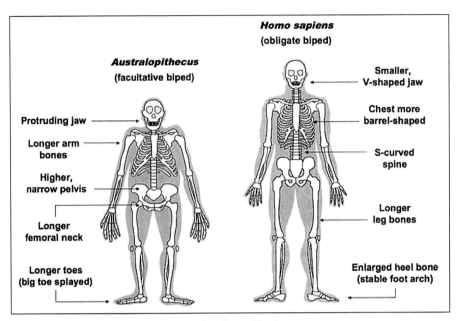

Image: Wikipedia, public domain

Chimp brains are over 90 percent developed by age three. Based on comparisons, however, Australopithecine brains are only 75% developed by the age of three, showing a slowdown of the child development process had already begun to evolve. This means hominins were adapting longer childhoods, in which offspring had time to learn survival strategies.

Chimpanzees and many other primates have brains with a deep furrow at the rear called the *Lunate sulcus*. In apes, the Lunate sulcus divides brain regions related to vision from the rest of the neocortex, where more complex thought processing occurs. Human brains lost this deep furrow, and their neocortices grew much larger than the vision-processing region (*occipital lobe*) at the back of the brain.

An *endocast* – a mold made from the inside of the skull – shows the surface of Selam's brain. A reorganization was occurring in Australopithecines, as the furrow called the Lunate sulcus was slowing moving backward to make way for expansion of the neocortex, the thought-processing region of the brain. Australopithecines had already become smarter than modern-day chimpanzees. They were still very ape-like, however: it would require another million years of evolution before these developments would give rise to modern humans.

In 2010, Drs. Shannon McPherron and Zeresenay Alemseged announced evidence of animal bones scraped by tools nearly three and a half million years ago, suggesting that Australopithecines had already learned to use tools, but their conclusions are highly controversial. Nearly all anthropologists agree such the development of such innovations would take at least another 800,000 years, and a substantial increase in brain volume.

The Green, Green Grass of Home

When the Earth's seasons stabilized, and the planet cooled and dried, animals which relied solely upon the forests for their diet went extinct, while others survived by evolving the ability to exploit other food sources. Herbivores evolved physical adaptations allowing them to graze upon the tough grasses which covered the newly-deforested terrain. Pressured by change, our ancestors, which had previously survived upon soft forest fruit, were among the African animals which evolved to survive in the new environments. New apemen began to appear all over the continent.

In Eastern Africa between 2.7 million and 1.2 million years ago, *Paranthropus boisei* adapted to eat a tough-to-chew but abundant plant-based diet, including nuts, roots and tubers. A 2011 study at the University of Utah on carbon isotope deposits in the teeth of 22 different Paranthropus specimens from East Africa shows that the species relied primarily upon grassy plants. By examining carbon isotope ratios in the teeth, Oxford's Dr. Professor Julia Lee-Thorp and researchers from Chad, France and the US, discovered these individuals had lived primarily upon C4 plants – dry-climate grass species which use a special form of photosynthesis that involves storing characteristic 4-carbon molecules.

---

*Feed the World - Plants typically take in six molecules of water through the roots, and six molecules of carbon dioxide along with sunlight through the leaves, converting them into the molecule $C_6H_{12}O_6$ (plant starch), and shedding six oxygen molecules in the process. This is how carbon is **fixed** (stabilized in useful forms) through photosynthesis. Glucose and other sugars are stored for later energy use, and cellulose is used to make cell walls.*

*Normally, plants breathe by opening their **stomata** (pores) to allow carbon dioxide to diffuse into their cells. In hot, dry weather, however, they must close them to keep from dehydrating. By opening their stomata in the heat, plants risk dehydration in order to breathe. They can conserve water by keeping their stomata closed, but cannot get sufficient carbon dioxide – so instead they take in oxygen, of which comparatively little is needed to bind to special photosynthesizing molecules. This is **photorespiration**, oxygen absorption in times of insufficient carbon dioxide.*

Photorespiration is inefficient however, because it results in toxic molecular byproducts which must be broken down and discarded. This extremely inefficient process occurs in 95% of the world's plant species – C3 plants, plants which rely upon the "standard" photosynthesis, that first evolved in an atmosphere devoid of oxygen.

*Evolutionary solutions exist for plants in the hottest conditions. **CAM plants** (desert species like pineapples) only open their stomata at night, storing carbon dioxide in **malic acid** molecules for use later, during the day. **C4 plants** – grasses which also include corn and sugar cane – are comparatively very efficient at water use during photosynthesis. They take in carbon dioxide and use enzymes to concentrate it in 4-carbon molecules, moved inside the leaf to special **bundle sheath** storage cells. This reduces or eliminates the loss of carbon during photorespiration, when stomata are closed and oxygen is taken in instead of CO_2.*

C4 plants inhabit hot, dry environments, and have a very high water-use efficiency, allowing twice the photosynthesis per water gram as C3 plants, though their metabolism is inefficient in shady or cool environments. Less than 1% of Earth's plant species are classified as C4.

According to Dr. Lee-Thorp, "We found evidence suggesting that early hominins, in central Africa at least, ate a diet mainly composed of tropical grasses and sedges. No African great apes, including chimpanzees, eat this type of food, despite the fact it grows in abundance in tropical and subtropical regions. The only notable exception is the savannah baboon, which still forages for these types of plants today. We were surprised to discover that early hominins appear to have consumed more than even the baboons."

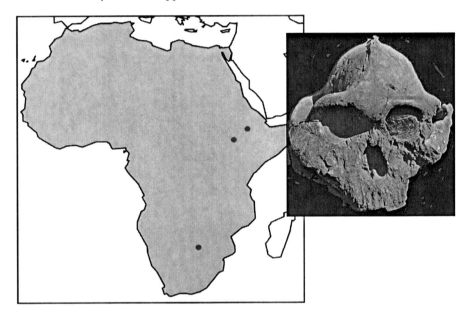

The finding shows an early dietary shift for these hominins, one way in which early humans adapted to survive in open landscapes with few trees. This adaptation enabled their move from the earliest ancestral forests, allowing them to exploit new environments much farther afield.

Fossils from three extinct specimens have came from two Djurab Desert excavations. Although this area is now dry and hyper-arid, in Australopithecus bahrelghazali's era, it would have been a network of shallow lakes, thick with reeds and sedges, with wooded grasslands and floodplains in the regions beyond.

It was previously believed that ancient human ancestors developed harder tooth enamel, larger grinding teeth and powerful jaw muscles to eat hard nuts and seeds, but this research indicates the early hominin diet diverged from that of apes much earlier. Since tropical grass leaves are too abrasive and tough to break down and digest, these human ancestors probably subsisted on the grass and sedge roots and bulbs.

"Based on our carbon isotope data we can't exclude the possibility that the hominins' diets may have included animals that in turn ate the tropical grasses. But as neither humans nor other primates have diets rich in animal food, and of course the hominins are not equipped as carnivores are with sharp teeth, we can assume that they ate the tropical grasses and the sedges directly."

Three species of this genus – *P. aethiopicus, P. boisei* and *P. robustus* - seem to have descended from the Australopithecines into a side group that eventually went extinct. The Australopithecines themselves would also eventually go extinct, after giving rise to the earliest humans, such as Homo habilis, with which Paranthropus would share the Earth for a time.

The most significant anatomical differences between Australopithecus and Paranthropus were primarily in the cranial regions. Paranthropus developed massive, muscular jaws and mohawk-like bony *sagittal crests* on the tops of their heads to anchor huge *masticatory* (chewing) muscles, and huge molars to help grind tough plant fibers. Paranthropus had evolved into highly-specialised vegetarians to ensure their survival. This helped in the short term, but being specialists in a changing world doomed the genus to extinction, because of intense cooling and drying during an Ice Age.

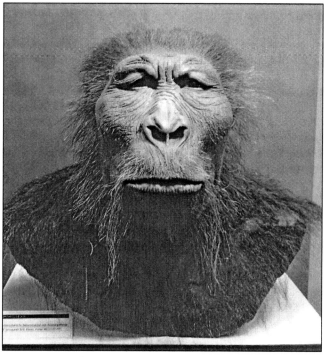

Image: Scientific reconstruction of Paranthropus boisei, Westfälisches Archeological Museum, Herne. Photography: Lilly Undfreya, Creative Commons Attribution 3.0 Unported license.

Middle Ground

Over the millennia, several hominid species came and went, each with gradually more human features – Australopithecus, about 4.4 to 2.3 million years ago; *Kenyanthropus*, about 3.5 million years ago; and Paranthropus, about 2.7 million years ago.

So what drove the evolution from apelike Australopithecus into the Homo genus, with its bigger brain and sophisticated tool use?

It was almost certainly the impact of climate change. Two and a half million years ago, Africa's climate became drier, shrinking the rainforests in which early hominids lived, both on the ground and in trees. Australopithecines were relatively defenseless as larger predators began to emerge in the open savanna.

Tremendous adaptive pressure for new survival skills brought about the evolution of the first true humans like *Homo habilis*, who took to life on the plains, diverging further evolutionarily from the remaining tree dwellers, which would remain largely unchanged as modern apes.

Sophistication

3.4 million years ago, a genetic copying error resulted in the duplication of the *SR-GAP2* gene, thereby changing the course of hominin evolution forever.

This duplication allowed developing neurons to migrate further and sprout a greater number of connections. Freed from constraints, they grew in complexity, enabling the information exchange between a larger number of neighbouring cells. At the same time, infant skulls became more flexible, allowing them to accommodate larger brains.

A million years later, this "daughter" gene was in turn duplicated again, producing the "granddaughter" gene SRGAP2c. The SRGAP2 duplications dramatically changed brain development at a time which coincides with the first use of tools among hominids, when the Australopithecine and Homo lineages diverged.

SRGAP2 is among the few genes (about 30) which duplicated in human DNA after our divergence from the other great apes, at the time the Homo genus split from the australopithecines, according to University of Washington human geneticist Dr. Evan Eichler and Scripps Institute's Dr. Franck Polleux.

All three SRGAP2 gene variants currently coexist in modern humans, helping drive brain development, enabling advanced cognitive functions like language and conscious thought.

This isn't mere speculation. Splicing this DNA into the brains of mice causes the rodents to sprout neurons with thicker, longer, more plentiful spines, root-like outgrowths and substantially increasing processing power. These neurons also migrate into position more quickly than in unmodified mice. The granddaughter copy, however, doesn't augment the original gene's function, but actively *interferes* with it, slowing the development, and thus allowing neurons more time to wire a more complex brain.

In the mutant mice, the specifically affected neurons – *pyramidal neurons*, the major neurons of the cortex – took much longer to sprout their full complement of *dendritic* spines. This delayed spine maturation had an unexpected effect: pyramidal neurons ultimately formed many more spines by the time they had finally matured – just like human pyramidal neurons.

A related discovery in 2012 by The Scripps Research Institute found a special set of stem cells with the unusual built-in ability to determine their fate from the start. Previously, it was believed that all cortex neurons came from one type of *radial glial cell*, or *RGC*. However, the massive human cortex is due in part to these special human *Cux2-positive RGC* stem cells. These unique precursor cells give rise to brain regions which distinguish humans from, for example, amphibians.

The cerebral cortex is where higher brain functions occur, sensory data is integrated, and conscious thought emerges, including decision-making, planning and judgment. Within these larger upper layers, close to the brain's outer surface, neurons integrate information coming in from the senses, and connect across the two lobes of the brain.

These upper layers are relatively young in terms of evolution, having greatly expanded during primate evolution, bestowing upon humans unique abilities for abstract thought, reflection, future planning and problem-solving.

Among mammals, the cerebral cortex is comprised of six distinct anatomical layers, each made up of different varieties of excitatory neurons. These layers aren't uniform like a cake, but more closely resemble the layers enfolding an onion. The innermost layers are comprised of neurons connecting the neocortex to the spinal cord and the *brainstem*, which helps regulate vital functions like breathing, while the comparatively larger upper layers, close to the brain's outer surface, contain neurons which integrate incoming sensory information.

Wired

Both human and chimp brains evolved from a common ancestor, making them appear superficially similar, but there are several distinct differences. Usually brain evolution is thought of as a mere expansion, but a much greater complexity is also at the heart of human brain evolution.

Studying post-mortem brain tissue, a team of UCLA researchers under Dr. Daniel Geschwind applied gene sequencing and advanced analysis to detect differences in genetic activity among humans, chimpanzees and rhesus macaques, a shared ancestor of both species.

The combined techniques enabled the team to zero in on precisely which changes had emerged between humans and chimpanzees: they're found among three brain regions: the *frontal lobe* (executive centers), *hippocampus* (navigational and memory-generating organ) and *striatum* (motivation/auxiliary movement planning center).

By tracking gene expression – specific proteins produced – the scientists were able to search the three genomes for regions where DNA diverged between the species. What they saw surprised them.

The frontal lobe changed most dramatically in humans, with a "striking increase in molecular complexity", while the hippocampus (memory generator and navigational center) and striatum (motivation and slow, deliberate movement control center) remained relatively more similar among all three species. In the frontal lobe, the human brain switches genes on and off in a much more complex, rich variety. Among changes to the specific genes and expressions they found:

> *The biggest differences occurred in the expression of human genes involved in plasticity – the ability of the brain to process information and adapt. This supports the premise that the human brain evolved to enable higher rates of learning.*

In particular, the *CLOCK* gene behaves very differently in human brains. This gene is the one of two master regulators of mammalian *circadian rhythms* (daily sleep-wake and metabolic cycles – *BMAL1* is the second), and its disruption is a part of the underlying pathology of mood disorders such as depression and bipolar syndrome.

The team also found humans have a greater number of connections among gene networks featuring the *FOXP1* and *FOXP2* (*forkhead transcription factor*) genes, central to the unique human ability to produce and understand speech.

Meaty Matters

Humankind also has carnivory to thank for its evolutionary success. When human ancestors began to hunt and eat meat, the upgrade in their diet allowed women to *wean* (stop breast-feeding) children at an earlier age. This in turn gave women more time to give birth to a greater number of children during their reproductive lives, contributing to the gradual spread of humans across the world.

A research team at Sweden's Lund University compared nearly 70 mammalian species and discovered clear patterns in the connection between meat consumption and faster weaning. The average length of breast-feeding is two years and four months, compared to that of our closest relatives, the chimpanzees, which suckle their babies for four to five years, and have lifespans half that of humans, on average only 60 years.

This previously puzzling difference between humans and great apes, appears to hinge on the simple fact that our species is carnivorous (deriving 20% of our diet from meat), as opposed to gorillas, orangutans and chimpanzees, which are herbivorous or omnivorous.

Mathematical models show infants of all species stop breast-feeding when their brains have attained a specific developmental stage between conception and full brain-size. Carnivores, which subsist on high-quality diets, are able to wean earlier than either herbivores and omnivores.

Learning hunting was another significant evolutionary step, requiring communication, planning and tool usage, all of which necessitated larger brains. Adding meat to the diet allowed such bigger brains to develop.

A skull fragment discovered at Olduvai Gorge in northern Tanzania indicates that human forebears ate meat at least 1.5 million years ago. And, according to Dr. Charles Musibaof the University of Colorado, "...1.5 million years ago we were not opportunistic meat eaters, we were actively hunting and eating meat."

The skull fragment was that of a two-year-old hominin suffering from *porotic hyperostosis*, a nutrient deficiency which makes bones soft and spongy. Says professor Musibaof, this indicates that meat had become so vital to the hominin diet that lacking its nutrients caused dangerous pathological conditions. The evidence indicates the child's diet was deficient in iron and vitamins B9 and B12, and it seems to have died from malnutrition.

Musiba believes the shift from scavenging, plant-eating creatures to meat-eaters provided the protein necessary for the evolutionary spurt in brain growth: "The brain is a large organ and requires a lot of energy. We are beginning to think more about the relationship between brain expansion and a high protein diet."

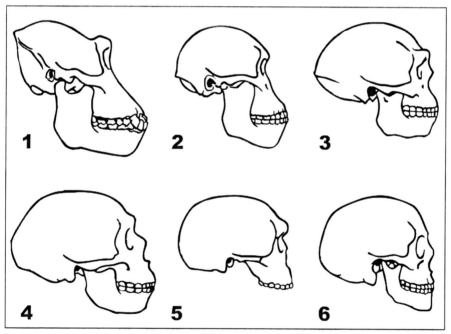

Hominid crania. Skulls of 1. Gorilla 2. Australopithecus 3. Homo erectus 4. Neanderthal (La Chapelle aux Saints) 5. Steinheim Skull (Archaic Homo sapiens) 6. Anatomically modern Homo sapiens. Wikipedia, public domain

Handy Man

Northern Tanzania's Olduvai Gorge is a favorite of fossil-hunters. A 30-mile stretch of river snakes through a deep ravine with four distinct strata of soil. Bed I, the oldest, is around two million years old. The world's most famous anthropologists, Louis and Mary Leakey, had been excavating the site for some thirty years, and turned up some astonishing finds: 20-million-year-old *Proconsul nyanzae*, one of the oldest apes, and scattered prehistoric tools, but frustratingly little evidence of who had made them. When war broke out, the Leakeys were forced to abandon their work, but eventually returned in the 1950s to resume.

In 1959, Mary Leakey unearthed the upper teeth and skull of an ancient hominin deep in the sediment. This was *Paranthropus boisei*, with its odd finlike sagittal bone crest. At 1.75 million years, it was the oldest hominin ever found. But a year later, Leakey and her son Jonathan would stumble across an even more spectacular find: one of the first true humans that ever lived. They had found their mysterious toolmaker.

In the 2.5-million-year-old layers of dirt, scattered among the bones were the world's first stone tools. These were relics from the dawn of humanity. The bones were of the elusive toolmaker *Homo habilis* (Latin for *Handy Man*) the first of a new animal, an ancient human species living in the *Pleistocene*, from 1.5 to 2.5 million years ago.

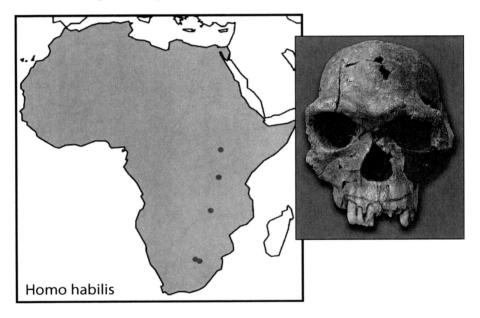

Homo habilis

An older species – *H. gautengensis* – was proposed in 2010, but its status is disputed, and thus H. habilis has remained the accepted oldest ancestor of modern humans – an ancestor of the more human Homo erectus. However, recent findings suggest the two species actually co-existed, and may have been separate lineages of a common ancestor, with H. habilis merely a side branch, and H. erectus the direct ancestor of humans.

In fact, fossil evidence suggests many early hominins coexisted for millennia, including Paranthropus boisei, H. habilis and H. erectus. But these less successful hominins gradually died out, and gradually ever more modern humans emerged, though some separate classifications are debated – *H. georgicus*, H. erectus, *H. ergaster*, the cannibal *H. antecessor*, H. heidelbergensis, H. neanderthalensis and H. floresiensis.

H. habilis used stone tools primarily for scavenging, cleaving meat from carrion. They were quite small, about 1.3 meters (4 ft. 3 in) on average, and were apparently rather poor fighters: many fossils show members of H. habilis were regularly dined upon by predatory animals like the large scimitar-toothed predatory cat *Dinofelis*. Perhaps this is why H. habilis was succeeded by our much hardier human ancestors *Homo erectus*.

Superficially, H. habilis was very unlike modern humans: squat, with long, lanky arms. However, it had lost the apelike snout, and its jaw jutted out substantially less than that of its Australopithecine forebears.

Homo habilis' brain had expanded from the Australopithecines to nearly double the size, about 600 cubic cm, with a sloping, elevated forehead to accommodate its growing cortex. It had also acquired that one very special, amazing ability – the ability to make tools.

These early *Oldowan tools* were rather crudely crafted at first: the toolmaker grasped a stone called the *core* and chipped it with a second called the *percussor*. This provided a sharp cutting edge which could pierce animal hide. But even such a crude tool as this required a cognitive leap, which experiments show even the most intelligent of modern chimpanzees are unable to duplicate after months of training.

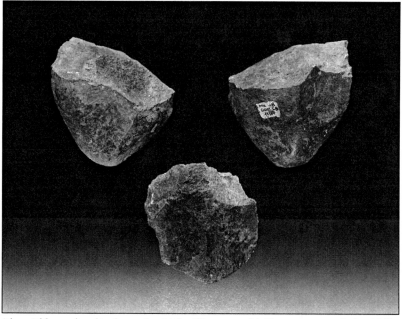

These Oldowan hand tools are about 1.7 million years old. They were unearthed at Melka Kunture, Ethiopia. Image: Didier Descouens, Attribution 3.0 license, Wikipedia.

The broad pad of the H habilis' thumb provided the necessary surface area for a fine, precision grip, and its dexterous hands allowed this apeman to craft its tools. Its teeth and jaws were too small to chew the same tough plants as its contemporary P. boisei, so food was scarcer for H. habilis. Because of this, H. habilis was an omnivore, eating nearly anything that crossed its path, particularly meat. H. habilis was ill-equipped to hunt, however, and had to resort to scavenging instead. It is likely these apemen learned to watch for vultures circling the remains of big kills – the carcass of a wilde-beest slaughtered by lions, or the remains of an antelope discarded by a leopard.

Meat is comparatively easy to digest and extremely calorie- and nutrient-dense. But snatching meat from big predators is a dangerous proposition, so quick wits were needed. To cope, H. habilis evolved the abilty to divert surplus energy from the body to the brain, allowing further brain growth.

Ancient scrape marks on animal bones show early humans began using primitive stone tools to smash them open and extract marrow. This was a highly nutritious food source unavailable to other creatures, full of fatty acids vital to brain growth and development. This further supplemented brain expansion, enabling our ancestors to create ever more complex tools.

It's almost certain that environmental hardship drove H. habilis to adapt and innovate. For nearly three million years, the African climate had been relatively stable, and early hominins from Toumai to Selam had changed very little in brain capacity for some three million years. Then about two million years ago, wild climate swings began to rack the African landscape, careening wildly between wet and dry conditions.

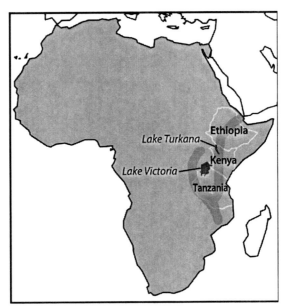

The Rift Valley, home of some of history's most important finds

The geological record clearly shows how violent climatic swings created freshwater lakes on the scale of Lake Victoria, which would fill the entire Rift Valley, then disap-pear in the span of a thousand years. The region was in constant flux, making living conditions terrible.

While in the longer scale of time, Africa was slowly drying out, it would periodically pulse with rapid climatic change, repeatedly cycling between wet and dry conditions. Flash flooding would alternate with brutal droughts, and rivers and forests would spring into existence, then wither into dry savannas in an evolutionary eyeblink. It was from this era of environmental upheaval that humanity sprang.

According to Penn State graduate student Clayton Magill:

> *The landscape early humans were inhabiting transitioned rapidly back and forth between a closed woodland and an open grassland about five to six times during a period of 200,000 years. These changes happened very abruptly, with each transition occurring over hundreds to just a few thousand years. Early humans went from having trees available to having only grasses available in just 10 to 100 generations, and their diets would have had to change in response.*

> *Changes in food availability, food type, or the way you get food can trigger evolutionary mechanisms to deal with those changes. The result can be increased brain size and cognition, changes in locomotion and even social changes – how you interact with others in a group. Our data are consistent with these hypotheses. We show that the environment changed dramatically over a short time, and this variability coincides with an important period in our human evolution when the genus Homo was first established and when there was first evidence of tool use.*

From *biomarkers* (molecules left by the waxy coating on ancient plant leaves) in lake sediments of the Olduvai Gorge in Tanzania, the team reconstructed the floral environment across specific time intervals, working forward from two million years in the past. Their findings show that the environment transitioned back and forth rapidly, between closed woodland and open grassland.

Says Penn State's Dr. Katherine Freeman, natural changes to the Earth's orbit were responsible for the dramatic shifts in the weather, driving changes to Africa's monsoon system. Her team's research found a clear link between environmental changes and planetary movement.

Water shortages led to food insecurity, which triggered major evolutionary changes. The wildly unstable African climate forced its inhabitants to adapt to dramatically different conditions. Those species which were unable to adapt – like the Australopithecines – went extinct, while craftier problem-solvers – like Homo habilis – survived. In other words, say anthropologists, humans evolved in response to variability. Change was the driving force of human evolution, and our unmatched adaptability has allowed us to flourish. We haven't adapted to any single environment, but to a variety of them. In essence, humanity is the product of climatic change.

The dramatic upheavals in climate continued for a million and a half years, driving our forebears down the path which would ultimately lead to you, the most intelligent creature the planet has ever known.

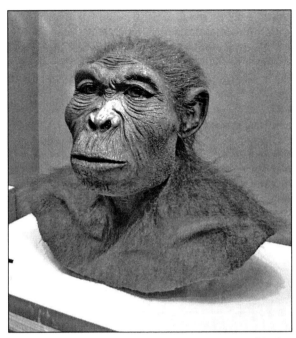

Image: Scientific reconstruction of Homo habilis, Westfälisches Archeological Museum, Herne. Photography: Lilly Undfreya, Creative Commons Attribution 3.0 Unported license.

Something Fishy

About two million years ago, there was a sudden puzzling, explosive growth in the size and complexity of the hominin brain. From an evolutionary standpoint, it makes little sense – growing a massive brain requires a huge caloric intake, and places a significant survival burden on both mothers and infants.

In 2004, researchers at eastern Lake Turkana in Kenya discovered the probable cause of this sudden surge in brain growth and complexity – the huge evolutionary leap that led to our eventual emergence.

For over four years, the international team had unearthed thousands of stone tools and fossilized bones of animal carcasses which had been butchered and consumed by hominins. Their findings show that early humans had begun eating a diet rich in aquatic proteins from the meat of turtles, fish, and even crocodiles, as well as fat-rich bone marrow.

Lakes and rivers were a plentiful source of small animals like turtles and fish, providing abundant protein without the risk of attack by dangerous predators. The happy side effect of this readily accessible, nutrient-dense food was that it was rich in fatty acids such as *docosahexaenoic acid (DHA)*, nutrients which would lift constraints on brain growth and help fuel brain evolution.

Lethal Weapons

Whatever the reasons for its first emergence, walking upright freed our hands for other, more complex purposes, including tool use. The bones and muscles of human hands allow us to grip and manipulate objects in ways no other primates can, indicating that as humans diverged from chimpanzees, our hands evolved away from locomotive use toward alternative functionality.

University of Kent anthropologists Stephen Lycett and Alastair Key seem to have confirmed Charles Darwin's theory that human hands evolved over eons of primitive tool use. Using stone tools matching 2.6-million-year-old artifacts from Tanzania, they showed how gradual hand evolution significantly affected tool efficiency. And over time, constant tool use led to gradual hand development.

Superior manual dexterity has given our species major survival advantages, enabling us to master tool-making. *HACNSI* (Human-Accelerated Conserved Non-coding Sequence 1) seems to be at the heart of this ability. HACNSI has existed in primates for millions of years, but mutated 16 times since the separation of hominids from our common primate ancestor. The genetic region functions as an on/off switch, activating embryonic development genes central to limb development.

Splicing the human HACNSI region into mouse embryos shows our mutated version acts upon forepaw development, in precisely the regions corresponding to human wrists and thumbs.

In addition to "opposable thumbs" which can move inwardly toward the palms – allowing precision gripping – we also have species-unique, extremely nimble hands compared with other primates. But it's a trade-off, according to Gladstone Institute's Dr. Katherine Pollard: "We can hold a pencil, but we can't hang from the limb of a tree comfortably like a chimp."

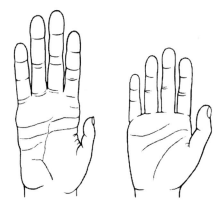

Chimpanzee hands (left) are built for gripping limbs, but poor at delicate manipulations. Image: Denise Morgan, 2012, University of Utah. Used with permission.

The human hand evolved not just to allow tool-making, but also specifically for fighting, according to University of Utah anthropologists Michael Morgan and David Carrier. The shape of the human hand, they say, makes an ideal weapon.

Most primate hands are adapted for climbing, with long palms and fingers, and short thumbs. With human hands, built for tool-making, it's the opposite – we have short palms and fingers, with long thumbs.

With its shortened fingers and palms, and longer, stronger, more flexible thumbs, human hands can not only delicately manipulate tools and other objects, but also clench into fists, something ape hands cannot do.

Drs. Morgan and Carrier say their experiments demonstrate that hand geometry is specifically adapted to deal damage in addition to crafting tools. In their study, the researchers gathered basic measurements, and then instructed a group of boxers and martial artists to hit a punching bag as hard as possible, using first a normal fist, and then an open palm. As the athletes struck from a variety of angles, an accelerometer attached to the bag monitored the force from each blow.

Next, they used pistons to measure the rigidity of various hand shapes, including a clenched fist, a fist with the thumb protruding outward, and a malformed fist, with the fingers uncurled but folded over the palm, thumb pointing outward, a chimpanzee's closest possible approximation of a fist.

The accelerometer attached to the punching bag showed that a closed fist provided the most damage because of its geometry, partly from the concentration of power in the small contact area of the knuckles, but primarily because of the rigidity imparted by bones arranged in a proper fist. This rigidity allows a punch with the potential to break bones.

Two factors are responsible: the precise length of human finger bones allows them to be curled tightly inward, leaving no space within a fist; and the thumb buttresses these curled fingers, adding to a fist's rigidity. When placed at the palm's side, the thumb is precisely the right length to provide this support.

Knuckles become four times more rigid when supported by the thumb, and thumb support doubles the force of a punch, transmitting force from the wrist via the thumb and index finger *metacarpals* (palm bones). Together these features give a human fist nearly 400% the rigidity of a chimpanzee-style fist; when chimps curl their fingers, a gap remains in the center of the fist, and the thumb is unable to add support.

These precise proportions make our hands perfectly suited for clenching into fists, weapons capable of delivering extreme damage while minimizing the risk of self-injury, protecting delicate hand bones and ligaments from harm. All this suggests that fists are indeed a direct product of evolutionary adaptation, instead of mere by-products of tool-making dexterity.

While manual dexterity was certainly a major factor in hand evolution, Dr. Carrier says that aggression also played a large role. Hominids capable of fisticuffs would have held a distinct advantage over competitors for scarce resources:

An individual who could strike with a clenched fist could hit harder without injuring themselves, so they were better able to fight for mates and thus more likely to reproduce.

The role aggression has played in our evolution has not been adequately appreciated. There are people who do not like this idea, but it is clear that compared with other mammals, great apes are a relatively aggressive group, with lots of fighting and violence, and that includes us. We're the poster children for violence.

Stand Tall

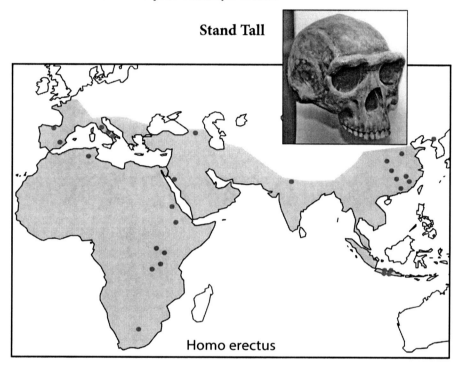

Homo erectus

In the grasslands and canyons of the Great Rift Valley of East Africa, two million years ago, a rather amazing creature was born. It was basically one of us, albeit with a slightly smaller brain and slightly larger jaw. It was the first of a remarkable species that would be the trailblazers who first departed Africa, and the first to use fire and hunting. They would colonize entire continents and create the first human societies.

Two million years after its emergence, Richard Leakey, the middle son of Louis and Mary Leakey, would make an extraordinary discovery. In 1984, while excavating near Lake Turkana, a remote inland sea in northern Kenya, his team came across one of the most extraordinary fossils ever found.

It was a nearly complete skeleton, with a skull, most of a spine and ribs, arms and legs. *Turkana Boy* was a member of the *Homo erectus (upright human)* species, which lived over one and a half million years ago. An examination of his teeth's daily growth shows he was eight years old when he died. At five foot three, Turkana Boy was already the size of a modern adolescent. This is because early hominins, like our chimpanzee ancestors, matured much more rapidly than we do, virtually skipping over childhood.

Our comparatively long and gradual childhood allows modern human brains to fully mature and absorb the lessons necessary for functioning in modern societies, but the brutal era of Homo erectus afforded no such luxuries.

Turkana Boy wasn't an ape, but a very early, true human. He had a more primitive skull than ours, with a lower forehead and significantly smaller brain. The decay of his jawbone indicates he had an infection that was likely fatal. Had he survived to adulthood, Turkana Boy would have reached about six feet - and needed a lot of calories to sustain such mass. This required high calorie food - meat.

The transition from hominoids to Homo was central to human evolution: legs grew thinner and longer, arms shortened, and brains expanded in the transition from apelike bodies to human ones. Homo erectus were the first hominins with the body proportions of modern humans – long legs and short arms compared to the torso, adaptations to a terrestrial life.

Endocasts show the species had brains twice the size of chimpanzees 1.8 million years ago. They would go on to become the longest-lived of the humans, colonizing all of Eurasia and reigning as one of the planet's most successful predators for two million years - about nine times as long as the modern human race's entire existence.

So how did a comparatively puny creature like Turkana Boy feed its massive, calorie-devouring brain?

Homo erectus had been faced with a dilemma: how does one kill a huge, dangerous animal, full of meat and fat, without dying in the process? The answer lay in two key innovations - endurance running and high activity in mid-day heat.

Originally scavengers, Erectus eventually evolved into fleet, carnivorous big-game hunters, working cooperatively in packs. They had thick, pronounced facial features, and the shape of their femurs shows they were swift - elite runners on par with modern Olympic athletes. Says Stony Brook University's Dr. John Shea, "If they were around today, chasing people around, we'd be in trouble. These guys were like wolves with knives."

Homo erectus had evolved to run, just like modern humans. When these early humans had shed their primate body hair, and evolved the ability to cool by sweating, it enabled a new technique for capturing prey: persistence hunting.

Because they're covered in fur, most animals run at a disadvantage in the midday African sun, and quickly overheat if they don't periodically stop to rest and cool down by *panting*. This limits their running to short sprints - ten to fifteen minutes at a stretch.

But hairless skin allows air to circulate freely, cooling the body as sweat transfers thermal energy into the air by evaporating. This feature makes humans excellent long-distance runners, among the best on the planet – if we need to, we can run nonstop, potentially even for days at a time.

Even today, this is how the Kalihari bushmen of Southern Africa continue to hunt, by running their prey down to a state of exhaustion – furred animals must eventually stop when heat stroke renders them helpless. It's believed this style of hunting first emerged with homo erectus two million years ago.

Homo erectus likely used weapons similar to those of the Kalihari bushmen, rocks, clubs, or spears thrown from a short distance. But the fossil record shows they favored the *Acheulean handaxe,* a razor-sharp stone cutting tool used primarily to slice limbs from prey. These handaxes were advanced and versatile tools chipped from stone – sharp, flat and symmetrical, used for chopping, cutting and skinning. They were also heavy enough to crack bone.

Homo erectus left behind thousands of half-finished Acheulean stone axes, which show it could gauge rock suitability, and recognize flaws which could potentially crack and ruin its handiwork.

Emory University's Drs. Dietrich Stout and Bruce Bradley believe the planning this required triggered evolutionary changes in the human brain. A million years of handaxe refinement prompted the growth of neural pathways which became language-processing centers.

Dr. Bradley is an experimental archeologist, who has perfected *flintknapping,* the technique behind hand-crafting prehistoric stone tools. An analysis of the process shows that, like language, the creation of chipped-stone implements requires thinking several steps ahead.

Chipping these hand axes into existence involves a mental two-step – counter-intuitively dulling a stone's edge to weaken it before chipping. The process is structured and rule-based, following an ordered progression, which requires keeping the final product fixed in mind.

Each strike on the stone must be performed in the proper sequence to create the final goal, a sharpened, flat blade. This is precisely the complex, sequential, abstract thought required for language production: words must follow proper sequences in a sentence, using the same set of mental skills required for crafting a stone tool.

MRI scans bear this hypothesis out: the same region of the brain activated during the construction of complex sentences lights up when contemplating how to chip out a stone handaxe. This region in the brain's left hemisphere is called *Broca's area,* and it deals with memory and executive functions, but also plays a central role in motor aspects of speech production, and is central to grammar usage and sentence processing.

Stone-tool-making draws upon the same language-processing neural pathways: chipping out Acheulean handaxes elicits a large amount of activity in Broca's area, the same region used to form complex sentences. According to Dr. Thierry Chaminade: "These areas of the brain are necessary both for language and stone-tool-making. These two things co-evolved."

His experiments show that Homo erectus' stone toolmaking paved the way for language, the most powerful human tool of all. Broca's area had already substantially developed in H. erectus, endowing humans with the potential for symbolic thought and speech.

For several hundred thousand years, early Homo erectus shared East Africa with Homo habilis, a lineage from which erectus seems to have descended. But Erectus would eventually evolve into our own species, *Homo sapiens*, by about 200,000-100,000 years ago.

Along the way, Homo erectus was the first to harness fire. This enhanced food palatability, safety and ease of digestion, and the fireside also provided light, warmth, safety and social interaction. According to Harvard University's Dr. Richard Wrangham, we know this because Homo erectus' smaller teeth and intestinal tract shows they were eating food made softer and more easily digestible by cooking.

But the act of gathering around the fireside would gradually transform humans into a cultural animal. Says Dr. Wrangham, "Humans have this wonderfully calm temperament compared to chimpanzees. Where did it come from? We were drawn to a common place, the fireplace." It's his contention that humans learned sharing and communication by sitting around the fireside together, waiting for their food to cook.

Most scholars agree Homo erectus was the first to leave Africa nearly two million years ago. This would be followed by wave after wave of successive ancient human populations, settling throughout Europe and Asia, and developing new adaptations to their regions.

One early wave to Indonesia probably gave rise to a group of the diminutive species Homo floresiensis; another took Homo erectus deep into China at least 700,000 years ago. A third wave headed for Europe, and would eventually evolve into the *Neanderthals* – our closest extinct relatives.

As progressively cooler global temperatures reshaped the planet, Homo erectus roamed steadily farther from its birthplace, following migrating animal herds, up through what is now the Sinai desert and beyond into the Middle East, then Eurasia. If a herd adjusted its range only one kilometer a year in the same direction, after 5,000 years, it would cross two continents.

Dmanisi, a tiny Georgien town about 75 miles southwest of the country's capital, is the first site H. erectus is known to have colonized outside of Africa. An initial find of ancient stone tools in 1984 intensified interest in Dmanisi's archeological potential, and in 1991, an international team of scholars joined forces to see what they could unearth.

Over the course of fourteen years, researchers uncovered 1.8 million-year-old remains of *Homo erectus georgicus*, an erectus subspecies whose ancestors had migrated over 4,000 kilometers. Five fossil skeletons were eventually recovered, members of a species with a primitive skull and upper body, but advanced spine and lower limbs.

By one million years ago, Homo erectus had colonized all of temperate Eurasia, aided by its intelligence, hunting and firemaking skills. The species went extinct in Africa and much of Asia about 500,000 years ago, but may have survived in Indonesia until about 150,000 years ago. This was long before the arrival of Homo sapiens, however, who only came to Indonesia about 40,000 years ago.

Perhaps the single greatest secret of Homo erectus' success was found buried in the Earth at Dmanisi – researchers had recovered the skull of an elderly, toothless Homo erectus man. His jawbones revealed he had survived two years without any teeth, which means his group had been feeding and caring for him the whole time – perhaps even chewing his food for him. Humans had learned to care for one another.

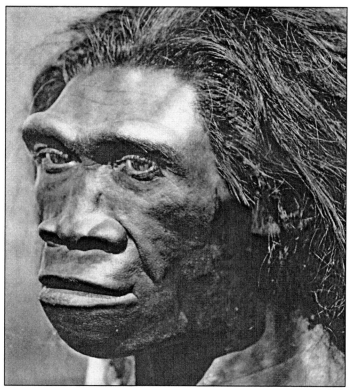

Homo erectus lived between 1.8 million and 300,000 years ago in hunter-gatherer tribes. It was a successful species for a million and a half years, with a brain size ranging from 900cc to 1200cc. Erectus developed tools, weapons and fire and learned to cook food. It travelled out of Africa into China and Southeast Asia, presumably wore fur and hide clothing for northern climates, and turned to hunting for food. Anatomically, only its head and face differed from that of modern man. Eerectus was sturdier in build and much stronger than modern humans, and had begun to develop the neural, muscular and skeletal structures necessary for speech, though it likely lacked the breath control for complex speech. Image: Homo erectus adult female, Smithsonian Museum of Natural History. Wikipedia, public domain.

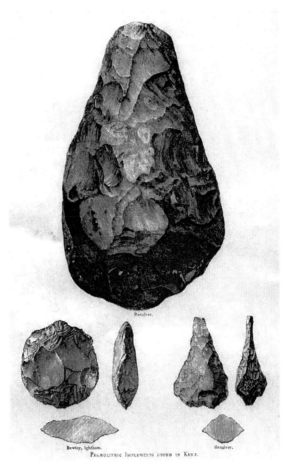

Acheulean hand axes, 1912,
Victoria County, History of Kent, public domain.

Form Follows Function

One result of mankind's rapid growth in brainpower was the ability to first conceive of and create tools. By comparing Stone Age tool-making techniques, British researchers have pieced together the puzzle of how human thought and behavior first emerged. Researchers at the Imperial College of London employed the skills of a flintknapper to accurately replicate primitive tool development, using sensor-equipped gloves and computer modelling to compare the precise physical techniques required to make two types of *Lower Paleolithic (stone age)* tools.

The progression from simple sharpened stones to stone axes was a major leap in development as the human cortex evolved in eastern Africa. Both flaked stones and hand-held axes require the same amount of manual dexterity to create, so hand coordination wasn't the impediment to advanced tool-making.

What was required was abstract thought – designs which sprang from the imagination. Refined hand tool manufacture meant primitive humans had first begun projecting ideas onto the outside world – imagining designs to use as guides in producing material articles. Stone hand axes are believed to be the first external manifestations of such abstract human thought.

Dr. Aldo Faisal believes the "massive technological leap" from crude rock tools to hand-held axes indicates a major leap forward in mental capacity. Ancient hand axes differed significantly from the materials from which they were derived, showing a mental design had been projected onto rock. This means primitive humans had developed the ability to imagine something that didn't exist in the natural world, to plan its creation, and then to render it from suitable materials they had chosen with a design in mind.

Over the Misty Mountains Cold

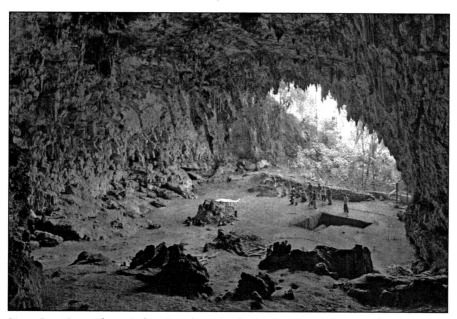

Liang Bua Cave, Flores, Indonesia, where the fossilized remains of Homo floresiensis were discovered in 2003. Image: Rosa Cabecinhas/Alcino Cunha, Attribution License 2.0 Wikipedia.

In just 2003, five thousand miles from the shores of Africa, on the Indonesian island of Flores, researchers made a baffling discovery: the bones of ancient, tiny humans, slightly more than three feet tall. They called the enigmatic new creatures *Homo floresiensis*. Because of their size, however, they soon earned the nickname *Hobbits*.

Homo Floresiensis lived between 95,000 and 12,000 years ago, sharing their island with pygmy elephants, giant rats, Komodo dragons, and other even larger giant lizard species. Modern Homo sapiens is thought to have reached this region by about 45,000 years ago, but would have had far greater intelligence – Hobbit brains were only about 400cc – only slightly larger than those of Australopithecines like Lucy, who had vanished nearly two million years earlier.

The Hobbit's face, feet, hands and legs were also comparatively primitive, but buried in the same cave with this creature were tiny but sophisticated stone tools, something far beyond the capability of Australopithecines. With Homo floresiensis' orange-sized brain, how it could have managed to craft such tools is a complete mystery.

It's been hypothesized that H. floresiensis was a population of hominins which underwent *dwarfism* – when a species is isolated in an region with limited food, evolutionary pressures favor the smallest members of the population, resulting in a slow size decrease over several generations; in fact, cow-sized pygmy elephants once lived on the very same island where H. floresiensis was found. However, the primitive tools and the creature's features have led some anthropologists to believe they evolved from Homo erectus. Another possibility is that Hobbits were from a migratory wave out of Africa before even H. erectus, by an unknown hybrid of Australopithecines and Homo erectus.

Your Superpower

One of most popular comic books in the world is Marvel Comics' *X-Men,* which tells about mutants with amazing superpowers. But your own personal, mutation-derived superpower is no less astounding. You possess the most potent, dangerous and subversive ability that has ever emerged through natural selection. It allows you to implant thoughts into the minds of others, instantly rewiring their synapses. Through thin air, you can alter the neural configuration of another's mind, and they can do the same to you, assuming they know how.

This power has given rise to the greatest of human achievements, and even led people to their deaths since the dawn of history. We're talking, of course, about speech.

Gusts of air you push across membranes in your throat are modified by the muscles of your larynx, mouth and tongue, allowing you to express an infinite range of ideas, memories, plans and emotions. These puffs of air can win you friends, allies, lovers, and wealth or, if you're overly rash, foolish or unlucky, get you jailed and even killed.

As a member of the animal species *homo sapiens*, you're blessed with a largely unique capacity for *social learning*; by observing and imitating, you benefit from the wisdom of others, and even improve upon it, choosing the best from among alternatives, leading to improvement and progress – a process called *cumulative cultural adaptation.* But your most powerful tool for social learning and cooperation, says Reading University Professor Mark Pagel, is language.

Language separates you from your genetically similar cousins, the chimpanzees, who cannot improve to any significant degree by watching and imitating, and so can never progress as a species, but will be forever consigned to using sticks to catch termites or rocks to break open nuts.

In the case of these relatives, communications are limited to a very narrow range of emotional states – very specific and limited sets of hoots, grunts and howls that, for example, signal an approaching predator, joy at seeing a companion or delicious-looking food, or rage at a potential competitor.

On the other hand, as a human, you can theoretically express an infinite range of meaning, not just statements of fact like "It's hot outside", but such abstractions as:

Burning rotted prehistoric life forms in our factories and cars spews heat-trapping gas into the atmosphere, threatening the very survival of every living creature on the planet, not to mention modern civilization and the safety of everyone I know and love.

It's unacceptable to me and I will not stand by and watch the slow death of all that is dear to me in the name of commerce and profit for the already obscenely wealthy. Instead, I'm taking daily steps right now to reduce my personal pollution, and to actively promote clean, sustainable alternatives.

Just reading those words has altered your synapses, leaving an impression upon you to motivate you toward action.

The Voice Of Your Genes

Language, says Dr. Pagel, is the voice of your genes. But it's important to remember that genes don't have "intentions". They also can't encode behaviors or thought processes. Genes can only encode the production of proteins such as signalling molecules, receptors, enzymes, and regulatory factors. So from what does this remarkable, incredibly powerful system develop?

Language's emergence may have come from a rapid change in human DNA brought about by lateral gene transmission, and biologists even know the specific gene sequence in which it occurred, one which gives rise to the third of three critical elements of human speech: lungs, a *larynx*, and *articulators*.

Lungs push air past the *vocal folds*. These membranes act like a vibrating valve that chops up airflow to produce audible sonic pulses. The membranes can be relaxed or tighted to change sound *pitch* – the speed of variations in air pressure – resulting in higher or lower tones.

Birds, reptiles and many other animals also possess lungs and a larynx, also used for communication, but it's the human *articulators* that allow greater range and precise control over these air vibrations, granting you powers of speech. Articulators such as your lips, tongue, jaw and cheeks use fine motor control to shape the sounds of air passing through.

This control is encoded primarily by a single gene – the human *FOXP2* gene on chromosome number 7. It's one of the most deeply conserved genes, meaning the DNA region has been passed down and maintained through the development of many species over millions of years of evolution, with little change, showing its importance for survival.

In mice – which share about 80% of human DNA – the FOXP2 gene exists, but with two different amino acids in the sequence. In chimpanzees – which share 95% of our genes – a single amino acid has been switched in the sequence, changing the protein's shape and function. The human version only emerged about 120,000 years ago.

FOXP2 produces a protein *transcriptional regulator*, which means it controls the first step in synthesizing proteins. This means FOXP2 switches genes off and on as body tissues are being produced, chemically signalling, in essence, the commands *"start making proteins"* and *"That's enough tissue growth for now"*.

Thus, FOXP2 alters tissue growth, enabling development of sophisticated muscles for the lips, tongue and lower jaw, muscles which allow the fine movements controlling the complex sound production of speech. Humans born with mutated forms of FOXP2 cannot control their lips, tongue and jaws sufficiently; nor can any other animal species.

Our superior vocal control gave us the physical mechanisms to progress from limited, primitive signalling calls which mean things like *"Lion! Lion!"* and *"Food! Food!"* to being able to articulate more sophisticated vocal sounds. This ability to create a tremendously sophisticated range of vocal expressions was a distinct advantage, when combined with the emerging brain circuits necessary to create and remember symbolic representations of reality.

Motor Mouth

A team of researchers at Princeton has discovered the roots of human speech in everyday primate behavior. The mouth and throat movements used to produce speech appear to have emerged from everyday, well-meaning expressions exchanged by primates: human speech mirrors the rhythm, development and internal dynamics of *lip smacking*, a friendly communicative exchange between primates like chimpanzees, baboons and macaques.

The mechanics of primate lip smacking are quite distinct from those of chewing, just as separate mechanics control human speech and chewing. The term suggests a smacking noise, but *geladas*, primates from the remote mountains of Ethiopia, sound extraordinarily like humans speaking when they communicate in this way.

Dr. Asif Ghazanfar of the Princeton Neuroscience Institute led a team which used x-ray films of adult rhesus macaques to demonstrate how lip smacking results in fast, loosely coordinated movement of structures like the lips, tongue and *hyoid* (a bone bracing the tongue, pharynx and larynx, allowing more varied sound production).

Lip smacking develops in the same way in rhesus macaques that speech-related mouth movements do in humans. Baby macaques smack their lips with slow, inconsistent rhythm, just as human infants at the same developmental stage babble. Upon reaching adulthood, however, macaques smack their lips with a distinct, faster rhythm, averaging 5 hertz (cycles per second), the same rhythm as in adult human speech.

Said Dr. Ghazanfar:

> *...we found that primate lip smacking and the facial component of human speech have the same frequency range, developmental trajectory and involve a similar interplay of*

the lips, tongue and hyoid. Lip smacking is performed by all Old World monkeys and apes, including chimpanzees, and is used in friendly, face-to-face interactions. They often take turns exchanging lip-smacking gestures. Because primate lip smacking has no vocal component, it might seem unrelated to speech, but human speech has two components: the source and the filter. The source component is when the respiratory system pushes air through a person's vocal cords to produce a sound. That sound travels up through the nasal and oral cavities and gets filtered by those cavities. We use our mouths, tongues and lips to actually change the shape of those cavities and, thus, those sounds. That filtering is a separate component with separate neural controls. Our work focuses on this filtering component.

...human speech originates from primate facial expressions that were eventually paired with vocal sounds to produce a primitive form of babbling..... the rhythmicity of those ancestral expressions led to the rhythmicity our faces produce when we speak.... Ultimately, our work suggests that the roots of human speech do not lie entirely in primate vocalizations or manual gestures, but are closely related to primate facial expressions.

For our study, we videotaped rhesus macaques of various ages producing lip smacks and used a computer algorithm to measure frame-by-frame the dynamics and rhythmicity of those lip movements. We compared those measurements with chewing movements. Incredibly, the pattern of lip-smack development in the rhesus macaques was identical to the pattern of speech development documented in humans. Moreover, chewing rhythms were basically the same for adult and juvenile primates just as in humans — about 2.5 hertz and without any developmental change. So, lip smacking in Old World monkeys, or at least rhesus macaques, has a similar developmental trajectory as human speech.

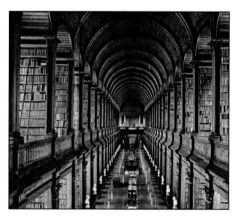

Miracles of language: Our hearing has evolved to be specifically attuned to human speech: it's most sensitive within the 60 Hz to 7kHz range.

Walk into the Library of Congress (the world's biggest library), and among the 850 km (530 miles) of shelf space, you will find some 130 million items. Open a book to a random page and read the first sentence. It's virtually certain you would not find that same sentence randomly searching any other book in the library.

In fact, at any given instant, you're capable of producing a sentence which has never before been said by any human in history. And yet, all those billions of sentences are simply combinations of little more than 100 phonemes – units of sound the human voice is capable of producing*. Yet you're able to both produce and understand this incredible variety of meaning instantly and effortlessly.

* English consists of about 47 phonemes, but as of 2005, the International Phonetic Association lists 107 letters, 52 diacritics, and four prosodic marks in all of human speech.

And Your Bird Can Sing

Human speech has two "layers" of construction – the flexible arrangement of words called the *expression layer*, and the specific core meanings of the words within the sentence, called the *lexical layer*. According to an international team of researchers from MIT and the University of Tokyo, the power of speech is derived from the ability to use both, but each layer has its roots in much more ancient communication systems in the animal kingdom. By combining both, we have a rule-based system that allows virtually infinite communication possibilities.

Animals other than humans can convey practical, basic information through a finite set of specific signals, without much capacity for elaboration. For example, bees dance in a very precise, limited sequence of motions to indicate to their fellows where food can be located; and many animals can utter warning cries and similar messages. Humans can also communicate vital information in this manner, but we share the additional ability of birds to recombine communicative building blocks, and add melodic, emotional nuances, changing the pitch, rhythm and stress of the sounds we make.

The authors believe humans combined these two modes of expression within the last 100,000 years, creating a uniquely powerful new means of communication. Because of this, the finite number of words we use can generate infinite meaning. This research echoes a supposition first proposed by Charles Darwin: that humans first communicated with a form of singing, and later integrated lexical components into their songs.

The difference between the lexical and expression layers can be demonstrated with the sentence "Tracy ate an apple". The *expression layer* enables rearrangement of the elements and the ability to change our tone into a rising pitch, to form the question "Did Tracy eat an apple?" But we're still using the same core components of the *lexical layer*: the subject Tracy, the verb eat, and the object, apple.

The researchers point out that birdsong and human speech are both built upon a finite number of stress and beat patterns. But there are other "striking parallels" between human and bird language, such as the critical stage of maturation for learning languages, as well as the regions of the brain used to produce language.

Fluent human speech incorporates precise, coordinated timing and movement of multiple articulators including the jaw, tongue, lips, and larynx.

Dr. Edward Chang, neurosurgeon at UCSF's Centers for Epilepsy and for Integrative Neuroscience, says this coordinated behavior is the most highly sophisticated human motor activity.

In 2013, his team revealed control of this incredibly sophisticated behavior is orchestrated by speech centers in the *sensorimotor cortex*, which controls the articulators while someone speaks. The sensorimotor cortex has a hierarchical, cyclical structure which exercises near-instantaneous, coordinated control over the jaw, lips, tongue, and larynx.

Dr. Chang recruited his volunteers from among UCSF surgery patients with incurable, severe epilepsy. Using implanted electrodes, his team observed activation patterns as the volunteers read a series of English syllables such as *bah*, *dee*, and *goo*.

Distinct brain patterns in the speech control regions of the motor cortex were found which correspond to specific vowels and consonants, and the activation patterns appear to be common to every human language.

Just as newborn humans must learn the sounds comprising human speech, songbirds are born without the ability to produce the songs they will sing in adulthood. The newborn of both animal groups must listen and imitate the sounds they hear.

The amniote lineage which led to both humans and songbirds split some 340 million years ago, but both groups seem to have evolved the ability to communicate through sound independently, using analogous brain structures which govern sound learning, imitation and mature production.

Duke University Neurobiologist Erich Jarvis says about 80 regulatory genes are responsible for brain activities governing the ability to speak, sing and to imitate sounds – in both humans and songbirds like hummingbirds, zebra finches, parrots and parakeets. This regulatory genetic network is not found in chimpanzees, non-singing birds (like doves and quails), or other species which don't learn to sing or mimic sounds.

Humans and vocally-imitative songbirds share a particular genetic pattern among roughly 40 genes in the human forebrain (the *anterior striatum*) and an analogous *area X* in songbirds, both structures involved in sound imitation. Similar matching patterns were found in a different set of 40 genes among regions involved in vocal production. In humans, this area is known as the *laryngeal motor cortex*, while in birds, it's the *robust nucleus of the acropallium*, or *RA nucleus*.

In the human brain, the motor cortex governs voluntary movement. A special region within it connects to nerve cells in the *brainstem*, atop the spine. These nerves send impulses to activate muscles in the *larynx*, the organ responsible for producing vocalized sound.

Analogous connections exist in songbird brains, suggesting the same ancient movement-controlling and motor-learning circuits evolved into language- and song-learning circuitry in both humans and songbirds. In humans, FoxP2 is the transcriptional regulator at the center of both the formation and function of this vocal control circuitry.

Mutual Growth

In 2012, scientists at the University of Edinburgh and Trinity College created computer-simulated brains which played against one another in the classic competitive game called *The Prisoner's Dilemma*, an ethical conundrum which allows the choice between cooperation or competition (see the later chapter entitled *The Moral Animal* for details).

50 artificial brains, each with up to ten internal processors and ten related memory nodes, were pitted against one another in these classic games. The games were treated as a series of elimination matches, simulating the way real life favors successful strategists, so the digital organisms which scored highest (minus a penalty for the size of their brains) were allowed to reproduce and populate the next generation of artificial brains.

The brains of these digital organisms were allowed to freely evolve, and the simulation showed how progress toward a cooperative society leads to a natural selection of bigger, more complex brains. As cooperation increased, the more sophisticated minds won out, while competitiveness weeded out the less sophisticated artificial organisms. Said Dr. Jackson:

The strongest selection for larger, more intelligent brains, occurred when the social groups were first beginning to start cooperating, which then kicked off an evolutionary Machiavellian arms race of one individual trying to outsmart the other by investing in a larger brain. Our digital organisms typically start to evolve more complex 'brains' when their societies first begin to develop cooperation. Our model differs in that we exploit the use of theoretical experimental evolution combined with artificial neural networks to actually prove that yes, there is an actual cause-and-effect link between needing a large brain to compete against and cooperate with your social group mates.

Bye Bye Love

Homo heidelbergensis

Deep in the heart of the Rhine Rift Valley, the ancient Celts chose the *Mountain of Saints* for their holy shrine in the 5th century BC. The stunningly beautiful site would later host a Roman legion in 40 AD, and still later come to be known as Heidelberg, celebrated for its beauty and beer. But the town's history is far, far older.

On the morning of October 21st in 1907, Daniel Hartmann, a quarryman known to the locals as Sand Daniel was digging in the sand outside the village of Mauer, when his shovel stuck something hard. Plucking the strange object from the end of his shovel, he saw that it was a oddly thick human jaw of tremendous antiquity. He set off for the nearby pub, where he breathlessly told listeners he had just found "Adam".

Professor Otto Schoetensack of the University of Heidelberg was summoned to examine the piece and was astounded – it was the mandible of an ancient human, over half a million years old, by far the most ancient human ever discovered in Europe. This was the first specimen of *Homo heidelbergensis*, an extinct human population which had flourished throughout the Old World from 700,000 to 200,000 years ago.

H. heidelbergensis were clever, aggressive and highly proficient big-game hunters, targeting horses, elephants, deer, hippos and rhinos. They were tall and exceptionally muscular, with the males growing up to six feet and nearly 200 pounds.

While omnivorous, they relied heavily upon meat, had brains about 93% the size of modern humans, and large faces with heavy and bony projecting brows. Several additional fossils would later turn up throughout Eurasia and Africa, along with stone butchering and hunting implements, including ceremonial spears.

400,000-year-old wooden spears preserved in a bog near Schöningen, Germany, were recovered alongside horse bones, constituting evidence of H. heidelbergensis hunting. These throwing weapons had been weighted at the ends, allowing them to be flung like javelins.

*The **Schöningen Spears** are eight throwing spears found in the mid-1990s by a German team of archeologists, led by Dr. Hartmut Thieme. The spears are each about seven feet long, and hand-carved from spruce trees. They were found in a German coal mine, buried in 300,000- to 400,000-year-old mud, and scattered among some 16,000 animal bones, mostly horse, and obviously butchered. Along with the spears were several wooden handles which appear to have held stone blades, various stone tools, and the remains of cooking fires.*

According to Dr. Thieme, at the time of its occupation, the region had been on the shore of a flat lake nestled among cool, open meadows and steppes. Along with the animal bones were the butchered remains of elephants, rhinoceroses, deer, cows and lions. Oxford studies have shown these species and even an extinct species of giant lions once roamed the northern hemisphere, including in Britain, Europe and North America.

A particularly severe Ice Age storm appears to have washed the remains into the low-lying region, then quickly buried them in mud, where they lay submerged for hundreds of thousands of years, until engineers drained the region to expose the coal for mining.

In the late 80s, archeologists working in northern Spain learned more of H. heidelbergensis' story.

The hills of Atapuerca contain a network of limestone caves long famous for ancient artifacts, including the bones of extinct prehistoric bears, and a primitive drawing depicting a horse's head dating from early Homo Sapiens. Juan Luis Arsuaga of the National Museum of Natural Sciences had been exploring a labyrinth of chambers and corridors deep inside these hills for years, coming across tiny fragments of prehistoric human bones. After two decades of searching, in 1997, he and his team finally found what they had been looking for, at the bottom of a 45-foot shaft. It was *La Sima de los Huesos*, the *Pit of Bones.*

They eventually unearthed 28 H. heidelbergensis skeletons, somewhere on the order of half a million years old – all adolescents. The question was, how and why did they come to be there? Professor Arsuaga believes they were laid to rest here by their kin.

500,000 years ago, Atapuerca would have made an excellent homestead, with sheltering caves overlooking a river from the hilltops. At that time, the Pit of Bones was open to the surface. It appears that Homo heidelbergensis had dropped the bodies into the pit as some sort of primitive burial, perhaps in a ritual. The evidence for this is in a hand axe of pink quartz, which could only have been brought from a distant site.

Naming the artifact *Excalibur*, after King Arthur's legendary sword, the team claim it constitutes an offering, and is thus the oldest symbol ever discovered. If true, it would mean complex thought had emerged, with symbolism and spiritual belief.

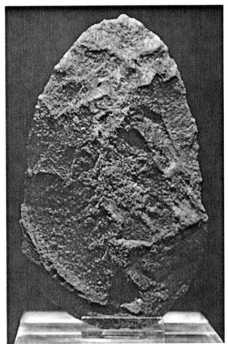

*The red quartzite handaxe dubbed **Excalibur** was the only stone tool recovered among the remains of dozens of prehistoric humans. Quartzite is said to be exceptionally difficult to knap.*

Says Dr. Arsuaga, the axe's unusual coloring and superior craftsmanship mean it was undoubtedly special, and part of an ancient funeral rite, suggesting the Atapuerca bodies had been deliberately laid to rest in the Pit of Bones. The remains come from a single group, dropped into the pit within the span of one year. Museum of Human Evolution, Burgos, Spain. Public domain image.

Almost all the bodies discovered in the Pit of Bones came from adolescents, with the exception of two adults and one child. All appear to have been the victims of some catastrophe, such as an epidemic, and many show indications of malnourishment, infection and abnormal growths. Some experts have urged caution before coming to conclusions, however, saying underground mudflows could have deposited the bodies into the pit, but if the bodies had indeed been dropped into this pit in a prehistoric funeral ritual, this would constitute the first clear evidence of symbolic thinking among early humans.

H. heidelbergensis resembled H. erectus with its jutting face and bony brow ridge (the *supraorbital torus*), low forehead which doesn't extend much above the brow ridges, and thickening of the top of the skull from front to back. It also had features in common with H. sapiens, such as a separation of the brow ridges over each eye, in contrast to the single continuous brow ridge of H. erectus, and a large brain case, more in line with that of H. sapiens. H. heidelbergensis tools were much more advanced than those of H. erectus – thinner, more symmetrical, and more carefully flaked.

According to Dr. Arsuaga, the evidence shows that "Half a million years ago, in these European populations, there was planning, there was consciousness, there was a human mind, and there was also symbolic behavior".

Comparison of Neanderthal and H. sapiens DNA shows our lines diverged from a common ancestor approximately 400,000 years ago – likely H. heidelbergensis. Nearby, at Gran Dolina, there are claims of an even older set of human remains said to belong to a previously unknown species called *Homo antecessor*, which may have lived a million years ago. As of yet, however, these conclusions are highly controversial.

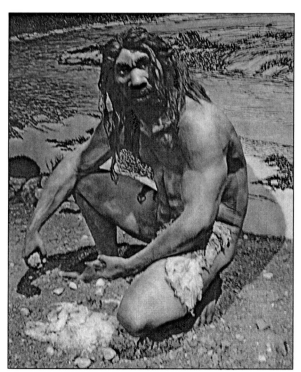

H. heidelbergensis, Jose Luis Martinez Alvarez, Wikipedia, Creative Commons attribution 2.0 license.

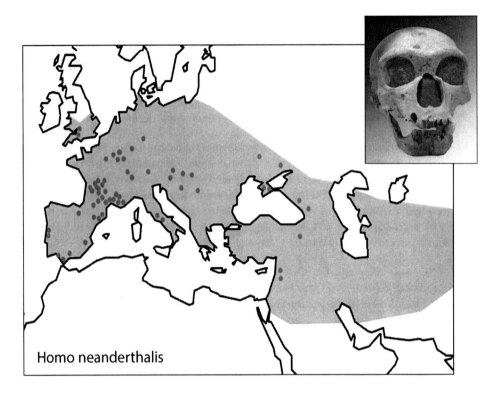

Homo neanderthalis

Us and Them

Neanderthals reigned as Eurasia's superpredators for over a quarter of a million years. They had superb hunting skills, brains larger than ours, and a lengthy track record of surviving the deadly winters of the Ice Age. They were once the most advanced humans on the planet – rugged and resourceful, adapted to the most punishing winters, until our arrival, when they suddenly vanished. The question still remains: what happened?

Fossils of over 400 Neanderthals have been recovered over a wide range, spanning the entire European continent from Portugal to Siberia, as far north as Germany and as far south as Israel. It's estimated that at their peak, there numbered around 70,000. They lived approximately 350,000 to 30,000 years ago, though the exact dates are currently in dispute.

The species was first discovered in 1829 in Feldhofer Cave in Germany's Neander Valley, a region which takes its name from 17th-century minister Joachim Neander. Neander is Greek for *New man*, while *thale* is German for *dale*.

The discovery of the *New Man of the Dales* predated Darwin's publication of the *On the Origin of Species* by some 30 years, and its announcement initially was met with bitter criticism from 19th-century religious fundamentalists, who were outraged at the suggestion that modern humans could have descended from another, more "primitive" animal species.

The Neanderthal body was shaped by cyclical Ice Ages. They were on average were four inches shorter than modern humans, and short limbed with heavy trunks, adaptations which reduced the surface area through which body heat could be lost. This trait is still found among modern Inuits. Neanderthals had robust bones, and would have been extraordinarily strong by today's standards, but, says Harvard University's Daniel Lieberman, Neanderthal anatomy from the neck down was structurally identical to ours.

Their heads were a different matter. Neanderthal skulls were much longer and lower than relatively spherical modern human skulls. Their faces were about 30% larger, with markedly bigger eyes, adapted to the lower light and long, dark nights of nothern latitudes. DNA analyses show many were red-headed and fair-skinned, an adaptation which would have helped generate vitamin D under comparatively weak northern sunlight.

Human skin color varies widely around the globe, ranging from very dark brown to a pinkish white. These differences are derived primarily from an organic molecule called **melanin**, *whose production is controlled by six genes.*

Melanin – from the Greek word for black – is a natural pigment used by most living organisms. In humans, the most common form is **eumelanin**, *a brown-black polymer. The other is* **pheomelanin**, *a red-brown polymer, largely responsible for generating red hair and freckles. Both light- and dark-skinned people have melanin, though amounts of these pigments vary by individual haplotypes. The number and size of melanin clusters also varies by individual.*

Fair-skinned people produce more pheomelanin, while dark-skinned people produce more eumelanin. Skin color is also affected to a lesser degree by the presence of subcutaneous fat and **carotene**, *a reddish-orange skin pigment, while hair color is determined by melanin.*

Melanogenesis *is the process by which specialized skin cells called* **melanocytes** *in the base of the epidermis manufacture melanin from the amino acid tyrosine. Melanocytes use photosensitive receptors to detect ultraviolet radiation, and respond by producing melanin a few hours after exposure. This pigment acts as a photoprotectant through the process called* **ultrafast internal conversion**, *dissipating over 99.9% of absorbed shortwave ultraviolet radiation (UVB) as heat. In this way, it provides a protective shield, preventing sunburn damage which can cause DNA mutations, with the potential for cancer. Those at highest risk are European Americans, who are 10 times more susceptible to* **melanoma** *than African Americans.*

If melanin completely shielded the skin from UV radiation, however, it would be harmful. Small amounts of ultraviolet radiation (UVB) must penetrate the outermost epidermis for the human body to produce vitamin D.

We synthesize about 90% of vitamin D in the skin and kidneys, when ultraviolet radiation acts upon a cholesterol-like chemical precursor. The other 10% of vitamin D is extracted from foods like egg yolks and fatty fish. Vitamin D is vital for the intestines to extract calcium and phosphorus from food, used for bone growth and repair, for preventing clotting, and for stabilizing heartbeat and the nervous system. It also helps promote the production of **cathelicidin**, *an antimicrobial the body secretes to fight fungal, bacterial, and viral infections, including common flu.*

Nature has selected for people with lighter skin in northern latitudes due to the comparatively weaker solar ultraviolet radiation. In these environments, dark skin is disadvantageous because it prevents the production of vitamin D, with the potential for illnesses such as **rickets** *in children, and* **osteoporosis** *in older adults.*

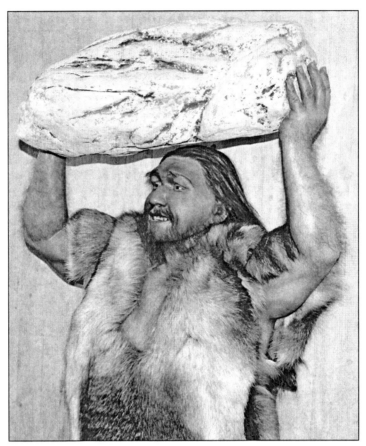

H. Neanderthalensis lifting a rock, Neanderthal Museum, Mettmann, Germany.
Image: Neozoon, Wikipedia, Creative Commons Attribution 3.0 Unported license.

Although typically portrayed as stupid, lumbering brutes, Neanderthals actually had brains larger than modern humans. The difference lies in how those brains were structured – Neanderthals had significantly more neural "real estate" dedicated to the *occipital lobe*, which processes vision, and to regions which govern physical movement, in contrast with the larger cortex with which modern humans come equipped.

Casts of Neanderthal braincases show their brains were less developed than ours in the *temporal lobe* (near the temples), a region which processes memory, hearing and language; and the *parietal lobe* (a top-rear brain region), where processing of arithmetic, abstractions and spatial relationships occurs. In these regions, modern humans seem to have distinctly greater development than Neanderthals.

Surprisingly, Neanderthals may have possessed a very rudimentary language, however. According to Dr. Jeffrey Laitman of the Mt. Sinai School of Medicine, the larynx, our voicebox, had slowly moved over time to a position unique among mammals, descending in the throat. This provides extra space which allows complex speech. It was a result of the gradual shift in the base of skulls that first began 160,000 years ago. By the time Neanderthals evolved, the anatomy was in place for speech, and, says Dr. Laitman, this indicates it evolved specifically for use in speech.

The *hyoid bone* in the throat is a crucial component of the larynx. Fossil finds show it had already developed in Neanderthals, indicating they were anatomically capable of producing speech. Says Dr. Margaret Clegg of the University College of London, their bigger lungs, huge noses and nasal passages would have endowed them with the tremendous booming voices of veteran opera singers. The modern human form of FOXP2 (which controls the development of speech articulators) also existed in Neanderthals, though the most important aspects of human language distinguishing it from other animal vocalizations are derived from cognitive, rather than physical, capacities.

Neanderthals had a gentler curve in the upper esophagus, allowing more rapid food consumption, but this would have made rapid speech such as ours difficult. So while they had the necessary FOXPRO genes, hyoid bone and larynx for speech production, it would almost certainly have been limited to very guttural, simplistic utterances.

Neanderthals hunted big game roaming the edges of great glaciers which covered most of prehistoric Europe and parts of Asia. They were omnivorous, living on large herbivores like bison, reindeer, horses and even woolly mammoths. Although chemical analyses of their bones showed they ate a very large amount of protein, examination of their fossilized teeth by three Smithsonian archaeobiologists in 2011 shows they also ate a great deal of cooked plant materials, some of them for medicinal purposes.

Material trapped in the fossilized dental plaque of five Neanderthals from Spain's El Sidrón caves was analyzed using mass spectrometry and advanced extraction techniques. The team discovered chemicals produced by wood-fire smoke, several types of cooked, starchy foods, and microfossils from two plants used as medicine in modern times.

Yarrow and *chamomile* are plants well-known as natural medicines. Since these plants are quite bitter, they would not have been selected for taste, and their use for medicinal reasons would be similar to behaviors seen among other animal species who self-medicate with herbs. Chamomile is used for its calming and digestive benefits, while yarrow is used for treating fevers, and as an antiseptic.

Artifacts excavated at the Grotte du Renne and Saint Césaire in France suggest Neanderthals may also have crafted bone tools and body ornaments after the arrival of modern humans, indicating that cultural diffusion took place between the two species, though these assertions are as yet controversial. They may also have fashioned dwellings out of animal bones: a site in Molodova, eastern Ukraine contains buildings constructed from mammoth skulls, tusks, jaws, and leg bones, with 25 inner hearths.

Based on morphological traits, Neanderthals seem to have been a side branch of humanity, the descendants of H. heidelbergensis, themselves descended from H. erectus, though they were eventually an evolutionary dead end.

Modern humans arrived in Europe some 43,000 years ago. Not much earlier than this, we'd been reduced to near extinction – a population of about 10,000, desperately struggling to survive, because of geological disasters and climate change.

Neanderthals, on the other hand, had been a very successful species for hundreds of thousands of years, until they suddenly disappeared from the face of the planet almost overnight about 30,000 years ago. They had much better eyesight than ours – the Neanderthal *occipital lobe* at the rear and bottom of the brain was significantly larger than that of homo sapiens. But though we were facing, stronger, hardier hunters with advanced sight and familiarity with the terrain, we were coming as conquerors. And there was no stopping us.

As Harvard University's Dr. Daniel Leiberman puts it, "Humans have a very intensive way of using the environment. Humans move into the Middle East, Homo erectus goes extinct. When humans move into Europe, the Neanderthals go extinct."

It's assumed that we were better able to organize and to invent than Neanderthals. Neanderthal brains were focused more upon vision and movement, leaving little room for the development of the social skills and creative problem-solving of modern humans.

Possibly our smaller frames also made us better equipped at hunting, and our human vocal abilities and cognitive skills enabled us to plan and cooperate more effectively. Whatever the reasons, we appear to have driven them to extinction. There are several theories as to why this may have happened, though the truth is probably a combination of factors: they needed to hunt frequently, as their large bodies and brains required twice the food of a modern human's. These metabolic needs would have intensified the survival difficulties they faced. With their bulkier bodies and larger brains, living in such a cold environment would have required about 5,000 kilocalories a day to sustain – over twice that of a modern human – about as much as one of us would require to race the Tour de France on an everyday basis.

Because of our trimmer, taller bodies, Homo sapiens had lower metabolic demands and an ever-improving arsenal, including projectile weapons, in the form of light, bone-tipped throwing spears. These enabled our ancestors to hunt a wider range of animals from a longer and safer distance, expanding our potential sources of food, with less personal risk.

As big game grew scarce, the hunting techniques of the Neanderthals were ill-adapted to catching smaller prey such as rabbits, which modern humans seem to have relied upon at the time. Our domestication of dogs also aided in hunting this smaller prey, according to Cambridge University professors Paul Mellars and Jennifer French.

Dr. Robin Dunbar, evolutionary psychologist at the University of Oxford, notes that Neanderthals had "developed a very confrontational and dangerous style of hunting, and were very dependent on a heavy meat diet".

"Modern humans (in Africa) developed the bow and arrow, as well as spear throwers, which allowed hunting at arms' length and often focused on smaller prey."

In contrast, Neanderthals hunted with heavy wooden stone-tipped spears used for thrusting rather than throwing. This meant Neanderthal hunters had to be within striking distance of their prey, making hunting very risky. The dangers are stamped clearly upon their bones: nearly all male Neanderthals showed signs of a violent existence, marked by multiple fractures, trauma marks and head wounds. Most of these wounds had healed, indicating they weren't the cause of death, but were a part of normal Neanderthal life.

Such patterns of injury most closely resemble those of rodeo wranglers, further evidence that Neanderthals hunted wild animals with sheer physical force, charging and pouncing upon their prey – or enemies. Neanderthal lives were nasty, brutish and short; their remains show that few lived beyond 30 years of age.

They lived in much smaller family groups than modern humans – 10 to 15, as opposed to our early bands of 150 or more. Nor did they exchange technology between their small bands, a failing which may ultimately have led to their demise. Smaller social networks likely made it harder for Neanderthals to cope with the harsh prehistoric Eurasian environments: they simply had fewer friends to turn to in times of need.

However, archeologists have found evidence that they did care for their sick and infirm: one Neanderthal man with a withered arm had been cared for over the course of at least two decades. His injuries indicate that, while he was incapacitated, he was fed and tended to for over a year as his worst injuries stabilized.

We Are Family

Some scientists suggest we simply absorbed the Neanderthals into the modern human population through interbreeding; DNA extracted from Neanderthal bones shows that our genomes are nearly identical, but according to Ed Green of Germany's Max Planck Institute, most modern humans carry a specific allele of the *microcephalin D* gene, which entered the human species 37,000 years ago. This gene is said to be Neanderthal in origin, showing our ancestors interbred thousands of years ago.

In fact, he says, all non-Africans carry between one and four percent Neanderthal DNA, and these genes contributed to our immune systems, likely helping us survive exotic illnesses as we spread across the planet.

DNA is passed down from parent to child, so geneticists can look for *signatures* of interbreeding in the DNA of people alive today. These markers are *single nucleotide polymorphisms*, genetic regions which differ from person to person by only a single DNA base that have been passed down over millions of years.

Harvard geneticist David Reich found many identical SNPs in the DNA of ancient Neanderthals and contemporary Europeans and Asians. By sampling the DNA of modern people worldwide, his team was also able to determine when and where these SNPs first arose.

Humans actually have two separate genomes in every cell (with the exception of blood cells, which don't have nuclei): most genetic material is housed within the cell nuclei, but in every cell's cytoplasm are approximately 1,700 mitochondria, which contain their own shared, separate DNA, and replicate independently from the rest of the cell. This mitochondrial genome is very small – only 37 genes and 16,569 nucleotide bases long.

But while nuclear DNA is a mixture from both parents, mitochondrial DNA is only passed down from mothers to children, so it remains unmixed and unchanged down the generations. Because of this, we know that a single African woman alive 170,000 years ago (popularly called *Ancestral Eve*) passed down her mitochondrial DNA to every human being alive today. This means that all the other women alive at Eve's time either had only sons, no children, or their children died without children of their own. (It also means that, if one goes far enough back, we're all Africans. So much for "white power".)

But there's more to the story, of course. DNA analyses show humans and Neanderthals are so closely related that some scientists consider both to constitute a single species. According to Dr. Svante Pääbo, a palaeogeneticist at the Max Planck Institute in Leipzig, Germany, whose team sequenced the Neanderthal genome, Neanderthals, "[were] a form of humans that are bit different than humans are today, but not much".

Any human whose ancestors developed outside of Africa has between one and four percent Neanderthal DNA in his or her genome. Because of this, we know humans and Neanderthals interbred and produced hybrid children at least 45,000 years ago.

A set of *human leukocyte antigen* (HLA) *class I* genes are the most significant benefit humans gained from this genetic merging. This is a group of about 220 immune system genes on chromosome six. The HLA proteins the genes produce assist the immune system in spotting evidence of cell abnormalities such as infection or cancer.

These genes encode *antigens*, tiny signallers on cell surfaces used to attract the immune system's killer T-cells to destroy infections. HLA antigens on the surface of cells are also used by the body to recognize its own cells versus foreign cells – an extreme difference in antigens is why transplanted organs are sometimes rejected.

HLA genes vary depending upon geography, shaped by natural selection to fight diseases specific to particular areas. Dr. Jeffrey Wall of the University of Southern California says that Neanderthal genes helped humans evolve and survive by adapting to the northern environment. These acquired genes helped protect against local diseases as humans spread out across the planet.

Dr. Svante Pääbo of the Max Planck Institute for Evolutionary Anthropology in Leipzig, Germany, says that every human alive today of non-African descent also carries DNA from a newly-discovered race of hominins called *Denisovans*.

DNA from a 40,000-year-old finger bone found in a Siberian cave provided the genetic link between Homo sapiens and the Denisovans.

1 HOMO HABILIS ~ NICKNAME: Handyman LIVED: 2.4 to 1.6 million years ago HABITAT: Tropical Africa DIET:Omnivorous – nuts, seeds, tubers, fruits, some meat; 2 HOMO SAPIEN ~ NICKNAME: Human LIVED: 200,000 years ago to present HABITAT: All DIET: Omnivorous - meat, vegetables, tubers, nuts, pizza, sushi; 3 HOMO FLORESIENSIS ~ NICKNAME: Hobbit LIVED: 95,000 to 13,000 years ago HABITAT: Flores, Indonesia (tropical) DIET: Omnivorous - meat included pygmy stegodon, giant rat; 4 HOMO ERECTUS ~ NICKNAME: Erectus LIVED: 1.8 million years to 100,000 years ago HABITAT: Tropical to temperate - Africa, Asia, Europe DIET: Omnivorous - meat, tubers, fruits, nuts; 5 PARANTHROPUS BOISEI ~ NICKNAME: Nutcracker man LIVED: 2.3 to 1.4 million years ago HABITAT: Tropical Africa DIET: Omnivorous - nuts, seeds, leaves, tubers, fruits, maybe some meat; 6 HOMO HEIDEL- BERGENSIS ~ NICKNAME: Goliath LIVED: 700,000 to 300,000 years ago HABITAT: Temperate and tropical, Africa and Europe DIET: Omnivorous - meat, vegetables, tubers, nuts; 7 HOMO NEANDERTHALENSIS ~ NICKNAME: Neanderthal LIVED: 250,000 to 30,000 years ago HABITAT: Europe and Asia DIET: Relied heavily on meat, such as bison, deer and musk

321

Run to the Hills

According to University of Bordeaux paleoanthropologist Dr. William Banks, "The colonization of Europe by anatomically modern humans... resulted in competition with which the Neanderthal adaptive system was unable to cope."

2010 research showed modern humans were living in Italy and the United Kingdom 41,000 to 45,000 years ago, but an international study in 2012 suggested that Neanderthals may have gone extinct before we ever arrived, posing a conundrum in light of our shared DNA.

In addition to radiocarbon dating, a new technique of *ultrafiltration* was used to wash out modern contaminants before dating. This removed smaller molecules, leaving only large *collagen strands* for more accurate measurements. Researchers screened over 200 fossilized bones from 11 Neanderthal sites, looking for traces of collagen, the bone protein most suited to radiocarbon dating. Out of these, only six yielded meaningful data. The bones were not of Neanderthals however, but of other animals whose remains were found in the same sediment layers as the Neanderthal remains.

The new findings set the age of the last known Neanderthals at 45,000 years ago. Oxford Professor Thomas Higham says this changes the picture of our early prehistory:

> *The picture emerging is of an overlapping period [in Europe] that could be of the order of perhaps 3,000-4,000 years - a period over which we have a mosaic of modern humans being present and then Neanderthals slowly ebbing away, and finally becoming extinct. What our research contributes is that in southern Spain, Neanderthals don't hang on for another 4,000 years compared with the rest of Europe. And the hunch must be that they go extinct in the south of Spain at the same time as everywhere else.*

Clive Finlayson, director of the Gibraltar Museum, takes issue with the findings, suggesting that the sites chosen for eligible samples skewed the data. It seems clear that some genetic mingling took place between our species and theirs; it is possible, however, that this occurred outside of Europe, within the Mediterranean or Middle East, further back in time, perhaps 80,000 to 90,000 years ago.

In the spring of 2013, Dr. Silvana Condemi of the University of Ai-Marseille may have found a definitive answer. Her team had retrieved the skeletal remains of a Neanderthal-human hybrid who had lived in northern Italy 40,000-30,000 years ago. The mandible was unearthed from a rock-shelter called *Riparo di Mezzena* in Italy.

Studying the jawbone via DNA analysis and 3-D imaging, her team concluded that its mitochondrial DNA was Neanderthal in origin. Mitochondrial DNA is only passed down from mothers, leading to the conclusion that a female Neanderthal had mated with a male Homo sapiens.

Said Condemi, by the time modern humans arrived in the area, the Neanderthals had already established their own *Mousterian* culture, which lasted some 200,000 years. Numerous flint tools, such as axes and spear points, have been associated with this culture. These artifacts are typically found in rock shelters and caves throughout Europe. This indicates "...a slow process of replacement of Neanderthals by the invading modern human populations, as well as additional evidence of the upholding of the Neanderthals' cultural identity."

Earlier fossils indicate that Homo sapiens lived in a southern Italian cave as early as 45,000 years ago. This means that modern humans and Neanderthals coexisted for thousands of years. The newcomers would likely have been rather unwelcome, however, and for a very good reason: Condemi's findings suggest that modern humans may have been raping female Neanderthals. We may also have committed genocide, or come bearing diseases which further imperilled the Neanderthals. One researcher even suggests we cannibalized them, though evidence for this consists of only one set of knife-scarred bones.

Whatever the truth may be, we do know their numbers declined, and by the end, they were struggling in Ice Age Europe, squeezed down to final footholds in the southernmost regions of Spain and Italy. Their final refuge appears to have been the Rock of Gibraltar, where the last of the species died 45,000 to 30,000 years ago in *Gorham's Cave*.

Once thought to have been our ancestors, the Neanderthals are now considered an evolutionary dead end. But, according to Cambridge Professor Sacha Jones:

> *They show us a different way to be human. It's a separate evolutionary path that went its own way, shared much of our own evolutionary history, shared many features with us, but also developed their own distinctive features and went their own way, with their own ways of adapting, their own ways of coping with the environment. So they're a fascinating experiment in how to be a human being.*

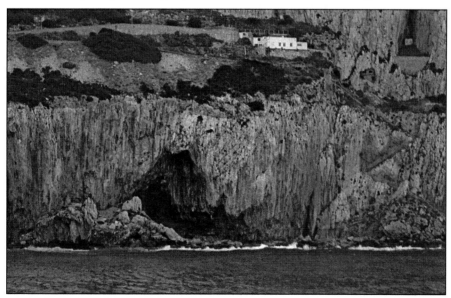

Gorham's Cave, the last known Neanderthal refuge, on the east face of the Rock of Gibraltar. Image: Tyson Lee Holmes, Wikimedia Creative Commons Attribution 3.0 Unported license.

Last in Line

In 2004, radioactive argon dating showed a pair of fossilized skulls unearthed in 1967 to be 195,000 years old. The skulls of *Omo I* and *Omo II* were buried in rock sediment which had formed from the overflowing Nile River in south-western Ethiopia. Dr. Richard Leakey made the find, but dating techniques at the time were too unsophisticated to accurately pinpoint their age. However, these are now the oldest known members of Homo sapiens – anatomically modern humans. The find also fits with genetic analyses of modern populations, which show Homo sapiens first emerged in Africa approximately 200,000 years ago.

Omo I was male, tall and slender, about 5'10" and 155 pounds, with a touch of Neanderthal to his features, while Omo II was also male, slender and moderately tall, at about 5'9". According to University of New Mexico anthropologist Osbjorn Pearson, "...these early modern humans were...much like the people in southern Ethiopia and the southern Sudan today". He adds that "without a doubt", Omo I is an anatomically modern human, although Omo II has a more primitive skull. Both lived around the same time and location. Anthropologists also found stone hand axes, picks and spearlike objects on the site.

Abundant fossils of large Nile fish on the site show conditions were much wetter in the region at the time, and big game was plentiful, including hippos, antelope, giant forest hogs, giraffes, elephants, zebras, rhinos, and many other hoofed mammals. Very few remains of predators were found, suggesting few, if any, large predators competed with these first humans. Dr. Leakey's team believes the region's human inhabitants practiced a *seasonal settlement* strategy – following migrating big game.

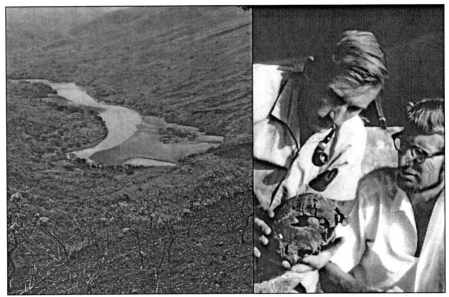

The Omo River, where modern humans lived in southwest Ethiopia. Right: Drs. Richard Leakey and Paul Abell examine the 195,000-year-old skull of Omo I. A nearly complete skeleton of an adult male Homo sapiens was recovered from the site in 1967. Public domain images.

Children of the Sea

Since the year 2000, a remarkable new branch of science has emerged called *genetic anthropology*. Combining DNA and fossil evidence, researchers can now track the movement of modern human populations across history. We now know that Homo sapiens first appeared about 200,000 years ago, and that we nearly went extinct twice. The first time was about 140,000 years ago, when nearly all of Africa was stricken by a megadrought and grew into an uninhabitable, continent-wide desert.

Race is a figment of your imagination. DNA analyses show that every human alive today shares the same mitochondrial DNA. Mitochondrial DNA is only passed down by mothers, and our ancient common maternal ancestor has been called Mitochondrial Eve. We know she lived in Africa about 140,000 years ago. She wasn't the only ancient Homo sapiens to have borne children, but only her line survived until the present day.

Furthermore, according to the U.S. Department of Energy's Human Genome Project website: "DNA studies do not indicate that separate classifiable subspecies (races) exist within modern humans. While different genes for physical traits such as skin and hair color can be identified between individuals, no consistent patterns of genes across the human genome exist to distinguish one race from another. There also is no genetic basis for divisions of human ethnicity. People who have lived in the same geographic region for many generations may have some alleles in common, but no allele will be found in all members of one population and in no members of any other. Indeed, it has been proven that there is more genetic variation within races than exists between them."

Forced to adapt quickly or perish, our earliest forebears were squeezed onto the coasts and highlands in a few scattered locations. There were about five locales able to support hunter-gatherer populations.

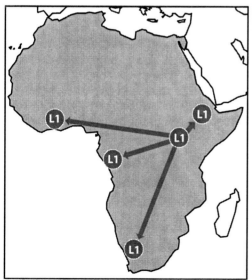

Four hunter-gatherer groups of H. sapiens – traced by their shared *L1* mitochondrial DNA – spread to the coastlines on the Cape of Good Hope, Congo Basin, Ivory Coast and northeastern Ethiopia.

The transition wasn't easy: DNA analysis shows every human alive today comes from a very tiny population of survivors – our genetic diversity comes from as few as 600 breeding individuals. Geneticist Spencer Wells says this population crash left an indelible stamp upon our genes through a *bottleneck effect*:

Humans, although on the surface seem to be so different from each other, actually have remarkably little genetic diversity. We're 99.9 percent identical. Look at other apes, like chimps or gorillas or orangutans. They have between four and ten times as much diversity at the DNA level. The lack of diversity in human DNA is a clue to a crisis that may have wiped out whole populations. Everyone alive today is a descendant of these individuals....That's how a bottleneck works. And everybody alive today is a descendant of that small number of individuals who made it through the bottleneck.

Life along the coastlines forced our ancestors to find new sources of food and the means of acquiring it. But as we've seen repeatedly, adversity drives evolution, and in the case of our ancestors, we adapted by becoming all the more clever, improving our technology and developing culture. Adaptability kept us alive. We started living in coastal caves, depending upon the sea for our livelihood, hardening our tools by fire and making body ornaments.

An international team of researchers led by Arizona State University's Dr. Curtis Marean has pieced together much of this story from a remarkable discovery on the southernmost tip of Africa.

Dr. Marean analyzed climate data, human migration patterns, geological formations and sea currents to pinpoint likely sites for mankind's early years. One of these was South Africa's *Pinnacle Point*.

From Pinnacle Point, looking out over the deep blue of the Southern Ocean as the whitecaps crash eternally upon the rocks, it's easy to imagine time on a scale of aeons, back to where, on this very spot, human civilization was born.

At least one set of caves which sustained humanity through the megadrought has been found here, where our need to adapt drove us to new levels of ingenuity: here, we learned to predict the tides; to anticipate when shellfish would be exposed by watching the cycles of the moon.

This series of caves sheltered ancient H. sapiens some 164,000 years ago. Sand dunes would periodically seal the entrances, and they would again re-open thousands of years later, ultimately sheltering our ancestors over the course of some 100,000 years.

Here, Dr. Marean and his team began excavating in the year 2000, and have since unearthed over 1,800 stone implements, pieces of prepared red pigment and a mountain of remains of seafood consumed by our ancestors – mussels, clams, snails, and even traces of seals and whales.

It's quite probable that these caves sheltered the only survivors of the environmental devastation that had rendered nearly all of Africa uninhabitable.

Here we learned to survive on a diet of seafood, to create sophisticated stone weapons and tools, and to manufacture and wear body paint and jewellery. Together, these three activities signalled a major shift from a nomadic life of hunting and gathering into one of settled cultivation – the first settled human society.

Pinnacle Point provided us with nutrition to sustain our brain's expansion. The seafood diet was rich in the fatty acid *DHA* (*docosahexaenoic acid*), providing protein building blocks for increased brain size, complexity and function. The harsh climate and reduced food resources kept us tethered to the water, with its constant source of DHA.

This seafood diet nourished us while we developed new skills and fire-hardened tools and weapons. These would prove invaluable, helping us survive and multiply, before we began dispersing north, to migrate across the continents in the wake of the retreating Ice Age glaciers.

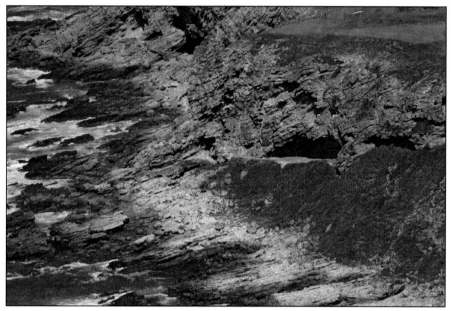

Pinnacle Point, Mossel Bay, on the southern coast of South Africa. The entrance to the main cave can be seen at the center of this photograph. Credit: Dr. Erich Fisher, Arizona State University. Used with permission.

Roam

Oxford University's Professor Stephen Oppenheimer describes what came next for mankind: between 135,000 and 105,000 years ago, Africa again grew significantly wetter, and the northeastern Sahara, Sinai, and Negev deserts became hospitable for migration. Fossils of snails in the northern Africa desert from 128,000 years ago show it had once again become habitable for a time. By following reliable water resources and animal herds northward, humans began once again to spread.

About 120,000 years ago, one group journeyed across a much greener Sahara desert, up the Nile River and into the Middle East. Just as ancient Homo Erectus had 1.7 million years earlier, humans would leave the cradle of Mother Africa, guided by the weather. At that time, two routes led out of Africa, one in the north and one in the south, and the climate determined which would be open at any particular time, directing early explorers where to go next, whether northward or eastward.

The first wave of modern humans exited Africa 120,000 years ago via the northern route. They were to meet with a grim fate: the only signs of that first group are fossilized bones found in Israel's *Qafzeh cave*. These are the earliest remains of Homo sapiens found outside of Africa, dating from 120,000 to 90,000 years ago. No trace of these people remains in the genetic record. Fortunately, however, a second foray would meet with much greater success, to spread and populate the modern world.

Salad Days

Over evolutionary history, the human diet changed radically, particularly with the advent of cooking, use of stone tools, and development of agriculture. Since dietary changes are difficult to track, researchers instead look for the genetic changes to human digestion.

Dartmouth biological anthropologist Dr. Nathaniel Dominy says a genetic change coincided with the dawn of agriculture, when we began to grow cereal grains. The rise of agriculture was a major point of transformation for the human race, spurring the building of larger settlements, innovations in cultivation and harvesting, an explosion of culture and, eventually, modern life.

Complex starches are hydrolyzed into simple sugars to fuel muscle contraction, organ and cell function, and *anabolism* – protein assembly for tissue growth and repair. To accomplish this, the human body relies upon high levels of the digestive enzyme *salivary amylase*. Chimpanzees have only two copies of the gene responsible for amylase production, *AMYl*, while humans possess from six to 15 copies, depending upon the individual.

Chimpanzees and other great apes primarily live on fruits and leaves, low-calorie foods which require almost constant foraging, but modern humans derive most energy from starchy grains or plant roots.

For neural growth, we are limited by our dietary need for *long-chain polyunsaturated fatty acids (LC-PUFAs)*, something our bodies can't naturally synthesize, and these substances aren't widely available in food. Early Africans first obtained these fatty acids from DHA-enriched marine foods. Then 85,000 years ago, the cluster of *FADS* *(fatty acid desaturase)* genes on chromosome 11 mutated, giving humans a digestive enzyme to convert plant-based LC-PUFAs into fuel for our hungry brains.

Once the trait emerged, intense natural selection caused its rapid spread throughout the entire population. This adaptation gave us the ability to exploit a greater variety of food sources, freeing us from dependency upon marine sources of DHA. It was an adaptation that would greatly aid our migration out of Africa in the *Great Expansion*.

When one considers all the mutations which led to such pivotal moments in human evolution, it looks like an unbelievable sequence of lucky accidents. But, says Dr. John Hawks of the University of Wisconsin Madison, it's only because we don't see the many mutations that were weeded out through billions of years of natural selection.

Those which conferred survival advantages were passed down through generations, while those that weren't advantageous didn't equip their owners to survive and pass the genes on through offspring. "It is only from today's viewpoint that the mutations that give us our current physical form appear to be the 'right' ones to have", adds Hawks. "It's hindsight, When we look back at the whole process, it looks like a stunning series of accidents."

*Agriculture was born with **forest gardening**, a low-maintenance food production system built around natural woodland ecosystems. It incorporates fruit and nut trees, vegetables, herbs, shrubs and vines useful to humans. The system originated along jungle riverbanks and in monsoon-region foothills. In a gradual process of shaping their surroundings, families would identify useful tree and vine species, then protect and improve them, while eliminating undesirable species. Later, foreign species could be introduced and incorporated into these gardens.*

*As techniques were refined, farmers developed **companion planting** – growing complementary crops side-by-side to increase crop productivity. Species could be intermixed, building woodland habitats in a succession of layers. There was a division of labor, with women tending to the crops and child-rearing, while men, with their stronger upper bodies, engaged in hunting and defense.*

*Forest gardening is still practiced widely throughout Africa and Asia, where it plays a critical role in food stability. In North Africa, **oasis gardening** makes use of palm trees, fruit trees and vegetables in a layered forest garden, but the most famous modern example is the **Chagga Gardens** on the slopes of Tanzania's Mt. Kilimanjaro. This farming system has continued for over a century, primarily because the Chagga continuously return nutrients to the soil.*

The Chagga are a diverse group of peoples living on Mount Kilimanjaro's slopes. As various groups arrived and settled there, they brought their own crops, such as maize, cassava and sweet potatoes. The rich variety of plantations slowly evolved into a distinctive type of land use, exploiting not just horizontal spacing on the ground, but also differing plant species heights, using trees for multiple growth levels.

The Chagga Gardens were inspired by observing the natural forest, which makes maximum use of its land, water, and light. Farming began with small parts of forest land, where useful plant species were found. Gradually, they replaced other parts of the natural forest with cultivated plants. The Chagga are now experts in combining a variety of plants which require varying amounts of light exposure and roots of varying depths.

Yams can tolerate shade from neighbouring trees, and use tree trunks for climbing support, and trees with the deepest roots allow crops to draw sufficient nutrients from the soil right beside them. Modern Chagga farmers grow up to 60 different tree species within areas the size of a football field, recycling nutrients and using cattle manure to fertilize crops.

These gardens are grown in different vertical zones. The lowest, at one meter or less, includes beans, taro, and grasses used to feed livestock. The next zone, at up to two and a half meters, contains coffee with a banana canopy above it. Above the bananas grow timber trees. An average plot can produce 125 kg. of beans, 280 kg. of coffee, and 275 bunches of bananas every year, while supplying timber and livestock fodder.

In the Light

Humans began heat-treating tools and weapons as early as 72,000 years ago in South Africa, using the stone called *silcrete*, which is easier to chip when heated, and results in sturdier, sharper blades, knives, and handle-mounted tools.

This sophisticated use of fire shows advanced intelligence, marking a turning point when Homo sapiens became "uniquely human," according to University of Cape Town archeologist Kyle Brown.

Dr. Brown's team has also uncovered hand-designed shell-bead jewellery, and the remains of *ochre*, a red-tinted clay used for body and cave painting. Ostrich-eggshell bead jewellery dating from roughly the same period was also discovered in Tanzania's Serengeti National Park by a University of Arizona team in 2004, as well as evidence of stone-tipped arrows and bow use.

A new type of symbolic consciousness was emerging. The first evidence of decorative art, made from naturally-occurring red ochre, was found at *Blombos*, another cave along the South African coast.

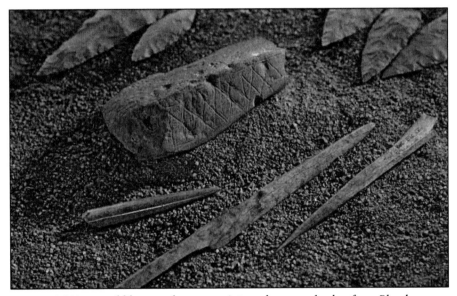

Image: 75,000-year-old bone tools, spear points and engraved ochre from Blombos cave.
Image: Chris Henshilwood, 2007, Wikipedia, attribution license 3.0

In Blombos Cave, Dr. Chris Henshilwood discovered 8,000 pieces of *ochre*, a soft stone which can be mixed with animal fat to make paint. This ochre had been transported from miles away, and fragments had been carefully prepared and meticulously engraved with geometric crosshatching designs. This is the earliest known example of the deliberate planning, production and storage of a pigment compound, serving, says Dr. Henshilwood, as an important benchmark of human cognitive ability. To this day, tribal *Ovashimba* women in Namibia Africa still cover themselves in such ochre-based body paint on a daily basis. But while the Blombos remains were 77,000 years old, even older evidence of civilization exists – carved bone harpoon tips, unearthed at three sites in Katanda on the Congo Republic's Upper Semliki River in the Western Rift Valley. Congolese still hunt catfish there with the same sort of harpoons.

Killer

Archeologists have managed to tracked human migrations by a rather grim method: tracing animal extinctions. In Europe and Asia, the arrival of H. sapiens coincides with the disappearance of the hairy mammoth, the cave lion and other large mammals. In Australia, most animals weighing over 100 pounds vanished within a few thousand years of the arrival of humans.

According to Stony Brook University's Dr. John Shea, the further from Africa humans migrated, the more pronounced extinctions became. Neanderthals were only one of several species that vanished after our arrival, gradually marginalized into the outskirts of Europe. After they vanished, we remained the only type of human on Earth for the first time.

Our species has spread across the entire planet, driving other hominins and many other species into extinction. The way our species has intensified exploitation of our environments is completely unique among Earth life.

Says Case Western Reserve anthropologist Dr. Donald Johanson:

> Homo sapiens is the most adaptable species in the human career, meaning that no matter what happens in the world, we have a way of adapting to it. Today, that way is called "culture." If glaciers came to Arizona where I live, we wouldn't be growing thick fur and thick skin, we would be building more fireplaces and heating systems.
>
> Culture is the storehouse of our complex ways of thinking and perceiving, and we pass it on to our children as surely as we pass on our genes. The ways in which cultural evolution and genetic evolution interact will be at the forefront of the research of tomorrow, because one thing is for sure, evolution is not stopping.

He Ain't Heavy

Both gene analyses and the fossil record show the first humans evolved 200,000 to 150,000 years ago, probably around South Africa, Namibia, and Angola, the modern-day homeland of the *San* tribesmen, commonly called the *Bushmen of the Kalahari*. Branches left Africa in what seem to have been two waves about 100,000 and 85,000 years ago, the first wave dying out, and the second spreading and eventually replacing earlier humans such as the Neanderthals and Homo erectus.

The San have unique genetic markers unlike anyone else in the world, showing they are direct descendants of the very first humans. There are about 85,000 alive today, mostly in remote regions of the Kalahari Desert in South Africa, Angola, Botswana and Namibia. About half live like our forebears in temporary wood shelters, caves or rocky overhangs in the Kalahari of southwestern Africa.

Their language makes use of unique *glottal clicks*, made by pressing the tongue against the palate and then flicking it forward and down. No other existing human language uses these sounds.

The San are among the world's last remaining hunter-gatherer societies, still living in the style of our common ancestors. Neighboring tribes call them *Basarwa*, which means *people who have nothing*, or *San*, meaning *vagabonds* or *those without cattle*.

As hunter-gatherers, the San live in small, highly-mobile, foraging bands. A modern San typically travels lightly, carrying a bow or hide sling, a blanket, and a cloak called a *kaross*, in which he or she carries food, firewood, and sometimes babies, smaller bags, and a stick for digging. A skin shoulderbag contains personal belongings, including medicines, poison, and arrows. They also sometimes carry clubs.

Women gather fruits, nuts and roots, while men hunt in excursions that can last for days at a time, primarily pursuing antelope, using spears and bows with poison arrows. They also enjoy leisure time by engaging in music, conversation, and dancing. Temporary shelters are fashioned from wood gathered in their travels.

Modern San hunt with arrows tipped with paralyzing poisons derived from plants, snakes, beetle larvae, crushed scorpions, caterpillars, or trapdoor spiders. Although they don't own animals or cultivate plants, the San have a deep knowledge of flora and fauna, including deep knowledge of thousands of plants for nutrition, medicine, and hunting.

Although they can fashion pitfall traps or snares made from plant fibers, the San prefer to hunt for their food, and San trackers are legendary for their ability to follow the *spoor* (tracks) of animals across any kind of terrain – even to the point of being able to distinguish the spoor of a wounded animal from a healthy one. They think much like forensic detectives, "getting into the minds" of their prey. This kind of mental ability is what made the human animal an unstoppable predator.

Their hunting methods are impressive: the study their prey's habits, and test the wind by throwing a handful of dust in the air. On open ground, they belly-crawl, sometimes disguising themselves with a small bush held before them.

Although respected elders or accomplished hunters may achieve a degree of leadership status, the San typically have no central authority, instead governing by group consensus, and settling disputes through discussion, until an agreement has been reached. They tend to be egalitarian, sharing possessions like meat and tobacco, and their land is shared among the group, with rights passed down through inheritance.

San are omnivorous, eating any available animal or vegetable food, including antelope, giraffe, lion, zebra, porcupine, snake, hare, fish, turtle, hyena, insects, eggs and honey. They boil or roast their meat, and use every part of the animal, tanning the hides to use for blankets. Water is scarce because the San are constantly mobile. It's usually acquired by scraping and squeezing roots, or by digging holes in the sand. When on the move, they sometimes carry water in ostrich eggshells.

Exodus

85,000 years ago, a second wave of humans left Africa, bands of beachcombers who crossed into the Middle East from coastal Djibouti and Eritrea. All of them carried common mitochondrial DNA from the *L3 haplogroup*, which would populate the entire planet outside of Africa over the next 85,000 years.

The straits called the *Gates of Grief* (from the Arabic *Bab-el-Mandeb*) is the Red Sea's narrowest point – about 12 miles wide. 85,000 years ago, global glaciation had locked vast amounts of seawater in ice, lowering sea levels by 80 meters and substantially narrowing the distance across the straits. Exposed undersea reefs formed stepping stones across the shallows into Yemen.

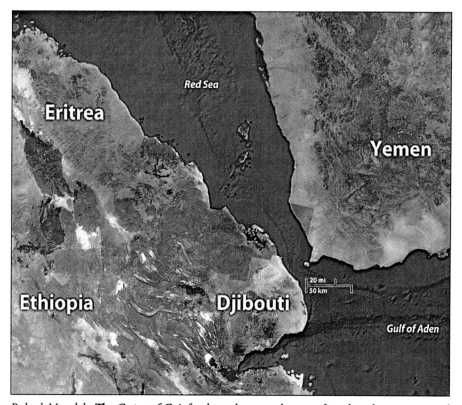

*Bab-el-Mandeb, **The Gates of Grief**, where the second wave of modern humans crossed out of Africa 85,000 years ago, when the channel was much narrower and shallower.*

Pushed by starvation, ancient Homo sapiens set out across the straits toward the forested mountains of Yemen visible to this day from the shores of Africa. Makeshift rafts may have been used to cross the deeper points, though they may not even have been needed at the time.

We now know that modern humans evolved in Africa, then split into two branches – one remained in Africa, while the other migrated into the Middle East and Eurasia:

Mutations are small glitches in the DNA sequence. When they're passed down to descendants, they can be used as *markers* to trace ancestral relations. Based on these markers, geneticists have traced our roots to a tribe of southern African hunter gathers called the *San*, near the South African-Namibian border.

The San carry markers in their DNA unique among humans, showing they are the world's oldest lineage. These are direct descendants of our oldest common ancestors – the group who stayed behind in Africa, while its other tribe members ventured into the Middle East and beyond, eventually spreading to populate the entire world.

One man among these travellers carried a non-coding mutation to a base pair on his Y sex chromosome. This *single nucleotide polymorphism* (SNP) is called *M168*. Since Y chromosomes are only carried by men, this mutation is passed down from fathers to their sons. The humans who successfully migrated out of Africa were all descendants of the man who first evolved this mutation, and this Y chromosome marker has been carried out into the rest of the world, and passed down to every non-African alive today. Africans who remained behind belong to the lineages A and B, found nearly exclusively in Africa.

On the female side, DNA in the mitochondria is only passed down from mothers, and every non-African human alive today is descended from a single woman called *Mitochondrial Eve*, whose mitochondrial DNA carries a set of markers classified as *L3*. Thus, all non-Africans alive today are descended from the M168 - L3 lineage. The African tribes who remained behind would go on to father the L1, L2, L3, A and B lines, called *haplogroups*.

From a total population of about 3,000 humans, a very small group – about 600 – crossed the Red Sea. Outside of Africa, everyone alive today descended from this single genetic line – *mtDNA haplogroup L3*. Since that first exodus, their environments have shaped genetically distinct human populations, which can now be distinguished by 13 Y-chromosome markers.

The human genomic record shows that every non-African alive today is descended from this group, the *L3* line. This group would continue to push eastward into India, and beyond, hugging the coastline. Within 10,000 years, it had settled most of tropical south Asia, including India, Sri Lanka, Malaysia, Cambodia, Thailand, Viet Nam, Indonesia, Borneo and South China.

When humans first arrived in Asia, we came as small, tightly-bonded groups of Africans, bearing language, spears, handcrafting skills and artistic talents. We lived in tribelike communities of 150 or more, and engaged in widespread networking, exchanging knowledge and technological innovations between our tribes, often using tokens like handcrafted jewelry, sculptures, totems, bead and bone artifacts. This allowed for a critical exchange of information, about – for example – domestic skills, navigational information such as game-rich hunting grounds, and which plants, and fungi were edible, medicinal or toxic.

There was a division of labor – with women performing the domestic chores, child-rearing, and foraging, gathering fruits, berries, roots and nuts, while the men hunted. It was likely a time of bounty. Then disaster struck – it was the second time humanity almost perished.

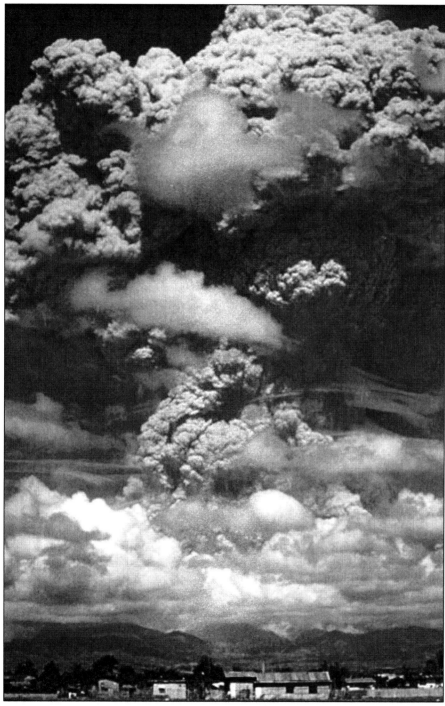

Pinatubo's eruption on June 15, 1991 was the largest in modern history. It ejected a cloud of volcanic ash 684 miles wide and 22 miles high. The aerosol cloud spread across the globe over three weeks, cooling the planet by 0.7 degrees Fahrenheit, over the years 1992 and 1993. 73,000 years ago, the Toba eruption would have looked similar, only 200 times as large. Image: United States Geological Survey, D. Harlow, public domain.

The Day Mankind Almost Died

74,000 years ago, the *Toba volcano* in Indonesia exploded in the biggest supereruption known to science, reducing the once-lush Indian landscape to a desert. The apocalyptic blast of toxic gas and dust generated continent-wide acid rainstorms, cross-continental deforestation, buried India, Pakistan and Malaysia in *five meters of ash*, and blanketed all of South Asia and its oceans in a six-inch layer of volcanic debris.

The supereruption is thought to have plunged Earth into a volcanic winter for a decade and triggered a 1000-year-long Ice Age. The disaster was so extreme it threatened our species with extinction. Humanity suffered a dramatic population crash, to less than 15,000 survivors, and studies show Eastern African chimpanzees, Bornean orangutans, Central Indian macaques, cheetahs, and tigers were also all reduced to near-extinction.

The human race just barely managed to survive. This, anthropologists believe, drove the intense natural selection which led to our modern culture and highly social nature – extremely inhospitable conditions forced innovation upon the human race. The *Great Leap* in advancement included the emergence of musical instruments, drawn images, carved arrowheads, bone needles, and other tools.

The extreme environmental crises imposed hardships which forced creatures to quickly adapt for survival. For humans, this meant banding together and learning to cooperate as never before. According to Edmund Baer Bolles, author of *Babel's Dawn*, women, as the household stewards and baby caregivers, developed *distributed attention*, a special kind of cooperative behavior, which allowed them to collectively care for their children and carry on other maternal survival activities.

Such collective pooling of primitive mental power, says Bolles, "...got us through the dangers of the extinctions that were wiping out our evolutionary cousins" and gave rise to spoken language and our highly social nature.

From this period onward, human creativity seems to have exploded, with early humans beginning to craft elaborate clothing, tools, decorative and ceremonial objects from shells, bone, animal hides, wood and natural pigments. Sharing of ideas and emerging language appear to have spurred neural adaptation that turned the human brain into an instrument capable of infinite creativity.

Images

Cultural traits – art and music, religious practices, and sophisticated tool-making appeared perhaps 73,000 years ago, but really blossomed about 50,000 years ago, in the *Upper Paleolithic* or *Early Stone Age*, according to archeological records.

These findings show that humans had begun planning ahead, inventing, establishing social and trade networks, adapting to changing environmental conditions, and using symbols to represent reality in cave paintings, burials, and jewellery-making to convey status or group affiliation.

John Hoffecker at the Russian Academy of Sciences has studied the earliest known European H. sapiens settlements, from 45,000 years ago. Here, bone and ivory needles show humans had invented sewing, and were fashioning fur clothing to survive Ice Age Russia's bitter winters. Hoffecker's team also unearthed mammoth ivory carved into the head of a small figurine, thought to be the oldest piece of art ever found.

In 2012, a team of Oxford and Tübingen researchers published data on additional ancient European artifacts found in Geißenklösterle Cave in Southwestern Germany. These artifacts are some 43,000 years old, from the dawn of the *Aurignacian culture*, the first to create a diverse range of art figurines, music and other key innovations.

Geißenklösterle is one of many caves in the region in which significant ancient items have been found – personal ornaments, figurative art, mythical imagery and musical instruments. In nearby *Hohle Fels*, archeologists found equally ancient flutes carved from bird bones and from mammoth ivory.

These objects predate any found elsewhere in the world, including artifacts from Italy, France, England and other regions. They also confirm the *Danube Corridor hypothesis*, which proposed that when modern humans migrated to Europe, they rapidly moved up the Danube River before an extremely cold climatic phase called the *H4 event*, 40,000 years ago.

Ice Ages – *The Earth goes through a series of cyclical warming and cooling based on three celestial cycles, which all take place over different time periods, altering the amount of warmth transmitted to us by the Sun. Oxford University's Dr. Stephen Oppenheimer calls these the **100,000-year stretch**, the **41,000-year tilt** and the **23,000-year wobble**.*

*As the Earth circles the Sun annually, its orbit forms an **ellipse**, more the shape of an oval than a circle, at some points closer to the Sun. Every 100,000 years, this ellipse shortens and fattens until it's almost circular, varying as much as 11.35 million miles, and affecting the Earth's climate.*

Meanwhile, the Earth's axis of rotation is tilted at a 23.5-degree angle toward the Sun, like a top which doesn't spin upright, giving us the seasons – the planet shows first the northern face and then the southern face to the Sun in a single circuit. This angle fluctuates between 21.5 and 24.5 degrees within a 41,000-year cycle. The more extreme its tilt, the greater the seasonal variation in heat from the Sun. We're currently at a neutral point between extreme tilt angles.

*In addition to spinning at an angle toward the Sun, the planet also engages in an **axial precession**, making a slow pirouette within its orbit every 22,000 to 23,000 years, just like a spinning top.*

*The overall effect of these combined movements is that the planet gradually changes which face is presented to the Sun during its orbit. Because of this, within the next 11,000 years, June 21 will become mid-summer in Australia and mid-winter in North America and Europe. This is called the **precession of the equinoxes**.*

*These three **Milankovitch cycles** are completely out of phase with one another, but combine in their effects to alter Earth's climate in cycles spanning great stretches of time.*

With a Little Help From My Friends

Humans tend to cooperate more than most species, including closely-related primates. According to psychologists, we have an intrinsic *altruism*, a willingness to help others, sometimes at a significant cost or risk to ourselves. The conventional wisdom has long been that such self-sacrifice grants a survival advantage to one's genes by helping close kin survive.

However, in 2012, Max Planck Institute researchers said numerous experiments show it's a much simpler matter of mutual self-interest: survival considerations force cooperation upon us, and we act altruistically toward others simply because we need them.

The scientists present a detailed account of the two-step process behind the evolution of cooperation, beginning with small hunter-gatherer groups. The behavior gradually grows in complexity and becomes embedded into cultures as larger societies develop:

Early hominids were forced to cooperate when foraging for food, and this gave each individual a direct stake in his partners' welfare. This interdependence led to the evolution of unique behaviors which other primates don't possess: fair division of spoils, communicating plans and tactics, and a need for each individual to recognize his or her place within the acting group. Partners most likely to succeed were those best at coordinating with their fellow foragers and doing their fair share of the work.

Subdivisions

The growth and increase in complexity of societies led to even greater interdependence among members, triggering a second major evolutionary step. Faced with competition from other groups, our ancestors further developed these human-specific cooperative skills and impulses on a larger scale. People began to identify with groups in their societies, even if they didn't personally know other members. The new sense of membership and belonging led to cultural *norms* (codes of conduct), conventions, and institutions which encouraged and rewarded feelings of social responsibility and group identification.

Long ago, Charles Darwin wrote about how groups with altruistic members were more likely to prosper, survive, and proliferate. Aggression toward competitive outgroups benefits an individual's own group, helping it to grow relatively stronger, and in this sense, aggression becomes an indirect form of altruism – showing loyalty toward an individual's own group.

Dr. Carsten de Dreu of the University of Amsterdam says that, if this principle is true, neurobiological traits must have evolved to promote altruism toward an individual's own group and defensive aggression toward competitors. His experiments show that, on a neurological level, a significant force in such altruistic behavior – and the strength of ingroup bonding and aggression toward competing outgroups – is the so-called "bonding hormone" *oxytocin*.

Oxytocin is known to increase mutual affection, and is released in significant quantities during orgasm, when a mother interacts with her newborn, while stroking a pet, and even when one simply looks at an object of affection. So how does one explain extreme variations in altruism among individuals, from Adolph Hitler to Mahatma Gandhi? Neuroscientists believe this depends upon differences in size and activity of a brain area used to comprehend the perspectives of others. The discovery also provides an explanation for the stability of one's altruistic tendencies over time.

Those most adept at understanding others' intentions and beliefs are more altruistic than those less skilled at the task. The *Temporo Parietal Junction* (TPJ) corresponds to exercising this ability to understand the perspectives of others; the University of Zurich's Dr. Ernst Fehr has demonstrated that relative size and activation of the TPJ relates directly to individual differences in altruism.

Subjects' brains were scanned while they played a game in which they chose how to divide money between themselves and anonymous partners. The more generous subjects had a larger TPJ in the right hemisphere when compared with stingier subjects.

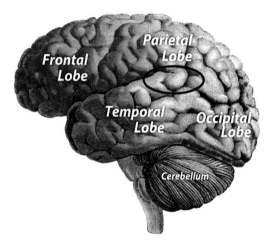

The experiments also showed TPJ activation levels corresponded to each subject's generosity levels – the maximal amount each subject was willing to sacrifice to increase his or her partner's payoff.

TPJ activity was highest during the most difficult decisions, when the personal cost was just under an individual's "cutoff value" – than during easier decisions which involved very low or very high costs.

Co-author Yosuke Morishima says TPJ development determines each person's individual *setpoint* (default level) for altruism, while *activation levels* of the TPJ predict what an individual believes to be acceptable costs for helping others in any given situation. The team also believes their findings indicate altruism can be developed, resulting in corresponding synaptic growth.

Old Friends

According to studies at Duke University, friendship is a product of natural selection. In early 2013, Duke University researchers released details of a two-year study on heritability of social interactions in a 90-member troop of free-ranging Rhesus macaques, and say natural selection affects offspring behavior.

Highly social Rhesus macaques tend to have descendants who are also highly social. Their ability to play fair and respect relationships wins them more reproductive success, resulting in a greater likelihood their offspring survive to maturity, according to Dr. Lauren Brent, who led the study. "Natural selection appears to be favoring pro-social behavior."

The monkeys under observation are descended from a 1938 release of Indian macaques on the uninhabited island of Cayo Santiago, off Puerto Rico's eastern coast. 75 years of pedigree data and genetic analysis have been combined with sophisticated social network maps in the study, in which observers largely just watched and provided provisions; otherwise, the macaques had no human contact.

Researchers in the field learned to identify each of nearly 90 monkeys on sight, logging interactions between them over the course of two years, observing grooming, proximity and aggression. From their observations, they built maps of the friendships and pro-social and anti-social interactions among the troop. What they consistently found was that the monkeys with the strongest friendships lived the longest and had the most babies, passing along their prosocial traits to their offspring.

According to UCal medical genetics professor Dr. James Fowler, this "landmark study" shows the positive behaviors which build social networks are heritable, something that's also seen in human studies.

Aggression didn't show much heritability, though it did influence reproductive success: the most aggressive and the most passive rhesus monkeys had better reproductive success than monkeys in the middle.

The team also conducted genetic analyses of blood samples, focusing upon two serotonin-related genes, one which synthesizes serotonin and one which transports it. These two genes have been widely studied in humans, in the course of developing modern antidepressants.

Variabilities among these two genes were closely aligned with differences the team observed in grooming behaviors among the monkeys. Said Dr. Brent, "We can see that some of these behaviors have a genetic basis, from what we know of the pedigrees and the network map. But we've only scratched the surface of figuring out which specific genes are associated with each behavior."

According to Dr. Michael Platt, director of the Duke Institute for Brain Sciences and the Center for Cognitive Neuroscience: "We know that neural circuits for a variety of things like social behavior, food and mood are under the influence of serotonin signaling, in both humans and monkeys."

While genes alone can't determine an individual's social standing, social success is derived from a combination of temperament and social skills, which seem to have a genetic basis. "This is just the first two genes. We'll hopefully be moving on to sequence the entire genome of each animal" to find even more associations, he added.

Walkin' the Dog

Penn State University paleoanthropologist Dr. Pat Shipman says that, rather than a simple novelty, our eons-long tendency to domesticate animals is, "...a hugely significant force that has shaped us and been instrumental in our global spread and success in the world." As she points out, from a purely evolutionary perspective, taking care of animals you aren't going to eat doesn't make much sense – it requires a significant investment in time and energy to care for a member of another species, and humans are the only mammal species to do this on a global scale.

She says the human/domestic animal connection began 2.6 million years ago, when Ethiopians first began chipping stones into useful tools, which required the mental ability to predict changes to an object's properties. Prior to this tool-making, says Dr. Shipman, humans had been mainly vegetarian, but at this point, animal remains began to appear in human settlements with cut marks, indicating meat had become part of the human diet.

Meat and fat helped speed up the evolution of the relatively massive human cortex, and, since landing a single game animal provides food for a much longer period than foraging for fruits, vegetables and nuts, it was very nutritionally advantageous – but it also put the first human ancestors in direct competition with other predators in their ecosystem.

In place of the evolutionary advantages of most carnivores, however – raw physical power, speed, claws and sharp teeth, or heightened senses for hunting – humans began to form blades from stones – an "...evolutionary shortcut to becoming a predator", as Dr. Shipman puts it.

Our ancient forebears had to contend against 11 predator species at the time – lions, cheetahs, leopards, four types of hyenas, now-extinct wolf-like dog forebears, and three species of sabretooth cats. The competition was fierce (pun intended). Since nearly all these prehistoric predators far outweighed the earliest ancient humans, scavenging freshly-killed antelope or other prey was a very risky proposition.

Within a little under a million years, five of these 11 predators became extinct, but humans managed to survive due to three qualities, says Dr. Shipman:

- we worked in social groups

- we had tools, allowing us to quickly remove meat and retreat to safety

- we could closely observe and recognize the habits of other animal species.

Predators must maintain small numbers, or they quickly exhaust their region's food supply. Becoming predators – and thus needing ever larger hunting grounds – led to the first human expansions out of Africa: fossil records show early hominins had been confined to Africa from the first appearance of Australopithecus 6 million years ago, until about 2 million years ago, when Homo erectus first made a dramatically rapid territorial expansion into Asia.

As consciousness emerged and the first human art appeared, it's apparent one of the most important topics in the lives of our ancestors was animals. Depictions of their colors, shapes, habits, postures, locomotion and social habits are in abundance. But pictures of people, ceremonies and social interactions are rarely found in such early art; and plants, water sources, geographical features, even less so.

What's more, there are no depictions of survival skills such as fire-building, tool-making or shelter-building, demonstrating the central importance of animals to early human life. Because of this evidence, she believes the emergence of early language was centered around the need to communicate animal-related information – warnings about nearby predators, or useful hunting information.

The first domesticated animals were probably accidental, she believes, but the advantages they conferred quickly led to their popularity. One can easily imagine scrap-scavenging dogs choosing to stay in close proximity to human settlements, where rudimentary acts of kindness led to interspecies companionship. Skulls from the first domesticated dogs date from about 32,000 BC throughout eastern Africa, where they helped with guarding, herding, hunting, pest control, transport, and companionship. Some 24,000 years later came the first domestic cats, appearing in North Africa and the Middle East around 7,500 BC.

It wasn't until 4,000 BC that humans first began taming horses however, according to archeological records; herd animals like goats, yaks, water buffalo, sheep and cattle soon also proved indispensable, providing wool, milk, meat and physical labor to support cultivation. To Dr. Shipman, this was the third great leap in human evolution: modern humans only truly emerged after first mastering tool-making, then language, and, finally, animal domestication.

The animal-human connection is so fundamental to our basic natures, she contends, that it's a pity we're driving so many other species into extinction at a historically unprecedented rate.

Mystery Men

For decades, evolutionary biologists have been predicting a boom in discoveries of new human species in Asia, and a 2011 discovery has proven them right.

Although the unusual skull of the *Red Deer Cave People* was first excavated in 1979 from a cave in south-western China's Guangxi Province, it was only fully analyzed in 2011. According to the University of New South Wales' Dr. Darren Curnoe, the bones are just 11,500 years old, and belonged to a completely new, previously unknown hominin species. This means that, unlike the Neanderthals, the *Red Deer Cave People* survived the worst part of Earth's most recent ice age.

The skull possesses an unusual mixture of primitive features similar to those of our ancient human ancestors, along with modern traits common to modern Homo sapiens. With its thick bones, prominent brow line, short, flat face and sunken chin, the skull is "anatomically unique among all members of the human evolutionary tree," according to Dr. Curnoe.

Curnoe and his Yunnan University colleague Ji Xueping have since found additional evidence of the new hominin elsewhere, at Malu cave in Yunnan Province. They named the new hominins based upon their appetite for roast venison.

Radiocarbon dating of charcoal found in the fossil deposits places the remains at between 14,500 to 11,500 years of age. This would mean Red Deer Cave people lived after all other prehistoric human species such as the Neanderthals had gone extinct. The dating would make the Red Deer Cave hominins even more recent than Homo floresiensis, who died out 13,000 years ago.

Because the Red Deer features are so different from that of modern humans, Dr. Curnoe believes they are members of an entirely different evolutionary line that evolved in East Asia in parallel with the human species, just like Neanderthals.

London Natural History Museum archaeologist Dr. Chris Stringer believes they might be related to the mysterious Denisovans, identified by a 40,000-year-old tooth and finger bone from a Siberian cave. Because DNA analysis has shown that Denisovans had mated with direct human ancestors, Stringer suggests Red Deer Cave People may be the product of that lineage.

Oxford University's Michael Petraglia also points out that 8000-year-old human skeletons with unusual archaic features have been recovered in India and south Asia. DNA analysis has proven difficult, but Curnoe's team is continuing attempts.

Solitude

Cooperation evolved as a result of *ostracism*, the use of social exclusion as a punishment strategy. According to new research. Dr. Tatsuya Sasaki of Austria's International Institute for Applied Systems Analysis says experiments with game theory show that excluding people from a group indirectly rewards the punishers, thereby encouraging the behavior and promoting group cooperation.

"Imagine a pie," says Dr. Sasaki. "The fewer people sharing it, the more pie goes out to those who receive it. But refusing to share the pie out of simple greed goes against natural moral instincts. There must be a justification, for example, someone refusing to contribute in making the pie – a *free rider*, in game theory parlance. If you punish free riders with social exclusion, it increases the payoff for the punishers."

Social exclusion also promotes cooperation – denying free riders a piece of the pie makes people more likely to cooperate, which ensures they get to participate in enjoying the rewards.

According to Dr. Sasaki, "Punishment is a common tool to promote cooperation in the real world, and social exclusion is a common way to do it."

It's not just humans that use this strategy. From vampire bats to chimpanzees, many non-human animal species foster community cooperation by isolating freeloaders.

Humans also use social exclusion to enforce societal rules. For example, says Sasaki, drunk drivers are punished by having their licenses revoked, in essence excluding them from the driving "community".

What is Life?

Evolution is a never-ending process, and one which just as surely affects us as the countless life forms which have gone before. So what does the future hold for the human animal? We already have some glimpses into a future that is beyond imaging.

We are unique among animals species in that we can participate in guiding our own evolution. Book two will explore the frontiers of medicine in greater depth, but we are already in the midst of a radical transformation in what it means to be alive:

For example, in May, 2010, American genetics engineer Dr. Craig Venter created the first entirely synthetic life "... totally derived from a synthetic chromosome, made with four bottles of chemicals on a chemical synthesizer, starting with information in a computer". His synthetic DNA was then transplanted into a bacterial cell, which replicated normally.

This is the culmination of a quiet revolution that has been underway within the last four decades, since biochemist Herbert Boyer and medical doctor Stanley Cohen were awarded a half-million-dollar Lemelson-MIT Prize for the 1973 transplantation of genes from one organism to another. Since their breakthrough, *recombinant DNA* has become the basis of the biotechnology industry, used to create everything from food to medicines, fuel and materials.

Biotechnology applies engineering principles to nature. To use the analogy of a desktop computer, if living cells are the hardware of life, then DNA is the software which runs it. That software can now be customized to produce entirely new lifeforms.

Custom DNA can be virtually assembled and tested on a computer, then assembled in the real world from swappable gene modules, just as a computer program can be assembled from subroutines using a programming language like visual C++. And, just as authorship of a computer game or word processor can be protected through copyright laws, genetic "software" – i.e. genetically-engineered life forms – can be patented.

Individual genes express proteins which perform specific subroutines like cutting, binding, detection, etc. These genes constitute modules which can be chemically synthesized by a commercial lab or extracted from living organisms, then reassembled into a completely new DNA "program" which can perform complex tasks, such as producing a custom protein like insulin, or altering a living organism to produce nutritionally-enhanced vegetables or even goats that excrete spider-silk in their milk.

Because DNA is a common code constructed from four nucleotide sequences and shared by all life forms, it can be recombined – the DNA from one organism mixed with that of another. Here's how the process works:

A bacterial cell typically contains at least one *plasmid*, a small loop of DNA separate from the cell's main cluster of nucleoid DNA. In the process called *transformation*, this plasmid is treated with an enzyme to allow the insertion of a customized gene. Human DNA is often inserted, and bacteria can be induced to absorb this modified DNA, turning them into custom protein or DNA factories.

STEP 1: Growing the culture – A bacterial colony – often E. coli – is grown in a shallow glass petri dish within *growth medium*. This medium can be either liquid broth or solid gel *agar* made from pre-digested milk or meat, algae gelatin, beef or yeast extract, and salt. The growth medium is incubated at 37 degrees, so large numbers of bacteria can be rapidly produced.

E. coli are selectively bred with a resistance to an antibiotic like ampicillin. This immunity can quickly spread through *conjugation*. During conjugation, one bacterial cell creates a *pilus*, a protein transferral tube that it inserts into another bacterial cell. It then sends across a plasmid DNA loop, giving the recipient bacterium a "software upgrade" to its DNA.

This is one way in which antibiotic resistance – the ability for bacteria to manufacture antibiotic-destroying enzymes, alter their membranes, or other defenses – can spread. Bacteria can also scavenge DNA remnants from dead microorganisms, or be themselves infected by jumping genes, small pieces of DNA called transposons, which hop from DNA molecule to DNA molecule and become permanently integrated into the host's genome.

STEP 2: Isolating the DNA – First, the cells of the bacteria colony are *lysed* – split open. There are three methods commonly used:

Commercially-purchased enzymes such as *cellulase* or *lysozyme* (created from snail gut yeast or chicken eggs) can break down cell membranes.

Alternatively, *sonoporation* uses sound wave vibrations to break apart cell membranes and release cellular components. In this process, the bacterial culture is placed in a test tube filled with water, and an ultrasonic probe is placed inside which vibrates at high speed. If the mixture is cooled with ice, this process doesn't cause *denaturation*, the structural breakdown of proteins.

Beadbeaters are machines which resemble blenders, used to disrupt cells through mechanical force. Chilled cultures in test tubes containing tiny steel beads are placed in an ice-filled chamber and agitated at high speed. The vigorous vibration causes cells in the solution to physically break apart. The resulting liquid can then be strained through a filter with a hand-held plunger, or placed in a *gel box*, where electrical charges separate DNA molecules according to their natural charges.

STEP 3: Extracting the Desired Genes – Specific genes are extracted from DNA using a *restriction enzyme*. Restriction enzymes arc naturally-occurring proteins in microorganisms which function as a defense mechanism against foreign DNA borne by invading viruses. These protective enzymes cut up foreign DNA in the process called *restriction*, while the host's DNA is protected by a modification enzyme marking it through methylation – the addition of methyl groups to the DNA molecule.

There are over 600 restriction enzymes for sale commercially, but over 3000 have been studied extensively, and are regularly used as tools in laboratories.

Each restriction enzyme recognizes a specific nucleotide sequence known as a *restriction site*, where it severs both sides of the DNA strand. The enzyme *EcoR1* (pronounced *echo r one*), for example, has a precise shape which allows it to travel along the DNA double helix, scanning for the nucleotide base sequence GAATTC, where it then cuts the plasmid, opening the molecule and allowing a customized sequence of DNA to be inserted. Exposing DNA to the enzyme EcoR1 separates DNA with a staggered cut, called "sticky" because the overhanging open ends easily bind to other Ecor1-cut DNA fragments.

As a simpler alternative, customized lengths of *single-stranded DNA* (ssDNA) can be chemically synthesized in laboratories.

STEP 4: Splicing the DNA – The customized DNA is spliced into the plasmid *vector* (host) using another enzyme called *lygase*, which acts as genetic glue. In a solution, the customized DNA sequence and the open ends of the cut plasmids naturally match up by matched base-pairing. Thus, the engineered gene naturally inserts itself into the open plasmid ring. The plasmid is then resealed by adding the enzyme *DNA ligase* to the solution.

Live E. coli and the pool of recombinant plasmids are mixed in a suspension of calcium chloride at freezing temperatures. Rapidly raising and lowering the temperature creates *heat shock*, a condition in which the cell membranes become temporarily permeable to DNA, and some of the E. coli cells absorb the recombinant plasmids.

STEP 5: Isolation and Growth – The E. coli are then placed upon a petri dish filled with growth medium, into which an antibiotic such as ampicillin has been added.

Because they come from selectively bred bacteria, the customized plasmids contain genes making them immune to the antibiotic's effects, so all non-immune E. coli are destroyed, leaving only the engineered bacteria. The colony of surviving E. coli is incubated at 37 degrees. When these cells replicate, they create identical copies of the customized DNA, producing whichever proteins the customized genes express.

If you'd like to try your hand at it, you can download free gene-designing software from www.dna20.com, and have your designs synthesized in the lab and delivered directly to your door – just like ordering a pizza.

Plasmid-based genetic cloning is limited to accommodating external DNA of about 10,000 base pairs, but a typical human gene is on average about 27,000. Because of this, bioengineers have begun to use a variety of vectors in place of plasmids, including viruses; *phages* are one variety of virus which only infect bacteria, though they are notoriously difficult to use.

Cosmids – a mixture between plasmids and phages – can hold up to 30,000 base pairs, enough for an average-sized gene, but for larger genes, in 1997, bioengineers created a new type of vector called a *Bacterial Artificial Chromosome* or *BAC* for short. These are artificially-synthesized lengths of DNA which can hold up to 300,000 base pairs, and are more convenient to use, because they have been prepackaged with tools that simplify the process, such as antibiotic resistance genes, and convenient base-pair-matching ends with which the cloned DNA can easily bond. The plasmid for creating a BAC vector is a special *F plasmid* (fertility plasmid), used by bacteria to transfer DNA via conjugation during environmental stress.

In the spring of 2013, Professor John Love at the University of Exeter, announced the successful development of E. coli which produce *diesel*, nearly identical to conventional diesel fuel. It means the E. coli-derived fuel can be used in current engines, pipelines and tankers without any modifications. This is just the start of many amazing innovations to come, not the least of which will be modifying the human animal's own genome.

The Long and Winding Road

From our distant origins, human civilizations have emerged, flourished and vanished, and human creativity and mental capacity has brought us to where we are today, an age of innovation that would seem nothing short of godlike magic to our ancient forebears, were they alive today to witness it.

Everything from the refinement of penicillin to the launching of the International Space Station (where, for a modest $20 million US, you can spend ten days in Earth orbit) has its humble roots in the grasslands of Africa, seven million years ago, when the first hominin stood and began to walk on two feet.

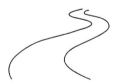

PART II: MIND

Neurons

Congratulations. You're the proud owner of the most complex structure known in the universe.

Three pounds of gelatinous tissue half the size of a head of lettuce control everything you do at a rate faster than any supercomputer, processing 100 trillion instructions every second. In fact, your brain is so complex and powerful that in a single second it can perform as many calculations as every computing device currently in existence on the planet – every integrated circuit chip, calculator and giant supercomputer – *combined*. Wire them all together, and they can execute, in *MIPS* (millions of instructions per second), about 6.4×10^{18} instructions per second – roughly the same amount as your brain.

It will take some time before synthetic computers will be able to compete. In late 2012, the US Department of Energy's Oak Ridge National Laboratory debuted *Titan*, the world's most powerful supercomputer. Titan is said to perform 17.59 *petaflops* – 17,590 trillion calculations – a second. Titan system contains over 18,000 multi-core CPUs, each coupled with its own graphics processor. It fills 200 metal cabinets, covering 404 square meters (4,352 ft²) of floor space, at a cost of $97 million.

This tremendous beast of computing power can't even come close to what your brain can accomplish. Your own brain, in terms of sheer processing alone, leaves it in the dust, outperforming the fastest and most massive supercomputer ever built by some 500%. But your brain is much, much more powerful in many other ways as well, ways in which neuroscience is just starting to understand.

Each neural impulse occurs in tens of milliseconds; and every second your brain fires millions of impulses in patterns over circuits distributed throughout its mass. But rather than through point-to-point transmission, your brain functions through *liquid computing*, similar to water rippling after a pebble is tossed into a pool. These waves don't immediately disappear, but instead overlap upon and influence each other's activation, spreading across your neural network at very high speed. This mode of functioning makes your brain much more powerful than any synthetic computer.

Most of its staggeringly powerful capacity has emerged by the time you're only three years old – child educator Maria Montessori suggested that if the development of an adult brain were compared with that of a child's, it would take 60 years to achieve what a child's brain does in those first three formative years.

Brain development commences within the first month from conception, as the brain and spinal cord start to form within the embryo.

By the sixth month, almost all the billions of neurons which will populate a mature brain have formed, new neurons generating at an astounding average rate of over 250,000 *every minute*. After forming, these neurons rapidly migrate to regions of the brain where they will function.

They differentiate into specialized roles, and begin to form synaptic connections with other neurons, enabling communication and information storage. Synapses will continue to form throughout life, but by the time a child is ready to be born, most of its neurons have migrated to brain regions where they will function for life.

A newborn is starving for sensory stimulation, novelty, and social interaction, all of which will alter the "wiring" of its brain significantly. Prior to birth and just afterwards, there is an initial *blooming* of neurons, far in excess than what will be kept for life. This results in tremendous potential for an infant's developing brain, but also makes that brain noisy and inefficient, with redundant connections. Because of this, the initial proliferation is quickly followed by a *pruning* stage, and unused synapses are eliminated, until the brain has an optimal number of synapses for efficient operation.

Stimulation through experience plays a central role in determining which synapses will be selected for elimination or retention. These stimulating experiences will activate specific synapses, triggering the growth which will consolidate synaptic connections. Unactivated synapses will progressively retract and wither.

In this manner, the developing brain becomes adapted to the everyday needs of the newborn's environment, and after a mere six months, its brain will have reached 50 percent of its mature potential. By age three, it will have reached 80 percent.

A three-year-old child has approximately 10^{15} synapses (one quadrillion), reduced through synaptic pruning over time, a process that largely stops by adulthood. Frequently used synapses are retained, while those rarely called upon are eliminated. By adulthood, the number of synapses will have largely stabilized at between 10^{14} to 5×10^{14} (100 to 500 trillion), depending upon the individual.

Your brain is about 60% fat – the fattiest part of your body. It weighs between 2 and 4 pounds, and consumes 25% of your body's blood and oxygen. It contains an estimated 10^{11} (one hundred billion) neurons, which are constantly shaped and reshaped by your experiences.

Almost all these neurons communicate by sending chemicals across the tiny gaps of your synapses. Through these microscopic connections, each neuron can contact thousands or even tens of thousands of other neurons, and every second of your life, your brain is changing, forming a million new connections, strengthening and reorganizing others. The complexity is staggering: each of your one hundred billion neurons has an average of 7,000 synaptic connections.

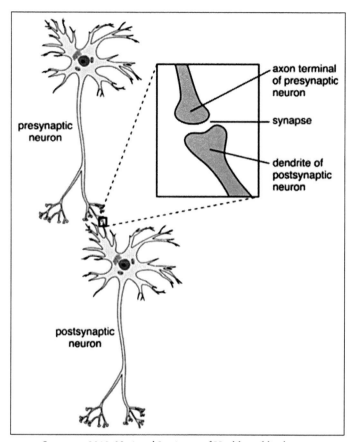

Synapses, 2010, National Institutes of Health, public domain

Support Cells

In addition to neurons, your brain is made up of *glial cells*, which nourish, perform repairs, provide structural support, regulate biochemical balance and remove toxic waste. There are approximately 10 to 50 times as many glia as neurons in a human brain.

Glial Cells – The Greek name *glia* means *glue,* but glial cells are actually multifunctional – holding neurons in place, supplying them with nutrients and oxygen, killing dangerous pathogens, removing dead cells, and assisting in neural repair. The most common glial cells are *astrocytes,* star-shaped, multipurpose support cells which dispose of damaged or dead tissue, form scar tissue and secrete a protective protein called *metallothionein* that clears away metal ions and *free radicals* – ionized organic molecules which leech electrons from your body's cells or distrupt molecular stability. *Microglia* digest dead neurons and *pathogens* – microscopic foreign invaders such as bacteria and viruses).

Glial cells further protect your brain by forming the *blood-brain barrier,* which prevents toxic substances in your bloodstream from entering your brain. Recent experiments have also shown glial cells help control neurotransmission, releasing chemicals

351

like *glutamate* into synapses. Glial cells also produce electrical insulation for neurons in the form of a fatty substance called *myelin*, which prevents signal leakage.

New understanding - Contrary to the long-held view that they only act as support cells in the brain, scientists have only very recently learned that astrocytes actually play an active part in how neural signals are distributed. Just as the transistors and wires powering your electronic devices are mounted on a base called a "motherboard", the neurons in your brain need a base material too.

According to Tel Aviv University's Dr. Maurizio De Pittà, astrocytes help control information flow between neurons and connect neuronal circuits across various brain regions. They integrate different messages transferred via the neurons and multiplex them (consolidate, transmit and re-separate them at the receiving end) throughout the brain's circuitry.

Astrocytes protect neurons by encasing them and forming borders between different brain regions, but they also transfer information very slowly, at about one-tenth of a second, as compared to the thousandth-of-a-second transmission of neurons. Thus, astrocytes produce signals which carry larger amounts of information over greater distances.

Astrocytes connect neurons differently than conventional synapses, by spreading information across different regions throughout the brain, or transferring it within regions. In this sense, astrocytes form networks beyond the neural and synaptic ones, simultaneously functioning to orchestrate information across different brain regions, just as an electrical motherboard operates in a personal computer, or a conductor ensures an entire orchestra works in harmony. Both communication systems are interconnected, and malfunctions in one system can critically influence the other.

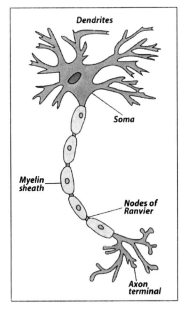

Neurons – like most of your body's cells, neurons have a main cell body – the *soma*, as well as typically several extensions at one end called *dendrites*, and a long tail at the other called an *axon*, extending into microscopic branches called *terminals*. Each of these terminals is capped by a *bouton* (button in French), which connects to a *postsynaptic* neuron. *Image: Quasar Jarosz, Wikipedia, Creative Commons Attribution 3.0 Unported license.*

Each of your estimated 100 billion neurons is connected to 5,000 to 200,000 partners, creating a huge number of potential pathways down which information flows. With roots and branches – axons and dendrites – growing in all directions, they interweave, forming a tangle of 100 trillion constantly-changing interconnections. Your brain is thus like a dense neural jungle, beginning as cell bodies, and later sprouting axons and dendrites.

According to pioneering neuroscientist Dr. V. S. Ramachandran:

The human brain is made up of one hundred billion neurons – and each neuron forms about a thousand to ten thousand contacts with other neurons – so the number of possible permutations and combinations of brain activity, that is to say, potential brain states, exceeds the number of elementary particles in the known universe.

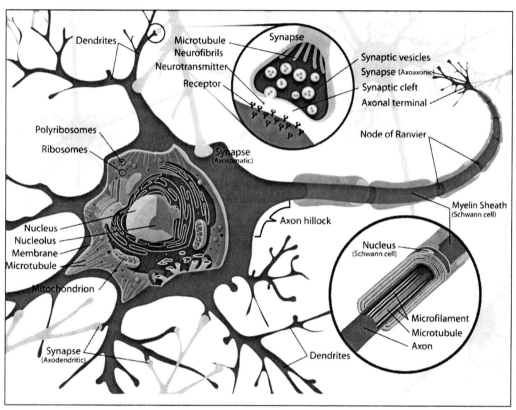

Image: Mariana Ruiz Villarreal 2008, Wikipedia, public domain

In response to your experiences, neurons constantly form new synapses or strengthening existing connections, with the average neuron connected to about 1,000 others. These synaptic connections shape your thoughts and behavior, as, simultaneously, every thought and action in turn physically reshapes those connections.

Everything you think and do relies on neural transmission – the world you perceive, and the way you mentally and physically respond to it is encoded into *action potentials*, the electrical signals which constitute your brain's basic information units, acting like a computer's *binary digits* – the electrical off and on states representing zeros or ones in a computer.

These neurons are the only type of cell in your body which will remain with you from birth until death; all your other cells will be completely replenished after about seven years. Neurons range from microscopically small to very large, some extending from your brain all the way down your spine. Half reside in the *cerebellum* (Latin for *little brain*), which sits just atop your spine and helps coordinate your movement and maintain your balance. Although they vary in size, almost all consist of a soma, axon, terminals and dendrites.

Neurons use electrochemical signalling, which means chemicals are used to trigger an electrical signal. These neurotransmitters are stored in tiny bubble-like packets called *vesicles,* each about one 100 millionth of a meter in size, in the axon terminals – the "roots" of the treelike structure of the nerve.

When activated by an action potential, these vesicles migrate to the neuron's membrane and fuse with it, spilling their neurotransmitters into the gap where neurons meet – the *synaptic cleft.*

Neurotransmitters fit matching receptors, like chemical keys in protein locks, and one neurotransmitter may match a variety of receptors. Fitting the neurotransmitter key (*ligand*) into its protein lock (*receptor*) opens a channel though the membrane and charged particles called ions are allowed to flow through, either into or out of the post-synaptic dendrite. Receptors can change whether the neurotransmitter is *excitatory* (increases the likelihood of firing) or *inhibitory* (decreases the likelihood of firing).

The soma is where most neurotransmitters are synthesized, though some of these signaling molecules are also made in the terminals which release them. The tendril-like extensions called dendrites are the main method by which neurons "learn", while axons and terminals are the main method by which neurons "teach" one another. Interestingly, however, there is no actual physical connection between neurons; their synapses join at a gap called the *synaptic cleft*, across which neurotransmitters are released.

Inside a typical neuron is a *cytoskeleton* which maintains its structure, comprised of protein strings that stretch and shrink as the neuron sends projections out toward nearby neighbors, constantly creating and breaking connections.

In the nervous system, the most important charge-carrying molecules are sodium and potassium ions, each with a single positive charge, and calcium ions, each with a double positive charge. The neural cell membrane is *semi-permeable*, meaning it allows some molecules to flow through, while controlling the passage of others into and out of the cell.

Proteins called ion channels are embedded in the membrane, and act like pores which open and close, allowing only specific ions through – sodium channels let sodium ions pass through the membrane, while potassium channels let potassium ions pass through. As the channels open or close, and ions pass through, it changes the polarity of the membrane. A few of these channels are constantly open, allowing a slow leak in and out of the cell, further helping to maintain the membrane potential.

When an electrical charge built up in the *axon hillock* reaches a threshold point, the neuron fires, and a charge called an *action potential* travels down the axon, away from the cell body.

This firing of the neuron is primarily the action of five components: sodium (NA+) and potassium (K+) ions, and three special proteins – potassium and sodium *ion channels*, and *sodium-potassium ion pumps*.

Neurotransmission

Nerves operate in a domino effect, with each neuron receiving an impulse and relaying it to the next. When dendrites receive an excitatory neurotransmitter, it adds to an ionic charge which builds to a threshold point, and the charge is released and shuttled down the axon, to be passed on to the next neuron in the chain. The entire process takes about seven milliseconds, faster than lightning striking. Here's how it happens:

> **1. Resting Potential** – Atoms try to reach stability, balancing the number of positive protons and negative electrons, until they reach a natural neutral non-charged state called *equilibrium*. Because similar charges repel one another, positively charged atoms called ions flow from the highest positive concentration toward the highest negative concentration. This ensures they travel in one direction at a time.
>
> Every cell in your body is surrounded by a membrane, which encloses *cytoplasm* (inner fluid) and cell *organelles* (substructures). When unstimulated, neurons are in a resting state, and the outer membrane is *polarized*, possessing a positive electrical charge on the outside of the cell, and a negative charge on the inside.
>
> Many positively-charged sodium ions (NA+) collect on the outside, but only a few positive potassium ions (K+) are contained on the inside, giving the inside a *resting potential* (negative charge) of about -70 millivolts. (One milliVolt is equal to a thousandth of a Volt, while wall sockets in your home carry 120 Volts.)
>
> Most of the tremendous amount of glucose energy your brain consumes is dedicated to maintaining this *polarity* – the resting potential of its neurons. Sodium-potassium *protein pumps* are constantly at work, each cycle pumping 3 NA+ ions outside the cell and 2 K+ ions inside it. This requires energy from *ATP*, the fuel molecule your body synthesizes from glucose (blood sugar) extracted from the food you eat. When at rest, fully 1/3 of the energy an animal consumes is used to power such sodium-potassium ion pumps in its body's cells.
>
> **2. Depolarization** – When a neurotransmitter is released from a dendrite, it binds to receptors on a postsynaptic neuron. This changes the molecular shape of proteins, opening sodium ion channels embedded in the membrane, allowing positively-charged sodium ions to flow into the cell. These ions make the inner charge more positive, and the resting potential starts to move toward 0

mV. When this depolarization reaches about -55 mV, a great number of sodium channels open, a large number of sodium ions rush in, and the neuron fires an action potential, a movement of sodium ions down the neuron's axon.

Whether a post-synaptic neuron is excited or inhibited depends upon which neurotransmitter it receives, and what kind of receptors the neurotransmitter binds to. Neurotransmitters which open Na+ channels excite neurons, triggering impulses, whereas neurotransmitters which open K+ channels (allowing potassium ions out and thus increasing the inner negative charge) inhibit this firing.

3. Propagation – Transmitting an action potential down the axon requires reamplification along the way. The axon is made up of segments like links of sausage called *Schwann cells*. A sheath of fatty myelin insulates each Schwann cell, so that ionic charges cannot leak out, strengthening the signal and speeding its passage tenfold.

A different kind of sodium channel called a *voltage-gated ion channel* is embedded in the membrane along the length of the axon, and as the name implies, this gate is opened by a change in voltage. When an action potential passes by, these gates open in response to the change in polarization, allowing positive sodium ions to pour into that segment of the axon, repeating the signal. Briefly, the membrane's polarity has reversed – the outside of the axon segment becomes negative, the inside positive. The change in polarity triggers the opening of the next sodium channel down the axon and so on, *propagating the signal*; the restrengthened charge moves to the next segment of the axon.

4. Repolarization – After the inside of the cell has been flooded with positive sodium ions, the membrane's potassium ion channels open. This allows positive potassium ions (K+) from within the axon to flow outward toward the temporarily negative region outside the axon, reestablishing the outer positive charge, and causing the sodium channels to reclose after the signal has passed by. Sodium-potassium ion pumps return the neuron to its resting potential of -70 mV, awaiting the stimulus of neurotransmitters to reactivate it.

5. Neurotransmitter Release – The impulse reaches terminals at the end of the axon, depolarizing the membrane, and ion channels open, allowing calcium ions (Ca2+) to flow into the cell. These calcium ions "push" fluid sacs called vesicles toward the membrane, releasing their contents, chemicals called neurotransmitters into the gap between neurons called the synapse. This neurotransmitter binds with protein "receptors" on the postsynaptic (receiving) neuron.

6. Reuptake – After a nerve fires, neurotransmitters shake free from receptors, and are either broken down by enzymes or are sucked back into the terminal boutons in the process called *reuptake*, allowing them to be recycled. The entire process occurs in only a few thousandths of a second, after which the cell returns to its *resting potential*, ready to receive and send another ionic signal. This neurochemical transmission is constant, every sleeping and waking moment of your life.

Information Flow

Like all the cells in your body, neurons maintain a different concentration in ions on both sides of their cell membranes. This polarity is maintained by the flow of ions through the numerous sodium and potassium ion channels embedded in the membrane of the neuron.

When at rest, the balance of ions inside and outside the neuron is carefully controlled, so the neuron maintains a constant negatively-charged internal state. Maintaining this *polarization* – the difference in charges between the inside and outside of the neuron – is the primary reason your brain consumes so much food energy.

ATP energy molecules – produced from food – supply power to protein pumps, which push ions across the membrane to maintain its polarization – the relatively negative inner charge. To fire a neuron, this natural negative charge must be overcome.

Many positively-charged sodium ions occupy the *extracellullar fluid* outside the neuron, with only a few inside. A smaller number of positively-charged potassium ions occupy the *intracellular fluid* inside the neuron, while only a few are clustered outside. When ion channels are open, they allow the passive flow of ions from the area of highest concentration to that of lowest concentration. Ion pumps require energy to push ions toward the area of high concentration, against their natural repulsion.

Neurons maintain their resting state mainly by pumping out positively-charged sodium ions. Protein sodium-potassium pumps are constantly at work, expelling three sodium ions (Na+) for every two potassium ions (K+) pumped into the neuron. This unequal pumping results in more potassium ions inside and more sodium ions outside the cell.

This keeps sodium ions concentrated outside the neuron, and potassium ions inside. The membrane is polarized, with a greater positive charge on the outside (typically 0 milliVolts) than on the inside (typically -70 milliVolts when at rest). As a neuron becomes less negatively charged, it's said to be *depolarizing*. When it returns to its resting potential of -70 milliVolts, it's said to be *repolarizing*.

In a resting state, potassium channels are more permeable than sodium channels, so more potassium ions slowly leak outward, than sodium ions leaking inward. This also helps keep the inside face of the membrane more negatively charged than the inside.

Excitatory neurotransmitters open sodium channels, so positively-charged sodium ions (NA+) flow *into* the cell, gradually reducing its negatively-charged inner environment – *depolarization*.

Inhibitory neurotransmitters open potassium channels, so *positively-charged potassium ions (K+)* can flow *out of* the cell, leading to *hyperpolarization* – an even greater inner negative charge, making the neuron less likely to fire.

Here's how a signal is transmitted – either a sensation travelling from your body to your brain, or from your brain to your body, typically triggering a muscle contraction:

There are three different types of sodium ion channels: 1) those which open when a ligand binds to them (*ligand-gated ion channels*); 2) those that open in response to a physical stimulus like pressure, vibration or a temperature change (*mechanically-gated ion channels*); and 3) those that open in response to changes in membrane potential (*voltage-gated ion channels*).

After a ligand-gated or mechanically-gated ion channel allows sodium ions in, it slightly depolarizes the membrane from -70 millivolts to -55 millivolts. This threshold level of depolarization opens voltage-gated ion channels, allowing a much heavier flood of sodium into the neuron, and there is a voltage "spike" – the action potential.

When sodium ions rush in, it depolarizes the membrane in the area where the stimulation occurred. If the depolarization is strong enough (-55 millivolts), it depolarizes adjacent areas of the membrane, triggering the opening of voltage-gated Na+ ion channels, spreading the depolarization.

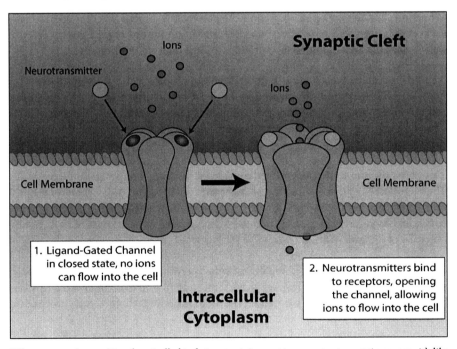

When a neurotransmitter chemically binds to a protein receptor on a postsynaptic neuron, it's like fitting a key into a lock. It opens a channel in the cell membrane through which ions flow. These are **ligand-gated ion channels.**

As membrane depolarization spreads down the membrane to open nearby voltage-gated ion channels, more sodium ions rush in. This works like a domino effect, as voltage-gated ion channels open progressively further down the axon. After opening, however, these channels have to "reset", ensuring the signal travels only one direction.

Sodium channels require a brief *refractory* (recovery) period after activating, and during this time they cannot reopen until they "reset". This ensures that action potentials can only travel forward, but not backward.

The action potential *propagates* down the axon, as sodium channels open in response to membrane depolarization. The leading edge triggers adjacent sodium channels, sodium ions rush in, and leads to another depolarization spike, triggering the next sodium channels down the axon until the action potential reaches the terminal boutons and triggers neurotransmitter release.

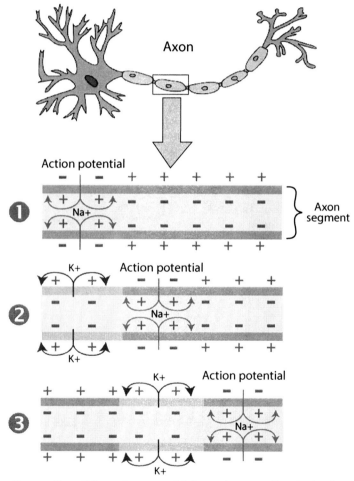

Propagation of the action potential down the axon. Depolarization of the membrane opens adjacent voltage-gated sodium channels. Closing of the sodium channels and expulsion of potassium ions in the wake of the impulse repolarize the membrane.

Slight depolarization won't open the channel; it requires stronger depolarization to reach a threshold value of -55 millivolts for these gates to open. When sodium channels open, sodium ions are attracted toward the relatively negatively-charged and sodium-scarce interior of the neuron, and flood through the membrane into the neuron, momentarily causing depolarization.

When this happens, potassium ions are pushed out of the cell through potassium channels. Thus, the sequence is in two steps: first sodium ions rush in, causing massive depolarization, then potassium ions rush out, causing repolarization - a return to the negative inner state.

The sodium channels close, no longer allowing sodium ions in, while the potassium channels remain open, allowing more potassium ions out. During this repolarization, the membrane potential drops back down to -70 millivolts. This is the *refractory phase*, during which the channels cannot reactivate.

This temporary switch in the membrane's potential is called the action potential. The depolarization-repolarization cycle is nearly instantaneous, occurring in only two milliseconds (0.002 seconds), as the voltage rises to about +30 millivolts. The short firing time allows rapid burst firing of action potentials. If the neuron does not reach the critical threshold voltage of -55 millivolts, voltage-gated ion channels will not open, and there is no rush of sodium ions to trigger the nerve impulse. Thus, neuron either fire or not – an *all or nothing* operating principle.

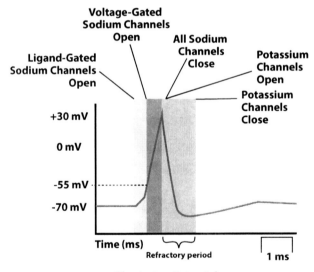

The Action Potential

Larger axons usually transmit more quickly. An increase in axon size allows a higher concentration of the sodium ions causing the depolarization wave along the axon. However, to conserve space, smaller axons can be optimized by insulating them with myelin, fatty molecules wrapped around the axon which concentrate action potentials by preventing leakage of depolarizing ions.

Blocks of insulating myelin have gaps between them called the *Nodes of Ranvier*, sites where the ion pumps and sodium and potassium ion channels are concentrated. This arrangement allows action potentials to "jump" from node to node, greatly speeding up transmission.

Myelin sheaths are critical for neural functions. Their degradation by the autoimmune illness called *Multiple Sclerosis* results in a gradual loss of function in brain, spinal cord and optic nerve axon bundles. The result is a tragic loss of coordination, muscle control, vision and speech, eventually ending in death.

When the action potential has travelled the entire length of the axon, it will come to the terminal boutons, in which sacs of neurotransmitter are housed. The membrane of the boutons is studded with voltage-gated calcium channels, which open in response to the membrane depolarization, calcium ions enter the bouton, and these push the sacs outward and downward toward the synapse. Here they fuse with the membrane, spilling their contents into the synaptic cleft, the gap between the presynaptic and post-synaptic neurons.

Thousands of dendrites on a single neuron can receive activations simultaneously. The inhibiting (-) charges and excitatory (+) charges accumulate, and once the charge in the *hillock*, reaches a high enough *threshold voltage*, the ion charge travels down the axon. The voltage or strength of this fired electrical charge is very small – up to 30mV (less than .3% of a nine-volt battery) – and it can be fine-tuned by other chemicals called *neuromodulators*; *agonists* can increase transmission, while *antagonists* decrease it.

But neurons are like guns; they either fire or they don't – and like computers, they transmit a *binary* (two-state) signal, either on or off. So the *intensity* of a signal is determined by *frequency* – the speed of firing – and the number of neurons involved in a signal transmission. High frequency neural firings in a short time create a strong signal. Neurotransmission is virtually identical throughout all animal species, so animal studies are generally considered applicable to humans.

Receptors are protein molecules to which other molecules bind, usually embedded in and protruding from the surface of cell membranes. A given receptor acts like a lock into which a chemical key called a *ligand* fits. Just as with locks, receptors are very specific, responding only to the appropriate chemical "keys".

These keys (ligands) – neurochemicals, hormones or foreign chemicals – may be circulating in the bloodstream, in a synapse, or even floating through the air, water or soil before they bind with a receptor. They can be simple molecules or as complex as a vanilla extract molecule, which binds to *olfactory receptors* in the nose, triggering perception of vanilla's fragrance.

Large proteins like the *hormone insulin* (a blood sugar regulator) or even DNA and RNA strands can also act as ligands – chemical keys fitting into receptors. Your body even has receptors which respond to electromagnetic radiation – heat-activated receptors in the *epidermis* (upper layer of the skin), as well as photoreceptors in the *retinas* (rear surface) of your eyes which convert photons into nerve impulses.

Receptors are found mainly on cell membrane surfaces throughout the body, even among simple one-celled creatures like bacteria. Generally, they function as switches for every cell in the body. Specific receptors tend to be found only with specific types of cells in specific types of tissue making up specific organs.

Receptor structure tends to be the same within a species as well – the receptor for the hormone *insulin* is identical from person to person, unless there are differences due to genetic mutations; insulin, the ligand for the insulin receptor, is also identical from person to person.

Receptors are also found within cells, on the surfaces of organelles like mitochondria (cellular energy processors) and ribosomes (protein assemblers). They initiate chemical processes and functions within every cell of every living creature, including plants, animals, fungi, bacteria, etc.

A single neurotransmitter may activate up to 50 different types of receptors, each responding differently, for example:

- as a direct chemical channel: the activated receptor opens a gate in a cell membrane, allowing ions to pass into or out of the cell (and changing the balance of charges between each side of the membrane)

- as an indirect chemical channel: the activated receptor triggers the release of chemical messengers inside the postsynaptic neuron, which sensitizes response to a neurotransmitter.

- as a trigger for growth: the activated receptor send signals to the cell nucleus, triggering an increase or decrease in protein synthesis.

A receptor protein can bind to more than one ligand, and when the ligand and receptor molecules bind, they form a new substance called an *active complex*, which functions like a *potentiometer* – an adjustable controller like a dimmer switch control ling a room's lighting. This active complex is able to change the receptor protein's structure to alter its function – activating it, switching it off, reversing its function, and even producing a range of states in between.

Making the Connection

Learning and memory are based upon new dendrite and receptor growth, and upon synaptic reinforcement. Altering the strength of synapses, and hence the ability of neurons within a connected network to activate one another, leads to long-term *memory*: when a neural circuit is stimulated rapidly or repeatedly, it prompts structural changes to the synapses, making the neuron *hyper-responsive*, also called a *potentiated* state. As a result, less stimulation is needed in the future to trigger the affected neuron. Thus, the potential for firing of the neuron has increased. This lasting increase in firing potential is called *long-term potentiation* – synaptic reinforcement that is the basis of lasting memories and learning.

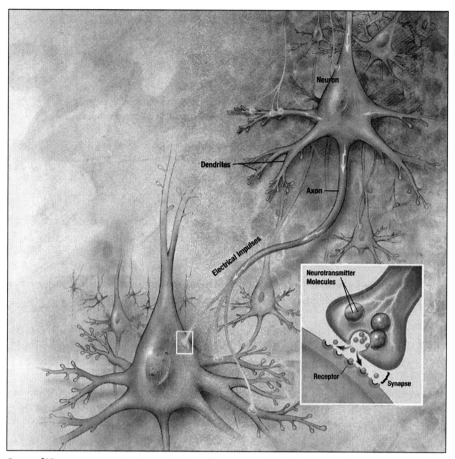

Steps of Neurotransmission *Image: National Institutes of Health, 2010, public domain.*

This strengthening of the connections between neurons is a physical adaptation as result of multiple firings – repeated experiences or thought processes. The connection becomes physically reinforced, and the neurons sprout new dendrites and receptors. This strengthens the communication pathways of that circuit, ensuring the information it contains requires less stimulation to access in the future.

An second class of nerves exits, which can directly transmit electrical signals, using *electrical synapses.* These are uncommon, priamrily found in the eyes. These electrical charges lose energy as they travel, so they are only effective for short distances; however, they are much faster than indirect (neurochemically-based) signalling.

They conduct electrical energy (as opposed to neurochemicals) between two adjacent neurons joined by an extremely tiny space called a *gap junction*, about 3.5 *nanometers* (billionths of a millimeter) wide, one-tenth of the distance of a chemical synapse. This charge in electrical synapses does not the opening of ion channels, but is a direct electrical transmission between two neurons. So while most neurotransmission is a two-step process (electrical signals triggering chemical signals triggering electrical signals and so on and so forth), electrical neurons send impulses directly between neurons, but don't play a large role in the human nervous system or brain.

Chemistry

*"In proportion to our body mass, our brain is three times as large
as that of our nearest relatives. This huge organ is dangerous and
painful to give birth to, expensive to build and, in a resting human,
uses about 20 per cent of the body's energy even though it is
just 2 per cent of the body's weight. There must be some
reason for all this evolutionary expense."*
– Susan Blakemore, Meme, Myself, I,
New Scientist Magazine, March 13, 1999

In response to your environment, your brain signals your cells to take action through two types of chemical messengers – *neurotransmitters* and *hormones*. Thus, your body has two main communications systems:

- **the nervous system** – very fast electrochemical signalling, which is single point to single point, occurring within milliseconds and fading quickly

- **the endocrine system** – hormones are chemical signalling molecules which circulate through the blood stream, taking much longer, occurring over seconds (like adrenaline) or days and even months (like growth hormones).

The previous chapter dealt with the mechanics of the nervous system – impulses moving down axons, triggering neurotransmitter release to activate other nerves, these messages travelling across synapses in a point-to-point relay system.

In the endocrine system however, glands secrete chemical messengers called hormones into your bloodstream, which circulate through your body about once every seven seconds, acting more like your body's broadcast system, sending messages throughout the bloodstream to be picked up by the appropriate receivers (cell receptors), and triggering changes in your body's state. Hormonal messages circulate throughout your body and only activate cells with receptors that match the specific hormone.

Some chemicals (like adrenaline) function as either neurotransmitters or hormones, depending on how and where they're used, and are thus called *neurohormones*. Like a lock and key, both neurotransmitters and hormones can only attach to receptors which chemically match them.

Neurotransmitter Chemistry

Neurotransmitters are the basis of all brain functionality, essentially lighting up your brain's cells with activity. Each delivers a different, specific chemical message, with a different result, which varies based upon the receptor receiving the message. There are both excitatory and inhibitory neurotransmitters, but some may switch this function, depending on which part of the nervous system they're operating upon.

NAME	POSTSYNAPTIC EFFECT	LOCATION	FUNCTION
Acetylcholine	Mainly Excitatory	Nervous system, brainstem	Muscle trigger, cognitive function
Dopamine	Excitatory & Inhibitory	Brain	Motivation, learning, movement
Endorphins	Inhibitory	Brain spinal cord	Pain suppression, pleasure
Epinephrine	Mainly Excitatory	Adrenal glands	Fight or Flight response
Norepinephrine	Excitatory	Brain Adrenal glands	heart rate, stress response
GABA	Primary Inhibitory neurotransmitter	Brain spinal cord	controlling anxiety
Glutamate	Primary Excitatory neurotransmitter	Brain spinal cord	Memory & Learning
Serotonin	Inhibitory	Brain, spinal cord, stomach	Regulating mood, sleep, pain, eating

These chemical signals are the critical means by which the brain and body's neural circuitry functions, and imbalances can result in severe behavioral, mental or motor problems. Over 100 neurotransmitters have been identified, and it's believed more exist. Some excite the nervous system, increasing activity; others inhibit it, decreasing activity. Some participate in generating muscle contractions, resulting in movement, while others engage in reporting sensations like pain, or in generating or modulating thought and emotion.

Thus, neurotransmitters are chemical communicators exchanged between the neurons in your brain and body, causing an action or reaction from a nerve or group of nerves, and enabling control of all your bodily functions.

Neuromodulators differ from neurotransmitters in that they induce long-term changes to post-synaptic neurons. Endorphins are one example, neuromodulators which reduce or eliminate the perception of pain perception.

Some neurotransmitters – chiefly *serotonin, dopamine* and *norepinephrine*, play a critical role in psychological well-being. Norepinephrine and serotonin activate or deactivate various brain regions, influencing your state of arousal and readiness to respond to your environment. Their production relies on an adequate supply of amino acids from proteins in your diet. Failure to eat the right proteins can lead to *depression*, anxiety, and possibly neurodegenerative diseases.

Depression is usually treated with medications which increase circulation of these *monoamines* – dopamine and norepinephrine – as well as serotonin. These monoamines are also behind the uplift you get from eating chocolate – or hanging out with your friends.

When neurotransmitters are no longer needed in the synapse, they are deactivated, usually by being reabsorbed into the bouton during reuptake, recycling them for later use. Many antidepressants rely on blocking this reuptake process, allowing neurotransmitters to linger in the synapses. However, seizures can result from excessive neural discharging, one of the reasons neurotransmitters must be removed from the synapses.

Hormones

While neurotransmitters are chemical messengers for your nervous system, hormones are chemical messengers for your body, circulating through your bloodstream. Hormones are primarily secreted by *endocrine glands* in your brain and body, the *pituitary, adrenal, pineal, pancreas, thyroid* and other glands.

These biochemical signals trigger a state change in cells or organs. They regulate body functions like growth and digestion, energy levels and sexual urges, physical reactions to emotions, and help regulate automatic life processes like heartbeat and blood pressure. Only minute amounts are required to alter cell function.

Every multicellular life form creates hormones, including plants. In vertebrates, they're released into the bloodstream (usually) for transportation, or transferred from cell-to-cell. When a cell has the appropriate receptor, the hormone will bind to it, triggering its effects within the cell. The same chemical can function as a neurotransmitter in your brain, but as a hormone in your body – circulating in your bloodstream to regulate organ functions. One example is *epinephrine* (previously called *adrenaline*).

Emotional responses are initiated by the autonomic nervous system through neurotransmitter release in the CNS, and through hormonal release into the bloodstream, resulting in changes in blood pressure, heart rate, respiration, perspiration, etc.

Neural Networks

The human nervous system has two main divisions:

- **Central Nervous System**, the brain and spinal cord, where all nerve signals are integrated and controlled;

- **Peripheral Nervous System**, nerves throughout the body, which 1) transmit sensory information from the body to the brain and spine, and 2) transmit motor control commands from the brain to the muscles, glands and organs. This is further subdivided into the somatic and autonomic nervous systems (please refer to the following illustration).

HUMAN NERVOUS SYSTEMS

CENTRAL NERVOUS SYSTEM - Brain and spinal cord

SOMATIC NERVOUS SYSTEM - nerves relaying sensation to the brain from the body and motor control messages to the body from the brain

AUTONOMIC NERVOUS SYSTEM - The sympathetic, parasympathetic and enteric nervous systems. All its functions are automatic and involuntary

Sympathetic Nervous System - Activates the fight-or-flight response when there is a threat, whether real or imagined

Parasympathetic Nervous System - Produces the opposite effects of the sympathetic nervous system - a "rest and digest" state. Acting in opposition, these two nervous systems maintain the body's homeostatis (balance)

Enteric Nervous System - controls the digestive system directly. Over 90% of the body's serotonin and 50% of the body's dopamine is produced within the gut.

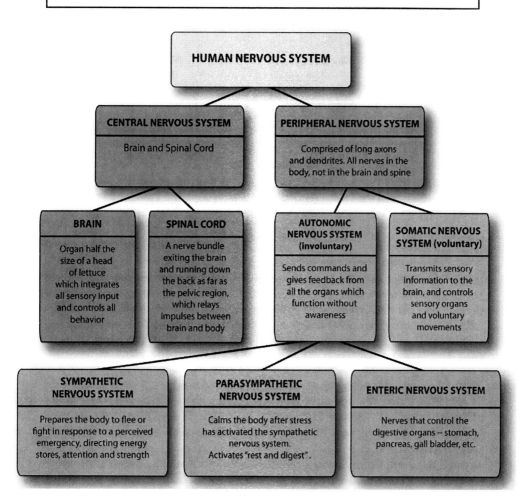

I. Central Nervous System

The Central Nervous System is made up of your brain and spinal cord. Because it has very little capacity to regenerate or repair itself after damage, its parts are well protected by the hard bone of your skull and spine. Your brain is also protected by tough inner membranes, and both your spinal cord and brain float within a nutrient-dense liquid called *cerebral spinal fluid*. This clear liquid and the various messenger chemicals within it are distributed through horn-shaped cavities in the brain called *ventricles*, which feed your brain a constant supply of oxygen and glucose from your bloodstream. Your brain is further protected from toxins in your bloodstream by a layer of glial cells called the *blood-brain barrier*.

Your CNS is responsible for regulating basic functions – breathing, heart rate, pulse, hunger, maintaining *homeostasis* (chemical and temperature balances), sensory input, *motor* (muscle movement) output, emotions, memory, personality – and generating your most complex ideas and thoughts. Your brain communicates with your body via 31 pairs of spinal nerves and twelve pairs of cranial nerves which constitute the CNS.

Information exits your skull and brain en route to your spinal cord through a single large hole called the *foramen magnum* (big hole) into the *medulla oblongata*, a region of your brainstem that controls automatic life functions. The exceptions to this information flow are the *cranial nerves,* which carry information to and from sensory organs in your head and muscles that operate organs such as your tongue and throat.

In your medulla oblongata, cranial nerves 8-12 exit , and this area deals with respiratory functions such as coughing, hiccupping, sneezing, and heart rate. Sensory and motor nerves cross over, switching sides, so the right side of your body is controlled by the left region of your brain and vice versa. Why this feature – called *decussation* – evolved is still one of the great mysteries of modern science.

The Spinal Cord

Your spinal cord has two major functions: generating simple behavior and transferring information. It's central to *reflex actions* (reactions to your environment without your conscious intervention), providing communication between your brain and body through your nervous system. The CNS has three kinds of nerves, gathered in bundles called *tracts. Dorsal tracts* relay sensory information to your brain from your body, and *ventral tracts* send muscle-activating messages to your body from your brain, while *interneurons* connect the two types, in roots joining along your spinal column.

In the following illustration, you can see the CNS in red, and the PNS in blue. There are 31 spinal nerves in pairs, one above each vertebra of your spinal column. These nerves either send messages from your body to your brain (*afferent nerves*) or from your brain to your body (*efferent nerves*). These 31 pairs of spinal nerves – motor paired with sensory –travelling out of your spine's *vertebrae* (bones in the spinal column) from the base of your skull down. Spinal motor neurons synapse with sensory neurons at the spine. *(Image: Central and peripheral nervous systems, Wikipedia, public domain)*

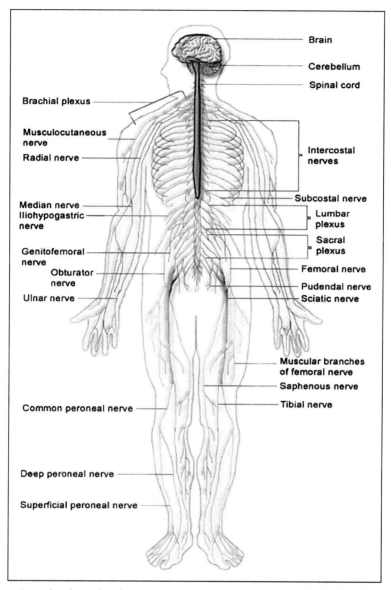

Central and Peripheral Nervous Systems, 2010, Paul Sherman. Public domain.

II. Peripheral Nervous System

Your peripheral nervous system connects your central nervous system to your body. Compared to the CNS, the PNS is relatively unprotected, and exposed to potential toxins and injury. These nerves project to your body to operate organs, muscles and glands, and receive sensory impulses to relay to your spine and brain. Your peripheral nervous system is further subdivided into the *somatic* and *autonomic nervous systems,* including the *cranial nerves,* which connect directly with your brain.

Cranial Nerves

Your peripheral nervous system includes 12 paired *cranial nerves*, connecting your body to your brain, as opposed to your spinal cord. A thirteenth pair may exist for pheromone detection, tentatively named CN0 (cranial nerve zero).

Cranial nerves perform several different functions, including *somatic* (body sensing), *visceral* (organ controlling), motor and sensory (sight, smell, hearing, taste and balance). The first two – the olfactory and optic nerves – branch out from the forebrain, atop the brainstem, but the rest (cranial nerves 3 through 9) branch out from the brainstem.

These ten nerve pairs control hearing, eye movement, facial sensations, taste, swallowing, and other movements using the face, neck, shoulder and tongue muscles.

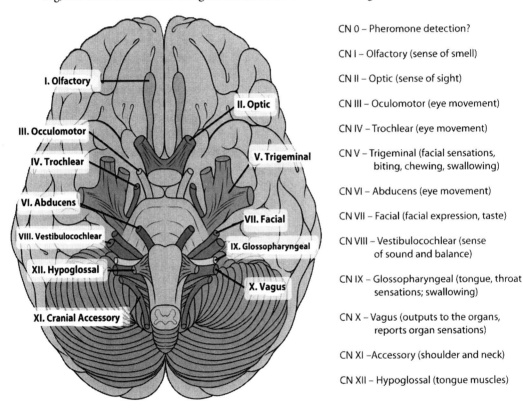

CN 0 – Pheromone detection?

CN I – Olfactory (sense of smell)

CN II – Optic (sense of sight)

CN III – Oculomotor (eye movement)

CN IV – Trochlear (eye movement)

CN V – Trigeminal (facial sensations, biting, chewing, swallowing)

CN VI – Abducens (eye movement)

CN VII – Facial (facial expression, taste)

CN VIII – Vestibulocochlear (sense of sound and balance)

CN IX – Glossopharyngeal (tongue, throat sensations; swallowing)

CN X – Vagus (outputs to the organs, reports organ sensations)

CN XI –Accessory (shoulder and neck)

CN XII – Hypoglossal (tongue muscles)

Brain Human Normal Inferior View, 2009, Patrick J. Lynch, Creative Commons

Cranial Nerve Ten, the *Vagus nerve* (*Wandering* Nerve in Latin) travels from your brainstem deep into your body, through your neck, chest and abdomen, where it innervates your *viscera* (inner organs). This is critical to your survival, sending input to your lungs, heart, digestive tract, including your liver, stomach and intestines. It also controls your vocal cords.

The vagus nerve gets its name from its wandering throughout the body, as it weaves through the abdomen and branches into other nerves extending through the limbs and organs. It regulates many bodily functions, including heart rate, breathing, swallowing, speaking and digestion. Because of its relationship with digestion, it's thought to help regulate feeding, through *satiation* (feelings of fullness and satisfaction after eating). Activating the vagus nerve reduces heart rate and blood pressure.

Incoming vs. Outgoing Signals

1. *Sensory (afferent) nerves* – transmit signals from your body to your brain, relaying impulses from *stimulus receptors* in your organs, skin, muscles, and tendons, information about your internal and external environments. Sensory neurons transmit information about temperature, pain, touch, vibration, and *proprioception* (the relative position of your body parts in space).

   Receptors in your skin, joints, tendons, and even your hair follicles transmit signals to your spinal cord, up to your brain's main sensory relay center, the *thalamus*, and to the *cerebellum*, which helps coordinate balance and movement. Proprioceptors in your muscles, tendons, and joints send information to your CNS about the orientations, relative positions and movements of your body parts, allowing you to maintain balance, and helping your cerebellum and other brain regions monitor movement and coordination.

   Visceral (internal organ) *nerves* signal your brain – usually unconsciously – about states of digestion and the health of your internal organs.

2. *Motor (efferent) nerves* – transmit signals from your brain to your body, triggering muscle contraction or organ and gland function. *General Somatic Motor Nerves* operate skeletal muscles responsible for movement. *Branchial Motor Neurons* transmit via your brain and cranial nerves to operate organs such as your larynx (voice box) and pharynx (for swallowing).

   Interneurons (also called relay neurons) form a connection between other neurons, relay messages between sensory and motor neurons. This allows for reflex reactions which don't require the intervention of your brain's higher-level computing power.

Reflex Arcs

Reflex arcs are neural loops which control automatic reactions, reflexively protecting you from threats. In a reflex pathway, a motor neuron connects to a sensory neuron, allowing for a very fast response. Hard-wired refle arcs are neural links to the spinal cord in a loop. Pain receptors trigger sensory nerves travelling to the spine, where they link through an interneuron to motor nerves, which immediately contract, drawing back an injured limb before the brain ever engages, in responding to stimuli such as contacting a flame.

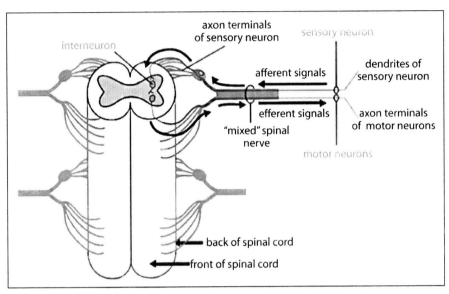

Spinal Nerves, 2010, National Institutes of Health, public domain

IIA. Sensory-Somatic Nervous System

Your sensory-somatic nervous system operates on a conscious level, receiving sensory stimuli and executing body movements. Voluntary movements are controlled by efferent nerves which stimulate muscle contractions. These movements are controlled by *motor patterns* which seem to be stored primarily within the posterior frontal cortex and the cerebellum.

Your body contains three types of muscles: *cardiac*, which control your heartbeat, *smooth*, which control your organs, and *skeletal*, which control voluntary movement.

Skeletal muscle cells are made up of hundreds of bundles called *sarcomeres*. Each sarcomere is composed of two special proteins, assembled in microscopic threads of *actin* and *myosin filaments*. Actin protein filaments are shaped like braided rope, while myosin protein filaments look like bean sprouts on a stem. These proteins are flexible, and can be chemically stimulated to act as *molecular motors*.

Muscles maintain a relaxed, non-contracted state until motor nerves transmit *acetylcholine*, triggering contraction. Acetylcholine is excitatory, triggering a calcium ion release in muscle cells. This activates energy release from the chemical fuel *ATP*. ATP releases a phosphate from the myosin protein, changing the protein's shape. The *heads* of the myosin molecules latch onto the surface of actin filaments and swivel, dragging the ropelike actin fibers inward. Millions of these molecules activating at the same time contracts a muscle fiber. And as hundreds of thousands of muscle cells contract simultaneously, it tugs on the tendon and bone, causing movement. Please see the following illustrations.

372

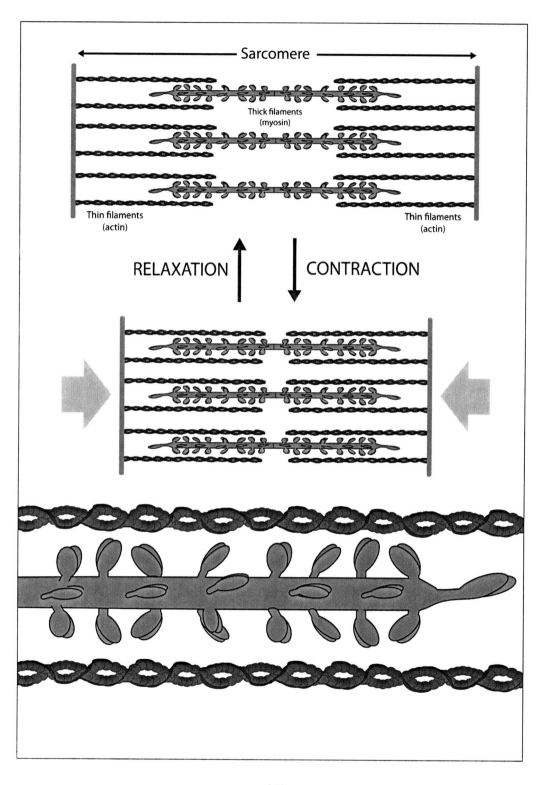

Sarcomere

Thick filaments
(myosin)

Thin filaments
(actin)

Thin filaments
(actin)

RELAXATION

CONTRACTION

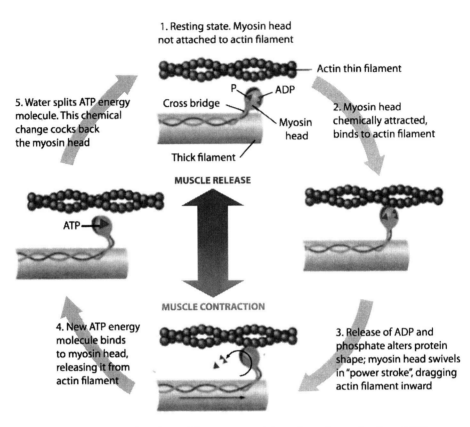

1. Resting state. Myosin head not attached to actin filament

Actin thin filament

5. Water splits ATP energy molecule. This chemical change cocks back the myosin head

Cross bridge

P. ADP

Myosin head

2. Myosin head chemically attracted, binds to actin filament

Thick filament

MUSCLE RELEASE

ATP

MUSCLE CONTRACTION

4. New ATP energy molecule binds to myosin head, releasing it from actin filament

3. Release of ADP and phosphate alters protein shape; myosin head swivels in "power stroke", dragging actin filament inward

Cross-Bridge Cycle, adapted from Human Phsyiology, Stuart Ira Fox, 1995

Force and range of motion are limited by opposing muscles which maintain safety. For example, to swing your forearm, you biceps and triceps work in opposite directions; when your biceps contract, your triceps relax, and vice-versa.

IIB. Autonomic Nervous System

Your ANS regulates internal organs outside your conscious control, monitoring your internal environment and making adjustments to maintain homeostasis and manage life functions. Its actions are almost entirely involuntary (as opposed to the sensory-somatic system) and includes: heart rate, digestion, respiration, salivation, perspiration, pupil diameter, urination, and sexual arousal.

The ANS is subdivided into the opposing *sympathetic* and *parasympathetic systems,* as well as the *enteric nervous system.*

In 1920, Nobel Prize-winner Otto Loewi discovered that vital organs can be controlled by electrochemical stimulation, and that nerve impulses are transmitted by chemical messengers. In his groundbreaking experiments, Dr. Loewi removed two live frog hearts, one of which had the *vagus nerve* attached. He found that applying electricity to the vagus nerve slowed the first heart's beating.

374

He then took some of the liquid bathing the first heart, applied it to the second heart, and found its beating also slowed, thereby showing the neural signalling was being controlled by some kind of chemical messenger. That heartbeat-slowing chemical was found to be acetylcholine, the first neurotransmitter to be discovered.

The cardiac system is controlled by the medulla of your brainstem, through activation of two nerves running from the medulla down to special contracting muscle tissue in the heart called the *sinoatrial node* (SAN) – the heart's pacemaker.

The sympathetic *accelerator nerve* speeds it up when stimulated by norepinephrine, and the parasympathetic *vagus nerve* slows it down when stimulated by acetylcholine.

Your brain's master regulator – the *hypothalamus* – responds to emotion and stress, including exercise by activating the *pituitary gland*. The pituitary releases hormones into the bloodstream which indirectly control heartbeat via the medulla and the accelerator and vagus nerves.

ANS activity is largely involuntary, but 2013 experiments by Dr. Maria Kozhevnikov of the National University of Singapore showed that core body temperature can be voluntarily controlled by Tibetan *g-tummo* meditation, a powerful technique examined in *The Path Book 2*. Skilled practitioners of yoga and meditation can significantly alter many autonomic functions, including heart rate, pain sensitivity and oxygen consumption.

The two main branches of the ANS (sympathetic and parasympathetic nervous systems) work in opposition to one another upon your body's organs. This is how your hypothalamus maintains homeostasis, through regulating your internal states; the SNS usually triggers excitatory responses, and the PNS usually triggers inhibitory responses. Both systems are constantly engaged, even while you're at rest. The balance between them constantly changes in response to internal and external stimuli to maintain an optimal state of homeostasis.

The hormones epinephrine (formerly called *adrenaline*) and norepinephrine (formerly called *noradrenaline*) primarily activate your sympathetic nervous system, speeding up your heart rate and breathing, while the hormone acetylcholine primarily activates your parasympathetic nervous system, slowing them down. These automatic biological responses are controlled by your hypothalamus and pituitary gland, and are triggered by your emotional responses to your environment.

Both epinephrine and norepinephrine are chemically very similar, and both are central to your body's fight or flight response to stress. The main difference between them lies in their structure. Epinephrine contains a methyl group in place of a hydrogen atom in norepinephrine. This chemical difference makes them act slightly differently when binding to receptors in the nervous system and muscles. Both chemicals act upon adrenergic receptors in the body.

The *fight or flight response* to stress is mediated by these adrenergic receptors, proteins which modulate blood pressure, and trigger muscle contractions and chemical secretions. Physical responses which involve adrenergic receptors include contraction of smooth muscles and heart muscle; constriction or dilation of the blood vessels; inhibition of secretions including saliva, insulin, and histamines; and promoting an increase in body secretions. The pounding heart and rising blood pressure in response to stress are partly due to adrenergic receptors acting upon the body.

Norepinephrine is secreted by neurons in both the brain and adrenal glands, but epinephrine is only produced by the adrenal glands. This means that norepinephrine acts within the brain, but its chemical derivative epinephrine, doesn't. When you undergo physical or emotional stress, the adrenal glands excrete both hormones to provide a response. Epinephrine is a hormone released into the bloodstream by the adrenal glands in response to sympathetic nervous system arousal. It increases heart rate and triggers the discharge of sugar from the liver into the bloodstream.

When you're frightened, anxious, nervous or angry, your SNS triggers your fight or flight response, speeding up your heart rate, and releasing glucose into your bloodstream for energy in preparation for quick action, dilating your veins to deliver glucose-rich blood quickly to your muscles, and slowing your digestion.

Enzymes quickly break down norepinephrine in your synapses however, so the effects on your organs are almost instantaneous and quickly fade, but the adrenal glands release much slower and longer-lasting epinephrine into your bloodstream, making it take longer to calm from the effects of epinephrine acting as a hormone in your blood.

After the stress has passed, your hypothalamus uses your PNS to calm your body, bringing your system back into homeostasis and initiating the storage of glucose and fat for later energy release. The PNS is mainly activated by your vagus nerves (tenth cranial nerves), and restores normal bodily functions after sympathetic nervous system activation – the SNS prepares your body for dealing with danger; the PNS calms it, reversing these changes after the danger has passed.

Acetylcholine is the main neurotransmitter which creates calming, recuperative functions, and triggers conservation of glucose for tissue repair and future energy needs. Acetylcholine constricts your pupils, slows heart rate, dilates your blood vessels, and stimulates your digestive system. Some neurons additionally use nitric oxide (NO) as a neurotransmitter.

Your *enteric nervous system* is the most neural-dense region, located in and monitoring your digestive regions on a subconscious level, regulating organs, including the esophagus, stomach, intestines and colon. This is also the basis of your *gut feelings* – an intuitive sense particularly highly-developed among the Japanese, who use this "belly sense" to *read the air* of those around them. Several phrases in the Japanese language which have no equivalent in English are related to such concepts. For example, someone who is "out of touch" with the collective emotional state of everyone around him is said to be "KOO-key Yoh-may-NY" (空気読めない) – "unable to read the air".

Soldiers suffering spinal war wounds which sever the connection between the enteric nervous system and brain become unable to read their own fear and anger – body sensations of their bodies, particularly in the stomach and intestines – seem to be a critical part of "feeling" emotions. Injuries to the conscious, rational region of the brain, the *prefrontal cortex*, on the other hand, which *interprets* emotions, leaves them unable to sense or rationally decide how to act upon emotions tied to risk and conflict – the mental link between their higher thinking and emotions has become disconnected. Thus, emotions are a complex interaction between your digestive and central nervous systems, affecting your entire body profoundly.

Endocrine System

THE MAJOR ENDOCRINE GLANDS

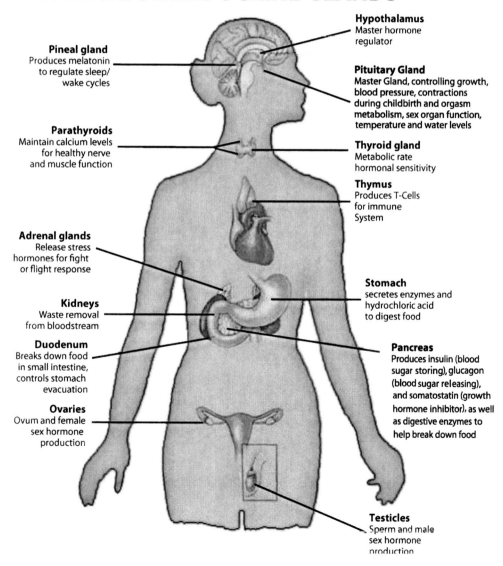

Hypothalamus
Master hormone regulator

Pineal gland
Produces melatonin to regulate sleep/ wake cycles

Pituitary Gland
Master Gland, controlling growth, blood pressure, contractions during childbirth and orgasm metabolism, sex organ function, temperature and water levels

Parathyroids
Maintain calcium levels for healthy nerve and muscle function

Thyroid gland
Metabolic rate hormonal sensitivity

Thymus
Produces T-Cells for immune System

Adrenal glands
Release stress hormones for fight or flight response

Stomach
secretes enzymes and hydrochloric acid to digest food

Kidneys
Waste removal from bloodstream

Duodenum
Breaks down food in small intestine, controls stomach evacuation

Pancreas
Produces insulin (blood sugar storing), glucagon (blood sugar releasing), and somatostatin (growth hormone inhibitor), as well as digestive enzymes to help break down food

Ovaries
Ovum and female sex hormone production

Testicles
Sperm and male sex hormone production

Your endocrine system is a network of glands in your body which secretes hormones – signaling chemicals – into your bloodstream to help your body function. *Endocrine glands* are small but critical organs which synthesize, store, and secrete hormones that regulate growth, reproduction, homeostasis, *metabolism* (energy consumption and use), and responses to external stimuli.

Like the nervous system, the endocrine system is a biochemical communication system. However, it uses blood vessels instead of nerves to deliver hormone "messages" to cells throughout the body. Delicate balances in this hormonal system must be maintained, or diseases can result; hormonal underproduction or overproduction can wreak havoc upon the biological system. The system is controlled by your brain's master regulator, the hypothalamus, using the pituitary gland to release hormones into your bloodstream, which control other edocrine glands throughout your body. In concert with this network of hormone-releasing glands, your hypothalamus and pituitary maintain the critical biochemical balances keeping you alive:

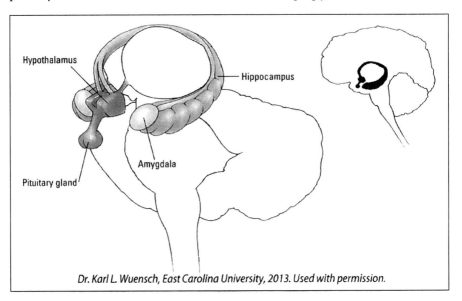

Dr. Karl L. Wuensch, East Carolina University, 2013. Used with permission.

The *Pineal Gland* maintains your body's internal clock by secreting sleep-inducing *melatonin*. It looks like a tiny pine cone (hence its name), and is located between the two hemispheres of your brain, near its center.

The *Pituitary Gland* produces six hormones which regulate growth, the production of sex hormones, *oxytocin* (which builds social bonds, increases trust, and truggers contractions during pregnancy and orgasm) and *vasopressin* (which increases blood pressure, prevents urine buildup in the kidneys and triggers male territorial aggression).

The *Adrenal Glands*, also part of your endocrine system, are found atop your kidneys, and produce the stress-response hormones epinephrine, norepinephrine and cortisol, which trigger fight or flight changes in your body in response to possible danger.

378

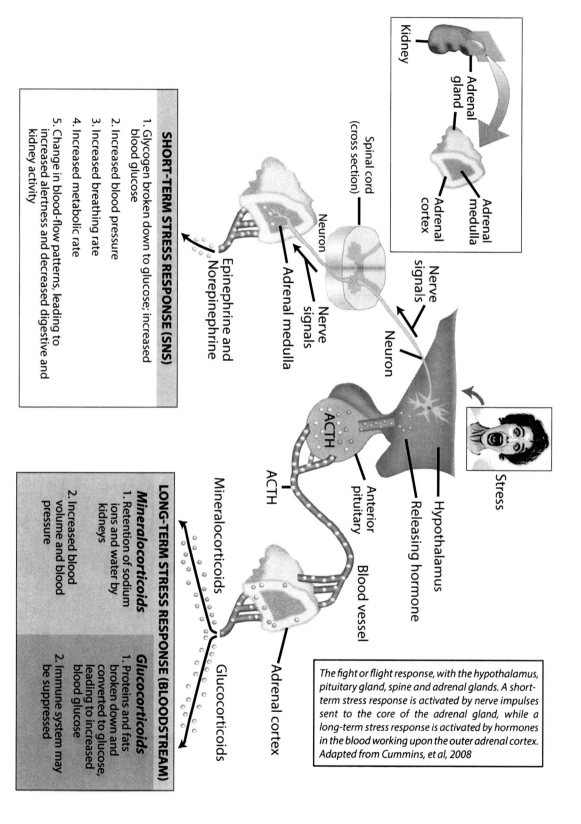

Kidney

Adrenal gland

Adrenal medulla

Adrenal cortex

Spinal cord (cross section)

Nerve signals

Neuron

Neuron

Neuron

Nerve signals

Adrenal medulla

Nerve signals

Epinephrine and Norepinephrine

Stress

Hypothalamus

Releasing hormone

Anterior pituitary

ACTH

ACTH

Blood vessel

ACTH

Mineralocorticoids

Mineralocorticoids

Glucocorticoids

Glucocorticoids

Adrenal cortex

SHORT-TERM STRESS RESPONSE (SNS)

1. Glycogen broken down to glucose; increased blood glucose
2. Increased blood pressure
3. Increased breathing rate
4. Increased metabolic rate
5. Change in blood-flow patterns, leading to increased alertness and decreased digestive and kidney activity

LONG-TERM STRESS RESPONSE (BLOODSTREAM)

Mineralocorticoids

1. Retention of sodium ions and water by kidneys
2. Increased blood volume and blood pressure

Glucocorticoids

1. Proteins and fats broken down and converted to glucose, leading to increased blood glucose
2. Immune system may be suppressed

The fight or flight response, with the hypothalamus, pituitary gland, spine and adrenal glands. A short-term stress response is activated by nerve impulses sent to the core of the adrenal gland, while a long-term stress response is activated by hormones in the blood working upon the outer adrenal cortex. Adapted from Cummins, et al, 2008

Neuromodulators

Hormonal neurons in your CNS differ from neurotransmitter-producing neurons in several ways. Hormonal neurons are mainly concentrated in the central brain regions and brainstem atop the spinal cord, regulating the most basic and critical automatic functions. While their numbers are small, their axons exert a profound influence, projecting throughout the brain.

A single one of these neurons can influence over 100,000 others, by secreting neuromodulators into the extracellular spaces instead of directly into a synaptic gap. While these neuromodulators affect other neurons more slowly, the effects last longer than those of simple neurotransmitters passing from single neuron to single neuron within milliseconds in the brain.

By affecting multiple neurons, these neuromodulators help control signal flow, instead of engaging in direct neuron-to-neuron synaptic transmission. *Acetylcholine, dopamine, histamine* and *serotonin* are the primary neuromodulators, which spread throughout your nervous system, affecting a wide area of neurons. By performing a dual function as neuromodulators (the brain's hormones) and as neurotransmitters, these neurochemicals can affect a greater variety of cells and at greater distances than simple nerve-to-nerve transmission. Neuromodulators are also not broken down or reabsorbed like neurotransmitters, thus remaining for extended periods in the *cerebrospinal fluid* which bathes the brain and spine. In this way, neuromodulators can influence overall activity levels throughout your entire nervous system.

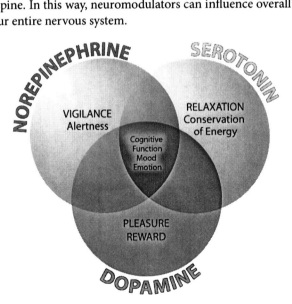

Mood Controllers

Dopamine and serotonin are chemically very closely-related, distributed throughout your brain and body. Both are synthesized from amino acids, and they're two of the chief means of modulating and stabilizing your moods, and for assuring that your central nervous system functions properly. If either becomes depleted, your moods and ability to think will decline, affecting your appetite, *libido* (sex drive), and motivation.

An imbalance between the two – too little or too much of either or both – will eventually lead to illness. A lack of dopamine saps your motivation and robs you of the ability to feel pleasure, while a lack of serotonin leads to depression, anxiety and aggression. Too little dopamine also underlies Parkinson's disease, while too much dopamine or glutamate may underlie *schizophrenia* – severely disorganized thought and speech, abnormal emotional responses, auditory hallucinations, and paranoid or bizarre delusions.

Dopamine and serotonin work in harmony throughout your body, each independently regulating specific separate brain functions. An imbalance in one increases the chance of imbalance in the other. Psychiatrists look for a means of restoring the balance in these neurotransmitters to treat mood disorders like depression, but the wisdom of earlier focusing upon serotonin alone has come into question. Modern medications consider the connection between serotonin and dopamine for treating imbalances.

Monoamines

Complex chemicals like neurotransmitters and hormones are assembled from components called *precursors*. Among these precursors are some amino acids. The neurotransmitters norepinephrine, epinephrine, dopamine, melatonin and serotonin are all *monoamine neurotransmitters*, because each contains a single amino acid. There are two classes, based on the amino acid used to make them:

Catecholamines

One vital precursor is the amino acid *tyrosine*, one of 20 essential amino acids your body needs from your diet, used by RNA to assemble proteins. The *catecholamines* – dopamine, norepinephrine and epinephrine – are all synthesized from tyrosine, found in almonds, avocados, beans, pumpkin and mustard seeds. B- and C-vitamins, iron and copper are also essential to the synthesis, contributing to over 100 chemical reactions in amino acid production.

Enzymes in your brain convert tyrosine into *L-DOPA* and then dopamine, and in the brainstem and adrenal glands, dopamine is used to synthesize norepinephrine and epinephrine. Dopamine, norepinephrine and epinephrine are called catecholamines because each combines a catechol molecule with parts of the amino acid tyrosine:

Catechol   Dopamine   Norepinephrine   Epinephrine

Dopamine is associated with the anticipation of pleasure and natural rewards, forming the basis of motivation, while norepinephrine and epinephrine promote focus, attentiveness, and the stress response. While dopamine and norepinephrine are neurotransmitters in the brain, they can also act as neuromodulators in the central nervous system, affecting neurotransmitter sensitivity and effectiveness. Both can also act as hormones, circulating through the bloodstream to affect organs and tissues. Norepinephrine and epinephrine are best known as fight-or-flight hormones, released into your bloodstream by the adrenal glands when your brain triggers a response to stress.

The Catecholamine Theory of Mood was first proposed by Dr. Joseph J. Schildkraut in 1965, who suggested that depression comes from catecholamine deficiency and mania comes from catecholamine excess.

According to this model, drugs which destroy catecholamines can cause depression, while drugs which increase catecholamines can alleviate it.

Indoleamines

L-tryptophan is another of the 20 essential amino acids in your diet used to synthesize neurotransmitters. Your brain and digestive system use tryptophan to synthesize serotonin, the mood-stabilizing neurohormone, and melatonin, regulator of your *circadian rhythms* (sleep-wake cycles).

Foods which provide the highest concentrations of tryptophan include milk, Swiss cheese, ham, turkey, soy products like tofu, black-eyed peas, and nuts and seeds such as walnuts, almonds, sesame seeds, and pumpkin seeds.

Melatonin is synthesized by the pineal gland, as well as in the intestines, while serotonin is synthesized in your intestines and the *raphe nuclei* of your brainstem, which sit atop your spinal cord and regulate sleep, breathing, heartbeat and other important automatic functions.

L-tryptophan

serotonin   melatonin

Neuropeptides

Neuropeptides are short amino acid polymers in your nervous system which act like specialized neurotransmitters. They help control mood, energy, appetite and pain and pleasure perception. They also help modulate thought and memory formation, in repairing scar tissue and in controlling your immune system. They are generally secreted by glands in your brain and body. The list of known neuropeptides is long, but chief among them are *endorphins, ghrelin, insulin, orexin, oxytocin, substance P* and *vasopressin*.

Endorphins are your body's natural *opiates*. The name comes from endogenous – self-made – morphine, because they provide a sense of calm, well-being and *analgesis* – pain relief. Endorphins function in the same manner as opium-poppy-derived drugs like heroin and morphine, binding with *opioid receptors* to shut down pain and anxiety. Endorphins are released during laughter, aerobic exercise, and other positive or pleasurable moments. They are produced by your hypothalamus and pituitary gland to soothe, stop pain signals, and help boost mood.

Ghrelin primarily triggers appetite when your stomach is empty, but is also involved in stimulating growth and in learning. In fact, ghrelin has several roles, such as stimulating increased concentration of additional hormones, which include cortisol. These multiple mechanisms enable ghrelin to speed up food intake and boost weight.

Three hormones in particular – ghrelin, *orexin*, and *leptin* – act upon your brain to control your appetite. Ghrelin stimulates appetite, while leptin suppresses it. Ghrelin levels fluctuate before and after you eat, increasing prior to meals and decreasing afterwards.

Secreted by your stomach, ghrelin influences fat metabolism by promoting its storage during food scarcity. It's made up of 28 amino acids, and is produced by stomach lining cells, as well as the pituitary, hypothalamus and the blood-sugar regulating *pancreas*. Together, ghrelin and leptin work in concert.

Binge eating (out-of-control), also known as *hyperphagia*, has been linked to malfunctioning in these hunger signals. Ghrelin levels depend upon your nutritional and hydration status; thus, it affects both your hunger and your thirst. Ghrelin helps to regulate fluid intake, so drinking water when you're hungry can dampen ghrelin signals to a degree, helping you control hunger.

Insulin is a hormone which regulates energy use, triggering the absorption and conversion of *glucose* (blood sugar) into long-term storage forms such as fat. The hormone *glucagon* works in opposition to insulin, triggering the *release* of glucose into your bloodstream to provide you with energy. Together, both regulate your blood sugar levels.

Leptin comes from the Greek word for *full*; it's produced by fat cells, and released in your brain, providing you with a feeling of satisfaction. While ghrelin whets your appetite, leptin provides satiety signals which diminish it.

Orexins are a pair of excitatory hormones that promote wakefulness, and seem to play a major role in sleep regulation, integrating metabolic and circadian rhythm systems. Orexin-producing neurons strongly excite brain regions used to control alertness and wakefulness, such as the dopamine, norepinephrine and acetylcholine systems. Orexin also increases food cravings.

Oxytocin is both a hormone in your body and a neuromodulator in the brain. It's central to stimulating feelings of closeness to other creatures, and plays a central role in both female reproduction and in fostering parental behaviors. It also plays a major role in *pair bonding* between lovers, in social recognition, and inducing contractions, during both labor and orgasm.

This "love molecule", is both a neurotransmitter and a hormone, found in high concentrations in the limbic systems of social animals. MDMA, better known as "ecstasy", causes a massive surge in oxytocin, resulting in the "feel-good" "chummy" effects of the popular club drug. Its promotion of bonding, protectiveness, maternal care and trust seem to arise from its dampening activation of the amygdala, the brain's "alarm-inducing" organ.

It's primarily secreted by your pituitary gland and helps control the *hypothalamic-pituitary-adrenal axis,* the activity of three major glands which respond to stress by activating your fight or flight response. Oxytocin inhibits the release of stress hormones like *cortisol,* creating a sense of calm contentment, and reducing fear and anxiety.

Animals with high oxytocin levels tend to be monogamous, suggesting it may be involved in faithfulness. Its production can be triggered by contact with a beloved human or even a pet. Social interaction, particularly with loved ones and pets, and sexual intercourse both result in the release of oxytocin, and it's therefore believed to promote social interactions which promote species survival.

Prairie voles are interesting creatures in that they're one of the few truly monogamous animals on Earth, and experiments have shown they have very high concentrations of oxytocin. When oxytocin receptors are blocked, however, these creatures instead become promiscuous.

Substance P is both a neurotransmitter and neuromodulator, controlling sensitivity to other neurochemicals. It appears to be chiefly responsible for transmitting sensations of pain when there is tissue damage from an injury, but it's also a powerful *vasodilator* (widening blood vessels), and may play a role in regulating insulin levels.

Vasopressin is a peptide hormone found in most mammals. Produced mainly by your hypothalamus and excreted by your pituitary gland into your bloodstream and brain, vasopressin functions as an *antidiuretic* (preserving your body's water supply). It also increases blood pressure, and helps your body maintain homeostasis, regulating blood water, glucose, and salt levels.

In men, vasopressin also promotes family protectiveness. Both its function and its chemical construction are similar to oxytocin. For example, it helps triggers birth contractions, and, when released during sexual activities, promotes pair bonding.

Vasopressin also appears to play a major role in triggering male-to-male aggression, and a less clear role in regulating circadian rhythms. Scientists at the Johns Hopkins School of Medicine in Baltimore also reported in 2008 finding a monogamy-promoting gene in humans, which expresses vasopressin receptors.

Steroid Hormones

Steroid hormones are created from the fatty molecule *cholesterol*, by the *gonads* (sex glands – the testes and ovaries), or by the adrenal glands. They are circulated in your bloodstream and are *lipid-soluble,* meaning they can dissolve in fatty substances like cell membranes, which they can diffuse across. Inside your body's cells, they bind to receptors suspended in the cell's cytosol or on the surface of the cell nucleus.

Steroids binding to outer membrane receptors trigger *signaling cascades,* chemical chain reactions which regulate cell functions. Those binding to the cell nuclei trigger genetic activity, such as sexual development or metabolic functions.

There are hundreds of naturally-occurring steroids in plants, fungi, insects and animals. In humans, they control sexual development, immune system function, metabolism, and salt and water balance. The primary steroids in humans include cholesterol, and various sex and metabolism-related hormones.

Functions

Acetylcholine – In your body, this is the most common neurotransmitter. Here, acetylcholine is excitatory, triggering muscle contractions, and stimulating the excretion of hormones from your hypothalamus, endocrine and digestive systems.

Neurons directly connect with muscle cells, releasing acetylcholine. This binds to receptors on muscle fibers, triggering a chemical sequence that results in muscle contraction. Most insecticides, exploit acetylcholine, by limiting its breakdown. It then remains and accumulates in the synapses, causing uncontrolled muscle spasms and rapid death.

Acetylcholine is also the main neurotransmitter governing the parasympathetic nervous system, where it acts as an *inhibitory* neurotransmitter to slow heart rate, and promote digestion, bladder function and other restful body maintenance activities.

In the brain, acetylcholine is transmitted mainly from the *cholinergic* system in the brainstem, out to the higher brain regions which control memory, thought, and emotion. It's therefore thought to be involved in cognitive functions, particularly memory. Extensive damage in these regions is found among Alzheimer's patients and this regionally-specific destruction is thought to underlie the tragic loss of memory.

It has also very recently been discovered that acetylcholine is released in your brain during learning, and plays a major role in the neural restructuring known as *synaptic plasticity*. Within the brain, it arouses your cortex, and assists in the boosting of synaptic potential associated with memory traces.

It's involved in wakefulness, attentiveness, anger, aggression, sexuality, and thirst, among other things. *Synaptic plasticity* is the ability of the neural connection (synapse) to become stronger through use or weaker through disuse. It also comes from an increase or decrease in the number of receptors in the synapse, the amount of neurotransmitters released into the synapse, and the sensitivity of neurons responding to those neurotransmitters.

Anandamide – People had been using the opium poppy and its extracts for thousands of years for both pain-killing and – unfortunately – recreational purposes, long before scientists learned the brain and body created its own painkillers, called endorphins or *endogenous opioids*.

Nearly every cell in your body can synthesize the neurotransmitter *anandamide*, which means *blissful amide* in the Sanskrit language. Anandamide binds to the same receptors as *tetrahydrocannabinol (THC)*, the active ingredient in marijuana. Since its discovery in 1992, it has been found – unsurprisingly – to play a role in stimulating appetite, apparently helping produce the pleasurable sensations from eating, but it also plays roles in promoting sleep and reducing pain.

Mild euphoria, relaxation, and heightened visual, auditory and tactile sensitivity are some of the effects of marijuana, whose active ingredient Delta-9-tetrahydrocannabinol (THC) mimics anandamide by binding to cannabinoid receptors found throughout the brain. When THC binds to CB1 receptors for anandamide, it modifies enzyme activity, affecting potassium and calcium channels to inhibit neurotransmitter release, reducing the general excitability of the brain and CNS.

Long-term marijuana use can lead to loss of these CB1 receptors in brain arteries, reducing bloodflow to the brain, reducing its supply of glucose and oxygen. This results in memory loss, impaired learning and attention deficits.

BDNF – *Brain-derived neurotrophic factor* is a protein *neurotrophin* – a nerve growth factor, which stimulates nerve and synapse growth, differentiation, and *neurogenesis*.

In your brain, BDNF is involved in neurotransmission, but plays a key role in learning and memory, particularly in fear-based conditioning and memory tasks involving spatial navigation and memory. It's critical in inducing the formation of memories and guiding synaptic development, mainly in the brain's memory-forming region called the *hippocampus*, but also functioning in the cortex and deep core known as the *forebrain*.

Cortisol – Another stress hormone, cortisol increases blood sugar in response to stress, suppresses your immune system, and helps regulate your use of fats, proteins and carbohydrates. It's produced by your adrenal glands when you're under stress.

Dopamine – Dopamine is one of the most important neurotransmitters and neuromodulators, helping control signal flow between neurons throughout the central nervous system, and by cells in your cardio-pulmonary system, and even your kidneys; various cells respond in different ways to dopamine, depending upon their location. It's involved in controlling movement and aiding information flow, particularly within your frontal cortex, the area responsible for conscious thought and integration of brain functions creating emotions, morality, judgment, and behavioral control.

This neurotransmitter gives you feelings of empowerment and energy when you perform survival-promoting actions, and this motivates you to repeat them. Survival is promoted by repeating behaviors which lead to the greatest rewards, so dopamine functions as a training signal in brain regions responsible for learning new behaviors.

Its other functions include regulating cognition, motor activity, mood, attention and learning. While comparatively few neurons actually secret dopamine, its influence is far-reaching as a neuromodulator throughout your CNS, and it's central to all motivated behavior in living organisms, including amphibians, birds, fish, insects, mammals and reptiles.

Dopamine is commonly thought of as your brain's *chemical reward*, creating pleasurable sensations, and thereby motivating you to repeat the pleasure-inducing behaviors. However, recent findings suggest it's actually a source of interest, energy, and dynamic excitement, motivating humans and other animals to seek out resources necessary for survival, and to pursue novelty and intellectual interests which bring fulfilment to life. Specific feelings of pleasure are probably more the result of *endorphins* (a contraction of *endogenous* – from within your own body – *morphine* – from Morpheus, the Greek god of dreams).

When dopamine is abundantly available in the synapses, it makes you feel superhuman. Without it, however, animals become listless and even *catatonic*, completely unmotivated – to the point of starving animals even ignoring food placed in front of their mouths.

This is why, for example, laboratory rats will press levers endlessly until they collapse from exhaustion just to trigger dopamine release in their brains – and why humans will trade their safety, happiness, homes, bodies, even their families for a hit of the drug they're addicted to.

Food, sex, cocaine and amphetamines are all addictive because they trigger dopamine release in your brain's primitive *mesolimbic reward pathway* – a neural circuit we'll revisit later. Understanding and mastering the principles by which it operates is no less than the single, fundamental secret to life, as you'll see.

Dopamine is also critical for controlling movement and posture, attention and focus. It helps regulate mood and plays a central role in *positive reinforcement* (reward-based learning) and addictions. Too little dopamine production can result in Parkinson's disease, the motor-control affliction affecting Michael Fox, while too much dopamine (or glutamate) may underlie *schizophrenia*.

Learning and Movement – Deep in your brain's core lie the *basal ganglia*, central to motivation, reward-based learning, automatic behaviors (like driving a car) and the planning, selection and coordination of slow, deliberate movement sequences (the cerebellum orchestrates rapid, coordinated *ballistic* movements).

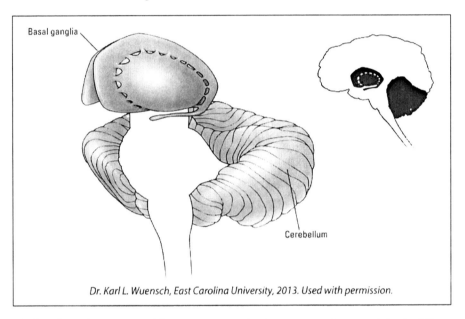

Dr. Karl L. Wuensch, East Carolina University, 2013. Used with permission.

The *basal ganglia* are part of the ancient inner brain structures humans inherited from reptiles – and still share with them. They form complex feedback loops between brain regions for motor control and those which interpret and integrate all of your senses into a single *percept* of the world around you, allowing you to initiate, stop, smoothen and correct movement.

When dopamine is at healthy levels, it also smoothly manages the transmission of sensory input between your cortex and *thalamus* (the main sensory relay station between your body and brain), and helps regulate automatic movements which no longer require conscious thought (such as walking).

Dopamine is mainly synthesized in these basal ganglia regions, though its neurons project extensively throughout the brain, via pathways which modulate the flow of other neurotransmitters. Cocaine and amphetamines are addicting because they hijack these dopamine pathways, which energize and enliven your brain and body, heightening stimulation and neural activity.

Your basal ganglia are essentially under the control of dopamine, which forms a sort of primary *power switch* for the region. This allows your basal ganglia to help control the initiation, smoothness, and precision of movement.

Movement is controlled using a series of *motor programs* – complete movement sequences which rely upon dopamine for proper execution. When you suffer from dopamine deficiency, your movements can become stiff, delayed and uncoordinated, while an excess can cause uncontrollable movements, such as tremors, tics and spasms.

Memory – Dopamine in your cortex improves memory through enhanced signal flow, but only to a certain point. When dopamine exceeds optimal levels, it can actually degrade memory formation.

Attention – Dopamine also plays a part in focus and attention. Sensory stimuli can trigger dopamine release, which draws your attention to a specific sound, sight, smell, taste or feeling.

Additional functions – Dopamine receptors are found in your brain and your cardiovascular system's blood vessels, within your heart and between your heart and lungs, helping to regulate blood flow and blood pressure. Dopamine receptors are also found in your kidneys, to help regulate urine production and excretion of excess sodium, and, if you're a woman, in areas of your hypothalamus which control milk production.

Dopamine also helps stimulate the pituitary gland to produce and secrete *growth hormone*, building muscle, burning fat and improving mobility. If hypothalamus dopamine secretion is blocked, it can interfere with the pituitary gland's production of human growth hormone, and with the adrenal glands' production of adrenaline. Inadequate dopamine protection of the pituitary can reduce male sex drive, decrease sperm count and cause impotence.

Epinephrine (adrenaline) – A hormone produced by your adrenal glands and released into your bloodstream during fear or stress, which stimulates heartbeat, metabolic rate and blood pressure, contracts blood vessels, dilates air passages, and releases glucose for ready muscle use during the fight-or-flight response to perceived danger.

When epinephrine is secreted into your bloodstream, this prepares you for rapid action when your life is threatened, boosting oxygen and glucose supplies to your brain and muscles, and temporarily suppressing nonessential processes such as food digestion and your immune system.

Among epinephrine's effects are: increasing heart rate and blood volume, dilating your pupils, and constricting *arterioles* (tiny blood vessels) in the skin and gastrointestinal tract to minimize potential blood loss, while simultaneously dilating arterioles in the muscles, to maximize available power.

Epinephrine also increases the conversion of *glycogen* (stored sugar polymers) into glucose (quick-burning sugar) in the liver, in this way elevating available system energy. It further triggers a cascade causing the enzyme *lipase* to start breaking down lipids in fat cells to free up more quick energy. As we saw earlier, epinephrine is derived from norepinephrine, which is in turn made from dopamine. All use the dietary essential amino acid tyrosine as their chemical precursor.

Estrogen – estrogens are a group of compounds necessary for development and maintenance of female sexual characteristics, and for sexual behavior and reproduction in humans and other animals. Named after the monthly human estrous cycle of fertility, they are produced by the ovaries, when stimulated by the hypothalamus and pituitary gland.

> *The Best Time to Ask for a Raise? Estrous* occurs just before *ovulation, when an egg is ready for fertilization. In a groundbreaking 2007 study, it was discovered by University of New Mexico's Dr. Geoffrey Miller and Brent Jordan that, contrary to centuries of conventional scientific wisdom, human women appear to go "into heat" just like other animal species, and human men appear able to sense it. The tip earnings of female exotic dancers rise significantly when they are in estrous and those who are on the pill (and therefore don't ovulate) earn significantly less than naturally-cycling women, a finding that may have profound implications for social interactions.*

GABA – *(gamma-aminobutyric acid)* This is the most common inhibitory neurotransmitter in your brain and spine. In fact, GABA is the primary inhibitory neurotransmitter in all mammals, where it modulates neural excitability throughout the central nervous system. Together GABA and its excitatory twin *glutamate* are used by more than 80% of the neurons in your brain and constitute its most important inhibitory and excitatory systems. GABA produces relaxation and lowers *inhibitions* – behavioral self-control – governed by your prefrontal cortex. GABA's effects are heightened by alcohol, barbituates and tranquillizers, while its release is inhibited by caffeine.

> *Yoga: Your Natural Antidepressant* – *GABA is an endogenous antidepressant, a naturally-created neurochemical that helps dampen neural activity, which is why most anti-anxiety drugs bind to GABA receptors. People suffering from mood and anxiety disorders tend to have decreased GABA. To improve mood and lessen anxiety, drugs which increase GABA production are regularly prescribed.*
>
> *But these positive effects can also be obtained through the practice of yoga, according to studies by Dr. Chris Streeter of the Boston University School of Medicine: GABA levels increase after yoga. In fact, yoga appears to have a greater effect on mood and anxiety than walking or other exercise, apparently because of GABA increases in the thalamus, according to The Journal of Alternative and Complementary Medicine. These findings may point to safe alternative treatments for depression.*

You're constantly bombarded with sensory input and need to filter out unnecessary data, so the inhibition of signals may be even more important that excitation. Because of this central importance in brain function, GABA contributes to a wide variety of basic functions, including motor control, vision, and regulating anxiety.

In your body, GABA regulates muscle tone and the growth of embryonic and neural stem cells. Interestingly, GABA is synthesized in your brain using glutamate as a precursor, meaning your brain converts its primary excitatory neurotransmitter into its primary inhibitory neurotransmitter.

As your brain's primary inhibitory neurotransmitter, GABA is used in about 35% of all your synapses, and is second only to glutamate as the most prevalent neurotransmitter in your brain.

It's most highly concentrated in your basal ganglia – which largely governs movement and motivation – and your *limbic system* – the emotion-generating system which includes your amygdala and hippocampus. GABA concentration in your brain is 200-1000 times greater than that of the monoamines (dopamine, serotonin, epinephrine, norepinephrine melatonin, etc.) or acetylcholine. Drugs used to treat epilepsy and calm the trembling of *Huntington's disease*, (a dopamine-deficiency nerve disorder) work by increasing GABA in the brain.

Glutamate – Derived from breaking down *glutamine*, an essential amino acid found naturally in many foods, glutamate is excitatory, promoting signal transmission and memory formation, and is by far the most common neurotransmitter in the CNS. It's central to long-term potentiation, the synaptic reinforcement that is the biological basis of long-term memories.

As the brain's primary excitatory neurotransmitter, glutamate stimulates neural activity throughout the CNS, and is involved in almost all brain functions, including thought, memory and learning. It also helps regulate brain cell metabolism, development, survival, elimination and synapse formation and elimination. Problems in making or using glutamate have been linked to many mental disorders, including autism, obsessive-compulsive disorder (OCD), schizophrenia, and depression.

Glutamate receptors are found throughout your brain – most nerve and glial cells have glutamate receptors. However, excessive amounts are toxic, destroying neural receptors through overstimulation, so glutamate is almost exclusively found inactive within synaptic vesicles.

Glutamate is also the basis of the fifth human flavor known as *umami* – Japanese for *savory* – a sort of rich, meaty flavor used in a number of Asian dishes in the crystallized form of the food additive *monosodium glutamate* (MSG). It's found naturally in a number of foods, including meat, poultry, fish, eggs, and dairy products – particularly Roquefort and Parmesan cheese. The Japanese derive it naturally from the dried seaweed they call *kombu*, although in the west it's usually commercially extracted from yeast and added to nearly every supermarket product, including ice cream. One of the reasons humans may crave it (a love which is knowingly exploited by food manufacturers), is that glutamic acid is the main free amino acid found in human breast milk.

Glutamate plays a central role in synaptic plasticity, and is thus critical to learning and memory: long-term potentiation begins at glutamatergic synapses in the *hippocampus* (your brain's memory-generating center), and is made permanent in various regions throughout your cortex.

Glutamate also functions as both a point-to-point neurotransmitter and as a neuromodulator, able to act excitatory upon a large range of neurons simultaneously.

Making Memories

The holy grail of neuroscience has long been the *engram* – an actual physical form of a *memory trace* – an association stored as a neural circuit. In the year 2000, Dr. Eric Kandel may have discovered it, winning a Nobel Prize for his research. Using *aplysia* sea snails, he showed how the responsiveness of the neural connection – the synapse – is physically altered by repeated and rapid stimulation of a neural pathway.

Repeated, rapid stimulation of two neurons promotes the growth of new synapses between them – new dendrites sprout, giving, for example, two neurons with a single shared synapse additional new synapses between them. In addition, the sending (presynaptic) neuron becomes more sensitive, requiring less prompting to fire, and the receiving (postsynaptic) neuron sprouts more receptor proteins to which neurotransmitters can bind. It can also include an increase in neurotransmitter vesicles, as well as a greater probability of vesicle release, and a strengthening of the physical neural scaffolding.

The protein called *beta-arrestin* is a scaffolding protein supporting neural connections, found in 2012 to play a major role in memory formation within the hippocampus. Although this is being tested for its effects upon sufferers of Alzheimer's disease, it may be effective for people at any age. It provides the energy driving the formation of new synapses, the neural connections which are the basis of learning and memory in the brain.

When you learn, neurons send out tendril-like connections called dendrites that create new synapses. This is a link between two bits of sensory data, perhaps linking a name to the sight of someone's face, for example.

Within the brain, new synaptic connections are constantly being formed, dendrites being produced and using *contractile proteins* to stretch out and connect from one neuron to another. Learning causes repeated, rapid neurotransmission which attracts these dendrites, and strengthens existing synapses, the process called long-term potentiation. But because the physical capacity of the hippocampus is finite, older, unused connections are disassembled in the process called *long-term depression* (LTD), allowing new memories to form in place of older, unused ones.

Beta arrestin helps control synaptic plasticity and LTD by regulating the actin cytoskeleton, a network of filament-forming proteins which comprise neural backbones, and are central to forming new synaptic connections, and disassembling unused ones.

Says lead author Dr. Iryna M. Ethell, beta-arrestin provides energy to the "puppeteer" which is the neural cytoskeleton. This cytoskeleton controls the "puppet strings" which are the dendrites stretching out to form new connections. When beta-arrestin is in short supply, it impairs normal learning in laboratory animals, as new synapses are unable to form.

In 2010, Dr. Z. Josh Huang of Cold Spring Harbor Laboratory published research of how dendrites go about finding a partner. As new dendrites probe about for potential connections, they send a sort of preliminary message transmission between the two neurons to test the compatibility of a possible connection. The process called *cellular adhesion* next brings the two cells into physical contact.

As Dr. Huang explains it, "...the cortical neuron's strategy is to initiate synapse formation with almost any nearby target and then to test it, by trying to communicate using synaptic transmission. Most of these tentative connections don't prove to be correct and will be eliminated. Only those between functionally compatible neurons will be validated and strengthened."

Cell-adhesion molecules act as neural glues making this preliminary connection, and the pre-synaptic and post-synaptic neurons act like a zipper, locking together via these adhesion molecules, according to Dr. Huang.

Synaptic plasticity is the ability to strengthen or weaken these synapses based upon use. A synapse which fires repeatedly and rapidly is strengthened through long-term potentiation (LTP), and one that is seldom used is weakened through long-term depression (LTD), its dendrites eventually retracting.

Long-term potentiation – the synaptic reinforcement which forms memories – increases the *amplitude* (strength) of synaptic signals in several brain regions. Triggering these special proteins strengthens synaptic connections.

The neurotransmitter glutamate is critical for Long-Term Potentiation – the bolstering of a neural pathway that turns a short-term piece of information into a lasting, permanent memory. Strengthening the junction between two neurons makes access to a piece of information easier – the neurons requiring less energy to fire. The name long-term potentiation is derived from the point that this increase in synaptic responsiveness – potentiation – lasts an extremely long time when compared with other processes affecting synaptic strength.

This neural strengthening, combined with growth of new synaptic connections, is the cellular basis of learning – a piece of data becomes fixed into a stronger pathway through which electrochemical signals can more easily flow.

Whenever any new task is learned, it's a difficult process, but as the signal crosses and re-crosses the same synaptic gaps regularly or at a high frequency, the neural pathway is reinforced, and that task becomes progressively easier. After multiple repetitions, using this neural pathway – and using your newfound skill – requires no effort, and you can do it any time you wish.

Thus, learning a new skill reorganizes your neurons, reinforcing and creating new connections across which signals can jump. Millions of new neural pathways are created each time a new task is mastered, and while repeated use of a connection makes it grow stronger; lack of use can cause a connection to be lost.

Two primary mechanisms appear to be at work in LTP: 1) there is an increase in neurotransmitter release and 2) the receptor proteins are altered on the postsynaptic neuron, increasing their sensitivity. After LTP, an altered neuron will produce a larger response, more easily than before. Stress plays a part - anger and fear in particular. Stress hormones trigger the release of extra glucose, available to the brain as fuel. And the brain's alarm center – the amygdala, located at the end of the hippocampus, boosts hippocampal activity.

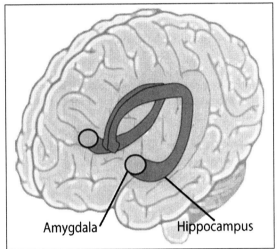

Amygdala   Hippocampus

In terms of memory, this can have two effects:

Heightened arousal can sear so-called *flashbulb memories* into the brain, and disrupt the memory of more neutral (non-emotional) events. Because of this, stronger emotions create stronger, longer-lasting memories. This is thought to be the power behind *PTSD* – post traumatic stress disorder - suffered by victims of traumatic events such as natural disasters or war.

The process is triggered by the release of the neurotransmitter glutamate in the hippocampus, the brain's memory-management organ. Glutamate activates two main types of receptors – "normal" *AMPA receptors*, and special secondary *NMDA receptors*. Both these receptors are distinctly different proteins, and are often found on the same synapse.

Weak stimulation of the presynaptic neuron releases a small amount of glutamate into the synapse, acting upon AMPA receptors, and the postsynaptic neuron is only slightly depolarized. When two glutamate molecules bind to the AMPA receptor, it undergoes a change in shape similar to the opening of a clam shell. This opens an ion channel within the AMPA protein, acting as a pore in the neural membrane, allowing sodium ions to flow into the cell, while potassium ions can flow out. But if glutamate transmission is repeated strongly and rapidly enough, it depolarizes the receiving neuron's membrane enough to activate the second, special type of glutamate receptor.

A neuron

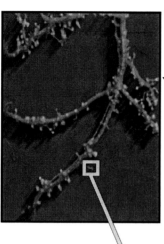

LTP IN THE SYNAPSES

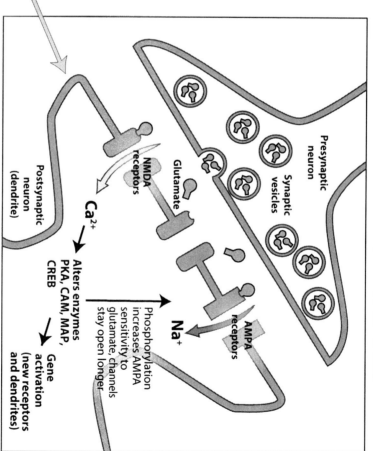

Presynaptic neuron

Synaptic vesicles

Glutamate

NMDA receptors

Postsynaptic neuron (dendrite)

Ca^{2+}

Alters enzymes PKA, CAM, MAP, CREB

AMPA receptors

Na$^+$

Phosphorylation increases AMPA sensitivity to glutamate, channels stay open longer

Gene activation (new receptors and dendrites)

When an ionic charge travels down the axon, it triggers glutamate release from synaptic vesicles. Glutamate binds to AMPA receptors, opening the channels to allow sodium ions to flow into the cell and build up a positive charge.

After a threshold voltage is reached, secondary NMDA receptors become unblocked, allowing a large amount of calcium ions (CA2+) to flow into the post-synaptic nerve's dendrite. Calcium activates several enzymes, triggering multiple effects which increase neural sensitivity - new dendrites and receptor proteins are synthesized, AMPA receptors are altered to enhance ion flow, and nitric oxide is emitted to trigger increased neurotransmitter release from the presynaptic neuron.

Because glutamate only remains in the synaptic cleft for a very brief time, the AMPA receptor quickly recloses, causing only slight depolarization of the postsynaptic membrane. However, if stimulation occurs at a rate of 100 Hz, for at least one second, the depolarized membrane doesn't have time to repolarize again, and a threshold voltage will build.

Normally, the secondary NMDA receptor is blocked by magnesium ions, preventing free ionic flow through its channel. However, when AMPA receptors depolarize the postsynaptic membrane to its threshold voltage, it expels the magnesium ions blocking the NMDA channel.

Unblocked NMDA receptor channels allow the free flow of large amounts of calcium ions, triggering signalling cascades within the post-synaptic dendrite. These calcium ions cause major changes in the post-synaptic neuron (and one change in the pre-synaptic neuron), primarily by altering the shape of six enzymes and thus activating them:

- *PKA* phosphorylates AMPA receptors, allowing them to remain open longer after glutamate binds to them.

- *CAM kinases* also phosphorylate the AMPA receptors, increasing their responsiveness to glutamate.

- *CaMKII* moves additional AMPA receptor proteins from storage sites within the neuron up into the membrane, adding to the number of receptors available to respond to neurotransmitters.

- *Nitric oxide* release signals the presynaptic neuron to increase its neurotransmitter release.

- *CREB* proteins increase gene transcription for new AMPA receptors, further increasing synaptic efficiency,

- *MAP* kinases build new dendrites.

Because memories need to be stable, special proteins called *SK channels* restrict NMDA receptor activity so synapses aren't in a constant state of construction – if neurons were constantly susceptible to change, memories could never be stabilized.

SK channels also restrict the ability to form new memories, however, a barrier which must be removed by acetylcholine. By shutting off this SK-channel restriction, acetylcholine allows NMDA receptors to trigger synaptic strengthening. This is thought to be the reason that acetylcholine-boosting drugs are the only known effective treatment for enhancing cognitive function after Alzheimer's disease has begun to develop.

While adding receptors potentiates the synapse, receptors are removed in long-term depression to weaken a synapse. Structural changes in dendrites also take place, dendrites strengthening or retracting based upon the amount of use a neural circuit receives. Synaptic plasticity in both excitatory and inhibitory synapses is dependent upon calcium.

Histamine – Histamine is a neurotransmitter which triggers *inflammation*, the tissue swelling that is part of your immune system's response to injury or the presence of foreign *pathogens*, disease-causing agents like viruses, fungi or bacteria. It's produced in white blood cells and body tissues, enabling white blood cells to pass through your capillaries – your body's tiniest blood vessels, which exchange water, gases, nutrients and waste between your bloodstream and the cells of your body.

Histamine is also the basis of allergic reactions, triggered when your immune system is hypersensitive, reacting to normally harmless *allergens* as if they were an invasive threat to the body. Drugs called *antihistamines* suppress this overreaction by your body's defenses. Common allergy triggers include specific foods (nuts, wheat, shellfish, milk and eggs), plant pollens, insect stings, latex rubber, and medications like antibiotics or painkillers. In some people, severe allergies can trigger *anaphylaxis*, a severe reaction that affects the whole body, and can be fatal.

Melatonin – A sleep-inducing hormone naturally found in animals, plants, and microbes. Varying amounts are produced during the day in response to light levels, thereby controlling your circadian rhythms. Melatonin is synthesized within the pineal gland using serotonin, derived from the amino acid tryptophan. In the pineal gland, serotonin is first acetylated and then methylated to create melatonin.

The *suprachiasmatic nuclei* are twin rice grain-sized neural clusters sitting at the rear of your hypothalamus, just above the point where your optic nerves join. When photoreceptors in the retinas of your eyes receive low light levels, it signals your suprachiasmatic nuclei that night-time has come, and your pineal gland secretes melatonin into your bloodstream, where it travels to the organs of your body. This is how melatonin takes part in governing the brainstem circuits which ultimately control your sleep-wake cycle.

Suprachiasmatic nuclei provide your body with its circadian rhythms. They act as a central rhythm-keeping system – tens of thousands of tiny neurons within each have rhythmic electrochemical activity, and the rhythm is synchronized by light via neural signals sent from the retinas of your eyes.

Information is relayed from the SCN to a variety of brain structures, along multi-neuronal pathways. During daylit hours, SCN excitation suppresses pineal gland melatonin production. When the sun sets, this inhibiting control gradually diminishes, allowing excitatory connections to increase melatonin secretion, allowing the pineal gland to be activated mainly by norepinephrine.

Studies conducted in 2001 at the University of Texas and in 2005 at the University of Göttingen, Germany have found melatonin to be a potent *antioxidant*, scavenging destructive *free radical molecules*, to protecting nuclear DNA. A joint 2007 study at the University of Granada, Spain and the University of Texas also found it reduces age-related neurodegeneration and free radical damage in mice. Decreased melatonin may underlie the high incidences of cancer among night-shift workers – just 39 minutes of exposure to an ordinary light bulb at night reduces melatonin levels by 50%.

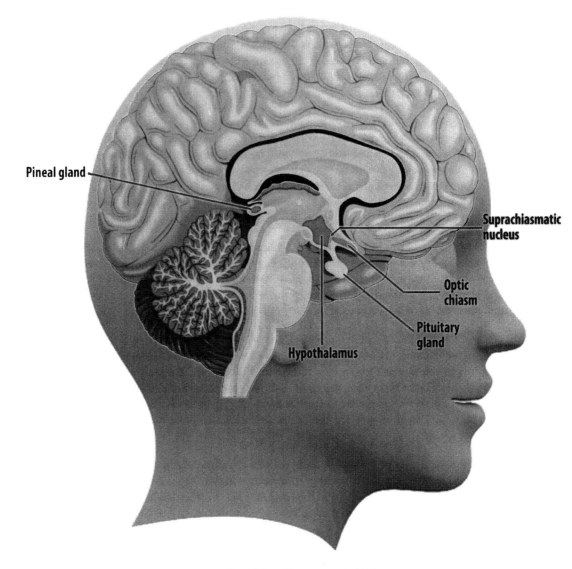

Pineal gland

Suprachiasmatic nucleus

Optic chiasm

Pituitary gland

Hypothalamus

Adapted from Thomson et al, 2008

Norepinephrine (noradrenaline) – is an arousal-inducing neurotransmitter, and stress hormone, along with cortisol, dopamine and adrenaline. It affects brain regions responsible for attention and impulsiveness, and mediates responsiveness of the *amygdala* (your brain's "alarm generator"). Norepinephrine and epinephrine are both stress hormones released by your adrenal glands into your bloodstream to engage your sympathetic nervous system in the fight-or-flight response, rushing oxygen to your brain, making your heart race, dilating your pupils, pumping increased blood to your muscles, and releasing a flood of glucose for action. Along with cortisol and endorphins, all these stress-response hormones suppress your immune system in order to direct all your energy to dealing with whatever threat you're facing. While beneficial in emergencies, over the long term, constant suppression of your immune system leaves your body wide open to a variety of illnesses.

Norepinephrine is also a neurotransmitter involved in mediating mood, and believed, like serotonin, to be connected to depression. Thus it plays a role in mood disorders like *bipolar disorder* (manic depression) as well as being important in controlling attentiveness, emotions, learning and wakefulness. It's concentrated in the brainstem, from where neurons project into the cortex, hippocampus, thalamus and midbrain. Norepinephrine increases excitation of the central nervous system, and is thus central to controlling attention and arousal in the brain.

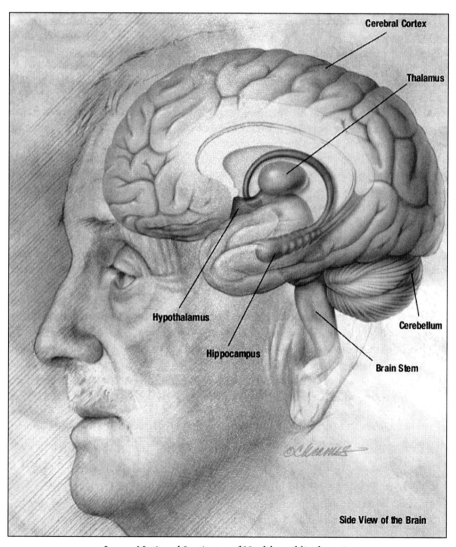

Image National Institutes of Health, public domain

Serotonin – Called the *molecule of happiness*, serotonin is far more than that – it sharpens your focus and improves your problem-solving abilities, radically improving your day. Sufficient serotonin can:

- Improve your aim in sports
- Boost your persuasiveness
- Help you sleep soundly
- Enhance your charisma and creativity

Serotonin levels are part of the reason some are better at maintaining calm in the face of adversity, exhibiting a self assurance and sense of control pver their own destiny. Your overall sense of well-being, capacity to organize your life, and ability to relate to others depends profoundly upon the *serotonergic system*. On the other hand, insufficient levels result in anxiety, fear, self-pity, insomnia, stress, and depression. Such deficits can be caused by a number of things, including poor diet, genetics and medications.

Serotonin is inhibitory, providing a mood-stabilizing source of calm, contentment and well-being, and is involved in memory, learning, pain perception, and regulating sleep, body temperature and appetite. In addition to depression, it appears to play a central role in taming aggression and impulsiveness. It also plays roles in regulating your gastrointestinal and cardiovascular systems.

Serotonin binds to *5-HT receptors*, located on neural and other cell membranes in all animals. In the central nervous system, serotonin helps mediate behavior and perception. Deficiencies may underlie *paranoia*, the unsubstantiated belief that others are your enemies, as well as depression, suicidal tendencies, impulsivity, and aggressiveness. Antidepressants work by blocking the *reuptake* (recycling) of serotonin by presynaptic neurons, keeping high levels in the synapse to stabilize moods. In your brainstem, serotonin helps regulate breathing and heart rate, and defects in this critical signalling may be the cause of *sudden infant death syndrome (SIDS)*.

For such a major component of brain functionality, serotonin is surprisingly minimal in your brain. Less than 2% of your body's total serotonin is located in the CNS, the rest found in your bloodstream and digestive system. You naturally have about 5 to 10 mg. of it circulating in your systems, with about 90% of that concentrated in your digestive system, where it regulates intestinal movement. The remaining 10% circulates in your brain and bloodstream.

In *Evolving Brains*, founder of the California Institute of Technology, Dr. John Allman, writes about the central role of serotonin:

> *Serotonergic neurons project in rich profusion to every part of the central nervous system (the brain and spinal cord), where they influence the activity of virtually every neuron. This widespread influence implies that the serotonergic neurons play a fundamental role in the integration of behavior. Our sense of well-being and our capacity to organize our lives and to relate to others depend profoundly on the functional integrity of the serotonergic*

system. There are only a few hundred thousand serotonergic neurons in the human brain, roughly one millionth of the total population of neurons in the human central nervous system. However, the serotonin receptors on the target neurons are remarkably diverse. Fourteen types of serotonin receptors have been discovered so far in the brains of mammals, located in different places and acting in different ways.

If one thinks of the structure of the brain as a house, the serotonergic neurons are located in the basement. Like the basement regulators of water and electricity, this set of neurons is fundamental to the functioning of the house, acting somewhat like the house's thermostat to maintain a comfortable equilibrium in response to outside variations.

The cell bodies of the serotonergic neurons occupy virtually the same location in the basement of every vertebrate brain. The serotonergic system was essentially in place 500 million years ago, and it has been amazingly conserved throughout evolution, yet it participates vitally in the most complex aspects of our thinking and emotions.

Serotonin is synthesized in your brainstem, projecting into your spine and *reticular activating system*, which controls arousal states, including your sleep-wake cycle. It functions like a "volume control" in your brain, influencing the effectiveness and efficiency of other brain signals and neurotransmitters. Your reticular activating system essentially activates your brain and body, bringing them into a state of wakefulness and maintaining that state, and the greater the serotonin availability, the greater the general neurotransmission, which improves your mood.

RETICULAR ACTIVATING SYSTEM

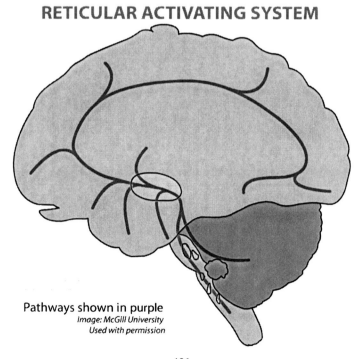

Pathways shown in purple
Image: McGill University
Used with permission

PRIMARY NEUROTRANSMITTERS AND PATHWAYS

Dopamine and Serotonin are two of the primary regulatory neurotransmitters in the brain. Although only a few neurons release them, each connects to thousands of others throughout the brain. Because of this, both exert a profound influence over virtually all mental and neural processes.

DOPAMINE

Dopamine is the basis of positive (appetitive) motivation among multicellular animals, including humans.

Its transmission in both the mesolimbic and the mesocortical pathways provides the positive stimulation that drives virtually all human behavior.

Eight dopaminergic pathways have been found, but three in particular play a central role in human behavior:

Mesolimbic and Mesocortical pathways
(VTA to Nucleus Accumbens, Amygdala, Hippocampus and Prefrontal Cortex)
. Memory
. Motivation and emotional response
. Reward and desire
. Addiction

Nigrostriatal pathway
(Substantia Nigra to Striatum)
. Motor control
. Damage can result in Parkinson's

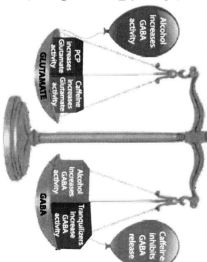

GABA (gamma-aminobutyric acid) and Glutamate are the major regulatory neurotransmitters in the brain. More than half of all brain synapses release Glutamate, and 30-40% of them release GABA.

Together, GABA and Glutamate regulate ion transmission - neural "traffic." GABA is inhibitory and glutamate is excitatory, so both neurotransmitters work together to control many processes, including the nervous system's overall level of arousal.

GABA, an inhibitory neurotransmitter, stops action potentials.

Glutamate, an excitatory neurotransmitter, starts or maintains the ongoing flow of action potentials.

Many drugs affect Glutamate, GABA or both, using them to tranquilize or stimulate the brain.

Dopamine Pathways / Serotonin Pathways

Frontal cortex
Striatum
Substantia nigra
VTA
Nucleus accumbens
Raphe nucleus
Hippocampus

Functions
* Reward (motivation)
* Pleasure, euphoria
* Motor function (fine-tuning)
* Compulsion
* Perseveration

Functions
* Mood
* Memory processing
* Sleep
* Cognition

NIDA

SEROTONIN

Serotonin is another neurotransmitter that is affected by many of the drugs of abuse, including cocaine, amphetamines, LSD, and alcohol. Serotonin is produced by neurons in the Raphe nuclei, whose neurons extend throughout the brain and transmit serotonin throughout the Central Nervous System.

Serotonin plays a role in many brain processes, including regulation of body temperature, sleep, mood, appetite and pain. Problems with the serotonin pathway can cause obsessive compulsive disorder, anxiety disorders, and depression.

Most of the drugs used to treat depression work by increasing brain serotonin levels.

Studies within the last decade have shown that people are born with varying degrees of serotonin sensitivity (genetically determined numbers of receptors), and that most serotonin is generated in the digestive system, and thus diet can affect serotonin levels.

Alcohol Increases GABA activity

PCP increases Glutamate activity
Caffeine Increases Glutamate activity
GLUTAMATE

Alcohol increases GABA activity
Tranquilizers increase GABA activity
Caffeine inhibits GABA release
GABA

Adapted from NIH and State of Utah Dept. of Education

402

The reticular formation is a sausage-shaped bundle of neurons at the core of your brainstem. Sensory data from the body passes up from the spine and through this region before travelling to higher brain regions like the thalamus and cortex. Its cells are *polysensory*, meaning information from multiple senses is integrated within its neurons. Information gathered from your senses is thus controlled almost entirely by serotonin transmission. It exerts its powerful influence indirectly, by modulating neural responsiveness to other neurotransmitters such as dopamine and norepinephrine.

This brainstem region is multitasking, regulating the sleep-wake cycle, filtering incoming stimuli, filtering out irrelevant background stimuli. As one of the evolutionarily oldest regions of the brain, it is critical for governing many basic functions among living organisms. Over 100 small neural networks in the region have varied functions, such as:

Motor control – Several motor neurons project into the reticular formation, where circuits help maintain tone, balance, and posture during movement, working with the cerebellum. The reticular formation relays visual and auditory signals to the cerebellum so the region can integrate visual, auditory, and vestibular signals and apply it to motor coordination. Motor nuclei in the region also enable the eyes to track objects, and generate rhythmic signals for muscles used in breathing and swallowing.

Cardiovascular control – The reticular formation contains cardiac and *vasomotor* (blood vessel constriction controlling) centers of the medulla oblongata.

Pain modulation – Many pain signals travel from the body to the cortex via the reticular formation, and from here, *analgesic* nerve pathways act upon the spinal cord to block transmission of some pain signals to the brain.

Sleep and consciousness – Your reticular formation projects to your thalamus and cerebral cortex, allowing it to exert control over which sensory signals reach your conscious attention. It's also central to helping generate varying consciousness levels, ranging from deep sleep to hypervigilance. Because of its necessity in maintaining consciousness, damaging the reticular formation can result in irreversible coma.

Habituation – Your brain learns to ignore unimportant, repetitive or constant stimuli, while retaining sensitivity to others. For example, you've become so used to wearing clothes that you no longer feel the sensation of fabric on your skin, and part of the reticular activating system includes nuclei which modulate awareness in the cerebral cortex.

In your brain, serotonin is released from neurons in the *raphe nuclei,* a cluster of neurons at the center of the reticular formation in your brainstem. The term *raphe* is Greek for a ridge or seam between two symmetrical parts. Like most of your brain, the raphe nuclei are grouped into pairs. These neural clusters are located in one of the evolutionarily oldest parts of the brain, the *reticular formation,* from where their projections spread throughout your brainstem, cortex and spinal cord.

Axons from the raphe nuclei extend almost everywhere throughout your central nervous system and brain. Thus, as a neuromodulator, serotonin profoundly influences neurotransmission and the sensitivity of neurons to other neurotransmitters. Thus, norepinephrine, dopamine, serotonin and other neurotransmitters operate synergistically to control your various brain functions.

Serotonin-releasing neurons in the raphe system are unique. Their neurotransmitter release is controlled by food intake – eating carbohydrates triggers increased serotonin production. Since serotonin is also central to functions like sleep onset, sensitivity to pain, blood pressure regulation, and mood control, people learn to eat carbohydrate-heavy snacks like pastries to feel better.

This tendency to use unhealthy food as if it were a drug is often at the root of weight gain. People may become overweight from trying to decrease life stressors, women suffering from severe PMS, sufferers of seasonal affective disorder (commonly known as "winter depression") and people trying to quit smoking. (Nicotine increases the secretion of mood-stabilizing serotonin just like eating carbohydrates, while nicotine withdrawal creates the opposite effect).

Since your body cannot normally synthesize serotonin, you have to obtain it by digesting proteins, which transport the precursor *tryptophan* in your blood to your brain, to be converted into serotonin. Tryptophan is abundant in foods such as wild game meat, seaweed, spirulina, soy protein, eggs, spinach, lobster, shrimp, crab and fish. For vegetarians, it's also found in pumpkin and sesame seeds, Parmesan and cheddar cheeses. Levels can and will fluctuate throughout the day, and can be boosted depending upon your diet.

Born Explorers – Natural levels of serotonin and its receptors vary between individuals. Dr. Allman believes individuals evolved with low serotonin levels and sensitivity to provide stronger motivations and a greater sensitivity to environmental risks and rewards. Conversely, individuals with higher serotonin levels are more stable, and less sensitive to potential hazards and opportunities.

Among natural monkey populations, this predisposes low-serotonin monkeys to become natural explorers, the first among their peers to discover new sources of food, and highly sensitive to danger, making them excellent sentinels that can warn of approaching predators.

This increased sensitivity to environmental risk and reward is probably at the root of the evolution of alarm and food calls that alert other group members that predators or resources are nearby.

While attracting attention to themselves with a warning call or venturing into unknown territory in search of food may be dangerous to these low-serotonin individuals, it greatly increases the survival chances of kin, and therefore the propagation of their shared genes. This sensitivity is potentially of great evolutionary benefit to the species, another evolutionary tradeoff, which may explain why so many humans suffer from mood disorders associated with low serotonin levels.

Studies have shown that exercise boosts brain serotonin and other beneficial neurotransmitters. A 1999 Duke University study found that engaging in just 30 minutes of physical activity five days a week substantially reduces the symptoms of major depression, increasing the body's sensitivity to endorphins and stimulating the production of norepinephrine.

The Journal of Psychiatry & Neuroscience has also reported that exposure to outdoor sunlight, even on a cloudy day, provides a boost to serotonin. Additionally, natural light also assists your body in the synthesis of *vitamin D*, critical for a number of biological functions, including helping to balance brain neurotransmitter levels.

Testosterone – This hormone, primarily responsible for the development of male sexual characteristics, is made from cholesterol by the *gonads* (testes and ovaries). It promotes sexual arousal in both men and women, muscle growth and strength.

Aside from the physical changes testosterone triggers, it also seems to shape cognition to a degree, and personality to a much more significant one – among toddler humans and even across primate species, males prefer playing with trucks, and females with dolls, before socialization can ever play a part in behavioral formation. Testosterone levels also affect competitiveness, faithfulness, sexuality, and even mental aptitude (in terms of spatial-rotational mental visualization).

Testosterone and Social Status – *According to Yale University biologist Dr. Stephanie Anestis, the amount of testosterone in male chimpanzees correlates with their social status – those with the highest levels of testosterone in their urine are the aggressive, dominant alpha males, and those with the least are the dominated beta males, on the receiving end of aggression. But such a specific link between aggression and testosterone hasn't yet been conclusively established in humans.*

In animals, such social status comes with a price – high levels of testosterone are evolutionarily expensive – depleting resources that could be used for the immune system and other vital functions to fuel competitive and dominant behavior.

Testosterone levels fluctuate based upon social status. Engaging in male competition raises a man's testosterone levels, hearkening back to the ancient needs to fight for territory and mates: Dr. Richard Bribiescas of Yale University has demonstrated that winning male to male contests raises testosterone (encouraging future competitive behavior), while losing encourages withdrawal and reassessment. Surprisingly, the effects extend to sports fans whose team wins – they also see a rise in testosterone levels.

At the University of Texas, Dr. Pranj Mehta has been running a special version of an experiment called **the ultimatum game**. *Two players separated by a wall are given $100 to divide between them. Player 1 can anonymously propose how to divide it, while player 2 can choose to accept or reject the offer. If player 2 rejects, neither player gets anything.*

So player 1 can offer only $10 (and keep 90), but this is often rejected – which means that player 2 is turning down $10 which is free – in indignation at the perceived unfair division. Dr. Mehta has found that men with high levels of testosterone reject such offers much more frequently, and that the insula – a prune-sized part of the brain concerned with negative emotions and pain perception – activates strongly in response to unfairness.

He believes this is a desire to protect social status, the insula governing reactions to perceived threats to status. The insula and testosterone activate in response to such status threats in both men and women.

Testosterone raises libido and even changes who you are sexually attracted to. Women, as demonstrated through photo, sweat sniffing and even voice recording blind choice tests, can instantly and very accurately determine men's testosterone levels through some as yet undiscovered cues. Generally, they prefer lower-t partners for long-term mates, but when they're ovulating, prefer high-t ones, who tend to be more assertive and flirtatious, less likely to marry, and have a greater number of partners.

Interestingly, testosterone drives men to seek out mates, but upon marrying, testosterone levels drop. Upon divorce (in fact a year prior to divorce), however, these levels rise again. There's also an acute decline in testosterone when men have children. Even holding a baby doll can cause a marked drop in testosterone – possibly an evolutionary adaptation which ensures men will stick around to care for their children. Sleep has also been shown to affect testosterone levels.

The Effects of Drugs

It's never the actual drugs you take that make you feel calm, euphoric, or wired – it's their effects upon your neurotransmitters. These *psychopharmacological substances* trigger changes in the function of serotonin, dopamine, norepinephrine and other neurotransmitters, causing drug-induced moods and sensations.

Chemical synapses are the site at which most psychoactive drugs create their effects. Drugs like curare, strychnine, cocaine, morphine, alcohol, LSD, and a number of others act upon the synapses, with distinctly different effects. They are often restricted to synapses which use specific neurotransmitters.

Alcohol – One of alcohol's most obvious effects is in the reduction of inhibitions; normally reserved people become outgoing, and seem to lose their timidity when intoxicated. This is because of the drug's effects upon the *prefrontal cortex* in the *frontal lobes* of the brain, the region normally responsible for controlling impulses.

When drinking alcohol, their uninhibited, impulsive and sometimes reckless behavior mimics that of people who have suffered traumatic frontal lobe injuries. These effects seem to stem from alcohol's effects upon the dopamine and GABA systems: alcohol increases excitatory dopamine release in the frontal lobes, and may inhibit its breakdown in the synapses by the enzyme *monoamine oxidase*.

At the same time, it enhances the prefrontal cortex effects of GABA, inhibiting the activity of other neurotransmitters. The active ingredient, ethanol, binds to GABA receptors, causing prolonged opening of ion channels, essentially "locking up" post-synaptic nerves, so they cannot respond normally to stimuli from neurotransmitters such as glutamate. This impairs the function of the frontal lobes in logical decision-making and the prevention of socially inappropriate behavior.

Cocaine triggers a massive dopamine, serotonin and norepinephrine release, then blocks their reuptake, leaving these neurotransmitters lingering within the synaptic cleft much longer, and increasing their effects. Together, the trio conveys a sense of empowerment, energy, engagement, wellbeing, and enhanced focus and clarity.

Curare is a poison that stops acetylcholine from affecting post-synaptic membranes; this means muscles cannot activate, and the result is paralysis. Paralysis of the cardio-vascular system starves the cells of oxygen and they die within minutes.

Strychnine is a poison which blocks the inhibitory effects of the neurotransmitter *glycine*, causing the body to become hypersensitive to stimuli, resulting in overstimulation and uncontrollable, fatal muscle spasms.

LSD interferes with synapses that respond to serotonin, because both molecules are structurally similar. It's thought that LSD binds to 5HT receptors in the raphe nuclei, inducing a dreamlike state during consciousness.

Morphine and heroin bind with opioid receptors which normally react to endorphins, the nervous system's natural painkillers.

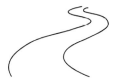

Brain

"Dollars and guns are no substitutes for brains and willpower."
– Dwight D. Eisenhower, radio broadcast, June 3, 1957

When a skull is opened, the brain inside has the consistency of thick, soupy porridge, until it is preserved with a fixative such as formaldehyde. Brain size, shape and organization vary slightly from person to person, though the specific trillions of connections is as unique as an individual's fingerprint. Thus, it's believed that individual personality are derived from this unique pattern of connections, called a *connectome*.

Every uninjured, physically healthy human carries identical brain substructures, but these are arranged and used slightly differently from person to person, an additional reason for our individual identities. And, for the record, it's a myth that you only use ten percent of your brain; in fact, every region of your brain is constantly active, billions of neurons constantly firing, even as you sleep.

In very broad terms, the human brain is comprised of a massive outer region called the *cortex* (or cerebral cortex) as well as a number of low-level subcortical internal structures, such as the medulla and brainstem (responsible for heart rate and respiration), the cerebellum (responsible for balance and muscular coordination), and the hypothalamus (which regulates chemical balances and ensures survival by triggering hunger, thirst and other basic drives). Your cortex, however, makes up fully 80% of your brain's mass.

Your brain uses more energy than any other organ in your body – about 25% of your total caloric intake. A great deal of that energy goes to feed the massive higher processing centers in your cortex, which handles your reason and other higher thought processes, and largely defines your personality.

Buried deep in the center of your brain are *ventricles*, four irregularly-shaped cavities that bathe your brain in cerebral spinal fluid (CSF), flushing metabolic wastes out of the CNS, cushioning your brain against physical injuries, and feeding it nutrients.

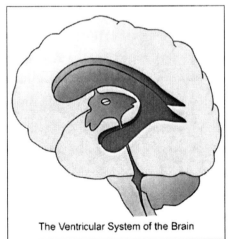

The Ventricular System of the Brain

Ventricles, Hopes Brain Tutorial, 2010, Stanford University. Used with permission

A ribbon of cells lining each of the ventricles called the *choroid plexus* produces *cerebrospinal fluid* (CSF) by filtering liquid from the bloodstream. This CSF is flushed out and recycled four times a day to remove waste, toxins and excess neurotransmitters.

The cells of the choroid plexus separate the ventricles from direct contact with the bloodstream's capillaries, forming a barrier between the bloodstream and the nervous system. This interface between two circulating fluid systems serves to both protect the brain from pathogens and toxins, and allows numerous exchange processes, supplying the brain with nutrients and hormones, and clearing away harmful substances. The choroid plexuses also participate in maintaining brain homeostasis.

A rich blood supply is delivered from the left and right *carotid arteries*, running up the sides of the neck. Brain cells make up about 80% of the brain's mass, submerged in CSF, which comprises the other 20%. This CSF is absorbed and completely renewed every six hours.

Your entire brain is divided by a deep central cleft into left and right hemispheres, joined by a thick, hard sheet of neural tissue called the *corpus callosum*, which allows communication between the two halves. Your corpus callosum (Latin for hard body), unlike the gelatinous consistency of the rest of your brain, is like a carrot, which would snap in your hand. This sheet of neural tissue relays and coordinates information between your brain's left and right hemispheres.

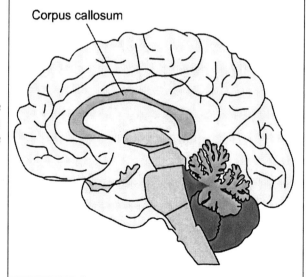

Corpus callosum

Corpus callosum, Hopes Brain Tutorial, Stanford University, 2010. Used with permission

A similar bilateral structure is echoed in many of your brain's substructures (as well as throughout the human body). Control of your body is reversed in your brain – your left hemisphere sends and receives data for your body's right side, and your right brain hemisphere does the same for your body's left side.

Your cerebral cortex (also called your cerebrum) is made of *grey matter* – the cell bodies on its surface. Gray matter is where the cells "talk" to one another – where the cell bodies and synapses are found. *White matter* is the axons connecting brain regions. Myelin is a fatty white coating on neural axons, giving the axon-dense region its color.

The cortex itself is folded and wrinkled to allow for greater surface area. This folded surface packs more neurons into the space, an organization not found in animals of lower intelligence, which only have smooth cortices. The deep grooves in the wrinkles are called *sulci* in Latin and the ridges are *gyri*. Below the surface of your cortex, neural axons extend downward, forming white matter, the bulk of your brain's material.

Cortex, Hopes Brain Tutorial, Stanford University, 2010. Used with permission

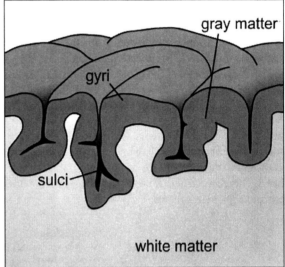

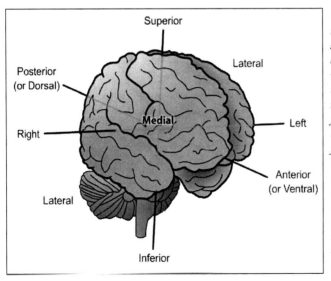

Which Way is Up? *In neuroanatomy, upward is* **superior** *or* **dorsal,** *and downward is* **inferior** *or* **ventral.** *Structures near the center are* **medial,** *and those away from the center are* **lateral.** *Anterior means frontal while* **posterior** *means rear.* **Rostral** *is toward the mouth (snout, beak, mandibles, etc.), while* **caudal** *is toward the feet. Image: Hopes Brain Tutorial, 2010, Stanford University. Used with permission.*

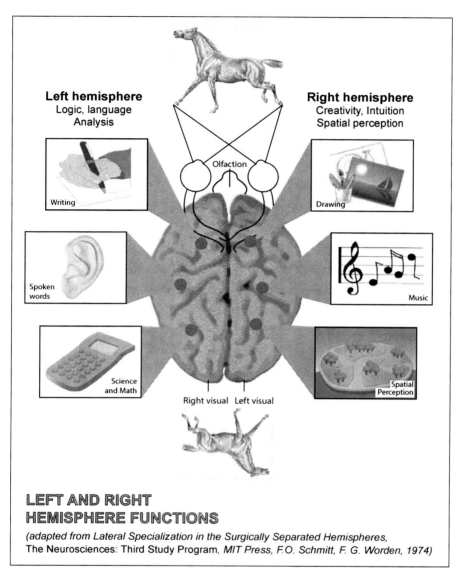

LEFT AND RIGHT HEMISPHERE FUNCTIONS

(adapted from *Lateral Specialization in the Surgically Separated Hemispheres*, The Neurosciences: Third Study Program, *MIT Press, F.O. Schmitt, F. G. Worden, 1974*)

The left hemisphere of your brain – if you're among the 90% of the population who are right-handers – is a little larger and deals mainly with language, math, logic and speech, and dominates cortical processing, while the right deals with creative functions, and plays a large part in interpreting visual information, pattern recognition, nonverbal thought, emotional and spatial processing.

Twin bands of neural tissue across the top of your cortex contain topographical maps of your entire body – nerve centers responsible for either the sensory input or the motor output of every part of your body.

The area has been well mapped; neuroscientists can electrically stimulate and induce sensations or involuntary muscle contractions in any specific region of your body using this topographical map.

411

Sensory homunculus

Motor homunculus

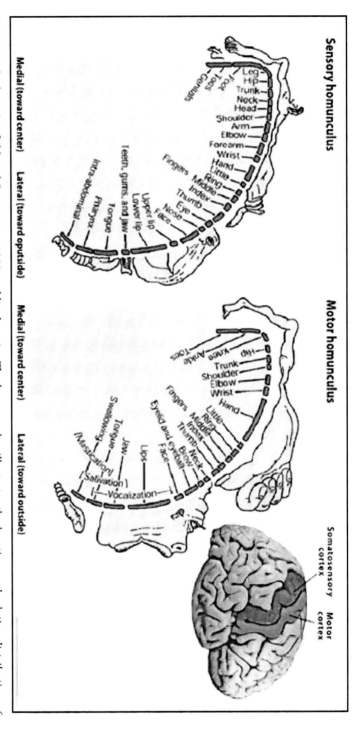

Medial (toward center)   Lateral (toward oputside)

Medial (toward center)   Lateral (toward outside)

Somatosensory cortex   Motor cortex

Homunculi, from Penfield and Rasmussen 1950, public domain. The homunculus illustrates the location and relative distribution of cortical space dedicated to various body functions. Your entire body is represented in an orderly arrangement of somatosensory inputs to these regions of the cortex. The relative area of cortex dedicated to a particular body part is related to how many nerves are distributed within that body part, so sensory input from your face and hands uses more cortical space than, for example, sensory input from your toes. Output from your motor cortex is organized the same way, with the amount of motor control corresponding to cortical surface area. Humans, as you can see, dedicate a great deal of the motor cortex to fingers and speech production.

412

Your entire brain is further divided functionally into four lobes, the largest of which is your frontal lobe, which is proportionally larger in humans than in any other animal. Most of your higher thought processes occur here. Since about twenty-five regions are referred to constantly throughout this book, please see the following illustrations.

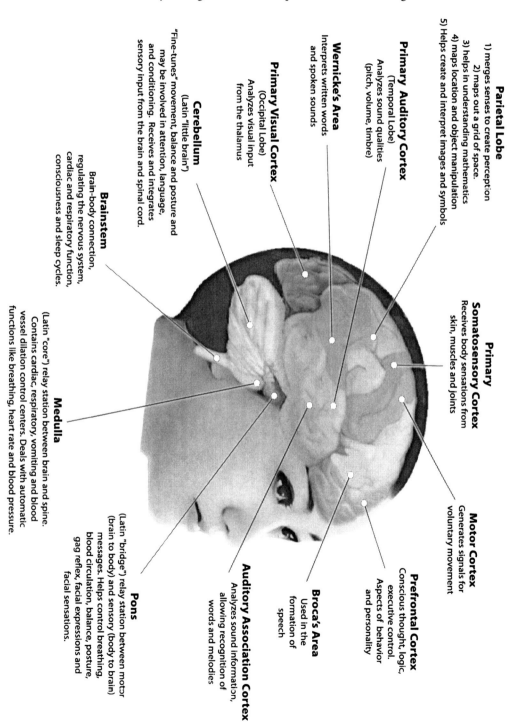

Parietal Lobe
1) merges senses to create perception
2) maps out a grid of space.
3) helps in understanding mathematics
4) maps location and object manipulation
5) Helps create and interpret images and symbols

Primary Auditory Cortex
(Temporal Lobe)
Analyzes sound qualities
(pitch, volume, timbre)

Wernicke's Area
Interprets written words
and spoken sounds

Primary Visual Cortex
(Occipital Lobe)
Analyzes visual input
from the thalamus

Cerebellum
(Latin "little brain")
"Fine-tunes" movement, balance and posture and
may be involved in attention, language,
and conditioning. Receives and integrates
sensory input from the brain and spinal cord.

Brainstem
Brain-body connection,
regulating the nervous system,
cardiac and respiratory function,
consciousness and sleep cycles.

Medulla
(Latin "core") relay station between brain and spine.
Contains cardiac, respiratory, vomiting and blood
vessel dilation control centers. Deals with automatic
functions like breathing, heart rate and blood pressure.

Primary Somatosensory Cortex
Receives body sensations from
skin, muscles and joints

Motor Cortex
Generates signals for
voluntary movement

Prefrontal Cortex
Conscious thought, logic,
executive control.
Aspects of behavior
and personality

Broca's Area
Used in the
formation of
speech

Auditory Association Cortex
Analyzes sound information,
allowing recognition of
words and melodies

Pons
(Latin "bridge") relay station between motor
(brain to body) and sensory (body to brain)
messages. Helps control breathing,
blood circulation, balance, posture,
gag reflex, facial expressions and
facial sensations.

MAJOR NEURAL STRUCTURES

Cerebral Cortex
Most highly evolved region; handles higher thought processes

Corpus Callosum
Sheet of neural tissue bridging the two brain hemispheres

Thalamus
Incoming and outgoing sensory "relay station" to cortex

Cerebellum
"Autopilot" motor system - coordinates balance and movement

Medulla
Responsible for regulating unconscious functions such as breathing and circulation

Hypothalamus
Regulates temperature, appetite, growth, thirst, and sex drive by controlling hormonal release

Pituitary gland
"Master gland" that regulates other endocrine (hormone-producing) glands

Pons
Involved in sleep and arousal (alertness) levels

Reticular Formation
Network of neurons related to sleep, arousal and attention

Spinal cord
Communication link between brain and body; involved in basic reflexes

The Brain's Main Subsystems

Cortex	**Frontal Lobe:** Front of the brain. Deals with reason, language, logic, motor skill planning, memory, coordinating multiregional brain function. At the rear of the frontal lobe is the motor cortex, integrating data from other lobes and using it to initiate muscle activity - the brain's sole means of output to the outside world. **Parietal Lobe:** Middle of the cortex. Processes sense of touch (tactile data) including pressure, touch, pain and body awareness. integrates visual and tactile information. **Temporal Lobe:** Bottom of the brain. location of the primary auditory cortex, which interprets sounds. Also involved in learning. **Occipital Lobe:** Back of the brain. interprets visual data from the retinas via the optic nerves.

Basal Ganglia	Starts and stops muscle movement. The brain's main learning system, producing dopamine, the "reward neurochemical" that motivates the search for food, sex and comfort. Main subcomponents include:
	
	Striatum: largest component, forms motivational loop with cortex.
	
	Caudate: task shifting, visual classification, feedback ("is this correct or incorrect")
	
	Pallidum: inhibits (quietens) other brain regions
	
	VTA (ventral tegmental area): main dopamine distributor through the brain, producing pleasure and reward seeking
	
	Substantia nigra: A motor center, helps start and stop movement by exciting the striatum and inhibiting the thalamus
	Learning occurs in two ways - successful behaviors are paired with positive brain states through the "Go" neural circuit
	       (and the situations are sought again)
	       - negative outcomes are paired with negative brain states through the "NoGO" neural circuit
	       (and the situations are avoided)

Limbic System	**Thalamus:** body's sensory "gatekeeper" or "relay center"; the thalamus also stimulates the cortex, increasing muscle motion **Hypothalamus:** Body's "appetite center" and regulator - maintaining body's hormonal, temperature and other balances. **Amygdala:** The brain's "sentry" or "alarm" bell - triggers fear or aggression when it senses danger **Hippocampus:** Emotional memory center and mental spatial "mapkeeper"
Cerebellum	The "mini-brain" that controls balance, muscle coordination, movement precision and timing. Using feedback from the body and brain's sensory systems as a guide, it "fine-tunes" motor activity.
Brainstem	Forms a stalk, connecting the brain to the spinal cord and thus to all the body's nerves. The brain-body "relay station", it conveys sensory input to the brain and motor output to the body; also acts as a "rhythm generator" for breathing, eating, heartbeat, etc. **Pons:** Controls arousal and aids in breathing control, autonomic (unconsciously controlled) functions and sleep. **Midbrain:** Controls eye movement, pupil dilation, hearing, and is associated with the motor system pathways. One component is the dopamine-producing substantia nigra, part of the basal ganglia, which starts and stops movement. **Medulla Oblongata:** lowest portion of the human brain, involved in autonomic functions such as breathing, heart rate, sneezing, coughing, swallowing, vomiting, and defecation. Helps transfer messages between the brain and spinal cord. **The Reticular Activating System (RAS):** a netlike configuration that helps control sensory/motor function and levels of arousal.

PRIMARY BRAIN SYSTEMS

Reticular Activating System (RAS)	Affects sleep, attention and arousal
Hypothalamus	Maintains *homeostasis (balance):* Affects heart rate, hunger, thirst, consciousness, body temperature, blood pressure, sexual behavior
Cerebral cortex	Affects speech, motor movement, sensory perception, hearing, vision, sensory discrimination, memory, language, reasoning, abstract thought and personality
Limbic system	Central to emotion and memory formation
Basal ganglia	Movement control and learning
Medial Forebrain Bundle (MFB)	Primary reward and pleasure circuit. A communication link between limbic system and brain stem.
Periventricular system (PVS)	Primary punishment circuit, involved in avoidance behavior
Brain stem	Regulates vital functions such as breathing, heartbeat, dilation of pupils, and blood pressure, as well as vomiting and other reflexes.

Detailed Architecture:
Hind- Mid- and Forebrain

Working our way upward and outward from the back and bottom, we're going to tour your brain, building it up region by region.

Early theories divided the human brain into three parts, based upon stages of evolutionary development. Dr. Paul MacLean, in *The Triune Brain in Evolution,* labelled the oldest and deepest part the *protoreptilian formation.* This area includes the autonomic nervous system, brainstem, cerebellum, and basal ganglia, now referred to as the *hindbrain.*

This deep reptilian core contains primitive instinctual behavior programs like exploration, feeding, territorialism, dominance, and sexual behavior. MacLean referred to it as the reptilian brain because its structures constitute nearly all of the brain structures of turtles, snakes and other reptiles which exist even in modern times.

This reptilian brain was not replaced by evolution, but was progressively built upon by two other structural expansions. Because we share these basic brain structures, we also share the same deep, pre-conscious and primally powerful behaviors of other, more neurologically primitive animals such as snakes.

416

Above the protoreptilian formation is the *paleomammalian* (old mammal's) *formation*, a subcortical structure common to all mammals, responsible for primal instincts, emotions and motivations below the level of awareness.

The final structure in triune brain evolution is the *neomammalian* brain, now referred to as the cortex. Its huge expansion allows for such things as language, abstract thought, creativity, planning, problem-solving, reflection and self-awareness.

The cortex also analyzes combined sensory information about the environment arriving from sense organs for sight, sound and touch. (Smell and taste are processed in the primitive subcortical regions, because finding nutritious food has been of primary importance to survival throughout evolutionary history). Thus, our final outer brain structure and most fundamental behavior patterns are thought to have first emerged about 225 million years ago.

The brain is also classified into three broad functional divisions, arguably reflecting these evolutionary stages. These very broad anatomical divisions are the *forebrain, midbrain* and *hindbrain*.

Your hindbrain is most like that of the simplest animals; it controls your respiration and heart rate, and coordinates the movement of each individual muscle (via your cerebellum). At the very bottom and core of your brain, this is the primitive center, with the structure and function of a reptile's brain, concerned with instinctive, aggressive, automatic self-preservation behaviors. The hindbrain's three primary regions work together to coordinate movement, balance, posture, and, overseen by the hypothalamus, help regulate sleep and unconscious vital body functions such as digestion, breathing and heartbeat. Its major functional regions are your *brainstem, pons* and *medulla oblongata*, in the area connecting your brain and spinal cord.

Your midbrain is the uppermost part of your brainstem, controlling your reflexes and eye movements. This is the physically smallest of the three regions, likened in structure and function to less-developed mammal brains, which contains an advanced sense of smell as well as the comparatively sophisticated learning and motivational systems underlying most instinctive survival behaviors.

Your forebrain is the most advanced region, with the most highly-evolved structures, shared by all primates (apes, gorillas and monkeys) and a few other species such as elephants and *cetaceans* – dolphins and whales. This is your cortex, seat of your reason, logic, creativity and your brain's executive control system. While this portion of your brain can exercise control over the less evolved inner brain structures, it can also be "led" by them, or even overwhelmed by them, as with addictions, impulsiveness, anxiety, obsessive worry, panic, depression or obsessive-compulsive disorders.

The cortex is the largest part of your brain (80% by volume), with folds and wrinkles increasing its surface area. The corpus callosum, as you'll recall, connects its right and left hemispheres. Each section of your cortex is specialized for specific functions, which we'll examine in greater detail later.

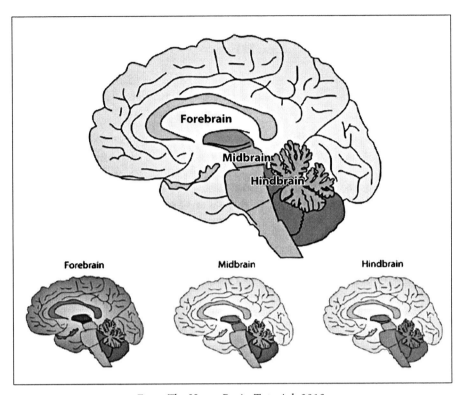

From The Hopes Brain Tutorial, 2010,
Stanford University. Used with permission

I. Hindbrain

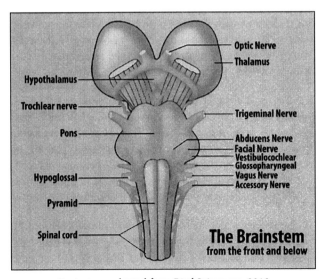

Brainstem, adapted from BirthInjury.org, 2010

Brainstem

This is the lower extension of your brain, where it connects to your spinal cord. Your brainstem is the pathway for nerve tracts passing up from your Peripheral Nervous System through your spinal cord en route to the higher functional regions of your brain.

Your brainstem includes, from the bottom upward, the medulla oblongata, pons and midbrain. These combined regions implement automatic functions critical for your survival, such as maintaining breathing, digestion, heart rate, blood pressure, and general arousal states, as well as regulating your body temperature, wake and sleep cycles, sneezing, coughing, vomiting, and swallowing.

Ten of the twelve cranial nerves connect to your brainstem. This is also your CNS's main gateway, conveying sensory input from your body to your brain and motor output from your brain to your body.

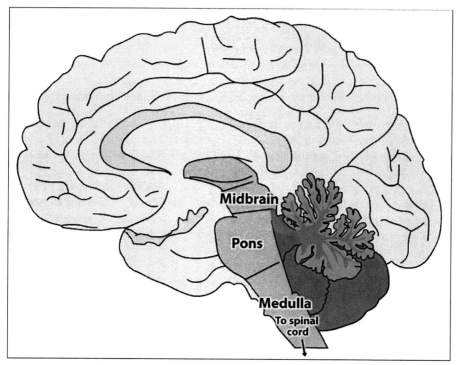

Brainstem, Hopes Brain Tutorial, 2010, Stanford University. Used with permission

Medulla Oblongata – Your medulla oblongata functions primarily as a gateway, where sensory and motor neurons run between your spinal cord and brain. It also contains your respiratory, *vasomotor* (blood vessel diameter control) and cardiac centers, as well as mechanisms for controlling reflex activities such as coughing, gagging, swallowing, sneezing, and vomiting. Cranial nerves 9 through 12 connect here, transmitting signals related to taste, mouth sensations, swallowing, tongue movement, back and neck muscles, and the vagus nerve, central to autonomic system function.

419

Reticular Formation

At your brainstem's core is the *reticular formation*, Latin for *net-like formation*, because the tissue looks spotty, like a net. This region is part of your *reticular activating system*, a finger-shaped area which acts as a kind of data gateway, blocking meaningless messages from coming in, such as the constant sensation of your clothes against your skin; or granting access to higher brain regions for important signals that require attention, such as pain.

The reticular activating system rises from the medulla through the pons and into the midbrain. It helps control vital functions such as breathing and heartrate, regulates sleep, attention, arousal and consciousness, and is highly integrated with the limbic system. These axons aren't fully myelinated until late adolescence, which is part of the reason children have comparatively short attention spans.

The RAS has deep connections, allowing it to modulate the entire brain and central nervous system. Because of this, it's thought to be the central coordinating point for information in the nervous system.

While the thalamus rigidly separates each sensory system, the RAS treats the senses as one overall system, providing arousal to activate wide regions of the cortex. The pre-frontal cortex can also send signals to the reticular activating system, instructing it to make the CNS more alert or more relaxed, depending upon the circumstances.

The region extends from your medulla up to your midbrain and thalamus. Its connections radiate throughout your cortex, as this system controls the degree of activity in your central nervous system, regulating arousal, and the transition from sleep-wake states to states of high attention, working with your thalamus – your sensory gateway into the cortex – to control the intensity of sensory signals reaching your higher brain centers. In this way the reticular formation controls sleep, wakefulness and varying degrees of alertness between. A number of neurotransmitters are involved in the reticular activating system's regulation of arousal, chief among them acetylcholine and norepinephrine.

In regulating arousal, the reticular formation serves to instantly activate other regions of the brain when you encounter something alarming, and to dull sensory perception when you need sleep.

Raphe nucleus

This cluster of neurons in the middle of your brainstem and reticular formation is your brain's main serotonin production center. Its name is derive from the Greek word for zipper and the Latin word for kernel, so-called because of its appearance and location in the middle of the medulla. Twenty percent of your serotonin is produced here, the remaining 80% in your intestinal tract.

This network of neurons has been present since the earliest vertebrates, and its structure has remained largely unchanged throughout evolution. In humans, neurons from this region project down the entire spinal cord, profoundly affecting the entire CNS.

Serotonin has a pronounced effect upon your entire CNS, and is central to mood stability, happiness, calm and well-being. It profoundly affects your cognition, sensory perception, sleep and appetite, dampens aggression and is central to *analgesia* (pain relief).

Pons

Atop your medulla is a bulging region of white matter called the pons (Latin for bridge), connecting your cerebellum and brainstem to your midbrain and other higher regions. The pons connects the twin hemispheres of the cerebellum and, together with the medulla, regulates breathing. *Ventral* and *dorsal respiratory groups* in your medulla's reticular formation, together with *pneumotaxic* and *apneustic centers* in your pons, regulate your rhythmic breathing, changing inhalation to exhalation and back.

Your pons helps your cerebellum control balance and posture, and its connections to your medulla make your pons the bridge relaying signals between your brain's most primitive regions to upper areas of greater sophistication and complexity. The pons additionally helps regulate bladder control and blood circulation.

Because of its connections to cranial nerves 5 through 8, your pons receives (and transmits upward) information about facial sensations, controls your facial expressions and some eye movement, and is the first point to receive auditory signals, which are then relayed up to your thalamus and beyond. During *REM* (dream) sleep, your pons activates a shutdown of twin *locomotor strips* connecting your medulla to your spinal cord. This shuts down motor signals to your limbs, preventing you from thrashing about in your dreams.

Locus coeruleus

Also in the pons is a region which regulates arousal and attention, the *locus coeruleus* (Latin for *blue spot*). While the adrenal glands produce norepinephrine in the body, this is the main site of norepinephrine production in the brain, used to arouse your sympathetic nervous system, particularly in the face of stress. It uses norepinephrine to stimulate your cortex, raising conscious awareness and altering your cognitive function, your hypothalamus arousing your body, your amygdala signaling alarm, your *basal ganglia* (the reward-processing center called the *nucleus accumbens*) stimulating your motivation, and your *thalamus* "turning up the sensory volume" on information which is most *salient* (important).

This excites extensive brain regions, stimulating wakefulness and attention, increasing sensitivity and excitability when there is something novel or interesting in your environment, or when heightened awareness is otherwise necessary.

Your hypothalamus uses the locus coeruleus as a major control center for homeostasis, and your prefrontal cortex, amygdala and cingulate cortex connect to this region, allowing emotional stress to trigger the fight or flight response. If your amygdala is the "tripwire" for your mental alarm system, your locus coeruleus is the "ringing bell". This region is responsible (with the pain-reporting *insula*) for generating the panic driving addicts to do anything for a fix. When addicts are deprived of their drugs, norepinephrine arouses anxiety, and panic sets in.

Cerebellum

Attached to the rear of your brainstem by three pairs of nerve tracts called *peduncles* (Latin for *flowers on a stalk*, the stalk here being your brainstem) is your cerebellum, which assists your *motor cortex* and *basal ganglia* in coordinating muscle movements, as well as helping you maintain posture and control balance while walking and standing. It operates through a trial-and-error correction process, providing constant, near-instantaneous feedback on precision and timing.

Like your cortex, your cerebellum has an outer, wrinkled surface, inner white matter, and deep nuclei below the white matter. While your cerebellum only makes up 10% of your brain's total volume, it contains over half of your brain's total neurons, arranged in highly regular, repeating units. These neural circuits can be modified, allowing for training and physical adaptation of motor circuits.

This area enables – for example – an Olympic skater to execute a flawless triple axel, or a world cup soccer champion to shoot a winning goal. But it does much more, helping to transform intent into activity, and to govern motor learning. Input from your body is integrated and analyzed, then sent upward for distribution to appropriate regions of your thalamus, basal ganglia and cortex. Command signals are sent from your cerebral cortex to your cerebellum, which acts as a comparator between intended movement and actual outcome to correct your movement.

Proprioception (limb position) messages gather here in the cerebellum, which sends nerve fibers down your spine to help modulate motor neuron function. Your cerebellum is divided into several distinct regions, receiving input from both your brain and spine, and sending output to motor systems. fMRI scans show the cerebellum is deeply involved in the planning and mental rehearsal of complex motor actions, and in consciously assessing movement errors. It influences movement by evaluating the differences between intentions and the outcome of actions, a system of monitoring and error correction that helps motor centers in your cortex adjust while movement is in progress and during repetitions of the same movement.

The region is concerned with precision, rhythm and timing aspects of correcting and coordinating movements, receiving input from your proprioceptors, which report changes in joint angle, muscle length, and tension, giving information about the positions of your limbs, trunk and head in space. Muscle and joint proprioceptors report in a direct pathway from spinal interneurons to your cerebellum, while also transmitting information about motor commands they are receiving from your motor cortex.

In addition, your cerebellum simultaneously receives input from your cortex, and, just as in the cortex, your entire body is mapped within your cerebellum, with twin maps receiving input from visual, and auditory receptors, as well as the *vestibular system* in your inner ear, where liquid shifting in your inner ear chambers is used to gauge your balance.

These different incoming perceptual streams keep your cerebellum updated with changes in the state of your body in relation to the environment and allow comparisons between the various signals. The cerebellum then sends signals back up to your motor cortex via the thalamus, and to your reticular formation (governing arousal states and the sensory gateway to the brain) and vestibular system (giving balance feedback), as well as having direct outputs to nuclei controlling motor pathways in your body, thus helping to modulate motor commands, including eye movements.

40 times as many axons input to your cerebellum as output from it, providing it with information about goals, commands, and feedback signals involved with planning and executing movement. As elsewhere in your brain, the *intensity* of signals fed to your cerebellum is encoded by *frequency* of firing.

The cerebellum's organization indicates it compares internal signals of intended movements with external signals of actual movements; and as a movement is repeated, the cerebellum generates corrective signals, in this way gradually reducing errors. In time, these corrective signals can be used to shape learned motor programs permanently.

Your cerebellum adapts by inducing *long-term depression* in the synaptic strength of selective outputs; the effect can last minutes to hours and is believed to underlie the cerebellum's role in learning motor programs. Low-frequency nerves called *climbing fibers* appear to detect errors in one movement and change the program for the next movement.

Altering the strength of specific synapses in this way allows corrections to eye or limb movements, generating an error signal that depresses incorrect active neural circuits, allowing error-free movements to emerge. This trial-and-error practice eventually leads to a productive behavior which can eventually be performed automatically.

In purely mental operations, the cerebellum's cognitive functions seem to resemble its motor functions, refining skills through repeated practice. fMRI scans indicate your cerebellum may govern your ability to judge elapsed time and to compare the speed of one moving object to another, as well as language tasks involving associating verbs with nouns.

Studies also show it plays a major role in consciously evaluating sensory information, and seems to be particularly important in acquiring and processing sensory information about tasks that require complex spatial and temporal judgments, essential for programming complex motor actions and movement sequences.

II. Midbrain

Your midbrain is a small but powerful region of gray matter between your brainstem and thalamus, with a number of functions. It controls eye movement, allowing the visual tracking of objects in your field of vision through cranial nerves 3 and 4, and helps process incoming auditory data on its way up to your thalamus and beyond. There are two directions of neural activity:

- *dorsal stream* – your brain signals your body, triggering muscle contractions;
- *ventral stream* – your body sends sensory perception signals to your brain for processing and interpretation

While physically tiny, this region is also essentially at the heart of virtually everything you do – the source of all your motivations and drives for survival, including addictions, habits, intensive love, pleasures and obsessions. Here are the *ventral tegmental area* and the *substantia nigra*, your brain's primary sites for synthesizing dopamine, the chemical engine of motivated movement and behavior:

Ventral Tegmental Area

Extending out from your midbrain are a cluster of neurons originating at the *ventral tegmental area* (VTA) (Latin for *rear covering*), These dopamine-signalling neurons extend throughout your brain in a number of areas including your prefrontal cortex and basal ganglia – the seat of most learning and of stopping and starting movement.

The ventral tegmental area in particular is packed with dopamine-releasing neurons which project into your brain's reward center – the *nucleus accumbens*. A squirt of dopamine makes you come alive, feeling energized, competent and capable, stimulating neural transmission throughout your basal ganglia and cortex.

This pleasurable energy is the basis of learning and motivation – and mastering your habits and thoughts puts you in control of this circuitry, as opposed to making you its slave. This circuit is at the very heart of self-mastery.

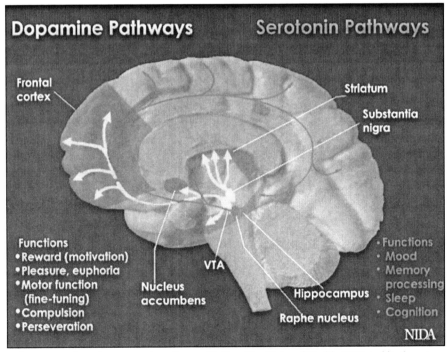

Dopaminergic and serotonergic pathways, National Institutes of Health, 2006, public domain

Substantia Nigra

Substantia nigra is Latin for *black matter*, because of the dark pigmentation of these neurons. This region is divided into two functional sections: the first sends dopamine to the *striatum* in your basal ganglia, areas mainly involved in habit formation, in initiating and stopping voluntary movement, and in *procedural memory* – the ability to act in complex ways that once required learning, but no longer require conscious thought, such as brushing your teeth or riding a bicycle.

The second region of the substantia nigra receives impulses from your basal ganglia to relay up to your thalamus and from there to higher cortical regions, such as your motor cortex, the cortical strip which controls and oversees voluntary movement.

Periaqueductal Gray (PAG)

This is a region of gray matter in the midbrain which is central to dampening pain signals. Directly stimulating the PAG triggers the release of pain-inhibiting *enkephalins*, ligands which block pain signal transmission through the spine to the thalamus. This is the same analgesic pathway used by opiates such as heroin, morphine and *oxycodone*, the drug conservative media star Rush Limbaugh was arrested for abusing.

- Pain and heat-sensitive nerves called *nocioreceptors* and *thermoreceptors* in your skin and organs report tissue damage or intense temperatures, sending impulses along a neural fast-track which bypasses most of your brainstem in a direct route from your spine through the PAG to your thalamus – the *spinothalamic tract*.

- Stimulating the PAG activates neurons which signal serotonin-producing raphe nuclei in your brainstem.

- This triggers a serotonin release down the entire length of your spine.

- The serotonin excites interneurons which release endorphins – your body's natural opiates.

- These endorphins bind to opioid receptors which inhibit the release of *substance P*, the neurotransmitter sending pain signals to your thalamus, *insula* and *somatosensory cortex*, where you first become aware of the sensations of pain. Thus, in extreme emergencies, pain signals can be naturally blocked from reaching your brain.

Drugs like heroin and morphine bind to these same opioid receptors, blocking transmission of *substance P*, which is how they produce their pain-numbing *analgesic* effect. The region may also constitute a hub where seven primal emotional response circuits converge, giving rise to reactions indicative of fear, rage, lust, separation distress, and other instinctive drives. Electrically stimulating specific PAG regions produces instinctive motor activities – emotional-response behaviors such as the back-arching, hissing, and hair-raising defensive display called *sham rage*.

III. Forebrain

In the most highly-developed part of your brain, the primary structures are:

- *the limbic system*, concerned with emotion, spatial-navigational, general memory and instinctive behavioral responses to the environment;

- *the basal ganglia*, your brain's primary motivation center, used for selecting, starting and stopping voluntary movements, habit formation, and *procedural memory* – the ability to perform activities without conscious effort, such as walking or riding a bicycle;

- *the cingulate cortex*, a multifunctional region that engages when your brain receives conflicting information, and when you intentionally refocus your attention or are controlling your emotions.

- *the cerebral cortex*, conscious-level, higher functional areas of your brain dealing with thought: logic, planning, imagination, language, reason, understanding and generating symbols, the interpretation of external events, self-awareness, self-control, object recognition and categorization, and more.

Limbic System

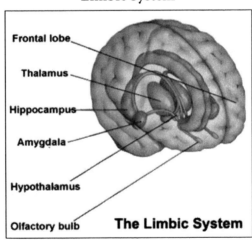

Frontal lobe
Thalamus
Hippocampus
Amygdala
Hypothalamus
Olfactory bulb **The Limbic System**

The first of these regions, your *limbic system* (from the Latin word for border) is comprised of a number of very important functional areas dealing with emotions, homeostasis, sensation, navigation and the formation of long-term memories. This area directly connects your most primitive, instinctive brain regions to higher-brain functions in the basal ganglia, cingulate cortex and cerebral cortex.

Let's look at its substructures in greater detail. Sitting atop your brainstem, your limbic system includes the *thalamus, hippocampus, amygdala, hypothalamus,* and *olfactory bulb.* Some neuroscientists also include the *insula* in this region.

Your sensory system brings you information about the world, and your motor system allows you to act upon it, but it's the limbic system that allows you to "engage" the world - that is, gives it meaning, allowing you to invest emotions in your experiences, to form memories about them, and to learn. This ancient collection of multiple sub-systems is the root of your unique personality, just as it is for other animals.

Of all your brain's subsystems, the limbic system is most easily modified by experiences in the world, as the primary seat of memory generation and learning. Here, the hippocampus acts as a memory-generator, an ancient neural structure that allows creatures to adapt to changes in the environment, improving their odds of survival.

This region is one of the first to fully form, reaching maturity by the age of five; con-versely, the *cortex* – seat of conscious thought and reason – doesn't fully mature until one's twenties.

Some psychologists say the limbic system controls as much as 90% of behavior. It does not involve rational or logical thought, shame or guilt, and is only concerned with three base-level drives:

- Promoting Survival

- Seeking Pleasure

- Avoiding Pain

Found deep in your forebrain's very core, within both hemispheres, your limbic system is the seat of your drives, from the sexual to the appetitive, from your need to bond to your instinctual fight or flight reactions, overseeing all the behavior that satisfies your cravings, desires and needs, as directed by the hypothalamus, your body's "want center" and master regulator. University of California psychologist Dr. Robert Ornstein describes the limbic system as responsible for "the four Fs" of survival: feeding, fighting, fleeing and sexual reproduction".

This deep inner structure has remained largely the same as in your ancient mamma-lian ancestors, and is therefore thought of as the *paleo-* or *old-* mammalian brain. The organs comprising this system serve a number of functions, in service of producing behaviors which promote survival and reproduction, and regulate autonomic and en-docrine responses to emotional stimuli. They also set arousal level, and are involved in motivation and reinforcing behaviors. Many of the areas are critical to emotional memory and have close connections with the primitive *olfactory system*, since your sense of smell is critical to survival.

Thalamus

Your *thalamus* (Greek for *chamber*), is made up of twin bulbs, each about the size of a robin's egg, sitting atop your brainstem. This paired structure is your brain's master switchboard, routing sensory information to your cortex from subcortical regions and back. All sensory input (except for your sense of smell) passes through this twin gateway between your cortex and the subcortical regions, including your midbrain, brainstem, cerebellum and spine.

Here, parallel sensory information is integrated and filtered – selectively inhibited and excited – before being passed on to your cortex. Your cortex also sends feedback to your thalamus, helping regulate its selective sensory signal-strengthening and -dampening.

This is the main gatekeeper for sensory information travelling from your cranial nerves and spine up to your higher brain centers, able to amplify, *attenuate* (dial down), or even block signals from travelling upward. As such, it's a critical relay station for all of your senses except olfaction, which has an additional direct link to your cortex. Along with the RAS, the thalamus also uses sensory filtering to direct your attention, and to shut out the world when you need sleep.

About 50 different types of neurons have been identified in the human thalamus, many specialized to transmit specific sensory information to appropriate processing centers in your cortex. Each of your senses has a dedicated region within your thalamus, and impulses reporting body sensations will be transmitted to your somatosensory cortex, while impulses reporting sound will be transmitted to your auditory cortex for analysis.

In addition to cranial and spinal nerves, all the limbic motivational, emotional-response and memory-management subsystems send input to the thalamus, suggesting it plays a role in these functions as well. Motor function information from the cerebellum and basal ganglia also pass through the thalamus en route to cortical executive motor control regions. Thalamic neurons primarily use inhibitory GABA or excitatory glutamate to selectively filter sensory perception, and their activity can be modulated from above or below – by both the cortex, and the brainstem.

Hypothalamus

If anything could be said to correspond functionally to Freud's idea of the *id* – the force of all our primitive, unrestrained desires, drives and impulses, it would be the hypothalamus, which controls the endocrine and autonomic nervous systems, using hormonal secretions to control biochemical states and generate desires such as hunger, thirst, sexual desire, and many physical responses to emotion. The most critical, unconscious survival mechanisms are controlled by circuits here and in the brainstem.

This area – the size of the tip of your little finger – is your body's master regulator, maintaining your homeostasis, chemically regulating your pulse, blood pressure, body temperature, blood sugar levels, digestion, breathing, hunger, thirst, pain response, sexual satisfaction, physical responses to stress, and immune system function. From deep in your brain, atop your brainstem and below your thalamus, it manipulates your body temperature, hunger, and thirst. Specialized neurons here sense whether the body contains adequate nutrients and stored body fat. These cells then send signals telling other brain regions to adjust food intake, metabolic rate, and physical activity— keeping your body's caloric intake in balance with the calories it burns.

The hypothalamus regulates the autonomic nervous system and the endocrine system, primarily to maintain homeostasis. Electrically stimulating specific regions of the hypothalamus elicits sensations of lust, pain, pleasure, hunger and thirst.

Among its duties are *osmoregulation* – maintaining the concentration of fluids and dissolved substances within bodily fluids. Specific functional regions include the *lateral* hypothalamus – the brain's hunger center; the *ventromedial* hypothalamus – its *satiety* center; and the *anterior* hypothalamus – the sexual regulatory center.

Osmoreceptors regulate thirst, motivating animals to consume water. When the concentration of water in the blood changes (becoming more or less diluted), the amount of water which diffuses into and out of osmoreceptor cells changes – they expand when more water is present and contract when it is deficient, sending signals from the hypothalamus to the pituitary. The pituitary then increases or decreases the hormone vasopressin in the blood, which in turn triggers water release or absorption in the kidneys, until water concentration in the blood is optimized.

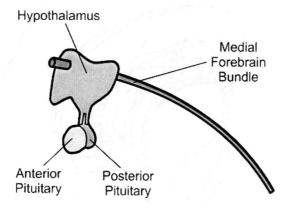

From The Hopes Brain Tutorial, 2010,
Stanford University. Used with permission

This organ is your limbic system's primary mode of output. Below and in front of your thalamus, your hypothalamus controls your so-called "master gland", the pituitary, which releases a number of hormones (body and brain-function-controlling chemicals) such as human growth hormone, vasopressin and oxytocin. As the source of ten vital body-controlling hormones, it helps regulate and control all your body's major functional glands, controlling autonomic functions through outputs to your brainstem, spinal cord and bloodstream, activating the sympathetic, parasympathetic and enteric nervous systems in response to the environment around you.

The five biological needs your hypothalamus regulates:

- Blood pressure and *electrolytes* (ionically-charged chemicals which conduct electricity – salts, acids, and bases)
- Body temperature

- Metabolism

- Sexual reproduction

- Immune system and other physical stress responses

Your hypothalamus has access to sensory information about essentially your entire body, with neural circuits that feed direct input from your visceral sensory system, olfactory system and the retinas of your eyes. Pain information from your viscera is fed directly from your spine and brainstem; change-sensitive neurons that monitor such variables as internal temperature, salt, glucose and other levels are found directly in your hypothalamus.

Hormones in the bloodstream bypass the blood-brain barrier to bind directly to hypothalamus nerves in regions called the *SFO* and *OVLT*. These structures read blood plasma concentrations of sodium and other minerals, and also contain neurons which control thirst. In the *preoptic area* thermosensitive neurons monitor temperature.

Neurons in the hypothalamus respond to steroids such as *glucocorticoids*, the hormones released by the adrenal gland in the stress response. It also contains specialized glucose-sensitive neurons which are important for appetite.

The hypothalamus receives significant input from the brainstem, and information on the status of internal organs from the vagus nerve. Its functions are mainly regulated by levels of monoamine neurotransmitters – noradrenaline, dopamine and serotonin.

The twin rice-grain-sized units of the suprachiasmatic nucleus connect to the anterior hypothalamus, controlling circadian rhythms in response to light stimulating the retinas, and this signal regulates melatonin synthesis to control night-time sleep.

Cerebral spinal fluid contains hormones such as appetite-regulating *leptin*, which binds to hypothalamus receptors, conveying nutrient levels: your hypothalamus strives to maintain biological *set points*; by comparing information about blood sugar, salinity, temperature, hormone levels and *osmolality* (the level of particles in a fluid, such as proteins or lipids in your blood) to these optimal set points, your hypothalamus can trigger hormonal and neurochemical releases to establish homeostasis.

When your hypothalamus detects a deviation away from one of these set points, it adjusts your autonomic and endocrine systems, and motivates behaviors to restore homeostasis. For example, if you're too hot, your hypothalamus will trigger a shift in blood flow from your internal organs to *cutaneous* (skin) blood vessels, triggering sweating, which evaporates water from your skin to cool you. At the same time, it will trigger discomfort – conscious urges for you to seek ways of cooling down.

When a threat is detected, your hypothalamus activates your pituitary, signalling your adrenal glands to secrete hormones which prepare your body for fighting or running.

The regulatory system, called the *hypothalamic-pituitary-adrenal axis* (HPA axis), is an evolutionarily ancient survival mechanism which is superb in the wild, but ill-adapted to modern human life, where the need to fight for flee for your life is no longer a daily possibility.

Chronic stress leads to overactivation of this system, with dire consequences that include the condition of constantly depleted energy called *burnout*. Potentially much worse conditions to which chronic stress is a major contributor include depression obesity, diabetes, and dendrite *atrophy* (wasting away) in your hippocampus, a possible central contributor to Alzheimer's disease. We'll look at stress – and strategies to deal with it – in depth later.

Different regions within your hypothalamus have neural clusters specialized to perform each of its varied functions, and one of the most centrally important to this book, which we'll focus upon later, is a major cluster of fibers running through your hypothalamus called the *medial forebrain bundle*, which connects your brainstem, amygdala, hypothalamus and cortex.

A part of this region forms the so-called reward circuit (*mesolimbic pathway*), in which the VTA transmits dopamine to your *nucleus accumbens*, enhancing brain function and generating intense feelings of energization and positivity. This same circuit has been evolutionarily conserved for half a billion years in vertebrates, motivating survival behaviors such as hunting, eating, mating, nurturing the young and competing for territory and resources.

A second cluster of fibers connects your hypothalamus to your *periaqueductal gray,* the pain mediator in your midbrain. When stimulated, this hypothalamus-PAG pathway triggers instinctive behaviors such as *lordosis*, female mammal arching of the pelvis for sexual mounting.

The hypothalamus also triggers your body's outer manifestations of emotion – governing ANS and endocrine responses to emotionally significant things in your environment. Direct stimulation of specific known circuits triggers every major emotional reaction, as you'll see in the section devoted to emotional circuitry.

Found in all vertebrate nervous systems, the hypothalamus is comprised of 15 distinct regions which read the body's conditions and direct neurohormonal secretions to maintain homeostasis, biological rhythms, and behavioral responses. The hypothalamus therefore responds to several internal and external signals, and is richly connected to many CNS regions, including the RAS and autonomic systems, cortex and limbic system, and particularly the amygdala, septum, and olfactory bulbs.

It responds to light for regulating circadian and seasonal rhythms; to olfactory stimuli, including odorants and pheromone signals; to steroid hormones, including sex hormones; to neurally-transmitted data, particularly from the heart, lungs, stomach, and reproductive organs; to blood-borne signalling molecules such as leptin, ghrelin, insulin, pituitary and immune system signalling molecules; to sodium and glucose concentrations in the blood; and to stress hormones and invading pathogens.

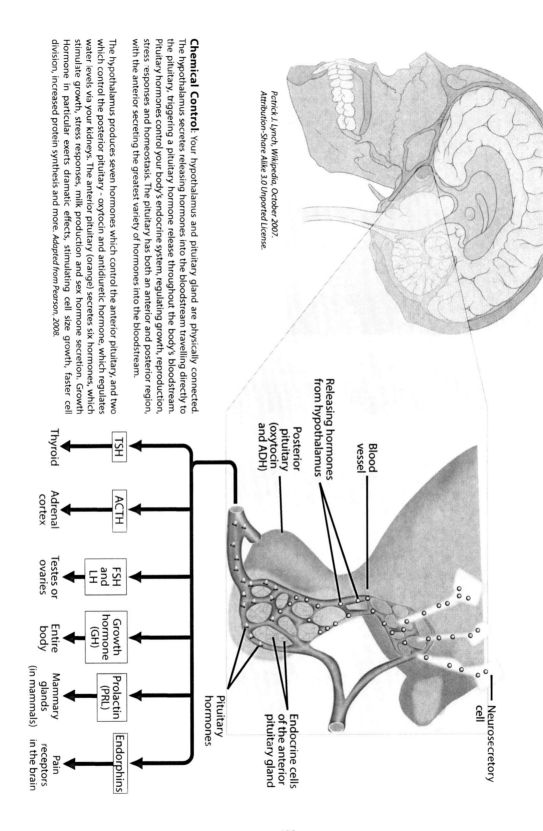

Patrick J. Lynch, Wikipedia, October 2007.
Attribution-Share Alike 3.0 Unported License.

Blood
vessel

Releasing hormones
from hypothalamus

Posterior
pituitary
(oxytocin
and ADH)

Endocrine cells
of the anterior
pituitary gland

Pituitary
hormones

Neurosecretory
cell

TSH	ACTH	FSH and LH	Growth hormone (GH)	Prolactin (PRL)	Endorphins
Thyroid	Adrenal cortex	Testes or ovaries	Entire body	Mammary glands (in mammals)	Pain receptors (in the brain)

Chemical Control: Your hypothalamus and pituitary gland are physically connected. The hypothalamus secretes releasing hormones into the bloodstream travelling directly to the pituitary, triggering a pituitary hormone release throughout the body's bloodstream. Pituitary hormones control your body's endocrine system, regulating growth, reproduction, stress 'esponses and homeostasis. The pituitary has both an anterior and posterior region, with the anterior secreting the greatest variety of hormones into the bloodstream.

The hypothalamus produces seven hormones which control the anterior pituitary, and two which control the posterior pituitary - oxytocin and antidiuretic hormone, which regulates water levels via your kidneys. The anterior pituitary (orange) secretes six hormones, which stimulate growth, stress responses, milk production and sex hormone secretion. Growth Hormone in particular exerts dramatic effects, stimulating cell size growth, faster cell division, increased protein synthesis and more. *Adapted from Pearson, 2008.*

432

To regulate body temperature, the hypothalamus stimulates heat production and retention, raising blood temperature, cools the blood through sweating and vasodilation. Fevers are the result of the hypothalamus elevating body temperatures. Prolactin and leptin, are sampled from the blood/CSF system through the choroid plexus, although how some other signalling molecules enter the brain is not entirely clear.

Pituitary gland

Your pituitary is a grape-sized master gland seated below and controlled by your hypothalamus. It lies in a small pocket of bone at the base of your skull, and is connected to your hypothalamus by the pituitary stalk. Known as the *master gland*, it controls other endocrine glands throughout your body, secreting hormones into your bloodstream.

The pituitary gland produces and secretes a number of controlling hormones, including *TSH*, *ACTH*, *FSH* and *LH*. ACTH stimulates the adrenal glands to activate the sympathetic nervous system for "fight or flight" responses. FSH and LH control gonad (testicles in men and ovaries in women) secretion of sex hormones, and regulate the production of sperm and ova (eggs). TSH stimulates the thyroid gland in the neck, which in turn controls metabolism (growth, repair and energy consumption).

Pineal gland

Your pineal gland is a cone-shaped neural cluster the size of an almond which secretes melatonin, your body's natural sleep aid. It's located behind your brain's third ventricle, where your hypothalamus uses it to regulate circadian rhythms by secreting melatonin into your blood.

Hippocampus

Named after the Greek word for *seahorse* because of its shape, this part of your limbic system is used for navigation, for helping regulate memory-based emotions, and for visual recognition. Your hippocampus is essential for recognizing context and spatial orientation. Most importantly, however, it reorganizes and creates new synaptic circuits which hold your memories – functioning as a sort of neural filing clerk, while the *amygdala*, to which it's connected, appears to attach emotional evaluations to those memories.

You hold information in your *working* (short-term) memory in your frontal lobe or sensory-processing regions of your cortex, but when that short-term information is deemed by your brain to be *salient* (personally relevant), your hippocampus will form long-term memories through the synaptic strengthening of LTP.

Long-term *episodic* memories are life experiences temporarily stored in your hippocampus. If you mentally replay those memories, they will eventually be transferred and become permanently wired into your cortex as long-term memories.

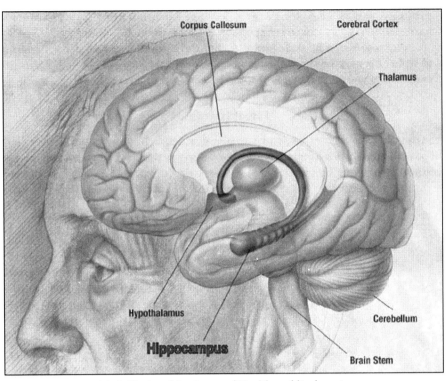

Corpus Callosum   Cerebral Cortex

Thalamus

Hypothalamus

Cerebellum

Hippocampus

Brain Stem

2010, National Institutes of Health, public domain

Alzheimer's disease and brain injuries to this region result in memory loss and disorientation. For example, in the condition called *anterograde amnesia*, when the hippocampus is damaged, a person can't create new memories, but can still carry on conversations, remember past events and use procedural memory skills, tasks which all rely upon non-hippocampal memory-storing regions of the brain.

Your hippocampus is *bilateral*, consisting of a pair of symmetrical, curved tails, with three layers of densely-packed *pyramidal cells* (so-called because of their triangular -shaped soma). The hippocampus has several two-way connections with various regions across your cortex, and receives input from your amygdala, thalamus, hypothalamus, raphe nuclei and locus coeruleus. It outputs to your hypothalamus, amygdala, and throughout your cortex, and is modulated by serotonin, norepinephrine, dopamine, GABA and acetylcholine.

Sensory information processed in various visual, auditory, tactile and somatosensory regions of your cortex converge here. Within your hippocampus, aspects of this information are gradually consolidated within appropriate regions of your cortex for permanent storage. The links between all these aspects of information are what constitute a memory of events in your mind, and their transfer into long-term storage occurs while you sleep. Retrieving memories re-fires many of the same neural paths you originally used when you sensed an experience and, therefore, almost re-creates the event for you.

A huge amount of data is necessarily discarded, as it would otherwise clutter your memory. But the amount of importance you attach to a piece of information – the emotional charge it carries for you – constitutes its *salience*. The greater the salience a piece of information holds for you, the stronger will be the synaptic links among the discrete parts of that information.

The hippocampus encodes navigational and spatial memories – allowing you to re-member your route to work, for example – making it a powerful evolutionary adapta-tion for vertebrate animals. Animals navigate through the use of *place cells* – indi-vidual hippocampal neurons that fire in strong bursts which corresponding to specific sites. These place cells activate to allow you to keep track of where you are.

Two types of hippocampus activity have been observed – *theta rhythm* firing patterns during navigation and exploration, and *spindle firing* patterns – sharp bursts of neu-rotransmission between the hippocampus and various parts of the cortex during deep sleep. Experiments indicate this spindle activity is the transfer of memories from your hippocampus into appropriate cortical areas for long-term storage.

Your hippocampus is so astoundingly powerful that no matter who you are, you can harness it to memorize entire libraries word-for-word, if you wish. Want to memorize a thousand-page textbook, or several of them? No problem, provided you're willing to invest the time and effort to learn how. You're going to look at how memory works in greater depth later, and how you can use it to build superhuman recall if you want. Literally any healthy person can do it, to a truly astonishing degree if one is simply willing to invest the time.

Insula

Folded deep within both hemispheres of your cerebral cortex – between the temporal and parietal lobes – is the *insular cortex* or *insula*. It's buried within the *Sylvian fissure*, the most prominent furrow in the cortex, which separates the frontal and temporal lobes in both cerebral hemispheres. The region is small – comprising under two per-cent of the cortex, but it has many two-way connections with the limbic system - pri-marily the thalamus and amygdala, as well as the cortex.

The insula is concerned with body awareness, particularly the anticipation of pain, disgust, revulsion and other unpleasant experiences before they occur; it's used to judge levels of pain severity, and to "read" physiological effects of emotions within your body, transmitting information on your inner states to your cortex – reporting sensations from your inner organs, including heartbeat and blood pressure.

The degree of warmth and coldness on the skin is assessed by the insula, as well as the severity of pain, and it engages when pain is anticipated or imagined. Other body sensations processed by the insula include the degree of fullness of the stomach and bladder, as well as itch, local oxygen status and sensual touch. Because of this, it is central to helping maintain homeostasis, and appears to be central in generating the craving sensations of addictions.

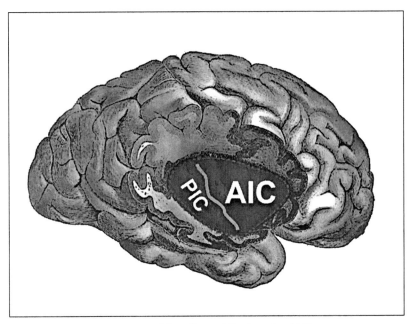

Image: Psychlopedia, public domain, 2009

The insula plays a major part in your sense of *empathy* – your ability to understand and share the emotions of others – and to experience compassion, laughter and crying. It's also involved in *norm violations* – giving rise to feelings of guilt, anxiety, shame or worry when you break rules or violate social taboos. It's thus very important to social interactions, effectively linking internal and external experiences in your mind.

Finally, because of its role as a "reporter" (to the cortex) of internal states, your insula participates in learning physical movement and motor control – coordination of hand and eye movement, swallowing, movement of food through the digestive system, and the coordination of mouth, larynx and lungs for speech, as well as the ability to formulate long and complex spoken sentences.

Because of its function in "reading" the body and physical responses to emotion, your insula is largely responsible for informing you when you're physically experiencing an emotion. It both sends and receives information through strong connective channels with your amygdala (your mental "sentry") and thalamus.

It reads signals from your senses and appears to integrate information from your amygdala, internal organs, olfactory and somatosensory cortices. It sends output throughout your limbic system, to the amygdala and the basal ganglia, as well as your *frontal cortex* (executive decision-making center), motor cortices, attention systems and *temporal lobe* (which deals with memory formation and the processing of *semantics* – the meaning of words, phrases, signs and symbols).

Its outputs also appear to help mediate cardiovascular stress responses, strongest in highly emotional people. Because of this, some scientists have suggested insular hyperactivity may play a role in heart attacks. It's been suggested that the increased anticipation of negative consequences associated with the insula may contribute to anxiety disorders and phobias, and fMRI scans seem to support this.

The insula appears to be intimately involved in decision-making, particularly when outcomes are uncertain. When considering possible negative consequences, the insula becomes highly active. It's thought that this activation is related to individual levels of *risk aversion* – activating the region may raise sensitivity to negative consequences, while inactivating or damaging the region is linked to increased risky behaviors.

The area also seems to come into play during moral decision-making. Often moral decisions require a choice between two alternatives – one that increases fairness, and another that increases profit at the expense of fairness. Increased insular activity is linked to a preference for greater fairness among the alternatives.

Amygdala

Amygdala, Hopes Brain Tutorial, 2010, Stanford University. Used with permission

The amygdala is a small brain region in the temporal lobe, behind your ears. It's located where parallel lines travelling through your eyes and your ears intersect in your brain's hemispheres. The twin amygdalae receive direct or nearly direct input from each of the various sensory systems processing your external world – inputs from visual, auditory, olfactory, touch, temperature, pain, and vestibular systems all converge within this region. Meanwhile, it sends outputs to all the emotional behavior systems, eliciting reactions to sudden danger such as freezing, elevated blood pressure and heartrate and stress hormone release.

437

In a sense, the amygdala is a loop, with sensory input from the external world flowing in, and commands to response control centers flowing out. It also receives information from higher-order processing systems like the prefrontal cortex and the association areas, which integrate information within the cortex.

Because it contains input from all the sensory systems, the amygdala receives a variety of information about the environment. It uses this information for association-based learning: if a sound immediately precedes a painful event, that sound becomes mentally linked to the painful event, and will trigger a protective response. If the sound immediately precedes the appearance of food, the sound becomes linked to a positive event. Thus, the amygdala helps control the formation of associations between neutral events and positive or negative reinforcing events, which stamp those experiences into powerful, lasting memories, creating *Pavlovian associations*.

These associations can then be used as a guide for adaptive behavior; if sometime in the past an animal found food in a specific location, the sights, sounds, smells and sensations associated with that location guide the animal towards the location again. With aversive stimuli, the same process occurs in reverse, driving an animal away from a location with negative associations.

These small neural clusters help generate emotional arousal, particularly fear and anger, but also, paradoxically, pleasure. The amygdala is one of the brain's primary emotional centers, helping to generate emotional memories. The amygdala colors all your perceptions, rating them as agreeable or disagreeable, instantly, instinctively telling your subconscious whether or not you like something, based on its potential as a reward or threat. Thus, your amygdala is your brain's emotional evaluator of outer experiences (sensory input) and inner experiences (thoughts).

When activated by norepinephrine, the amygdala focuses your attention, initiating emotional and behavioral responses to outside events, evoking emotional reactions such as fear, anger and sadness, particularly those involving aggression. This emotional arousal results in strong, long-lasting memories through long-term potentiation.

Latin for *almond* because of their shape and size, the twin amygdalae are your brain's alarm, a psychological sentinel which examines every situation for a potential threat. When a threat is perceived, your amygdala sends alarm signals throughout your brain, and your hypothalamus responds by activating your autonomic nervous system's flight or fight response.

Studies show the amygdalae are central to a circuit which controls fear-based learning, emotion generation and reward-based behaviors. This fear and aggression hub activates your natural fight-or-flight response to confront or escape from danger.

Your thalamus is directly connected to your amygdala, so sensory data is sent directly to the amygdala along a fast track, before it reaches your cortex and conscious mind through a more complex, circuitous route. This means your brain and body will react to a potential threat before you are even aware one exists.

Emotional memories you may not even consciously recognize can trigger a threat response without your awareness – your amygdala and hippocampus compare past events to the situation at hand, including memories from your infancy. Completely irrational survival instincts may be telling you your present situation poses a threat.

This subconscious, instinctive evaluation system classifies and assesses threats, and decides whether or not you like something within milliseconds. As psychologist Daniel Goleman puts it, "Our emotions have a mind of their own, one which can hold views quite independently of our rational mind".

In addition to the thalamus and hippocampus, the amygdala also receives direct input from the nearby *olfactory bulbs*, which is why smells can trigger strong emotional memories. It's made up of at least 12 functionally separate subregions, receiving information primarily from the thalamus and sensory cortex.

A special connection exists between the amygdala and the *nucleus accumbens* – the area in your midbrain which receives dopamine transmission to create positive sensations at the heart of motivation and learning. This circuit is central to *associative learning*, linking *gratification* – positive feelings of satisfaction – or *aversion* – the desire to avoid – with specific stimuli. Additional amygdalar output is sent throughout your brain, to your basal ganglia, brainstem, hypothalamus, *septum*, prefrontal cortex, hippocampus, and thalamus.

The basal ganglia are largely concerned with controlling movement, so the amygdala-basal ganglia circuit helps provide your ability to engage in behaviors expressing your emotion. The amygdala's connections to the adjacent hippocampus allow strong emotional-memory formation and associative/evaluative comparisons. Finally, its connections to your cortex and brainstem allow the amygdala to influence attention and perception.

In rats, at least, the amygdala contains receptors for *vasopressin,* linked to aggression and other fight or flight behaviors; and *oxytocin,* linked to a reduction in stress responses. These two hormonal signallers appear to strengthen or dampen amygdala activation.

Creatures with amygdalar damage no longer experience fear, and have difficulty learning from negative emotional experiences or forming fear- or other emotionally-charged memories. The amygdala also controls innate, inborn emotional responses, such as the instinctive fears of heights, snakes and spiders shared by most mammals.

This emotional mind is nearly the entire brain among non-mammalians such as birds, fish and reptiles, where snap evaluations can mean the difference between life and death. For you, it provides a kind of situational compass, helping you quickly (and usually quite effectively) choose between alternatives.

Dr. Antonio Damasio has studied many patients with injuries impairing this instinctive capacity to decide. He says emotional processes which guide behavior and decisions use *somatic markers* created by your amygdala. These emotional *best guess guides* reside in your *ventromedial prefrontal cortex*. They link your body (gut) sensations to choices, sending warning signals to steer you away from bad choices and toward good ones. When you can't decide through logical analysis, these somatic markers act as guides.

Salience

Your amygdala helps signal *motivational salience* – whether or not something's important enough for survival for you to act upon it. It gauges aspects of your environment such as noises, shapes, movement, facial expressions and behaviors, and informs you of potential threats and rewards. Novelty, uncertainty, intensity and/or emotionally-charged stimuli register as the most salient.

Your amygdala projects throughout your brain, receiving input from sensory networks, while also helping to modulate them and thus focus your attention. By determining salience, your amygdala affects where your attention and action are directed, and what is marked for long-term memory. When your amygdala registers something as salient, it directs other brain regions to focus upon it, collect more information, and engage in deeper processing.

The amygdala also helps generate *place-preference*, so animals seek out environments where rewards have previously been found and avoid those where punishments or potential dangers have been found. Such rewards can range from the simple (sweets) to the complex (sexual partners). Stimuli from the reward's environment become associated with that reward, and these environmental cues are given positive values, increasing the likelihood an animal will seek out and maintain contact with that place in the future, even when the reward itself is no longer to be found. It's the *basolateral complex* which integrates sensory input in the amygdala, associating rewards with place cues, while the hippocampus creates lasting memories of these associations.

Input from your amygdala, hypothalamus, and raphe nuclei can regulate dopamine released from your substantia nigra and ventral tegmental area as an excitatory signal when a reward-linked stimulus appears. When no reward is expected, inhibitory signals from the *habenula* block dopamine release. In this way emotions and emotional memories help to control behavior, through the limbic system's actions upon motor control and motivational-*reward circuits* in your basal ganglia.

Social Interactions

Charles Darwin first pointed out in 1872 that fearful, angry, and happy facial expressions are universal, with not just personal, but also social significance; recognition of facial expressions is critical for social behavior. Recognizing emotion in facial expressions engages the amygdala, as shown by PET and fMRI scans. Damaged amygdalae result in difficulty in interpreting such expressions.

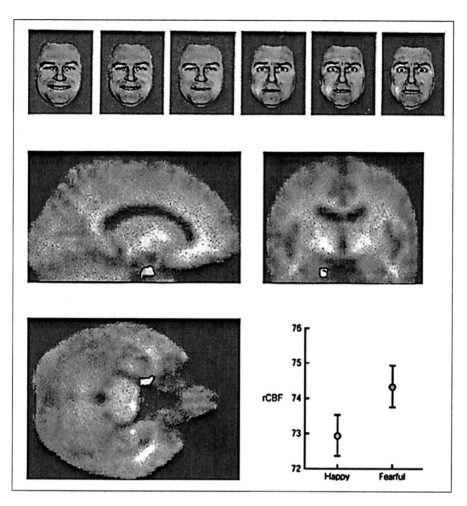

Amygdala in Processing Facial Emotional Expressions, 1998, Dr. R. J. Dolan, et al, Cambridge University. Used with permission. As subjects view various facial expressions ranging from happy to neutral to fearful, brain scans show strong activation of their amygdalae in response to fearful expressions.

The amygdala is central to processing emotional states, particularly fear and anxiety, and is related to several psychological disorders, including social anxiety, phobias, obsessive and compulsive disorders, paranoia, and post traumatic stress disorder. Psychopaths show reduced amygdala responses to fearful stimuli, while patients with borderline personality disorder have much greater amygdala activity than normal, appearing to have difficulty in classifying emotionally neutral faces, even reading hostility where none exists.

Emotional Memories

Moments with the greatest emotional weight tend to be deeply stamped into your memory, with the strongest, permanent effects. Through activation of your limbic system, emotional memories – as opposed to memories of dry facts or trivial events – are deeply imprinted into your psyche, and thereafter forever hold the potential to bias your perceptions of reality.

The more thrilling or distressing the event (the stronger the limbic arousal), the more vivid and lasting the memory becomes. From the standpoint of evolutionary biology, this ensures a creature remembers best those events with the greatest potential for benefit or harm.

Your limbic system is constantly scanning sensory data as you receive it, comparing this with your memories of previous events, but because the circuitry between your thalamus and amygdala is unsophisticated, little processing goes into making emotional snap evaluations, so your amygdala can be triggered by even vague similarities, at times leading to illogical but nonetheless intense responses to neutral events.

Traumatic events – situations so emotionally overwhelming the shock value has left a permanent, debilitating impression upon the psyche – can result in chronic worry, anxiety disorders, or in the illness known as *post-traumatic stress disorder*, where the amygdala repeatedly triggers danger signals, even when the threat is only imaginary, sending adrenaline rushing throughout the body. Neocortical, rational thought is by-passed, and over time the neural circuitry encoding the trauma strengthens, and its activation can becomes a permanently-ingrained aspect of personality.

The ability to withstand such stress varies from individual to individual and is be-lieved to be a result of genetics and events experienced during infancy, particularly in parent-child interactions. Those with the lowest stress thresholds can more easily fall victim to stress-triggered anxiety disorders.

These emotions trigger responses before the rational mind can engage, sometimes with an influence so intense it overpowers the neocortex, a process Dr. Daniel Gole-man calls *neural hijacking*. It's at times like these – when overwhelming instinctive responses have inhibited your rational mind – that you blow up at coworkers or lash out with hateful words or even violence toward another.

The reptile within you has seized control. As Goleman puts it, "The amygdala can react in a delirium of rage or fear before the cortex knows what is going on because such raw emotion is triggered independent of, and prior to, thought".

Alarm System Circuits

The amygdala plays a key role in your ability to feel emotions like fear and anger, and to detect these emotions in others, giving rise to fight or flight reactions in your body. It contains about twelve subregions, but the *lateral nucleus* is its main gateway, through which your amygdala receives warnings of danger from the outside world, either along a fast, direct but imprecise route from your thalamus or a second, slower but more precise route from your cortex. Startling sounds for example, first exit the auditory thalamus and enter the lateral nucleus of your amygdala.

This short, direct thalamus-amygdala route allows you to prepare for a potential threat before you've accurately assessed it, valuable in dangerous situations where a split sec-ond can become a matter of life or death: if you're walking barefoot and come across a green, coiled-up tubular shape, within milliseconds, the short thalamus-amygdala route will trigger a fear response, so you can leap out of the way or bash it with a walking stick if necessary.

At the same time, the signals are travelling along a slower route to your cortex, which carefully analyzes the object and will eventually inform you it's just a harmless garden hose.

Circuits from your prefrontal cortex – seat of your conscious thought and control – also connect to your amygdala, and are responsible for *extinction,* where fear associations gradually lose effect if they repeatedly occur without the fearful stimulus. For example, if a flash of light is paired with a shock, eventually an animal learns to fear the light flash – they've been *conditioned* to associate the light with pain.

Over time, however, if the light repeatedly returns *without* the shock, the fear gradually disappears. This is the basis of *behavior modification therapy,* where a patient is exposed to what he fears in situations gradually progressing from the least threatening to the most threatening, until he no longer fears the source: if you'd been bitten as a child, you might be afraid of dogs, but gradually learning to approach and eventually pet and feed them would ideally cause your fear to fade.

The prefrontal cortex-amygdala circuit also allows you conscious control over your anxiety or, if you allow yourself to worry and imagine disaster or threats which may or may not exist, the circuit can have the opposite effect – creating anxiety. This PFC-amygdala circuit governs the final stage of danger reactions, where, after the first instinctive emotional reaction, you're forced to choose a course of action to escape harm.

Since our brains have evolved over billions of years from more primitive survival systems, there are many more connections from more primitive subcortical, emotional and instinctive subsystems toward the cortex, seat of conscious thought and will, rather than in the opposite direction. This is thought to be why emotions have such a powerful effect and are sometimes difficult to control. And, while the amygdala is fully developed at birth, the PFC-to-amygdala circuit doesn't fully develop until adulthood, so children have much less control over their emotions than adults.

Vigilant Neurons

The amygdala evolved to integrate many of your body's alarm circuits. Thus, your amygdala is a polysensory analysis center. Multiple sensory inputs feed it information, warning of potential threats or rewards in the environment. This is the heart of the body's alarm system, governing reactions to salient events – things important for your survival – warnings of immediate threats, or of events signaling the presence of food, rivals, sexual partners, etc.

Specific amygdala neurons respond to each sense – auditory, gustatory, olfactory or somatosensory, as well as to visual stimuli, although visual neurons are the most plentiful in the amygdala. Additionally, some amygdala neurons respond primarily to faces. A great number of projections also travel from your amygdala to your hippocampus, many more than in the opposite direction, allowing for the formation of emotional memories.

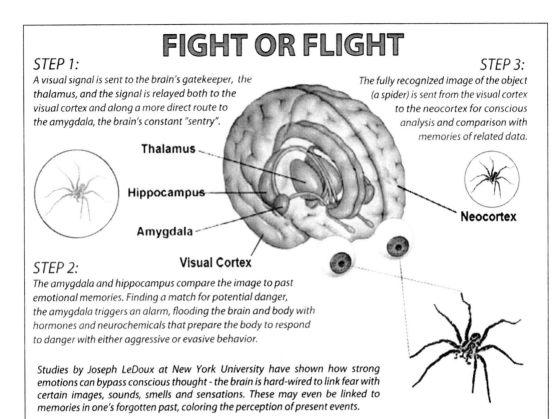

FIGHT OR FLIGHT

STEP 1:
A visual signal is sent to the brain's gatekeeper, the thalamus, and the signal is relayed both to the visual cortex and along a more direct route to the amygdala, the brain's constant "sentry".

STEP 3:
The fully recognized image of the object (a spider) is sent from the visual cortex to the neocortex for conscious analysis and comparison with memories of related data.

Thalamus

Hippocampus

Amygdala

Neocortex

STEP 2:
Visual Cortex

The amygdala and hippocampus compare the image to past emotional memories. Finding a match for potential danger, the amygdala triggers an alarm, flooding the brain and body with hormones and neurochemicals that prepare the body to respond to danger with either aggressive or evasive behavior.

Studies by Joseph LeDoux at New York University have shown how strong emotions can bypass conscious thought - the brain is hard-wired to link fear with certain images, sounds, smells and sensations. These may even be linked to memories in one's forgotten past, coloring the perception of present events.

The fight or flight response begins when a visual signal is sent to the thalamus. Most of this message is relayed to the visual cortex for processing, but a direct neural connection to the amygdala triggers a faster alarm response, sometimes generating intense emotions before we are even consciously aware of the reason.

Your amygdala also receives internal chemical signals of emotion – arousal of your autonomic nervous system, via your hypothalamus and brainstem. The hypothalamus activates your sympathetic nervous system, releasing stress hormones, altering heart rate, blood pressure, respiration and perspiration to create your physical emotional responses.

All sensory information is first routed through your thalamus, which then forwards the information to the appropriate sensory region – the visual or auditory cortex, etc., where it's evaluated and assigned meaning. But part of the sensory message from your thalamus also travels directly to your amygdala, bypassing the cortex. This short route is your *thalamo-amygdala pathway*, while the "long route" is your *thalamo-cortico-amygdala pathway*.

Because it's much shorter, your thalamo-amygdala pathway allows nearly instantaneous reactions to danger. This short route gives a very crude assessment of potential threats (e.g. "it's big and moving quickly!"). If a threat is detected, your amygdala triggers appropriate response circuits. Your cortex can confirm or refute the danger assessment moments later – moments which might have been fatal if you hadn't already reacted instinctively.

An Unexpected Encounter – *Meeting something fearful engages the same four instinctive reactions in all vertebrates, including humans: First the creature stops what it was doing. Next, it physically turns to face the source of the threat. It then stops all activity, to concentrate on mentally evaluating the threat. Finally, if the encounter is indeed a threat, the creature tries to escape or hide. If evasion is impossible, as a last resort it will try fighting to preserve its safety.*

Your brain is particularly adept at both pattern recognition and noticing contextual change – sudden, unusual movement, sounds, smells, etc., in the environment. This evolutionary advantage emerged to protect you from danger. Sudden changes in your environment – potential dangers – are filtered through your brain's first-line sentry – the reticular formation, then matched against known threats by your limbic system, and sensitivity to details about potential threats these environmental changes might pose are selectively heightened by excitatory signals from the thalamus, your brain's sensory gateway.

When your amygdala decides you've indeed encountered a threat, your hypothalamus puts your entire body on alert – your senses heighten, attention elevates, and energy floods to your musculature, while digestion and even your perception of time slow in the interest of ensuring your survival at all costs.

Your hypothalamus has triggered your sympathetic nervous system's fight or flight response with squirts of epinephrine and norepinephrine, elevating your heartbeat, readying your muscles with a rush of glucose to the bloodstream. Meanwhile, your enteric nervous system halts digestion, all of this occurring before you're even consciously aware you've met a threat.

It's these body changes which alert you to the danger – your cortex is sent an alarm by the fear circuitry of your amygdala, thalamus and somatosensory cortex. Only then do you become consciously aware of a strange noise, odd smell, or unusual shape in the distance. At this point, you focus your attention, and your cortex and amygdala further activate your sympathetic nervous system via your hypothalamus.

*Your cortex and hippocampus engage in a memory search for matches that can shed light on the threat, shutting down other thought processes, in what psychologist Daniel Goleman calls an **emotional hijacking** of your brain – in states of anxiety, worry, fear and anger, your abilities to focus, concentrate, remember and think rationality are impaired because your brain's neural and energy resources are being channeled into self-preservation – even when the situation isn't life-threatening and no emergency exists. If chemical imbalances or severe trauma have impaired this circuitry's functionality, it can overengage, leaving your cortex hostage to constant irrational fears, anger or worry.*

The thalamo-amygdala pathway is a sub-cortical pathway in which no cognition is involved, generating emotional responses before any perceptual integration or evaluation has occurred. Later, information which travelled via the thalamo-cortico-amygdala pathway and was processed by your cortex reaches your amygdala, informing it of the threat status of a stimulus.

Your cortex processes the information through several systems. Each of an object's aspects is analyzed – its size, shape, color, the sounds it makes, smells it emits, its position in space relative to you, etc. These aspects are all integrated in *association areas* of your cortex, and the data is fed back to your amygdala. The final, integrated mental representation of the object is compared with your memories by your hippocampus, which communicates directly with your amygdala.

Fearful Memories

Commands exit your amygdala from its *central nucleus*, en route to your hypothalamus. Between the entrance and exit – the lateral and central nuclei – a number of additional regions gather, process, and relay information, allowing each of these amygdala sub-regions to be modulated by emotion-influencing brain structures – the hippocampus, frontal cortex, hypothalamus, *septum* and reticular formation.

Your hippocampus is most directly and richly connected with your amygdala; since the hippocampus governs memory storage and retrieval, hippocampus-amygdala connections can generate strong emotionally-triggered memories. These hippocampal-amygdalar connections are the reason people or places connected to a traumatic event provoke anxiety.

The hippocampus processes sensory stimuli collectively, as opposed to in isolation, in this way organizing memory *context*. Because your hippocampus organizes memories within such a web of connected details, events are linked in your memory to the conditions in which they occurred.

Various input from systems such as long-term memory, internal balance, and auditory perception are integrated in your amygdala, and most of these incoming pathways are paired with outgoing ones. One important output is the *amygdalofugal pathway* (Latin for "fleeing from the amygdala"), which plays a central role in *associative learning* – such as learned fear responses, where a neutral stimulus like the sight of a flame is paired with an *aversive* (unpleasant) stimulus – such as the pain of a burn.

The amygdalofugal pathway also feeds information to the pleasure center called the *septum*, and to the hypothalamus, brainstem, cortex and basal ganglia, a nuclear center including the *mesolimbic reward pathway*, involved in learning, habit and motor control. Here in the basal ganglia, pleasant or unpleasant associations are created by connections between your amygdala and the *nucleus accumbens*, the target of your brain's dopamine "reward" circuit, which uses positive sensations to train you to pursue things promoting your survival.

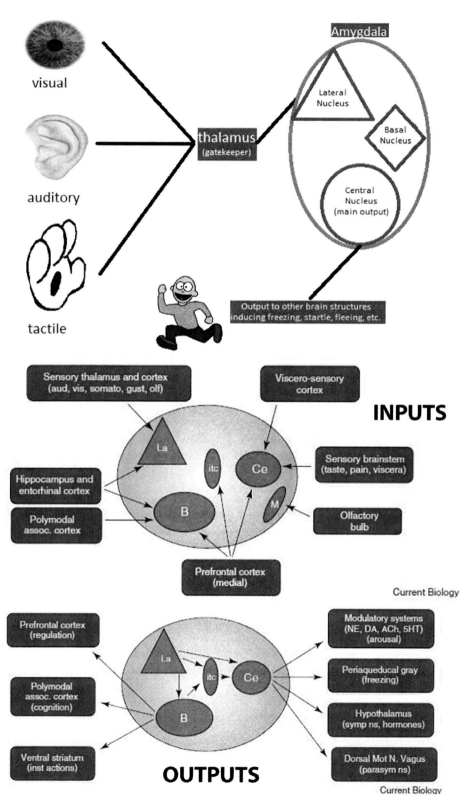

Amygdala, Dr. Joseph E. LeDoux, 2008, Center for Neural Science, NYU, New York, NY
Scholarpedia, 3(4):2698. doi:10.4249/scholarpedia.2698; Used with permission

Also via this circuit, automatic body responses to emotions like fear are controlled primarily by your amygdala's output to sympathetic nervous system arousal centers in your brainstem and hypothalamus. Here too, amygdala connections to your cortex, thalamus and brainstem influence attention, perception and memories of dangerous experiences.

When you undergo trauma, your amygdala's *implicit* (subconscious) memory system, and your hippocampus' *explicit* (conscious) memory system work to record different aspects of the event. After, your hippocampus allows you to remember contextual details, such as where and when the event happened, its sequence, and who was with you. Meanwhile, your amygdala will activate, tightening your muscles, raising your heart rate, etc.

Conscious *(explicit)* memories from your hippocampus, and unconscious *(implicit)* ones from your amygdala are the reason you can't remember traumatic experiences from when you were a baby – at that time, your amygdala was fully developed, and capable of recording unconscious memories, but your hippocampus was yet immature. Because of this discrepancy, sometimes childhood trauma can cause mental and behavioral problems well into adulthood, although no conscious memories exist to explain why.

Both your hippocampus and amygdala have many receptors which respond to stress hormones such as cortisol. Prolonged stress – long-term exposure to this cortisol – impairs LTP (memory formation) in your hippocampus, but *enhances* LTP in your amygdala, resulting in an increase in emotional sensitivity, and heightened implicit memory encoding, but impaired explicit memory encoding. You become better at remembering unconscious emotional memories, and worse at remembering practical, conscious ones.

Information on your body's emotional (chemical) states – particularly hormonal states related to fear and anxiety – enters your amygdala through a special set of nuclei called the *basolateral complex*. Memories will be encoded about these salient stimuli for future use – so new experiences can be compared to previous ones to predict outcomes. Information about related stimuli is also transmitted to your conscious mind (cortex) by organs whose homeostasis has been disturbed, via your vagus nerve, insula, and related structures.

2012 experiments at Cold Spring Harbor Laboratory show a special neural population in the central amygdala is central to the learning, control and memorization of these fear responses. The *lateral subdivision* region was previously believed to be simply a passive signal relay within the circuit, but Professors Bo Li and Z. Josh Huang learned it plays a much more active role.

"Neuroscientists believed that changes in the strength of the connections onto neurons in the central amygdala must occur for fear memory to be encoded," says Dr. Li, "but nobody had been able to actually show this." So if fear memories are stored in the central amygdala, how are those traces reactivated and translated into a fear response?

Mice undergoing fear tests were trained with *classical conditioning* to respond in Pavlovian fashion to auditory cues, trained to freeze at sounds they'd learned to fear. Dr. Li's team bred mice with light-sensitive proteins in the region's neurons, and very thin fiber-optic cables were implanted in the area. This allowed the researchers to activate the genetically-altered photosensitive neurons with tiny beams of laser light, a technique called *optogenetics*. The resultant behavior of the mice was then monitored.

The team discovered that two sets of neurons are central to fear-learning and memory activation. One subset enhances neurotransmitter release, while the other diminishes it. Experiences which condition animals to feel fear increase excitatory neurotransmitter release, while enhancing inhibitory neurons suppresses central amygdala activity.

Particularly important are neurons modulated by the hormone *somatostatin*, which alters neurotransmitter release. Fear-memory formation is impaired when *somatostatin-positive* (SOM+) neurons are deactivated. These SOM+ neurons are needed to recall fearful memories, and activating them drives fear responses.

Fear memories in the region modify the circuit in a way which translates into action – the fear response, according to Dr. Li. His group is now trying to determine exactly how these processes are altered in patients suffering from PTSD and other fear-related disorders, with the hope of developing drugs to alleviate the conditions.

Olfactory system

Unlike your other sensory organs, your olfactory bulbs bypass your thalamus, connecting directly to your limbic system. Because of this direct access to your amygdala and hippocampus, smells can trigger very strong emotional memories. The olfactory system, together with the amygdala and hippocampus, forms the basis of a powerful emotional learning and memory system, an evolutionarily ancient *rhinoencephalis – nose brain*.

This sensory apparatus is one of the first to have evolved, and is vital for survival: being able to recognize the unique airborne chemical signatures of creatures and objects as potential food, poison, mates or enemies is central to preserving one's existence.

Olfactory nerve clusters receive stimuli from nasal special receptors, directly communicating with your limbic system, so smells can trigger spontaneous emotions, with pleasant scents cheering or calming you, and unpleasant ones triggering revulsion, irritation or other unpleasant moods.

Septum

The *septum* (Latin for *an enclosure*) is a pleasure response center comprised of the *septic nuclei*, which receive input from your hypothalamus and hippocampus and return output back to the hypothalamus. Although its precise role is not fully understood, according to the University of Rio's Dr. Júlio Rocha do Amaral, "Inside it, one finds the centers of orgasm, four for women and one for men. This area has been associated with different kinds of pleasant sensations, mainly related to sexual experiences."

The septum was the first reward system area discovered by Dr. James Olds and Peter Milner in electronic brain stimulation experiments on rats during the 1950s. During their experiments, their subjects would self-stimulate their septums to the point of collapse and starvation. Stimulating the region in humans excites vagus nerves, which transmit internal body sensations to the cortex.

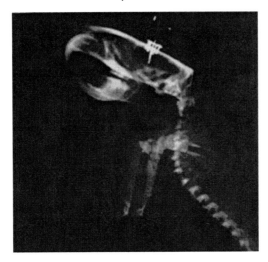

X-ray of a septal electrode, Olds and Milner, 1954. Public domain image.

The septum is the brain's primary pleasure center, but it also seems to reduce aggression markedly. Conversely, damaging the septum increases aggression, and can result in the violent set of behaviors called *septal rage*. Hypersexuality, hyperemotionality and increased rage reactions have all been reported following injury to the septum. Damaging the amygdala or hypothalamus markedly decreases this septal aggression, and can make even normally aggressive creatures extremely docile.

2011 experiments in Japan also show septal nuclei help categorize rewards according to salience, and studies show the septum also sets a tempo for neurotransmission, synchronizing neural firing rhythmically, as signals pass from brainstem through septum, en route to the hippocampus. The septal tempo is a *theta rhythm* – a frequency of 3-12 *Hertz* (cycles per second) a brainwave cycle associated with deep trancelike, meditative or dreamlike states. Maintaining this frequency locally, however, keeps neural activity within normal ranges, says University of Texas professor Luis V. Colom. Your neurons are in constant cross-communication, but if their chatter becomes overactive, it can "snowball" into the electrical chaos of an epileptic seizure. Ensuring that neurons fire normally prevents such *hyperexcitation* – the overstimulation of epileptic seizures – as well as *hypoexcitation* – the understimulation seen in afflictions like Alzheimer's.

Theta synchrony may also help maintain the health of brain structures, and may even be vital for memory formation. Some of the strongest brainwaves appear in the hippocampus, dominated by 4–10 Hz, the *hippocampal theta rhythm*. This is thought to be a *ready to receive* state for processing memories, vital for long-term potentiation. Some neuroscientists believe this theta rhythm also separates memory encoding from retrieval, helping your brain avoid interference from both processes occurring simultaneously.

Wirehead – *In 1953, two young McGill University scientists erred while implanting an electrode into the brain of a rat, leading to a revolutionary discovery. Drs. James Olds and graduate student Peter Milner were studying systems responsible for regulating arousal, by stimulating the reticular formation in the brainstem. But during the tests, something rather odd occurred. Whenever it was stimulated, one rat would return to the area of the cage where it had received the stimulation, apparently in hopes that the experience would be repeated. Every time it was stimulated, the subject would step forward and begin sniffing and searching while it moved. When this stimulus was switched off, it would immediately return to its normal behavior, and sometimes even step back. This was much different than any behavior which the scientists had previously seen: in all their other experiments, they were able to control rat movement by giving a tiny jolt to the brainstem whenever the animal turned in a certain direction.*

X-rays showed they had miscalculated their electrode's insertion point, placing it near the hypothalamus, in an area called the septum, and stimulating the region produced dramatic effects. To find out what had caused this behavior, the team devised a new experiment, in which the animals controlled their own electronic stimulation. They implanted silver wire electrodes 1/100th of an inch in diameter into the brains of 15 male rats, which were then placed in a **Skinner box**, *where they could give themselves a mild jolt of up to five volts by pressing a lever. A time delay switch cut off the current if the rat held the lever down continuously.*

Electrodes were placed in different regions in each experiment, so various forebrain, thalamus and midbrain sites could be tested, with mixed results. Several lower brain regions seemed to produce effects which the animals chose to repeat, but when the electrodes were placed in the septal forebrain, the effects were dramatic: the rats spent nearly every moment in the box frantically pressing the lever. In fact, the most active animal pressed the bar continuously over 7500 times before dropping from exhaustion. Some sites in the thalamus had the opposite effect, and the animals would do everything they could to avoid stimulation of these punishment centers.

By restructuring their experiments, the team could train animals to perform novel behaviors to receive rewards in the form of brief pulses of electronic brain stimulation. Their test subjects would run across long and painful electrified grids and even forego eating to press the lever. Drs. Olds and Milner concluded they'd found brain circuits which constituted a reward system.

In fact, they had found nothing less than the very heart of animal motivation. The system allows organisms to learn from experience, repeating behaviors with positive consequences, like finding food, water, friends and mates, and stopping behaviors with negative consequences, like exposure to extreme temperatures. Eventually, Olds and Milner mapped out a large system of neural centers rats preferred to self-stimulate, a neural "interstate highway" they called the **medial forebrain bundle** *(MFB). This multi-synaptic pathway connects regions from the lateral hypothalamus through the ventral tegmental area (VTA) and Periaqueductal Grey (PAG) with the Nucleus Accumbens (NA) and other regions in the limbic system, basal ganglia and cortex.*

It was later discovered that dopamine was the common neurotransmitter shared by these areas. Drugs which increase dopamine's effects within the reward system include amphetamine, cocaine, morphine and nicotine. They enhance the effects of electrical stimulation in the ventral tegmental area (VTA), hypothalamus, nucleus accumbens (NAc) and septum, by either increasing dopamine release or by blocking its re-uptake or breakdown in the synapses. This greatly reinforces repetition of learned behaviors such as lever pressing.

Basal Ganglia

Every voluntary effect you have upon the world is through muscle contraction.

Your brain has only one form of input and one form of output. Sensory stimuli, converted into electrochemical impulses, allow your environment to alter you. Conversely, muscle contractions, triggered by the same electrochemical impulses, allow you to alter your environment.

To accomplish the latter, premotor areas in your cortex plan movements, and the primary motor cortex oversees their execution. Impulses are sent from the motor cortex down *corticospinal tracts* to the peripheral nervous system, to activate muscle contractions. Before reaching the spinal cord, however, the cerebellum and a regulatory hub called the *basal ganglia* modulate these impulses, orchestrating all the individual muscle contractions into smooth movement sequences.

The basal ganglia are twin neural clusters which lie at the base of your forebrain, hence their Latin name, *basal* – at the base – and *ganglia* – swollen mass. They're located in the temporal lobes on either side of your septum and thalamus, outside and over the limbic system. They're central to motor control, emotions, thought and learning.

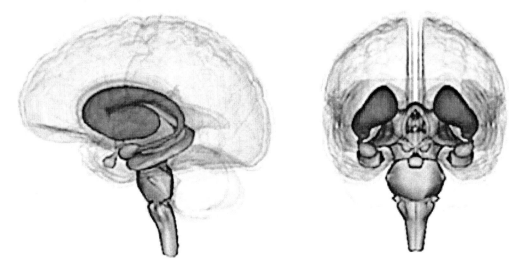

Basal Ganglia, Wikipedia Creative Commons, 2006, author unattributed

Basal ganglia functions haven't yet been fully mapped, but they unquestionably regulate movement – without their input, the cortex cannot properly direct movement, resulting in motor dysfunction such as *Parkinson's* or *Huntington's disease.*

They operate primarily by inhibiting motor regions of the thalamus, allowing selective amplification or inhibition of muscle-activating impulses transmitted from the motor cortex down the spine to the muscles. This region is arguably the most complex, and thus the next 25 pages are the most challenging (and most rewarding!) portion of this book.

The basal ganglia work hand-in-hand with the cerebellum, limbic system, thalamus and motor cortices, which plan and initiate movements. As in the rest of the brain, glutamate is the most *plentiful* neurotransmitter among the basal ganglia, though inhibitory GABA and modulatory dopamine and acetylcholine are the most *critical* neurotransmitters for basal ganglia function.

It was once believed that the basal ganglia only engage in selecting motor activity, but recent studies show they serve multiple functions, acting as *pattern generators* for both movement and thought – generating patterns of learning, habit and memory which eventually guide actions, according to MIT's Dr. Ann Graybiel. Connected with the cortex via multiple control loops, the basal ganglia "allow us to select what we'll do". Repeated activation of the same circuit eventually develops into a habit. the are modulated by reward-signalling dopamine from an area called the substantia nigra.

The largest basal ganglia region is the *striatum* (striped body), made up of the *caudate* (tail), *putamen* (stone/pit of a fruit), *globus pallidus* (pale globe), and *nucleus accumbens* (leaning cluster). The putamen is the basal ganglia's primary entry point into the striatum.

The cortex sends excitatory signals to the putamen, and dopamine in the striatum acts upon these signals to regulate movement and learning. Inhibitory signals exit the basal ganglia's globus pallidus, en route to the brainstem and thalamus, to modulate motor signals.

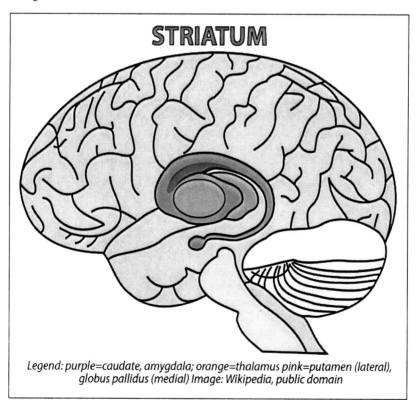

STRIATUM

Legend: purple=caudate, amygdala; orange=thalamus pink=putamen (lateral), globus pallidus (medial) Image: Wikipedia, public domain

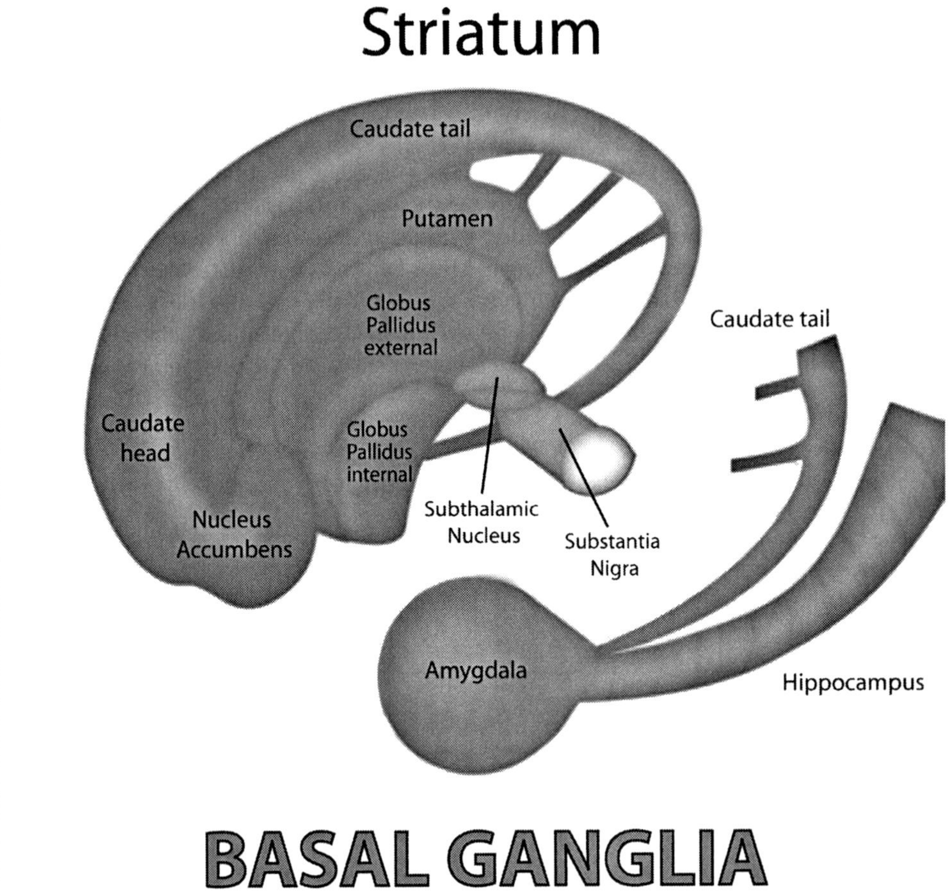

Striatum

Caudate tail

Putamen

Globus
Pallidus
external

Caudate tail

Caudate
head

Globus
Pallidus
internal

Nucleus
Accumbens

Subthalamic
Nucleus

Substantia
Nigra

Amygdala

Hippocampus

BASAL GANGLIA

Adapted from *Atlas of Functional Neuroanatomy*, 2nd Edition, Walter Hendelman, MD 2005

In the striatum, the apostrophe-shaped caudate starts just behind the frontal lobe, its tail curving backward toward the occipital lobe at the rear of the skull, near its base. This specialized region transmits messages to your *orbitofrontal cortex*, just above and behind your eyes. The caudate seems to inform you when something is amiss and needs to be corrected – warning, for example, *Turn off the stove!* or *Wash your hands!*

An overactive caudate seems to underlie the uncontrollable, ritualistic behaviors of *obsessive compulsive disorder* (OCD), while an underperforming caudate seems to result in several disorders, including ADHD and general lethargy. Medial to the caudate is the putamen, the peach-pit-shaped neural cluster, which acts as entryway to the striatum and seems central in coordinating *procedural memories* – automatic behaviors like brushing your teeth or driving a car. *Tourette's syndrome* – characterized by frequent outbursts or impulsive actions – is thought to arise from a dysfunctional putamen.

The putamen's primary function, however, is movement regulation. It communicates with the globus pallidus using GABA, acetylcholine and enkephalins. The globus pallidus itself contains both an exterior and interior region, and receives input from both the putamen and caudate, sending output to the brainstem and thalamus, which then relays signals back to the cortex.

There are two major regulatory pathways in the basal ganglia. Dopaminergic axons project into the striatum along these two main paths:

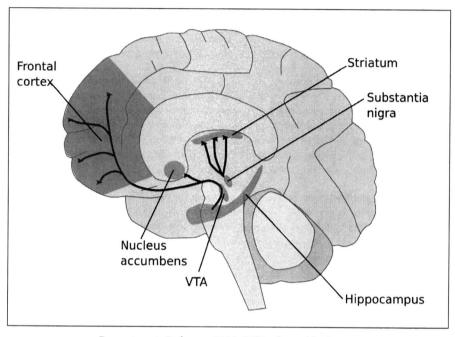

Dopaminergic Pathways, 2010, Wikipedia, public domain

1) in the *mesolimbic pathway*, dopamine axons project from the VTA to the nucleus accumbens of the *ventral* striatum;

2) in the *nigrostriatal pathway*, dopamine axons project from the substantia nigra to the *dorsal* striatum.

1. Mesolimbic Pathway

VTA neurons transmit dopamine from atop the brainstem through the *medial forebrain bundle* to the *nucleus accumbens* in the striatum. Stimulating this pathway gives rise to pleasurable sensations, and this is the basis of motivation in virtually all animals (including insects), working hand-in-hand with the limbic system.

VTA dopamine drives the mesolimbic pathway, signalling the limbic system when something significant has occurred. The frontal cortex is then alerted by signals forwarded along the *mesocortical pathway*.

*Within the striatum, dopamine released from the VTA and SN, and glutamate released from the thalamus and cortex both converge on special **medium-sized spiny neurons**.*

*Dopamine is used in forming habits and in the temporary "data holding space" of the frontal lobes called **working memory**. It regulates the flow of other neurotransmitters, altering the concentration and passage of ions across neural membranes, changing the ease of achieving depolarization, and thus ion channel opening and neural activation.*

Thus, in the cortex, limbic system and striatum, dopamine acts like a water spigot regulating the flow of neurotransmitters like glutamate, depending on both target neuron firing rates and the types of receptors being acted upon. Because dopamine can be released into the extracellular space, it acts as a neuromodulator, affecting many neurons simultaneously.

*Dopamine neurons fire in two ways, depending upon the status of cues and rewards. Normal, slowly increasing dopamine is released at a **tonic firing rate** of 5 Hertz (five times a second), probably acting as a motivation or expectancy signal. However, when an unexpected reward appears, dopamine neurons fire in a sudden **phasic burst** at four times the normal speed, 20 Hertz. This burst of dopamine secretion is thought to be a signal of **salience** – something highly important for survival. If an expected reward is not delivered, dopamine release dips below normal levels.*

*A dopamine **feedback loop** between the Hippocampus and VTA seems to control the encoding of **episodic memories** – memories of events. The VTA feeds dopamine to both the amygdala and hippocampus, signalling salient events "worth" long-term potentiation (memory formation). In return, the hippocampus can **disinhibit** the VTA, allowing greater dopamine release, probably when a salient cue stored in memory has been re-encountered.*

The striatum receives excitatory input from the cortex, sensory data such as the sight and smell of food. Dopamine functions as a training signal for this input – leading to new synapses which link the sight and smell with pleasurable sensations.

Remove dopamine from the system, however, and animals cannot learn or remember behaviors such as maze navigation, how to avoid danger, how to press levers for food, or recognize new objects in their environment; nor will they engage in normal eating, social interaction, or movement, all *behavioral adaptations* – the ability to alter behavior in response to environmental changes.

Dopamine amplifies or suppresses signals from the cortex – strong signals become stronger, and weak signals become weaker. Without this dopamine modulation, however, all sensory input is relatively equal, and the response is apathy – a complete lack of motivation, as well as an inability to create lasting memories.

The cortex sends excitatory glutamatergic signals to the striatum, where numerous dendritic spines project from *medium spiny neurons*. Dopamine regulates this region, with powerful effects, as shown on the following page: a single dopamine neuron can project multiple axonal branches that fill about 10% of the striatum. This dopamine is critical for driving life-sustaining behaviors.

DOPAMINE IN THE BASAL GANGLIA

Adapted from Palmiter, 2010 and Matsuda et al, 2009

A medium spiny neuron in the striatum, with many dendrite spines - the target of dopamine and glutamate

Cortical pyramidal neurons - long axons, fewer dendrites

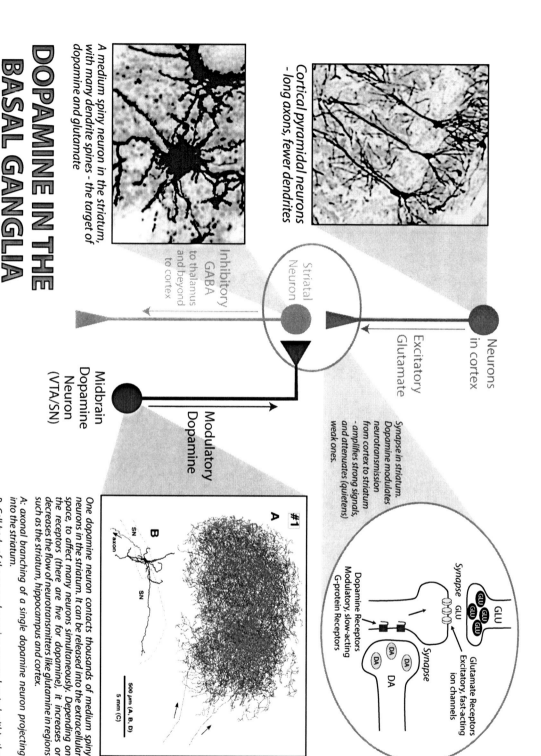

Inhibitory GABA to thalamus and beyond to cortex

Striatal Neuron

Excitatory Glutamate

Neurons in cortex

Midbrain Dopamine Neuron (VTA/SN)

Modulatory Dopamine

Synapse in striatum. Dopamine modulates neurotransmission from cortex to striatum - amplifies strong signals, and attenuates (quietens) weak ones.

Dopamine Receptors Modulatory, slow-acting G-protein Receptors

Synapse

GLU

GLU

Glutamate Receptors Excitatory, fast-acting ion channels

Synapse

DA

#1

A

B

SN

axon

SN

500 μm (A, B, D)

5 mm (C)

One dopamine neuron contacts thousands of medium spiny neurons in the striatum. It can be released into the extracellular space, to affect many neurons simultaneously. Depending on the receptors (there are five for dopamine), it increases or decreases the flow of neurotransmitters like glutamine in regions such as the striatum, hippocampus and cortex.

A: axonal branching of a single dopamine neuron projecting into the striatum.

B: Cell body of the same dopamine neuron located within the hindbrain (from the SN).

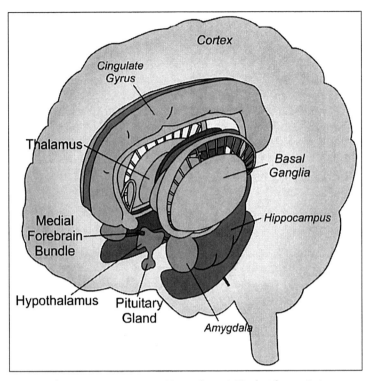

Limbic System, Hopes Brain Tutorial, 2010. Used with permission.

Mice genetically unable to produce dopamine will simply lie still, completely un-interested in exploration, interaction with others, nest-building, or eating, even if they've gone a day or more without food, and such food is placed right under their noses. Inject them with a dopamine precursor, however, and they come alive, acting just like normal mice. This precursor, *L-Dopa*, is used to synthesize dopamine in the VTA and substantia nigra, bringing dopamine-deficient mice rapidly to life.

Striatal activity – specifically dopamine excitation of the nucleus accumbens – ap-pears to be at the heart of learning, motivation and addiction. The pathway also plays a major role in depression, and in *schizophrenia*, a condition marked by severely dis-ordered cognition and hallucinations. Since schizophrenia is thought to be caused by excessive dopamine activation in the mesolimbic pathway, *antipsychotic drugs* work by blocking dopamine receptors.

The mesolimbic pathway is part of a larger pleasure-inducing circuit called the *me-dial forebrain bundle,* a bundle of axons interconnecting the cortex and limbic system, running from the VTA to the hypothalamus. The VTA and nucleus accumbens of the basal ganglia are the two major centres in this circuit, though it also includes the sep-tum, amygdala, prefrontal cortex, and parts of the thalamus. Each of these neural cent-ers participates in various aspects of behavioral response.

458

This is your brain's training center: the MFB is rich in dopamine neurons, so activating the region produces behavior-reinforcing positive sensations. Dopamine is released in high frequency bursts in response to smells, sights, sounds and sensations judged to be pleasurable, novel, interesting, hazardous or otherwise noteworthy. Stimulating the MFB alerts the hypothalamus and cortex of the presence of rewards. The hypothalamus sends responses to the ventral tegmental area and to the pituitary gland, resulting in hormonal releases throughout the body. Dopamine-signalling as a training mechanism has existed since the first nervous systems evolved, and is at the heart of learning and behavior in all animals, from fish to birds to mammals, and even worms and fruit flies.

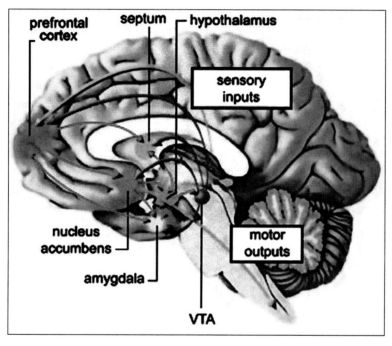

Six major areas interact in the medial forebrain bundle: the VTA, Cortex, Nucleus Accumbens, Amygdala, Hypothalamus and Septum. Bruno Duboc, McGill University, 2002. Used with permission.

The mesolimbic pathway is responsible for *conditioning* – a trained, automatic response to a repeated event – and the synaptic connections which encode it. These *stimulus-response associations* underlie the conditioning demonstrated by Russian scientist Ivan Pavlov, who trained his dogs to salivate in anticipation of food whenever a bell rang. Thus, the mesolimbic pathway is the basis of motivation and reward-based, *reinforcement learning.*

This reinforcement learning is the mental linking of a stimulus with a reward or punishment. For example, if a mouse finds a piece of cheese in a corner for the first time and eats it, it discovers that cheese tastes delicious, and this creates positive feelings of energy and contentment. Thereafter, every time it approaches the corner where it found the cheese, the mouse will link positive values (memories of delicious taste, energy and satiety) to the area.

Learning in both animals and humans is similar in regard to rewards such as food, or relief from aversive stimuli like pain. In *conditioning*, animals learn to mentally link a reward-predicting cue with delivery of a reward.

Eventually, dopamine releases shift, responding to secondary reward-predicting cues rather than the reward itself. This was the basis of the change in Pavlov's dogs, which could be trained to salivate at the ring of a bell instead of seeing or smelling food.

Synapses are formed which associate this stimulus – the sensory data – with the positive sensations. Afterwards, the learner subconsciously predicts good feelings will result from seeking satisfaction under the same conditions – the place where it first encountered the reward. The more frequently the environmental conditions and the reward are encountered together, the stronger the association (and the physical synaptic connections) will become.

Appetitive stimuli (rewards) are pleasant sensations, while *aversive stimuli* (punishments) are painful or otherwise unpleasant sensations. Surprisingly, both rewards *and* punishments trigger dopamine release, arousing the CNS and enhancing its function. Likewise, so do high-intensity or novel stimuli; all of these attention-arousing stimuli are *salient*, marked by the limbic system as holding important meaning related to survival.

Dopamine isn't released in constant, large amounts, but is instead released in response to excitatory signals. Salient stimuli trigger dopamine burst firing – for example, when a hungry mouse sees and smells cheese, it gets a burst of dopamine activation from its VTA into its nucleus accumbens. This stimulates the limbic system, cortex and central nervous system as a whole.

Dopamine within the VTA-NA circuit excites and enhances neural function throughout the central nervous system, creating feelings of elation, power and energy, and registering as a reward the limbic system commits to memory, mentally linking the reward with the sensory stimuli experienced at the time it was discovered.

VTA dopamine neurons burst fire into the nucleus accumbens in response to novel, subjectively relevant or intense stimuli, in anticipation of rewards such as food, sex or – in the case of addicts – drugs. This dopamine activity prompts the brain to link pleasant neurotransmission sensations with environmental cues (i.e. taking a drug), and addicts learn to expect these cues will lead to the same rewards in the future.

Researchers have found that humans can have varying degrees of sensitivity to dopamine, based upon genetics. People who express fewer dopamine receptors have normal higher brain functions such as memory and spatial navigation, but may suffer from general lethargy and apathy. Because of this, it's been theorized that people with dopamine deficiencies seek greater levels of stimulation simply to reach a baseline feeling of "normalcy". Their need for stimulation creates a susceptibility – a *predisposition* – to addictions to drugs, foods, behaviors, and almost certainly even neurochemical states created by certain emotions.

Conditioning is optimized by a short interval – optimally half a second – between the *conditioned stimulus* (e.g., a bell ringing) and an *unconditioned stimulus* (the sight and smell of food) which elicits a *response* (secretion of digestive juices in anticipation of eating). Repeating the sequence results in a *conditioned response*, so the CS – the ringing of the bell – triggers digestive juice secretion.

In *operant conditioning*, reinforcement changes mental responses, either increasing or decreasing their probability. *Negative reinforcement* – the removal of an unpleasant stimulus – and *positive reinforcement* – the presence of a pleasant stimulus – increase the probability of a response, while *punishment* reduces its probability. Separate clusters of neurons in the basal ganglia register this stimuli as either *appetitive* (positive) or *aversive* (negative).

In this way, visual and other stimuli become mentally linked to either rewards or punishments, assigned a positive or negative value. This value is used in the future to predict whether something is likely to hold a reward or a punishment, and the value attached to that particular stimulus can be updated every time it's encountered – how well did the reward meet expectations? If it didn't meet with expectations, a drop in dopamine levels constitutes an *error signal*, while a burst of dopamine constitutes a reward.

Based upon these predictions of reward or punishment, humans and other animals modify their behaviors to ensure they maximize rewards – *approach behaviors* – and avoid punishment – *avoidance behaviors*, thus ensuring their health and survival.

This means, in essence, that everything you want is, at its core, a dopamine release, which is why you want it. One might say dopamine and related neuromodulators – serotonin, oxytocin, endorphins – are the only things one truly enjoys in life.

When the mesolimbic pathway links pleasurable dopamine release to survival-enhancing behaviors, it drives learning and reinforces life-sustaining actions such as eating, drinking and mating. It's also responsible for addictions; many addictive substances artificially boost dopamine in this pathway's synapses, resulting in euphoria.

---

*In opposition to the pleasure circuit, the brain's **punishment circuit**, called the **periventricular system**, or PVS, is activated by aversive stimuli, resulting in fight or flight responses. The PVS includes the hypothalamus, thalamus, amygdala, hippocampus and aqueduct of Sylvius. The PVS functions using acetylcholine, stimulating the secretion of adrenal corticotrophic hormone (ACTH). ACTH then activates the adrenal glands, which release epinephrine and other stress hormones to prepare organs in the body for fight or flight. Stimulating this punishment circuit inhibits the reward circuit, supporting the observation that fear and punishment extinguish pleasure.*

*The MFB and the PVS thus constitute twin signalling systems which underlie all motivation. The **behavioural inhibition system**, or BIS, is a third circuit which involves the basal ganglia, septum, hippocampus, and amygdala. The BIS receives input from the prefrontal cortex and sends output via the brainstem – norepinephrine centers in the locus coeruleus and serotonin centers in the Raphe nuclei. Serotonin seems to play a central role in this system. The BIS engages when neither fight nor flight seem possible, leaving passive submission as the only remaining behavioural option. Prolonged activation of this behavioural inhibition in response to ongoing stress can be extremely damaging to health in the long run.*

Contrary to popular misconceptions, dopamine release in the medial forebrain bundle is more directly related to *anticipation* and *desire* than to the pleasurable effects of actually *obtaining* rewards. Dopamine neurons encode the *likelihood* of obtaining rewards, helping animals gradually improve their prediction skills, and thus the ability to obtain the rewards they seek.

fMRI studies of cocaine addicts show dopamine release to the nucleus accumbens increases just prior to cocaine use, indicating dopamine activation of the nucleus accumbens is the basis of reward *expectancy*. A number of studies have found such increased NA activity in anticipation of a range of rewards, including money and food.

Dopamine neurons fire in a more sustained pattern during reward *expectation*, and the intensity varies with the probability that the reward will occur. Interestingly, if a reward is 100% certain (or 100% *uncertain*), dopamine signalling vanishes: in other words, a certain level of *uncertainty increases* dopamine signalling – probably the reason the unpredictability of gambling gives addicts a high, and why a lover who is fickle may seem more interesting than one who is unswervingly faithful.

Dopamine also works in other previously unpredicted ways; for instance, it's also be released when *negative* stimuli are encountered. And when a reward is greater than anticipated, dopaminergic neurons fire more frequently; while with a lower than anticipated reward, they fire less. For this reason, many researchers believe dopamine may be related more specifically to desire than to pleasure. Physical pleasure itself seems to be derived more from the release of oxytocin and endorphins, although dopamine neuromodulation certainly plays a part.

> *The Anti-Reward Center: An as-yet little-understood subcortical region called the **habenula**, connected to your pineal gland, was found in 2007 to help mediate dopamine reward and punishment signals by strongly inhibiting VTA and SN dopamine release. The habenula is excited when a punishment or no reward is expected, and inhibited when a reward is expected – the opposite anticipatory mechanism of the mesolimbic dopamine pathway.*

2. Nigrostriatal Pathway

The second major dopamine pathway comprises the *basal ganglia motor loop*, which works with the motor cortex and cerebellum, helping govern movement, using modulatory dopamine from the substantia nigra.

The nigrostriatal pathway also works hand-in-hand with your cerebellum and motor cortex to create and manage *procedural memories* – activities you practice to the point they become automatic, such as brushing your teeth or driving a car. The formation of these memories appears to be independent of the hippocampus, instead being made through modifications to synapses in your cerebellum, basal ganglia, and motor cortex, all of which participate in motor control. Evidence for this independent memory system is that procedural memories are unaffected by the hippocampal damage which causes amnesia, but damage to the cerebellum or basal ganglia impairs these skills.

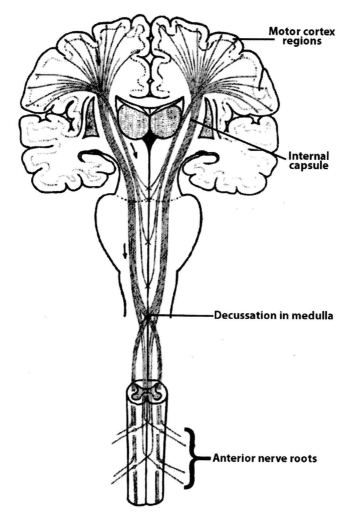

Motor cortex regions

Internal capsule

Decussation in medulla

Anterior nerve roots

To initiate voluntary movements, your motor cortex needs information from throughout your brain and body, including updates from your parietal lobe about your body's position in space, information from your prefrontal cortex about your intended goal and strategy for attaining it, and memories of past strategies from the temporal lobe, etc.

Movements more complex than automatic reflexes require the direction of the motor cortex and centers in the brainstem. The motor cortex orchestrates voluntary, purposeful movement, while the brainstem governs automatic movements like postural control. Both regions send motor control impulses to the spinal cord through descending pathways. Motor neuron axons from the primary motor cortex converge into a bundle called the **internal capsule**, which descends through the cortex, then follows the surface of the medulla. These motor neurons synapse directly with brainstem nuclei and the spinal cord.

Motor impulses travelling from the brain to the spinal cord through these corticospinal tracts cross over one another at the medulla, a process called **decussation**. This means that your brain's left hemisphere controls the right side of your body, while its right hemisphere controls the left. Meanwhile, an additional signal pathway – the corticobulbar tract – carries facial muscle control signals from the motor cortex to cranial nerves in the brainstem. Image: Gray's Anatomy, public domain.

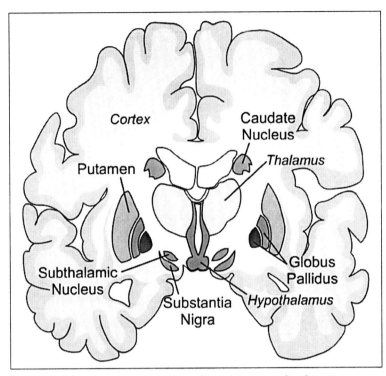

Image: Basal Ganglia, Hopes Brain Tutorial, 2010. Used with permission.

The basal ganglia's four functional regions form a motor control loop, receiving input from the motor cortex, and sending modulating signals back to the cortex through motor regions of the thalamus. The largest structure is the striatum, which receives motor-signal modulating dopamine from the substantia nigra and projects into the globus pallidus and subthalamic nucleus.

Cortical movement planning and execution neurons project to the striatum, then project to the globus pallidus, which projects to motor thalamus. The motor thalamus in turn projects back to the motor cortex. Thus, the caudate, putamen and globus pallidus act upon the motor thalamus, which acts upon the motor cortex, before it sends muscle activation commands to the pons, cerebellum and spinal cord.

The basal ganglia's motor loops are closed circuits, receiving excitatory input from the cortex, and projecting back out to it via the thalamus. The most significant input to the basal ganglia comes from the premotor cortex, used for planning, patterning and initiating movements.

The caudate curves along the lateral ventricle. Its most anterior region is the head, while its tail wraps around like an apostrophe, ending in a "ball" which is the amygdala. Medially – toward the structure's center – are the putamen and globus pallidus, shaped like a lens. Because of this shape, they are collectively called the *lenticular nucleus*.

The striatum's *putamen* is the entrance, and it's fed signals from three main sources: excitatory glutamine from the cortex; and dopamine from the *substantia nigra* and *ventral tegmental area* atop the brainstem (not shown above). The striatum outputs to the *globus pallidus* (pale globe). This relays motor selection and behavioral response signals to motor nuclei in the brainstem, to the motor thalamus, and beyond to the cortex.

There are two signal pathways through the basal ganglia, one directly outputting to the globus pallidus, and the other first detouring through the subthalamic nucleus. These pathways have opposing effects upon movement – one inhibitory and the other *disinhibitory*. A balance between the two is thought to regulate *muscle tone*, a balance of tension in the skeletal muscles. The opposing circuits also help coordinate and monitor gradual, sustained contractions related to posture and support, and in voluntary motor activity selection, suppressing unwanted or unnecessary movement.

> **Disinhibition** – *Inhibitory signals can switch off inhibitory circuits, "releasing the brakes" on neurotransmission. This principle is at work in the basal ganglia, where a circuit can inhibit the substantia nigra's (inhibitory) control of the thalamus.*

The caudate and putamen of the striatum constitute entryways into the system for both the direct and indirect pathways, receiving input from the entire cortex and the thalamus, but primarily premotor cortex regions. The substantia nigra and raphe nuclei also provide modulatory dopamine and serotonin input. Output from the striatum uses entirely GABA inhibitory neurons, signalling the globus pallidus and substantia nigra.

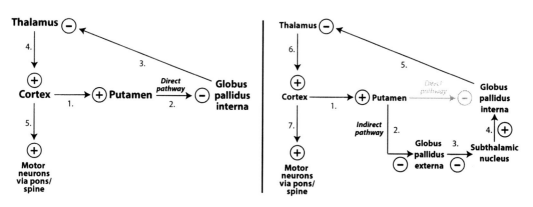

Direct vs. indirect basal ganglia motor control pathways

The Balance

In essence, your basal ganglia function as a complex *braking system*, using a balance of inhibitory and disinhibitory signals. This balance of signals, necessary to execute smooth movement, depends primarily upon dopamine and GABA. All input to the basal ganglia is excitatory, channeled through the putamen; all output is inhibitory, used like a selective braking system to control motor signals between the cortex, thalamus, and brainstem.

Basal ganglia neurons output GABA at a constant rate, ensuring regions of the thalamus and brainstem are under constant, tight inhibitory control. Cortical input can release this control, freeing the brainstem, thalamus and its motor cortex targets from normal inhibition. This process can also selectively allow some motor activities to occur while inhibiting others.

For example, if you swing a tennis racket in an inward stroke, you need to move your wrist and bicep. But there are additional muscles you don't need to engage, so your basal ganglia inhibits their motion, allowing you to focus upon just those muscles required to execute the movement – a function called *surround inhibition*.

Basal ganglia use many different neurotransmitters (acetylcholine, glutamate, GABA, dopamine), but the primary overall effect upon the thalamus, brainstem and motor cortex is inhibitory, and so inhibitory GABA plays the most important role in the basal ganglia, unlike the rest of the brain, where excitatory glutamate is most common.

The basal ganglia are responsible for helping select, initiate, inhibit, and fine-tune movement. This fine-tuning is managed by the looping circuits which integrate your internal input (cognition and intentions), with your external sensory input, and information about the positions of your body parts in space.

These circuits are connected to the cortex, thalamus, limbic system and other regions in a complex series of inhibitory (*GABAergic*) and excitatory (*glutamatergic* and *dopaminergic*) feedback loops, used not just for voluntary motor control, but also for motivation, habit formation and learning procedural memories – skills which eventually don't require concentration to execute, like driving a car.

There are two pathways to the globus pallidus, one direct and one indirect. These two pathways exert opposite effects upon motor activity. The direct path increases excitatory input to the cortex from the motor thalamus – *turning up* motor activity, while the indirect path decreases this excitatory thalamocortical input – *dialing down* motor activity. Thus, activating the direct pathway facilitates movement, while the indirect pathway suppresses it. The direct pathway sends signals directly from the cortex through the striatum to the GPi, increasing excitatory signals from the thalamus to the cortex.

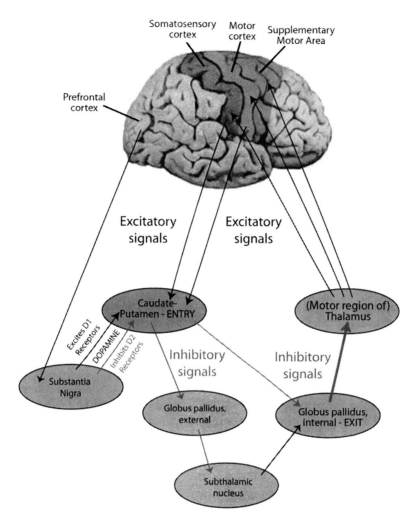

Somatosensory cortex · Motor cortex · Supplementary Motor Area

Prefrontal cortex

Excitatory signals

Excitatory signals

Caudate-Putamen - ENTRY

(Motor region of) Thalamus

Excites D1 Receptors

DOPAMINE

Inhibits D2 Receptors

Inhibitory signals

Inhibitory signals

Substantia Nigra

Globus pallidus, external

Globus pallidus, internal - EXIT

Subthalamic nucleus

BASAL GANGLIA MOTOR CIRCUITS

The cortex activates the striatum with glutamate. Striatal neurons send inhibitory GABA to the GPi. GPi cells also use GABA signalling upon the motor thalamus, but, because they have been inhibited, they ease up on their own inhibition of the motor thalamus. When the motor thalamus receives *less* inhibition, it increases firing to the motor cortex. Thus, the direct pathway turns the motor system up, resulting in increased muscle activation.

In the Indirect Pathway, the cortex activates the striatum with glutamate, which sends inhibitory GABA to the GPe, decreasing the inhibitory signals to the subthalamic nucleus. These subthalamic nucleus cells use excitatory glutamate to activate the GPi, which sends more inhibitory GABA signals to the motor thalamus and beyond to the

467

motor cortex. This *decreases* excitatory output from the thalamus to the cortex. The overall effect is that the motor thalamus receives *more* inhibition, and decreases firing to the motor cortex. Thus, the indirect pathway turns the motor system down, resulting in decreased muscle activation.

Neurons in the striatum are modulated by two important neurotransmitter systems. Each differentially affects both the direct and the indirect pathways, altering the amount of motor activity which is produced. Dopamine from the substantia nigra to the striatum *excites* striatal cells in the direct pathway by activating D1 receptors.

However, dopamine *inhibits* striatal cells in the indirect pathway, by activating D2 receptors. This means that the direct pathway – used to increase motor activity – can be excited by dopamine, while the indirect pathway – used to decrease motor activity – can be inhibited by dopamine. Because of the receptors, *dopamine's effects are the opposite in each pathway*, but the end result is that *dopamine increases motor activity along both pathways.*

A second group of *cholinergic* (acetylcholine-using) modulatory neurons act only within the striatum. They work in opposition to dopamine striatal signalling, inhibiting the direct pathway and exciting the indirect pathway. The end result is that *actylcholine decreases motor activity along both pathways.*

The Power to Choose

It's believed the basal ganglia engage in *motor selection*: your brain needs to determine which competing behavior pattern should be allowed control of the brain's shared motor system at any given instant. Two-way parallel loops from cortical and sub-cortical systems send competing excitatory signals to your basal ganglia. *Input salience* is compared, and the most salient inputs are *selectively disinhibited* – allowed to trigger motor activity.

In the ventral striatum, inputs arrive from structures in which intentions arise, such as the prefrontal cortex, amygdala and hippocampus, while in the dorsal (upper) striatum, input comes from regions which guide movements – the somatosensory and motor cortices. Thus, intent is integrated with action to produce action selection. This goal-directed behavior is a three-tier process, with selection required at each step:

1. goal selection

2. action selection to achieve the goal

3. movement selection to achieve the action.

Goal, action and movement selection are thought to arise from, respectively, limbic, associative (cortical) and sensorimotor circuit input to the basal ganglia. The basal ganglia's multiple control loops allow you to select actions, and repeated use of these specific chosen circuits results in the development of a habit, synaptic reorganization modulated by reward-system dopamine signals from the substantia nigra and VTA.

Thus, the nigrostriatal pathway constitutes an additional reward system: functional MRI studies on drug addictions clearly show the connection between motor control and learning circuits within the basal ganglia. For example, just watching another addict manipulating drug paraphernalia is enough to strongly activate the basal ganglia of cocaine addicts, not only in the mesolimbic pathway, but also the nigrostriatal pathway.

MIT's Dr. Ann Graybiel studies the progress of drug addiction within the brain, and she has discovered specific changes in gene activation which appear to underlie the extreme habits of drug abuse, obsessive-compulsive disorder, and Tourette's syndrome.

According to Dr. Graybiel, just a single shot of amphetamine leads to genetic changes in the basal ganglia, leading to increased transcription factor expression. These genetic changes are most apparent in tissue patches called *striosomes*, used to in controlling dopamine and possibly acetylcholine transmission, and the effects come primarily from two genes – *CalDEG-GEF1* and *CalDEG-GEF2*.

Genetic changes in the dopamine-acetylcholine system seem to be central to a wide range of drug addictions, particularly changes to genes in regions such as the striatum, which are central to both obsessive-compulsive disorder and drug addiction. Since the dopamine and cholinergic systems provide an opposing seesaw balance of control, changes in their function can have a major impact upon voluntary and involuntary motor activities and behaviors.

The Evolution of Goal-Oriented Behavior

It's been proposed that the complexity of the basal ganglia – with their interconnections throughout the frontal lobes, motor cortex, thalamus, hippocampus and amygdala – evolved to protect your brain and body from excessive overstimulation.

What's more certain is that together, your striatum and thalamus act as an interface between your most highly-evolved cortical motor centers, and the more primitive behavioral response circuits of your brainstem. The two structures – striatum and motor thalamus – evolved in tandem, gradually increasing interlinks between sensory processing and behavioral-emotional motor output.

The basal ganglia and hindbrain (brainstem, and cerebellum) have participated in motor control throughout vertebrate history, just as with modern humans. The human form of the system works in conjunction with the limbic system (amygdala, hypothalamus, hippocampus, septal area and related control regions) to govern primitive, instinctual responses to the environment.

The basal ganglia first evolved from primitive olfactory-amygdala circuits called the *rhinoencephalon* (Latin for nose brain), which are often considered an extension of the limbic system. The striatum was formerly subservient to the amygdala, and the entire forebrain, including the amygdala, hypothalamus, and hippocampus, was influenced by the olfactory system to a great degree, olfactory stimuli giving rise to basic behaviors like the "four Fs" – feeding, fighting, fleeing, and sexual intercourse.

Early in the course of evolution, the amygdala and striatum separated because of the increased need for complex movements. As sea animals began to evolve into amphibians and live on dry land, the amygdala and striatum had almost completely separated, but the connection still exists in humans, where the striatum's tail becomes the amygdala.

From this point, the amygdala and striatum continued to evolve separately, and the olfactory bulb and its related olfactory-processing neural structures expanded, allowing animals to adapt to a world where a finely-tuned sense of smell was vital for survival.

In humans, the amygdala and basal ganglia have evolved to work as a cohesive functional unit for governing defensive and other emotional behaviors which involve major body movements like kicking, flailing, or running, and kicking. The amygdala exerts a great deal of influence on the basal ganglia, which seem to have evolved from the amygdala to serve as a specialized emotional-motor interface so that amygdala/hypothalamus-generated needs and impulses can be acted on in a flexible way.

The basal ganglia are critical for such motor expression of social/emotional states as fleeing in panic, biting defensively, punching and kicking, or for conveying emotion through facial expressions, posture, muscle tension, and/or gestures. These emotional expressions are generated at a deep, fundamental anatomical level – universal expressions of happiness, sadness, and anger are easily identifiable throughout history and across diverse cultures.

> **The animal that eats its own brain** – It's not surprising that the evolution of a movement-control center plays such a major role in the human brain – according to Dr. Rodolfo R. Llinás, Chairman of the Physiology and Neuroscience Department at the NYU School of Medicine, the brain itself evolved from the need to govern motion. Along with triggering actual muscle contractions, movement requires intentions and predictions, which are, says Dr. Llinas, the basis of thought.
>
> As proof of his argument, he offers the example of tunicates like the **sea squirt**, a primitive, filter-feeding marine animal. Adult tunicates are all sessile, but before they settle down and permanently attach themselves to rock, their larval form swims about in search of the ideal spot to plant itself.
>
> A sea squirt larva has a rudimentary brain in the form of a cerebral ganglion, which controls its movement as it swims about in search of a permanent home. upon settling down, as the creature matures, it no longer needs a brain to guide movement, so it simply digests its own.

The basal ganglia's role as interface between the cortex and limbic system means disturbances in the basal ganglia can affect the functionality of both regions. Injury or abnormalities in the region, particularly diminished dopamine levels, can result in a number of cognitive, *affective* (emotional), or motor problems such as Parkinson's, Huntington's and Alzheimer's disease, *hemiballismus* (uncontrolled kicking and punching), obsessive compulsive disorder, or depression.

When Things Go Wrong: Parkinson's Disease

Damage within this region results in two types of problems, marked by either an increase in movement (*hyperkinesia*) or a decrease in movement (*hypokinesia*). *Huntington's disease* is a form of hyperkinesia – uncontrollable jerking, caused by deterioration of GABAergic cells in the caudate, while *Parkinson's disease* is an example of hypokinesia – impaired movement caused by the death of dopamine-producing cells.

The nigrostriatal pathway in the midbrain transports dopamine from the substantia nigra to the striatum. This dopamine-rich midbrain pathway below the thalamus is where Parkinson's disease occurs. Its color is derived from *neuromelanin*, an enzyme related to skin pigment. One region called the *pars compacta* sends dopamine signals up to the striatum. Parkinson's disease arises from the death of dopamine neurons in this region.

The second region of the substantia nigra is called the *pars reticulata*. It's comprised mainly of GABA neurons, and primarily controls eye movements. Dysfunction of the region is also involved in Parkinson's disease and in epilepsy.

The death of dopamine-producing neurons in the nigrostriatal pathway results in *Parkinson's Disease*; when about 75% have died, symptoms begin to appear, including uncontrollable tremors, slow, rigid movement, difficulty walking, and eventually *dementia*, the extreme loss of mental function usually associated with aging.

In 2013, researchers at Researchers at Washington University School of Medicine in St. Louis announced they had finally uncovered the cause of this tragic and mysterious illness. Drs. Gerald W. Dorn II and Yun Chen say that faulty mitochondria in the substantia nigra can build up, eventually reaching toxic levels. At that point, instead of making fuel, they begin consuming it, leading to neural death.

Under normal conditions, mitochondria are monitored, to ensure that dysfunctional or damaged ones are quickly found and destroyed. The problem arises with a special signalling protein called *mitofusin 2* (Mfn2). Mitofusin 1 and 2 are typically used to temporarily join mitochondria, allowing the conjugational exchange of DNA.

However, Mfn2 has an additional role in quality-control. Healthy mitochondria must actively work to keep a chemical switch turned off to prevent their own self-destruction, by importing and destroying a molecule called *PINK*. Dysfunctional mitochondria cannot destroy PINK, so it begins to accumulate. High levels of PINK cause phosphorylation of Mfn2 on the mitochondrial surface. This attracts a signalling molecule called *Parkin*, in the cell cytoplasm. Parkin binds to phosphorylated Mfn2, marking the faulty mitochondrion for destruction. The Parkin label attracts special organelles within the host cell, which consume and destroy faulty mitochondria.

When all the links within this quality-control system are functioning properly, damaged mitochondria are destroyed. However, mutations in PINK, Parkin and Mfn2 can all cause Parkinson's disease, as well as certain forms of heart failure, gradually killing heart muscles, and impairing bloodflow into the body.

When Things Go Wrong: Obsessive-Compulsive Disorder

Stress can come not just from external pressures – work, school, or social relationships – but also from internal pressures – your own personally objectionable or negative thoughts, moods and impulses. The caudate plays a central role in such mental activity, acting like an *automatic transmission* in your brain, allowing you to switch between mental tasks as needed. This process influences motor function, cognition, mood and behavior in several ways, including the development of *obsessive-compulsive disorders* – the persistent appearance of unbidden, unwanted thoughts (obsessions) and the drive to repeatedly perform rituals to banish these thoughts (compulsions).

It's estimated that 2.5% of the world's population suffers from OCD – some suffering only from obsessions, some from compulsions, but the majority suffering from both. The obsessions tend to be concerned with contamination or religion, coupled with cleansing rituals. Intrusive, unpleasant, violent and/or sexual imagery is common.

The compulsion component of the disorder provides a means of coping with these unwanted or disturbing impulses: by engaging in certain actions or repeating certain thought patterns, the sufferer is able to escape acting upon or consciously acknowledging personally objectionable thoughts, actions, or impulses.

Error detection circuits in the *cingulate cortex* (see below), which access the caudate can get locked in gear, with the result being persistent obsessive thoughts that can't be banished. The cingulate cortex seems to regulate error detection – so in OCD, one's cognitive "errors" are repeatedly brought to the forefront of consciousness. The end result is that a person becomes bombarded with very troublesome thoughts or feelings.

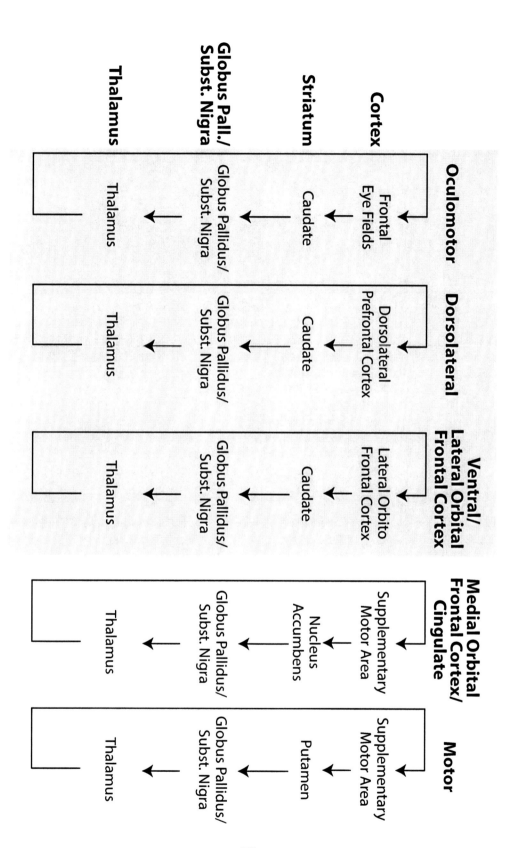

473

When the "executive control center" of your brain – the prefrontal cortex – receives an error detection signal from the cingulate cortex, it sends these signals to the caudate nucleus, which acts like an automatic transmission, shifting gears (attention and mental resources) after the problem has been dealt with. But mainly due to genetic traits, the caudate can become "stuck in gear", leading to a repeated rehearsal of these troublesome thoughts, bombarding conscious awareness.

Caudate damage seems to leave sufferers "stuck" on a theme or activity, with little self-awareness or ability to evaluate their *obsessive* or *compulsive* behavior. This low self-awareness seems to make them unaware of their own atypical behaviors which are obvious to others, and to impair their emotional depth and ability to see other viewpoints, making it difficult for them to maintain healthy relationships.

The caudate and cingulate cortex send messages to the *orbitofrontal cortex,* just above the eyes, which appear to inform the brain when something is amiss and corrective measures need to be taken, sending messages such as *Make sure the stove has been turned off!* and *Wash your hands!* Obsessive compulsive disorder (OCD) is thought to be the result of overactivation of this caudate function.

It's believed the frontal lobe has lost control over the caudate, or there's been a loss of inhibitory striatum influence on the frontal lobe. Obsessive-compulsive disorders have been linked to hyperactivity in the caudate – as well as reduced serotonin levels, resulting in the disinhibition and overwhelming of inhibitory control circuits in the basal ganglia.

These frontal lobe/basal ganglia inhibitory circuits are used to prevent someone from engaging in acts they find objectionable or "dirty." The frontal lobes control integration, inhibition and/or suppression of thoughts and emotions; caudate and frontal lobe dysfunction can therefore result in an inability to extinguish certain thoughts and actions, and these persistent, repetitive thoughts or actions can interfere with the ability to choose alternative responses. The end result is that the OCD sufferer repetitively dwells on a certain theme, thought, or action to the exclusion of others.

A homophobe who secretly harbors homosexual desires might *sublimate* impulses to act out on hidden desires, substituting another behavior, for example, rubbing, polishing and cleaning, thus symbolically cleansing what he perceives as "dirty" thoughts. Here, he engages the prefrontal cortex and basal ganglia in impulse inhibition and memory avoidance (repression).

Your caudate, cingulate and frontal lobes work together to prioritize information transfer in your brain. Experiments show the caudate also contributes to the short-term "scratch pad" type of memory called *working memory,* particularly in regard to planning and selecting motor sequences. Consequently, damage to the caudate can seriously impair frontal lobe function, supplying incomplete or biased information, making it difficult to prioritize, to organize, and manage simultaneous tasks. Damage seems to result in behavioral changes such as an inability to control emotions, impulses, thoughts and movements, or sometimes in an inability to experience embarrassment, guilt or shame, emotions used to help curb socially unacceptable behaviors.

> **Unable To Focus** – ADHD is the most common behavioral disorder diagnosed in children, said to affect about 2 million in America alone. It's characterized by hyperactivity, inattentiveness and impulsive behavior.
>
> In a 2011 study, Kennedy Krieger neuroscientists found preschoolers with ADHD have differences in their caudate structure. fMRI scans in studies of 4- and 5-year-olds with and without ADHD symptoms showed cortical and basal ganglia size differences, specifically in the caudate nucleus, associated with cognitive and motor control.
>
> According to Dr. Mark Mahone, lead author of the study, children with ADHD have significantly smaller caudates than children without ADHD symptoms. Smaller caudate volumes were also accompanied by parental reports of hyperactivity and impulsiveness. These differences in caudate development appear to be at the heart of the attention problems, hyperactivity and impulsiveness of ADHD, contributing to cognitive challenges and academic difficulties.

A caudate which *underperforms* seems to underlie a number of disorders, including ADHD, autism, depression, and the recently-discovered *PAP syndrome*, which involves a dramatic drop in motivation.

Because the caudate and frontal lobes are highly connected with the amygdala, in times of extreme stress – such as terror – a *catatonic* (frozen) panic state can result, as the amygdala overwhelms connections to the PAG, striatum and frontal lobes. This amygdalar-PAG-striatal circuit is central to and to predatory behavior, threat perception and responses.

This freezing reaction to extreme panic is probably linked to the act of playing dead as a survival mechanism. In these states of frozen panic, attention may become narrowed to the point at which the mind shuts down – little to nothing is perceived and cognitive ability vanishes temporarily. It's been suggested the accompanying physical numbing comes from a massive secretion of endogenous opiates, and that the paralysis and loss of the will to fight comes from overwhelming fear – an extreme overactivation of the amygdala, resulting in inhibition of the frontal lobe and striatum. The amygdala appears to trigger a complete arrest of motor and cognitive activity via the brainstem and striatum.

The airline industry refers to this as a *frozen panic state*, sometimes seen during air and sea disasters. In such mass disasters, 10-25% of victims become completely incapacitated in this way – stunned and immobile, unable to even take the smallest self-preserving steps, like trying to escape from a burning vehicle, even if they have no injuries preventing such an escape.

The evolutionary advantages of being able to shut down distracting pain or fear are obvious, but the evolutionary advantage of physical paralysis is less so. But by becoming immobile, animals in the wild often escape the notice of predators, or appear to be non-living prey, which many predators refuse to eat. It's also a signal of complete surrender, possibly ensuring a painless death. In such cases, a prey animal has given up attempts to fight or flee, allowing itself to be eaten alive.

The adaptive behavior of playing dead has also been observed in humans during war-time. Witnesses of atrocities sometimes collapse in a state superficially resembling death, remaining essentially catatonic for long periods, even though they're unharmed. As a result, they're sometimes mistaken for the dead, even by potential rescuers.

Cerebellum vs. Basal Ganglia

Movement is orchestrated by the interplay of three brain regions: your basal ganglia and cerebellum work at the bidding of your cortex to modify movement on a moment-by-moment basis. Two-way circuits connect the basal ganglia and cerebellum. The cerebellum's output region – the *dentate nucleus* – projects into the striatum, while the basal ganglia's subthalamic nucleus projects into the cerebellum through the pons in the brainstem. These reciprocal connections enable two-way communication between the basal ganglia and cerebellum, and both pathways also have parallel two-way connections with the cortex.

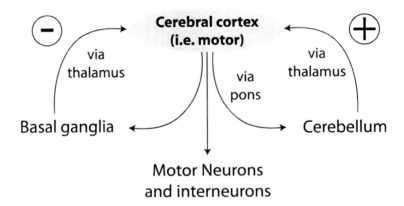

Both the basal ganglia and cerebellum simultaneously receive input from your motor cortex, processing and outputting it back through your thalamus, the gateway between the subcortical and cortical structures. Cerebellum output to your motor cortex is *excitatory*, while the basal ganglia's is *inhibitory*. Both systems are in balance, allowing for smooth, coordinated movement, and disturbances in either system are manifested as movement disorders.

Your cerebellum compares motor cortex intentions with actual motor outcomes, based on the position of proprioceptors in your trunk and limbs, correcting your movements on the fly. The cerebellum is also partially responsible for learning procedural memories – motor skills such as riding a bicycle. While the basal ganglia oversee the choreography of overall movements, the cerebellum coordinates every individual skeletal muscle.

The cerebellum is greatly involved in both planning and coordinating movement. It helps develop new motor programs which enable voluntary movements to develop with practice into rapid *ballistic* movements. Examples include speaking, writing, playing musical instruments, and most athletic skills. It's also responsible for maintaining steady, non-relaxed positioning of the hands, feet, trunk, head, and limbs.

Motor commands from the motor cortex to the spine are intercepted at the pons and relayed to the cerebellum, which appears to maintain an internal mental model of the body. This representation includes all the body parts and their positions relative to one other from moment to moment.

The cerebellum seems to use this mental model to simulate the actions initiated by the motor cortex before they are actually performed. It examines these simulated movements for errors, calculates corrections, then resimulates the action until a correct version is produced, at which point the commands are allowed to be relayed down to the appropriate muscles.

Voluntary motor movements which improve with practice are governed by the cerebellum, which has its own special nuclear center in the thalamus, receiving input from the motor cortex via the pons, and reciprocally to and from the basal ganglia.

The jerky movements and lack of coordination seen in alcohol intoxication come from suppression of cerebellar function (i.e. walking in a straight line). Prolonged, extreme alcohol abuse also eventually kills these cells, and, since neurons don't undergo mitosis (don't regenerate) after birth, this destruction is permanent.

The basal ganglia are important for overall postures and movements of the body, controlling slower, more gradual movements which are modified by sensory feedback while the movement is still underway. Damage to dopamine neurons in the basal ganglia results in Parkinson's disease, a progressive deterioration in the ability to walk, stand, and other movements of the body as a whole. Within the basal ganglia, the caudate acts as a central mechanism for automatic motor behaviors – this, again, is the region found to be malfunctioning in OCD patients.

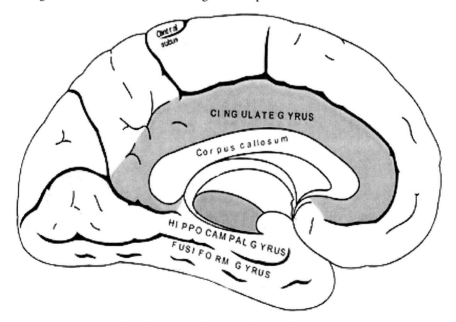

Cingulate Cortex, Gray's Anatomy, public domain

477

Cingulate Cortex

The *cingulate cortex* (also called the *cingulate gyrus)* is a band of tissue forming a *cingulum* – Latin for belt – surrounding the corpus callosum – the flat neural sheet joining your brain's left and right hemispheres in the medial region of your brain.

Wrapped around the corpus callosum and connecting the limbic system and prefrontal cortex, the cingulate cortex appears to monitor the brain for errors, to integrate emotion with cognition, to help regulate emotions, and to assist in inhibiting responses and making decisions. Researchers believe this brain circuit searches for information-processing conflicts, providing a kind of neural self-regulation.

It seems involved with shifting attention, and activates when you focus attention inward, or when you experience sadness, anxiety or phobias. Because the brain engages in constant, massive parallel processing, conflicting streams of information from different brain processing regions can sometimes interfere with one another, impairing performance. Tracking and avoiding such conflicts is necessary.

The cingulate also appears to mediate when emotions and rational thought compete for your brain's time and energy – the mind appears able to focus on one or the other, but not both simultaneously.

The surface of each person's cingulate cortex varies widely, and it's said that everyone has his or her own unique cingulate surface "fingerprint". Its functions are not yet fully understood, but fMRI and PET scans show it seems to govern the following functions:

- Detecting errors
- Constructing mental models of yourself and others
- Building trust in others
- Assisting in selecting responses
- Assisting in processing visuo-spatial information
- Integrating sensory information for emotion construction
- Modulating emotional responses to pain
- Switching between reward-based tasks
- Relaying signals related to pain perception and the *placebo effect*
- Helping the cortex regulate aggression

The cingulate cortex is functionally divided into four separate regions, with input from the amygdala, thalamus, and *parietal lobe* – the region of the cortex that unites spatial navigation data into unified perception, and constructs a virtual coordinate system of the world around you.

The cingulate outputs to autonomic motor systems in your brainstem and to your *entorhinal cortex* – the gateway between the cortex and hippocampus, a hub for widespread memory and navigational circuits throughout your brain.

The four functional regions of the cingulate cortex are:

Anterior, dealing with *affect* (emotion) and error/conflict monitoring

Medial, dealing with error detection, response selection and motor control

Retrosplenial cortex, dealing with short-term memory use

Posterior, dealing with visuo-spatial processing.

Anterior – considered by some to be functionally part of the frontal lobe, the *Anterior Cingulate Cortex* (ACC) plays a major role in directing attention and maintaining vigilance. It seems to coordinate attention processes between areas of the cortex which integrate all the senses (*association areas*) during novel or significantly difficult tasks.

The Anterior Cingulate Cortex directs your attention by inhibiting activity related to irrelevant stimuli. In this way, it's a major part of generating attention in the executive control system of the frontal lobes of your brain. When there are novel or complex cognitive tasks, the ACC coordinates attention control in the prefrontal, parietal and temporal association areas, acting as sort of a circuit switch. ADHD (Attention Deficit Hyperactive Disorder) may be a malfunction of this attention switching circuit.

The ACC is the most significant cortical inhibitor, mediating between cortical regions, so if conflicting stimuli demand attention, the ACC inhibits signals which need to be disregarded. Thus, the ACC appears to be a major attention switch, working in concert with the prefrontal cortex. When choosing among several possible goals or alternatives, the prefrontal cortex and ACC oversee the processes of choosing, accessing information in parallel processes from among cortical association areas.

This region is also involved in emotions, activating ANS responses to emotion through connections to the hypothalamus, brainstem, periaqueductal gray and two-way connections with the amygdala. It helps integrate sights, sounds, sensations, tastes and smells into emotions, and helps the PFC regulate aggression. The ACC is also an active component in detecting and monitoring errors, evaluating the degree of error, and suggesting appropriate corrective actions.

The ACC seems to be where visceral sensations (insula), arousal states (reticular formation), directed focus (ACC, thalamus, PFC) and emotion (limbic system) are integrated. Thus it seems to be a key center for generating a conscious experience of emotions - where a mental representation of the physical self in terms of autonomic arousal emerges. The ACC also seems to allow the prefrontal cortex to regulate emotion, aggression and other types of top-down control.

The ACC seems to be central to detecting conflicts between a creature's present functional state and new information with potential emotional or motivational consequences. When conflicts are found, the ACC relays this information to prefrontal cortex regions where potential responses can be weighed and selected.

More recently, researchers at Columbia University have used functional magnetic resonance imaging to show that a region in the ACC acts as a dampener on the amygdala, providing an emotional "on-off switch". The ACC's specific functions appear to include:

- *Thought/emotion integrator* – An amplifier and filter that integrates emotional and cognitive processing,

- *Performance monitor* – watches for errors, uncertainty and conflicts in thought-processing.

- *Paying attention* – monitors sensory input from the thalamus and chooses what we pay attention to, directing the thalamus for selective excitation and inhibition.

- *Decision-making* – assists the frontal lobes in assessing rewards vs. risks and conflicts, based upon past experiences. The frontal cortex uses this evaluation in selecting the appropriate response.

- *Response inhibition* – integrates prefrontal cortex input and detects and corrects errors in behavior.

- *Controlling and detecting emotions* – monitors emotion-derived sensations, pain, and physical arousal, and controls the voluntary suppression of such sensations.

Go/No-Go – *The Go/No-Go test is used to demonstrate the ACC's role in error and conflict detection. In this task, images are presented to volunteers in a continuous stream, and they are asked to respond with a choice between two alternatives. Go states require a response, while NoGo states require inhibiting responses. This leads to an increase in potential errors – errors the ACC watches for and attempts to correct.*

A Go-No-Go Error Awareness Task (EAT), for example, shows a series of color names, where the colors of the letters sometimes don't match the words they spell, causing confusion when rapid responses are required; for example, sometimes the word green is spelled out in red letters.

Volunteers are told to press a button if the font color matches the color name, and to hold off from responding if the same word is repeated or if the word and its color didn't match. If they made a mistake – pressing a button when they weren't supposed to – they then press a second button showing they are aware of the mistake.

EEG, skin conductance, eye movement, and fMRI scans of brain blood flow can all be measured during these tests, showing which areas activate upon discovering conflicting information (e.g. the word blue spelled out in red letters) or errors in their actions or thoughts. The Anterior Cingulate Cortex consistently lights up with activity whenever these tests are performed.

Medial – The MCC works with the basal ganglia in selecting responses with the highest salience, implementing these behaviors through spinal and cortex motor outputs to skeletal muscles. While the ACC seems to help direct *visceral* motor activation, the MCC is believed to help control *skeletal* motor activation.

The region also assists with working (very short-term) memory, reward anticipation, monitoring inner competition for resource control, and error detection. It outputs to the spinal cord, motor cortices and limbic system. fMRI studies show it has a major role in response selection, directing behavioral changes to changing rewards.

Retrosplenial – the hippocampus and thalamus are strongly interconnected with this region, where tasks which require holding small bits of information (e.g. phone numbers) in short-term working memory activate the RSC region of the cingulate and thalamus in a special circuit that seems central to working memory.

Posterior – This region works with the parietal lobe and hippocampus in forming *topographic* and *topokinetic* memory, the mental construction of visual maps used for navigation, and one's physical movement through those mental maps. It also deals with reward responses, and integrating sensory and motor information with established behavior patterns, below conscious awareness. Finally, it seems to help process emotional autobiographical memories and one's internal emotional outlook on oneself and others.

The cingulate cortex and related bundle of nerve fibers called the *cingulum bundle* are sometimes the target of surgery to alleviate chronic pain and remedy severe anxiety, major depression, and obsessive-compulsive disorder.

---

*Locked In Forever Alone – A dysfunctional cingulate cortex may lie at the heart of **autism**, where sufferers seem locked into an internal world, unable to fully relate to others. Autistic patients have difficulties in constructing mental self-concepts, impairing their ability to understand and relate to the world, according to 2006 fMRI research from the Baylor College of Medicine. In other words, they seem unable to understand the concept of themselves and others as separate beings in a social exchange, and never fully develop healthy social skills. Successful social interaction requires building mental models of oneself and other people, then using these models as guides for behavior.*

Paying Attention Sets Off a Symphony of Cell Synchronization

When your mind wanders, details can fade into the background, with the potential for missing them, but if something engages your attention, it stands out sharply in your mind. The mechanism underlying how attention thus sharpens perception has recently been uncovered by researchers at Northwestern University, who show that paying attention isn't just a matter of neurons responding more strongly (firing at a faster rate); a wide population of neurons responds in *synchronicity*, like an orchestra playing together, instead of individual musicians bleating and hooting randomly. Thus, attention makes a stimulus stand out by making your brain's responses to it more coordinated and coherent.

fMRI scans show that a region called the *intraparietal sulcus* is key for engaging attention: your cortex contains regions for processing sight, sound, olfactory, gustatory, somatosensory and motor information. Mediating between them is the intraparietal sulcus, which contains a miniature map of all of these neural circuits. Your brain's control centers (PFC and cingulate cortex) connect to this neural map, using it to switch your attention from one set of stimuli to another.

There are at least 13 duplicates of this miniature map of things you can pay attention to reproduced throughout your brain, all with connections to the intraparietal sulcus. Each map copy seems to do something different – one map processes eye movements, while another processes analytical information. These sensory maps representing reality appear to be a fundamental basis of how information is represented in the brain.

Cerebral Cortex

Think of your brain as a construction company: the CEO would be your cerebral cortex, the other subsystems acting as departmental heads reporting to the boss. Just as the CEO directs corporate strategy, your cortex analyzes and integrates incoming sensory data, ised for decision-making. Along the way, every employee affects the company, just as every synapse provides an opportunity to modulate signals – dampening or heightening them.

The mail room (relay stations in the brainstem) routes messages upstairs or deals with them locally. All this information is forwarded, examined and evaluated by the executive secretary – the thalamus – before being passed on to the CEO. The secretary can put through some phone calls or paper correspondence (excitatory signals) while putting some on hold (inhibitory signals). Feedback between boss and secretary is constant and two-way.

Just as the CEO (cortex) can direct his staff to concentrate on specific tasks, the cortex can use circuits in the cingulate, limbic system and basal ganglia to zero in on and select tasks which deserve special attention. These are like department heads who handle task scheduling and other functions the boss is unaware of and doesn't need to be concerned with. The hypothalamus acts as the building superintendent, ensuring all the plumbing, power and ventilation systems work efficiently.

The CEO decides how to respond to incoming information, sending orders to the motor cortices to take action, via the basal ganglia – "vice presidents" which implement the logistics of corporate strategy, based on company success and failure. When orders are sent to the cerebellum, it acts as a foreman, telling each individual worker (muscle) onsite what his individual task will be. The foreman gets feedback from his workers and measures progress against his blueprints (motor programs) to ensure instructions are being followed.

The Crowning Achievement

The human cerebral cortex has been called the crowning achievement of evolution. It's the outermost layer of the human brain, comprised of about 200 distinct regions, though for naming conventions, it was divided into 50 numbered areas in 1918, a system still in use today among neuroscientists.

The cerebral cortex has two hemispheres, each receiving information from the opposite side of the body. Its divisions – the lobes of the brain – can be easily distinguished by the deep fissures (sulci) which divide them. They are the *frontal lobe* (specialized for planning, judgment, movement control and other higher functions), the *parietal lobe* (specialized for processing touch and body sensations), the *occipital lobe* (specialized for visual processing), the *temporal lobe* (specialized for auditory perception), and, arguably, the *limbic system* (specialized for emotional processing).

There are two types of brain regions: *projection areas*, which either receive sensory input or send motor output; and *association areas*, which integrate and process multiple sensory data. Most of the cortex is devoted to either sensory processing or motor control processing.

The three regions in which all sensory input from the outer world (perception) is integrated into the experience called reality are the *association cortices*: 1) the prefrontal area, dedicated to executive functions; 2) the *parietal-occipital-temporal junction*, a *multimodal area*, in which all the senses are integrated; and 3) the limbic system, dedicated to emotion and memory. In other words, thinking as we know it primarily occurs within these regions, where perceptions converge into an overall *percept* of the environment, and evaluation and planning occur.

Within these association areas, long-term memories are thought to be created through protein synthesis, physical changes to the synapses connecting far-ranging regions of your cortex. To recap, your cortex is the physically largest part of your brain, second only to the cerebellum in neural density. Soma color the surface of the cortex a grayish-brown, hence the name gray matter. Beneath this layer are the long connecting fibers of the axons, comprising the lighter gray – so-called white matter. Your brain is divided into twin hemispheres, joined by a thick sheet of nerve tissue called the corpus callosum, which allows communication between the two halves.

This bilateral architecture is echoed in many of the brain's substructures, as well as throughout the human body. For right-handed people, the left hemisphere is more frequently activated for language, math, and logic, and the right hemisphere is more frequently activated for pattern recognition, nonverbal thought, and emotional processing. Communication between the hemispheres is through the large connective sheet of nerve tissue called the corpus callosum. The corpus callosum (which means hard body in Latin) is like a carrot which would snap in your hand, unlike the gelatinous consistency of most of the brain. This sheet relays and coordinates information between the two hemispheres.

Each hemisphere is divided by deep grooves called sulci into four lobes – major regions with specific known functions. The largest is the frontal lobe, which is bigger in humans than in any other animal. Most higher thought processes are conducted here. The folding of the cortical surface increases your brain's surface area, allowing more neurons to fit inside the skull and enabling higher functions – lower intelligence animals have smooth cortices. Each fold is called a gyrus, and each groove between these folds is called a sulcus.

If you recall the illustration of the homunculus, sensory data input and processing is organized sequentially across the surface of the cortex, with sight being granted the highest priority and therefore the largest amount of cortical "real estate". The body parts with the largest number of nerve endings – fingers, tongue, eyes – have the greatest amount of cortical surface area dedicated to them.

Sensory processing regions are arranged in side-by-side columns of nerve tissue, with each column responsible for reading and interpreting a small portion of the overall data that's coming in.

One tissue column will be dedicated to processing a certain portion of the visual field or a specific sound frequency, or a specific sensation in a specific region of the body; your cortex integrates, interprets and acts upon all this separate sensory data as a whole. Of course, all this processing is happening simultaneously, in what's called parallel processing, while the cortex is in the midst of managing speech, reasoning, emotions, learning, and movement planning.

The Cortex's Powerful Inhibitors

The neocortex is the uniquely human brain region which distinguishes us from other species. It's responsible for our sensory perception, conscious thought, language, reasoning, analysis, judgment and decision making.

The bulk of the cortex is comprised of excitatory *pyramidal cells*, but sparsely distributed among them are a special type of inhibitory neurons called *chandelier cells*, named after their resemblance to old-fashioned candlesticks. These unique cells are suspended individually among large numbers of excitatory pyramidal cells, the comparatively short branches of chandelier cells contacting their excitatory neighbors.

A single chandelier cell may synapse with as many as 500 pyramidal neurons, and is thus able to affect multiple neighboring excitatory pyramidal cells, causing chain reactions throughout the brain.

Though their operation is still not fully understood, it's thought that they operate by exerting a kind of "veto" power over messages exchanged among the much more numerous excitatory cells surrounding them. Recent experiments also suggest they play a vital role in balancing message flow, and in helping organize excitatory neurons into functional groups.

Unlike other inhibitory neurons, chandelier cells connect with excitatory pyramidal cells at a single location of extreme importance: the region called the *axon initial segment* (AIS), where a "broadcasting" pyramidal cell creates the message it's transmitting. Since one cell appears to be regulating the "broadcast" messages of 500 neighbors, each individual chandelier cell seems to play a vital role in coordinating and spreading messages throughout its region.

Chandelier cells are also found in the brains of other animal species, but in humans they are uniquely robust and complex, suggesting they play an important role in higher intelligence. Interestingly, the number and synaptic density of chandelier cells is significantly lower among schizophrenics, and epileptics also have abnormally-formed chandelier cells.

Cortical Lobes

Each cortical hemisphere has four lobes: *frontal, temporal, parietal,* and *occipital.* Each of these lobes serves very specific functions, but none of them functions alone; all are within constant cross-communication, integrating functionality throughout the enormous complexity of your brain.

Frontal

- Personality, behavior, emotions

- Judgment, planning, problem solving

- *Producing* language: speaking and writing (Broca's area)

- Body movement (motor strip)

- Self-control and conscious-level sense of self

Parietal (*rear and top of the skull*)

- Visual attention, touch, pain, temperature perception (somatosensory strip)

- Integration of senses into overall perception

- Spatial and visual perception

Occipital (back and base of the cortex)

- Processes vision (*color, light, movement*)

Temporal (*lateral, at the sides on the level of the ears*)

- *Understanding* language (Wernicke's area)

- Hearing

- Memory

- Sequencing, organization, categorization of objects

LOBES OF THE CEREBRAL CORTEX

Integrates sensory information, including motion perception and awareness of the body's orientation in space, language comprehension, spatial organization and perception

Processes visual information

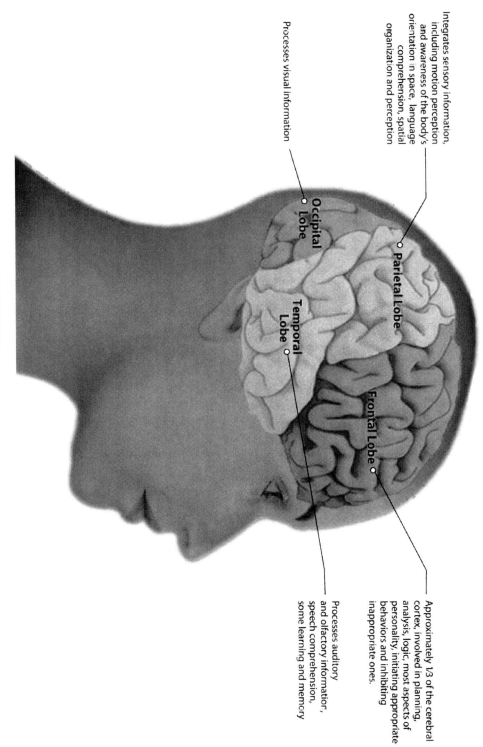

Occipital Lobe

Parietal Lobe

Temporal Lobe

Frontal Lobe

Approximately 1/3 of the cerebral cortex, involved in planning, analysis, logic, most aspects of personality, initiating appropriate behaviors and inhibiting inappropriate ones.

Processes auditory and olfactory information, speech comprehension, some learning and memory

Frontal Lobe

The frontal lobes are the largest part of your cortex, where your conscious thoughts and awareness reside. They are responsible for *cognition* – logic, analysis, planning, judgment, etc – as well as speech, attention, movement and emotional interpretation. This region is where you consciously analyze information and invent new concepts. It's also where you analyze and consciously recognize the biochemical changes in your brain and body called emotions. Part of this region also prevents you from acting upon impulses which are socially unacceptable. It's where you engage in voluntary social interactions and impulse control.

Perhaps more than anywhere else, differences in the frontal lobe account for individual differences in intelligence, self-awareness, planning and more, resulting in unique personalities. This is the site of *Broca's area*, where speech and writing are formulated, and it appears to be the seat of your short-term, "working memory".

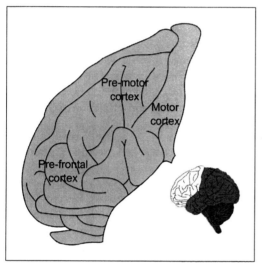

Frontal lobe, Hopes Brain Tutorial, 2010, Stanford University. Used with permission

Prefrontal cortex (PFC) – The most anterior region of the cortex is the prefrontal cortex, critical to higher cognitive functions and personality. The posterior or rearmost region of the PFC contains premotor and motor areas for initiating conscious movement; thus, your frontal lobes have a central role in planning and executing deliberate actions.

This is the seat of your brain's executive functions. Executive mental functions are usually voluntary, conscious mental processes, triggered when you're faced with a new or changing situation and have to choose from among a range of possible responses. These functions include:

- *Vigilance*
- *Selective attention*
- *Shift of attention*
- *Dealing with novelty*
- *Overcoming habit*
- *Judgment*
- *Planning*
- *Creativity*
- *Flexibility*
- *Comparison with events in memory*

- *Choosing goals*
- *Holding ongoing events in memory*
- *Choosing among alternative actions (sequence of muscle movements)*
- *Initiating actions and sequences*
- *Inhibiting unwanted actions*
- *Regulating ongoing action*
- *Recognizing self as initiator*
- *Monitoring outcomes*
- *Error correction*

At the top of this list of functions are cognitive tasks involving attention and conscious selection about what to focus upon. In the middle are tasks comparing what's happening in the moment with similar events in memory, selecting goals, and keeping these details in working memory. At the bottom of the list are mental processes which include tuning out interruptions, monitoring results, and correcting errors on an ongoing basis. This attention coordination is conducted by the ACC and *dorsolateral* region of the prefrontal cortex. The *dorsolateral prefrontal cortex* manages behavior prioritizing and adaptation to changes.

The *orbitofrontal cortex* specifically extracts cultural *norms* – accepted rules of behavior – from the social environment, allowing you to use these as behavioral guides. It also allows you to understand the consequences of your actions.

Choosing among alternatives involves weighing positive and negative outcomes. The anterior cingulate and dorsolateral prefrontal cortex interact with emotional decision-making regions of the prefrontal cortex such as the orbitofrontal cortex to decide between goals. The process is a complex comparison of a number of factors, requiring parallel processing throughout the prefrontal cortex and related regions. That is, no single region functions alone as a decision-making part of the brain. Regions of the PFC are also involved in using short-term (working) memory, and in retrieving long-term memories, and in controlling limbic system reactions to stressful events.

The motor cortex occupies the posterior frontal lobes, allowing voluntary movement and stimulating the muscles used to produce speech. Pre-motor and motor cortices plan, analyze and transmit motor information, working in tandem with the basal ganglia and cerebellum to coordinate movement.

Parietal Lobe

Located posterior to the frontal lobe and at the top of the brain, this region processes touch, vibration, pain, position sensing, spatial orientation, object recognition, integrates sensory information, and is key to hand-to-eye coordination. Its function is to integrate sensory input into your overall perception, and to provide you with orientation in three-dimensional space.

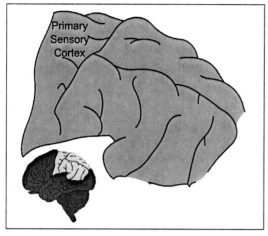

Parietal lobe, Hopes Brain Tutorial, 2010,
Stanford University. Used with permission

Your parietal and frontal lobes are separated by the *central sulcus*; the parietal lobe is posterior to the frontal and superior to the temporal lobes. This region contains the *primary sensory cortex*, through which sensations such as touch and pressure are processed. In addition, it has a key role in spatial orientation and information processing.

The parietal lobes construct a map of your body in space, combining all the input from your proprioceptive nerves about the position of your limbs and body. Your brain constantly updates this mental map to track the movement and position of your limbs and trunk in space.

The parietal lobe is also involved in abstract thinking – mathematical calculations, symbol interpretation, drawing and more. Since it's linked to visual systems, your parietal lobe assists you in such things as tying your shoelaces or kicking a soccer ball.

Parietal Lobe functions include:

- *Processing sensory information*
- *Localizing touch, pressure, pain, and temperature on the opposite side of the body*
- *Spatial processing*
- *Visual guidance of hands, fingers, eyes, and limbs, head*
- *Responses to eye movements*
- *Visual motor guidance for reaching and for grabbing objects*
- *Tactile recognition*

- *Information on limb position*
- *Localize objects around us*
- *Directing movement in space*
- *Detecting stimuli in space*
- *Distinguishing left from right*
- *Spatial cognition, such as reading and arithmetic*
- *Creating visual mental maps*
- *Reading Maps*

489

Temporal Lobe

The temporal lobes are at approximately ear level, and are responsible for distinguishing, recognizing and interpreting auditory and olfactory stimuli, and for memory formation. Temporal auditory processing helps you in learning and using language, in interpreting music and in reading.

Since the temporal lobe is where the hippocampus resides, it's also central to memory formation, storage and retrieval. In right-handed people, the right temporal lobe deals chiefly with *visual memory* (as with remembering faces) and the left temporal lobe deals chiefly with *verbal memory* (remembering words and names).

Wernicke's Area is located in the temporal lobe, processing incoming speech and allowing you to comprehend it. Your brain uses Wernicke's area to understand speech, *Broca's area* to create responses, and the motor cortices to stimulate the muscles controlling your larynx and mouth when you speak.

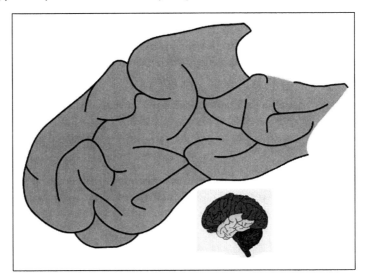

Temporal lobe, Hopes Brain Tutorial, 2010, Stanford University. Used with permission

Occipital Lobe

Your occipital lobe is posterior to your temporal lobe, and houses your brain's primary visual processing center. This hindmost region of the cortex controls vision, and analyzes, interprets and sorts visual data such as brightness, color and movement, assisting in the recognition of shapes and colors. Here, the visual cortex receives data from your eyes via the optic nerve.

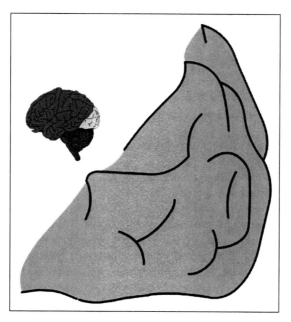

Occipital lobe, Hopes Brain Tutorial, 2010. Used with permission

Association Areas

In addition to the primary cortices for sensory input and motor output, there are *association areas* which don't receive direct sensory or motor feedback input from the thalamus, but integrate the information from each distinct cortical sensory mode and motor system – linking perception to action.

Each sensory cortex outputs data to a nearby *unimodal association area*, which integrates data for that single sense. For example, the *visual association cortex* integrates visual form, color, and motion information from separate pathways in the brain. These unimodal association areas then project to *multimodal association areas*, which integrate information from multiple senses. Lastly, these multimodal *sensory* association areas output to multimodal *motor* association areas adjacent to the primary motor cortex in the frontal lobe. Motor association areas can then use this integrated sensory data to help plot appropriate motor program responses, which are then implemented by commands from the premotor and primary motor cortex.

Multimodal association areas link sensory information to movement planning, and are therefore thought to house the highest brain functions – conscious thought, perception, and goal-directed action. They are used in the most sophisticated processes, like recognizing objects (apples, words, etc.). Information from the various senses converges upon these cortical regions, which integrate it into a polysensory event. The multimodal association areas are of major importance:

491

- The *posterior association area*, where the parietal, temporal, and occipital lobes meet, integrates information from several senses for perception and language.

- The *posterior parietal association area* is concerned with defining spatial relationships in the world around you, and with integrating all the separate elements of a visual scene into a single coherent whole.

- The *limbic association area* helps orchestrate emotions and memory storage.

- The *anterior association area*, near the prefrontal cortex, is concerned with planning movement.

All sensory information is processed along parallel pathways from receptors in specific sense organs to each of the primary sensory cortices. From there, the data from each sense is integrated within a unimodal association area. This integrated data is then sent to the multimodal association cortices in the posterior parietal and temporal cortices. These posterior association areas, which process *sensory* information, are linked with frontal association areas responsible for planning *motor* actions. The anterior association areas use integrated sensory information to help select motor programs for achieving goals, such as satisfying thirst by drinking.

What's the Frequency, Kenneth?
Brainwaves And States of Consciousness

Your brain can communicate between functionally specialized regions such as the limbic system and occipital lobe when several neurons simultaneously send signals in patterns similar to radio waves. The number of impulses per second is the frequency measured in hertz, or cycles per second, just as with electronic equipment, and these different frequencies support different functions.

If you picture your brain as a radio, tuning it to different frequencies brings different information to the forefront of your attention, and this is how important messages are selected from among the chatter of irrelevant signals.

Although these brainwave fields are found throughout the brain, they're strongest and most repetitive in the hippocampus and neocortex. Recently, scientists have come to the conclusion that this constant wash of overlapping, weak electrical fields throughout the brain, once thought to be unimportant, is fundamental to brain function.

California Institute of Technology neuroscientist Costas Anastassiou believes these fields represent an additional form of indirect neural communication. Through these fields, he suggests, physically unconnected neurons can communicate across the brain – a previously unknown form of neural communication independent of synapses.

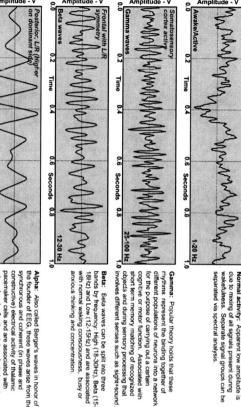
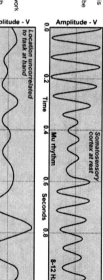
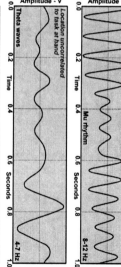
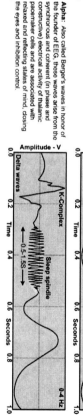

Awake/Active — Amplitude - V — 0.0, 0.2, 0.4, 0.6, 0.8, 1.0 — Time / Seconds — 1-20 Hz

Gamma waves — Somatosensory cortex active — Amplitude - V — 25-100 Hz

Beta waves — Frontal with L/R symmetry — Amplitude - V — 12-30 Hz

Alpha waves — Posterior, L/R (Higher on dominant side) — Amplitude - V — 8-12 Hz

Mu rhythm — Somatosensory cortex at rest — Amplitude - V — 8-12 Hz

Theta waves — Location uncorrelated to task at hand — Amplitude - V — 4-7 Hz

Delta waves — Children posteriorly, Adults frontally — Amplitude - V — 0-4 Hz

Delta waves — K-Complex — Sleep spindle — ← 0.5-1.5S → — Amplitude - V — 0-4 Hz

Normal activity: Apparent low amplitude is cue to mixing of all signals present during wakefulness. Separate signal groups can be separated via spectral analysis.

Gamma: Popular theory holds that these rhythms represent the binding together of different populations of neurons into a network for the purpose of carrying out a certain cognitive or motor function. Associated with short term memory matching of recognized objects and during sensory processing that involves different senses such as sight+sound.

Beta: Beta waves can be split into three bands by frequency: High (18-30Hz), Beta (15-18Hz) and Low (12-15Hz) and are associated with normal waking consciousness, busy or anxious thinking and concentration.

Alpha: Also called Berger's waves in honor of the founder of EEG, these waves arise from the synchronous and coherent (in phase and constructive) electrical activity of thalamic pacemaker cells and are associated with relaxed and reflecting states of mind, closing the eyes and inhibition control.

Mu rhythms: In the same band as Alpha waves. Mu rhythms are believed to reflect the electrical output of the synchronization of large portions of pyramidal neurons of the motor cortex which control hand and arm movement when inactive. Desynchronization can occur during movements by subjects as well as when viewing those movements in someone else.

Theta: Associated with drowsiness or arousal in older children and adults and with inhibition of elicited responses where a subject is actively trying to repress a response or action and found in young children in all wakeful states. "Hippocampal theta rhythms" are found in many mammals where "Cortical theta rhythms" are usually only recorded from humans.

Delta: Slowest and highest amplitude waves normally seen in adults during slow wave sleep and in babies that are both awake and asleep. Sometimes this has also been found during some continuous attention tasks.
FIRDA - Frontal Intermittent Rhythmic Delta
OIRDA - Occipital Intermittent Rhythmic Delta

Delta with K-complex and Sleep spindle: Sleep spindles (Sometimes called Sigma waves) along with K-complexes are defining characteristics of non-REM stage 2 sleep. Sleep spindles are thought to represent periods of processing inhibition used to keep the sleeper from waking, such as when a loud noise is heard while sleeping. Sleep spindles also occur at the onset of stage 2 sleep.

EEG-Brainwaves, 2010, Wikipedia, public domain.

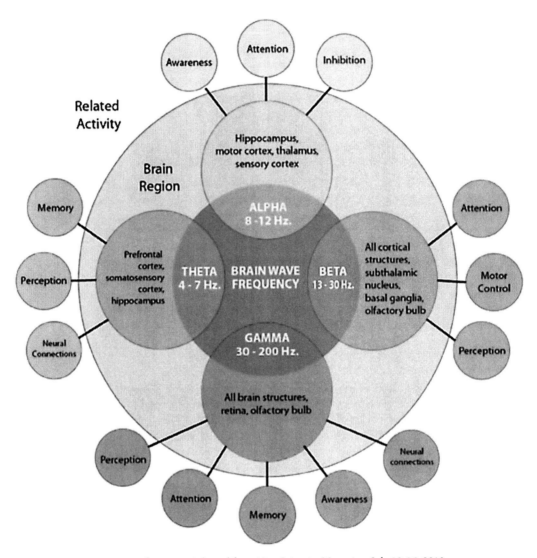

Brainwave functions. Adapted from New Scientist Magazine, July 10-16, 2010

These waves of rhythmic electrical signals result from clusters of neurons transmitting signals simultaneously, a unique form of *liquid computing* which bathes your brain in electrical fields, different frequencies washing across your brain simultaneously. This enables separate regions to communicate more efficiently than through discrete circuits one at a time. Neural circuits in different regions of the brain can link *transiently* (for brief periods) through this mechanism, without the need for physical proximity. Dr. Anastassiou's team has found that these weak fields alter individual neural firing and help synchronize firings among neural groups. He says this allows a significant increase in the amount of data transmitted, and likely plays a major role in many thought and behavioral processes.

Perhaps the answers to the mind's greatest remaining mysteries lie within these electrical fields. Scientists at the Max Planck Institute in Germany have discovered that, for example, to perceive something consciously, your neurons need to be firing in synchronicity, and, the greater the synchronicity, the stronger your perception will be – a sound will be more distinct, for example. These synchronized neural firings allow your mind to focus on one task over another at a given instant.

Brainwave frequencies are categorized into five bands of speed, each associated with a specific activity: *Alpha, Beta, Delta, Theta* and *Gamma.*

Delta waves (0 to 4 cycles per second) – the slowest brainwaves appear during the deepest, dreamless sleep, deeply relaxed states and trances. Delta waves increase as you "tune out" awareness of the physical world, and they are apparently associated with accessing information in your unconscious mind.

Theta waves (4 to 8 cycles per second) – thought to be central to learning and memory, and possibly in tracking location within an environment. These waves also appear to be connected with daydreaming, fantasizing and/or intuition, and with accessing the subconscious, emotions, memories and sensations.

Theta waves are strongest during moments of internal focus, including meditation, prayer, and spiritual states. They appear frequently in the cortices of young children, but among older children and adults, normally only appear during drowsy, meditative, or light sleeping states. Several types of mental illness show abnormally strong or persistent theta waves in the cortex. In awakened adults, excess theta waves are abnormal and may indicate a distracted, unfocused state, but strong theta wave activity is normal during sleep, and in children up to the age of 13.

Alpha waves (8–12 cycles per second) – appear during relaxed, calm awake states. This is the brain's default state when you're alert but not actively thinking. It increases when you close your eyes and breathe deeply, and decreases when you think or calculate. This is the most common brainwave frequency appearing in normal relaxed adults and teens over the age of 13, although alpha waves don't even begin to appear in humans until age three. Recent theories propose that these waves dampen activity in the cortex when regions aren't in use, or that they may have a role in coordination and communication across brain regions.

A subset of Alpha waves are *mu waves* that fall in the 8–13 Hz range and, through the use of special mirror neurons, are believed to play a critical role in understanding, empathizing with, and imitating the behavior and emotions of others.

Beta waves (12 to 30 cycles per second) – These waves are associated with active, busy, or anxious thinking and active concentration as well as with control of physical movement. These frequencies indicate active listening, thinking, problem-solving, judging, making decisions, and processing information about the environment. Higher beta wave frequencies appear to indicate agitation.

Gamma waves (above 36 Hz) – this is the only frequency range of brainwaves found throughout every region of the brain. It's believed that this frequency range is critical for coordinating processing between different brain regions. *Parvalbulmin (PV) neurons* are special fast-spiking sensory nerves found throughout the brain, which are named after a calcium-binding protein within them. They seem to be responsible for region-to-region gamma frequency signalling.

The Heart of Consciousness? Gamma Waves

As scientists try to unravel the mysteries of the human mind, at the core looms the central question: *what* **is** *consciousness?* They've long known that personality, thoughts and emotions are created by electrical and chemical transmissions through networks of nerve cells in the brain. But consciousness is much more than just a matter of isolated electrochemical processes. Part of it is a simple awareness, the knowledge that one exists, is alive, and has a unique, coherent, enduring identity, including emotions, memories and thoughts separate from the environment and unique among all other living creatures.

Thus, consciousness is basically a recognition of both the environment and oneself via sensations and perceptions. This self-awareness is shared by some animals with highly developed brains such as chimpanzees, dolphins and elephants, and can be demonstrated using Dr. Gordon Gallup Jr's *mirror test*: an animal shows self-awareness by recognizing when a dye has been placed on its own body and not the reflection in a mirror, and the animal responds by poking at the marking on its own body while looking at the mirror.

But the physical mechanism underlying consciousness itself may just now be coming into focus. The newest research is zeroing in on a specific range of brainwave frequencies, now believed to be the very basis of conscious thought. Brainwaves have long been monitored through *electroencephalography* (EEG), with electrodes placed on the scalp, but neurosurgeon Eric Leuthardt, in searching for physical causes of untreatable seizures for surgical removal, places electrode grids directly onto patients' brains – a process known as *electrocorticography* (ECoG). Because ECoG reads brainwaves directly from the brain's surface, it allows a more precise study of a wider range of brain activity than ever before.

Dr. Leuthardt and his team are able to monitor brainwave frequencies as consciousness fades and returns under the influence of anesthesia. A series of changes in the gamma band frequency range occur in a specific sequence as consciousness fades, and reoccur in reverse order as consciousness returns.

In Norway, another team of researchers has been studying the same frequency range to understand mental focus. Dr. Laura Lee Colgin and colleagues have discovered how brainwaves are used to focus and filter out distractions. Again, as with a radio, the brain tunes into specific frequencies to filter out all the distracting, irrelevant sensory "noise". Measuring brain waves in the hippocampus, Dr. Colgin's team found significance in the gamma wave range, and, like Leuthardt, believe it's the basis of consciousness.

Neurons act as switches, says Colgin, jumping between frequencies many times every second, sending or receiving either slow or fast waves in each state, but only one kind at a time per cell. This makes the tuning process very efficient – reception of irrelevant information is switched off, while cells are attuned to receiving and transmitting signals in the relevant frequency range.

Just like songs carried over radio waves, information is carried by gamma waves from one brain region to another. And, as with the different frequencies of radio stations, there are slow gamma waves and fast gamma waves. Lower frequencies, says Dr. Colgin, are used to transmit memories of past experiences, and higher frequencies to transmit information about events in the present.

In this manner, each neuron deals with a single piece of data each instant, and the different frequencies allow one to distinguish between the present outside environment, what's happening internally, and what has occurred in the past. Colgin and her team believe this frequency encoding scheme is fundamental to the brain's information processing. Because every neuron can "choose" from among several different kinds of signals at any given instant, it also shows the brain has a much greater complexity and flexibility than previously realized – it was long thought that each cell was specialized to receive only one type of information. Colgin also says that, based on her findings, the phrase *being on the same wavelength* with another person is a real and demonstrable social phenomenon.

She also suggests the inability to switch properly between these frequencies may be the basis of schizophrenia, where thoughts and experiences, reality and fantasy are confused, and patients have difficulty in distinguishing between, for example, voices from people who are present and voices from memories of movies they've seen. Their perceptions are confused, like a radio tuned between stations, she says. *Biofeedback,* which is used to help patients learn to control their brainwaves, may point to future treatment methods for schizophrenics.

The Root of Consciousness? A Primate Social Monitoring Network

An essential aspect of consciousness is the somatosensory system, granting the sense of who "you" are physically. The somatosensory cortex is located in the parietal lobe; trauma to the region causes radical personality changes from the loss of this sense. Patients with lesions in the area often, for example, suffer from the strange malady called *contralateral neglect,* consciously denying one half of their bodies belongs to them. If you hold up a victim's left arm, for example, he'll deny it belongs to him, fully convinced it belongs to someone else.

Your hippocampus, meanwhile, generates your *episodic* memory – your autobiographical awareness of who you are in terms of your past. There appear to be other anatomical regions responsible for consciousness as well: Romanian neuroscientist Constantin von Economo first discovered a strange new type of neuron in 1926 – long, spindly and much larger than typical brain cells. Named after their discoverer, *von Economo neurons*

(VENs) are 50 to 200 percent larger than typical neurons, with longer, spindly cell bodies and a single projection at each end with few branches.

They are comparatively rare, comprising only one percent of the neurons in the anterior cingulate cortex (ACC) and the insular cortex. But both these regions respond intensely to socially relevant cues – a frowning face, a wince of pain, or the voice of a loved one, including one's own baby's crying. VENs also activate during the experiences of love, lust, anger and sadness. These regions appear to be central to the *salience network,* which keeps track of the most personally important aspects of the environment, as well as monitoring the state of the body's sensations.

Dr. John Allman of the California Institute of Technology believes they're integral to a *social monitoring network,* which tracks social cues, allowing us to alter our behavior in response to them. VENs have since been discovered in a number of other social animal species, including chimpanzees, gorillas, elephants, dolphins and some whales.

Their size allows for extremely rapid signal transmission, and Dr. Bud Craig of the Barrow Neurological Institute in Phoenix, Arizona believes they function as a rapid information-relay system, allowing the gist of a situation to be transmitted quickly across brain regions, enabling fast reactions on the fly, a crucial survival skill.

Dr. Craig says the social monitoring network provides an ongoing self-monitoring system, a sense of *How do I feel at this moment?* with the ACC and insula receiving input from the body, then integrating that information into emotions via limbic system input, and projecting output to the thalamus and beyond to the orbitofrontal cortex, allowing rapid behavioral adjustment in response to the environment.

He has an interesting proposition – because the bigger brains of social animals require more energy to operate, efficient use of that fuel is vital. Thus, he proposes, the inward-monitoring system we call *consciousness* evolved primarily as a means of moment-by-moment calculation of energy use. *How am I feeling now?* translates, he says, into monitoring one's energy needs and expenditures. If it's true, consciousness itself may only have been an interesting byproduct of evolution, rather than its goal.

One form of dementia results from a die-off of VENs within the ACC and insula, and sufferers completely lose social awareness, empathy and self-control. Autopsies of autism and suicidal schizophrenia sufferers also show extreme anomalies in the number of VENs, suggesting the under- or over-sensitivity to social cues may derive from too few or too many VENs.

The State of Mind

In 1641, a brilliant French aristocrat, mathematician and philosopher by the name of René Descartes first tried to deduce what a "mind" is. He reasoned that it's difficult from within one's own mind to say with absolute certainty what is *real* – the senses can be deceived, so they cannot be fully trusted. He then proceeded with doubt as his yardstick – if something is *beyond* doubt, it must be real, he said. This became the basis of scientific method – falsifiability – which says, in essence, *something must be true if you can consistently show it's not false.*

The fact that Descartes was able to think at all – and therefore existed – was the only thing he was unable to doubt, which meant Descartes knew for certain he existed. He also recognized that humans (or at least he himself) were capable of creativity and emotions, unlike the animatronic statues popular in Paris at the time – even though such machines could be made to look and move like humans.

What this suggested to him was that logically, a mind was something robots and other physical objects couldn't possess, and so the mind must be something separate from the physical body. This notion of *dualism* – the belief that a mind can exist apart from the physical neurons that house it, that a consciousness or soul exists separately from the physical body – had existed for thousands of years in religions around the world, but this was the first time anyone had applied formal rules of logic to try proving its existence.

Modern science swung to the opposite extreme in the 1930s, when Harvard psychologist B.F. Skinner began to develop his theories of behaviorism, which suggested that the "mind" was completely illusory, that the illusion of having a mind, and all of human behavior, are the simple function of nerves firing in response to the environment. Over the next thirty years, Dr. Skinner's experiments led to behaviorism's popularity, and many believed human minds are nothing more than black boxes – machines which receive input and generate output. Freewill, emotions and consciousness, are, said Skinner, all just illusions designed to ensure survival.

Pure determinism – input *stimulus A* and inevitably receive *response B* – is no longer considered an accurate model of the human mind, but questions about consciousness remain – what is it? Is consciousness really nothing more than chemical signalling, or is there something apart from the physical brain, a separate mind?

Today, most scientists discount the notion that there can be an unmeasurable spiritual essence lying outside the physical realm. The mind is seen as just an incredibly complex transmission of chemicals and ionic impulses through a vast network of gelatinous tissue. A popular thought experiment runs thusly: supposing scientists were able to engineer artificial neurons to replace worn-out ones in the brain and body. If all the neurons in your brain and body were replaced, would your mind still exist? If there is nothing but artificial nerves in you, can the "mind" still exist?

In the end, consciousness may well be only an inward-looking sense, your brain monitoring its own functions along with the body. In terms of more practical definitions, however, consciousness is also a stale of alertness, one which can be monitored and measured: a Universily of Manchester team has invented a new 3D scanner that allows recording of a brain losing and regaining consciousness in real time for the first time in history. Using a technique called *functional electrical impedance tomography by evoked response* (fEITER), the machine can be used to construct 3D movies of a brain falling under the effects of anesthesia.

The device takes 100 scans a second, measuring electrical impedance (resistance to current flow) in a cross-section of the brain. So far, the team has examined 20 volunteers, essentially able to watch a 3D film of their brains' change in conductivity as they lost consciousness. The real-time 3D film shows that losing consciousness is like having a dimmer switch turn down neural activity, inhibiting communication across various neural networks in the brain. These experiments and others show some specific aspects of consciousness that may be useful in defining it:

- *Arousal* – being physically conscious

- *Awareness* – your knowledge and perception of the environment; this is distinct from an awakened state. It's possible for you to be physically awake, but unaware of things in your environment.

- *Self-awareness* – a sense that you exist as an individual in your world

- *Temporality* – an awareness of the passage of time

- *Memory* – storing and retrieving previous sensory experiences

- *Feelings* – sensations, emotions and desires

- *Intentions* – plans, motives and expectations

- *Thoughts* – ideas, beliefs, a sense of reason, inner imagery and the ability to manipulate symbols (as in speaking or writing)

An additional aspect of consciousness is self-consciousness. In the spring of 2011, Swiss researchers published research which indicates the sense of self-awareness resides in the temporoparietal junction (TPJ), the point where integrated sensory and motor signals allow you to track your position in space. Out-of-body experiences are commonly associated with brain damage to this region. This is also one of the neural regions enabling you to deduce the thoughts and motives of others.

As well as the ability to read the emotions of others, another central aspect of human understanding lies in logically deducing what's going on in their minds, a process called *Theory of Mind.*

Since you know you're capable of thought, and can observe others engaging in motivated behavior, you begin to logically assume from an early age that others think, using the same mental processes as you. Your own internal mental environment provides a logical basis for deducing what's going on in their minds.

The region which seems to control this understanding lies at this point where the temporal and parietal lobes meet in the right hemisphere of the brain, called the right temporoparietal junction (RTPJ). Cognitive Neuroscientist Dr. Rebecca Saxe's discovery of the region's functions was said to be "...One of the most astonishing discoveries in the field of human cognitive neuroscience".

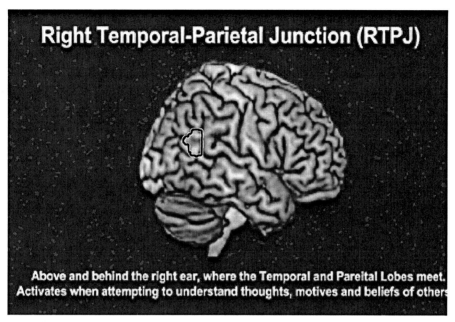

This specialized region activates when you attempt to understand the thoughts, motives and beliefs of others. Above and behind your right ear, it's the point where your temporal and parietal cortices connect. This region doesn't fully develop until sometime around puberty, explaining to a great degree the social naiveté often displayed by children. A number of studies show the more efficiently this region functions, the more compassionate people are when judging the responsibility of others for crimes and accidents which cause harm.

Free Will – Just An Illusion?

A recent study, some say, also brings into question the notion of freewill. UCLA studies in the 1980s and 1990s show a conscious decision is actually preceded by a subconscious one by 300 milliseconds, leading some scientists to once again conclude that humans have no freewill.

University of California professor Benjamin Libet ran a series of experiments in which volunteers watched a clock, and moved a finger whenever they chose, taking mental note of the moment on the clock they decided to move. Meanwhile, electrodes on their scalps measured brain activity.

Dr. Libet found his subjects' brains prepared for finger movement several hundred milliseconds before they made a conscious decision to move. An electrical potential built up in their brains half a second before they moved their fingers, which he called the *readiness potential*. Libet measured three points in time for each volunteer:

- The time for the readiness potential to build up

- The moment subjects reported the conscious wish to act

- The actual moment of the physical movement

He discovered the readiness potential occurred up to half a second (500 milliseconds) before the subjects took action, and the moment they reported making a decision was 300ms after the readiness potential and 200ms before acting. In other words, their brains had already activating muscles 300ms before the subjects consciously made a decision to move.

This means, says Dr. Libet, that the subjects' brains had reached a decision and begun to act upon it before they made a conscious, voluntary choice. He believes this shows that freewill does not exist – your subconscious mind acts, and reports what it's doing, and when you become aware of it, you then believe you're making a choice.

But the idea that these studies prove free will is an illusion is easily dismissed with a simple real-world situation: the musical *jam session*:

When highly-skilled musicians who have never met before gather to improvise, the music's key, tempo, theme, harmony, and time signature can fluidly, spontaneously change and be chosen at a whim. Every other musician participating in the session cannot possibly know in advance where the musical thread is going. They must respond in real-time, improvising upon the existing structure. Because the musical piece isn't predetermined, the improvisations they create on the spur of the moment cannot be predetermined.

And at the very least, the fact that the conscious mind is aware and involved in the decision at some point means we have the capacity to either approve or reject any action.

According to Dr. Michio Kaku, Professor of Theoretical Physics at City University of New York, Heisenberg's uncertainty principle disproves the a "clockwork" model of the universe – *Newtonian determinism* – and proves that free will must exist – it's impossible to predict anything with 100% certainty, so there's always a possibility of uncertainty in anything we do.

The Perceptive Animal

"If I, deaf, blind, find life rich and interesting, how much more can you gain by the use of your five senses?" – Helen Keller, The World I Live In, 1928

"Reality is what we take to be true.
What we take to be true is what we believe.
What we believe is based upon our perceptions.
What we perceive depends upon what we look for.
What we look for depends upon what we think.
What we think depends upon what we perceive.
What we perceive determines what we believe.
What we believe determines what we take to be true.
What we take to be true is our reality."
– Gary Zukav, Dancing Wu Li Masters:
An Overview of the New Physics, 1979

An Exploration Of The Senses

The way the human animal has evolved to learn about its environment is amazingly complex and elegant. Each sensory stimulus provides a wide range of data in different forms – intensity, timbre, frequency, color, position, movement, shape, etc. Before all of these aspects are integrated into a coherent, polysensory representation, each of these characteristics is processed within a different region of the sensory cortices, in a simultaneous, massive and continuous parallel processing.

Millions of discrete bits of multiple sensory input are reaching your brain at this very instant, being processed simultaneously along parallel streams of data, racing to and from your brain, up and down the information superhighway that is the bundle of nerves comprising your spinal cord. Each of your varied senses is receiving varied stimuli from your environment, then converting it into the same electrochemical impulses through the process of *transduction*. This conversion means that, ultimately, within your mind, your inner reality is just as powerful as your outer reality – the form in which thoughts and sensory stimuli are encoded is identical.

All your senses receive information about the world around you through specialized receptors, and that data is then converted into electrical signals for your brain to process through transduction. These electrochemical impulses travel through cranial and spinal nerves to the sensory gateway buried deep in your brain called the thalamus. Although the end result – transduction into electrochemical signals between your neurons – is the same for every sense, the means by which you gather that information about your environment is dependent upon each sense organ in question.

In the retina of your eyes, photons strike light-sensitive proteins and later their shape. In your ears, differences in sound pressure displace specialized cilia. In your nose, odorant molecules bind to receptors. However they are triggered, all of these stimuli are converted into neurochemical impulses, and your cranial nerves and spine channel each perceptual mode through separate pathways to your thalamus.

The thalamus processes and then relays this data to your sensory cortices for analysis and interpretation, and eventually your association cortices combine it to build a polysensory model of the world around you.

The system is two-way as well; your cortex sends feedback to your sensory organs, selectively exciting and inhibiting sensory input. This signal strengthening – excitation – and weakening – inhibition – allows you to selectively turn your attention to specific stimuli, just as, for example, your visual cortex automatically directs your eyes to track and focus upon objects moving within your field of vision.

Your thalamus acts as a sensory gatekeeper, relaying data to the appropriate cortical center, and receiving feedback from your cortex on which sense and which stimuli to enhance at any given instant. There are built-in safety mechanisms as well – if a flash of light is too bright, your irises automatically contract, and if a sound is too loud, your muscles in your inner ear tighten the tympanic membrane to protect the delicate bones and deeper structures within.

Your olfactory system is an exception among the sensory systems – it can bypass your thalamus, travelling in a direct route to your cortex. There's a very good reason for this; the olfactory cortex is an ancient structure, vital to survival. In the wild, if a creature eats something toxic or putrid, or fails to detect a predator's spoor, it can very quickly come to a nasty end.

Ultimately, however, every sight you see, every sound you hear, every feeling, taste and fragrance you perceive means specialized receptors have been activated and transduced the signal – converted it into an action potential, the same action potential that encodes every thought you generate and every memory you learn.

Think about what this means – the concept of transduction – the process of turning information about the outer world into the exact same form as your inner world of thoughts, plans, emotions and attitudes is an incredibly empowering realization – *to your brain, your inner (subjective) reality is every bit as powerful and influential – as your outer (objective) reality, perhaps more so.* It's all encoded, retrieved and stored in the same fundamental way – action potentials – ion movement across axons and electrochemical releases across synapses.

This also means you can easily misinterpret data that's coming in. Your personal biases of thought have a tremendous effect on what you perceive and how you interpret it. So, for example, if your habitual thought process is to believe that the world is a hostile, unfriendly place, your brain will reinforce that belief by selectively heightening or *tuning in* to information in your environment that validates your beliefs.

This is the basis of the *self-fulfilling prophecy*, where life gives you what you expect. A profound illustration of this is Stephen Crane's chilling short story, *The Blue Hotel*. In the tale, a man referred to as *the Swede* arrives in a small Nebraskan town, an environment alien to him. Because of his preconceptions about the "wild West", he feels fear, and expects danger.

Although there is no real threat to his safety, the Swede simply cannot see the truth because of his own overly anxious mental state; in the end, drunk and blustering, he begins to act wilder and wilder, eventually drawing death upon himself.

Similarly, in Fyodor Dostoevsky's *Notes from Underground*, a formerly respected civil servant spirals relentlessly into misery, paranoia and self-imposed exile because he is unable to see objectively how his internal negativity and fear both color and elicit the reactions of everyone around him.

Sight

Although humans have the most highly-evolved brains of any known creature on Earth, our eyes are not quite as powerful as some other animals. For example, the antelope has eight times the magnifying power, enabling it to spot dangers from a great distance. However, because of our status as predators, we have evolved *binocular vision,* with two eyes facing forward, slightly apart, allowing *depth perception,* the capacity to instantly calculate distances with incredible accuracy.

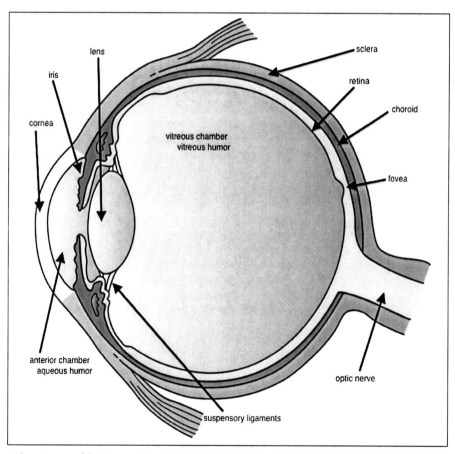

Three Layers of the Human Eye, 2013, Holly Fischer Creative Commons 3.0 Attribution License

Within the human eye, the *retina* is a thin, transparent, ten-layer organ of specialized nerves and receptor cells lining the eyeball's inner surface. Here some visual-processing occurs before signals are ever sent to the brain. The second-deepest layer contains special light-sensitive photoreceptors called *rods* and *cones*. In the illustration below, the inner surface of the eye is at the bottom, so light travels in an upward direction through layers of amacrine, ganglion, bipolar, horizontal and Muller cells, before striking photon-absorbing *pigment* molecules in the rods and cones.

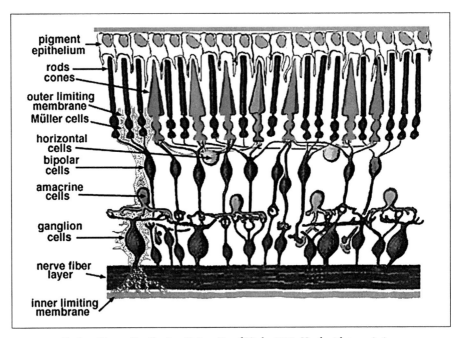

Retina, Moran Eye Center, University of Utah, 1995. Used with permission.

The pigment in rods is *rhodopsin* – an *opsin* protein combined with *retinal,* a vitamin-A chemical derivative. When the retinal portion of the rhodopsin molecule is struck by light, energy from the photon is transferred to electrons, which jump to a higher-energy state and alter rhodopsin's molecular shape. This triggers a chemical cascade, disinhibiting ganglion cells, which send an impulse down the optic nerve to a vision-specific region of the thalamus called the *lateral geniculate.*

Photoreceptors converge into bipolar cells, which connect to ganglion cells, which in turn connect with the optic nerve. Bipolar cells are normally inhibited by a steady flow of inhibitory neurotransmitters. When light activates cones and rods, however, this inhibition is relaxed, and excitatory neurotransmitters stimulate the ganglion cells. These fire impulses which travel down the optic nerve. Each ganglion in your retina is responsible for a portion of your visual field, receiving input from several photoreceptors or rods simultaneously. Changes in the intensity or frequency of light change the rate of electronic impulses sent by the ganglia.

Within each retina are about 120 million rods, the more sensitive of your photoreceptors, which respond to photon *amplitude* (intensity), and to varying shades of black, white, and grey. Rods are specialized for discerning shape and change – movement – even in near darkness. They're densely clustered at the periphery of your retina, which is why you're better able to see things out of the sides of your vision at night.

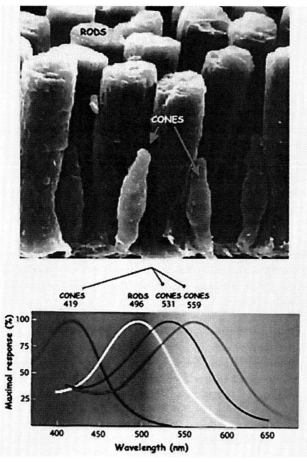

Rods and Cones, Moran Eye Center, University of Utah,
Health Services Center, 1995. Used with permission.

The second kind of photoreceptors in your retina are *cones*, of which there are about six million. They're densely clustered in a pinhead-sized area called the *fovea centralis* at the center of your eyes – the region most important for discerning fine detail, such as when you're reading. Cone density drops off significantly away from the fovea, providing only low-resolution, highly-compressed information at the outermost regions or the retina. Fully 50% of the signals your optic nerves receives are from the fovea; the remaining 50% are from the rest of your retina. The light-responsive chemicals in cones are similar to those in rods, combining retinal with *photopsins* in place of *scotopsins*.

Cones come in three varieties, each with a pigment specialized to absorb photons vibrating within a specific range of *frequencies* or *wavelengths* (color): *long* (red), *medium* (green), and *short* (blue) lightwaves. When cones disinhibit bipolar cells, and a ganglion fires, it sends the message *"There's a region of red (or green, or blue)."* The occipital lobe assembles these tiny regions of color, resulting in the millions of combinations your eye is capable of distinguishing. According to the international color standards consortium CIE, that number is approximately 2.3 million, but some scientists say the human eye can actually distinguish around 10 million distinct colors.

Each ganglion in the fovea only receives input from one or a few cones, allowing for more detailed perception. The *fovea* – the retinal region with the greatest visual acuity – is responsible for most color processing and spatial information. The rest of the retina's ganglia are mainly activated by rods and non-color-coded receptive fields specialized for perceiving objects which are moving or quickly changing. This means your retina is primarily designed to notice novelty or change, particularly in your visual periphery. Change prompts the brain to point the fovea at novel or changing stimuli for detailed analysis.

While signals from your retina are being processed, your occipital lobe sends messages back to your thalamus, providing feedback to control eye adjustment. Neurons in the visual cortex are also specialized to individually respond to a specific angle in your field of vision. As an object changes its orientation, the signal rates of each neuron will vary, depending upon whether or not the object's angle now matches their specialized angular sensitivity. These neurons are adjacent, so their synapses are interlinked, combining the data each processes. These neighboring neurons can also influence one another through *lateral inhibition*, via dendrite connections.

The network of retinal neurons analyzes photoreceptor signals in the eye before relaying this data to the thalamus, which can *attenuate* (dampen) consistent stimuli that's normal within your environment, so your cortex ignores these signals. This all happens instantly and instinctively, responses hardwired into you from 3.5 billion years of evolution, ensuring you don't miss the prey – or predator – that's entered your vicinity.

On its way to the cortex, visual data travels in parallel streams through regions responsible for various functions, including eye movement and focus. Image analysis is divided into parallel streams of varying function, and the tasks are completed simultaneously, allowing speedier analysis than if each task was carried out sequentially.

The primary visual centers of the brain are labelled progressively from V1 through to V5, and each region is responsible for processing a different aspect of vision: most of the V5 neurons process the image's color data, the parietal areas deal largely with the image's position in space, and the temporal regions analyze object contours.

Ten billion neurons reside in your visual cortex, which builds up a visual archive, a lifetime bank of stored images for comparison when interpreting what you see, a training process which takes years to develop. The incredible discriminatory power requires input from over 25 cortical regions however, each in some way dedicated to processing vision, using about a third of your brain's power, more than for any of your other five senses.

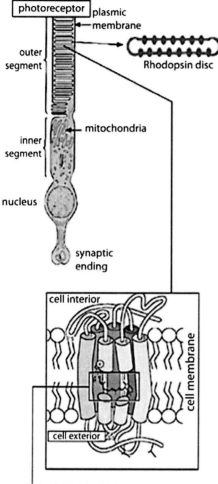

photoreceptor | plasmic
←membrane
outer segment
Rhodopsin disc
inner segment
mitochondria
nucleus
synaptic ending

cell interior
cell membrane
cell exterior

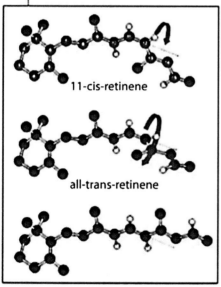

11-cis-retinene

all-trans-retinene

The lens of your eye focuses light particles – photons – onto your retina. Your retina is composed of:

1) light-**frequency**-sensitive red, green and blue **cones** (pictured) and 2) **movement** and **brightness**-sensing **rods**.

When photons strike light-sensitive **rhodopsin**, energy transfer to the electrons in **rhodopsin** causes a shift in the molecular structure. This triggers a chemical cascade, leading to a neural impulse along the optic nerve to the brain.

Retinal function is rather odd. In receptor cells (rods and cones) sodium channels are **open** by default – an constant state which of inhibitory neurotransmitter release. Photon activation of rhodopsin causes a chemical cascade which **closes** sodium channels, so **inhibitory** neurotransmitters **stop** flowing. This disinhibits bipolar cells, and they depolarize, releasing neurotransmitters that activate ganglion cells.

The ganglia send action potentials to the optic nerve, and ultimately the special vision-processing region of the brain's sensory gateway (thalamus) called the **lateral geniculate**.

Extremely optional biochemistry: There are three main functional molecules in visual receptor cells: 1) the pigment rhodopsin, made up of the protein opsin coupled with **retinal** (a slightly-processed form of vitamin A); 2) a tri-part molecule called **transducin**; and 3) deactivated **PDE** (phosphodiesterase). PDE is the "workhorse" of the retina, but it's inactivated by a pair of alpha subunits – one at each end of the molecule.

When a photon strikes rhodopsin, it alters the molecular shape. Retinal loses its attraction for the opsin protein, and detaches. The opsin protein migrates to transducin, where it phosphorylates an energy subunit called GDP, converting it into GTP. GTP can then remove the inactivating alpha subunit from one end of the PDE molecule, and thus activate it.

A second photon striking rhodopsin frees another GTP to remove the second alpha subunit from the PDE molecule, which is now freed to convert the sodium-channel ligand **cGMP** (cyclic GMP) into GMP.

Under NO light, (with no stimulation) cGMP-gated sodium channels are open by default, and sodium flows through, causing constant inhibitory neurotransmitter release. When light causes the chemical cascade, cGMP is converted into GMP, the sodium channels have no ligand to open them, and inhibitory neurotransmitters stop flowing. This releases constraints upon bipolar cells, which activate ganglions to fire a neural impulse. Source: Leslie Samuel, MS, "How Rods and Cones respond to Light", "Visual Processing in the Retina", Interactive Biology, 2011; Image: Rod Cell, McGill University, 2010. Used with permission.

The *fusiform* is an especially interesting area in the right temporal lobe, which contains neurons that respond specifically to faces and their features, reflecting the importance of social interactions to primate species. If the fusiform is damaged, it results in *prosopagnosia*, where the sufferer cannot recognize faces – even a spouse or close relative can walk past and the sufferer will not recognize them unless spoken to, and even if looking at photographs of the same person side-by-side, a victim of prosopagnosia cannot tell they're the same person.

Hearing

Your sense of hearing allows you to distinguish:

- **tone** – the colors of sound called *timbre*, based on combined variations in air pressure fluctuations, with a main tone and *overtones* that help shape each individual sound

- **attack** (onset) and **decay** (fading) of the *sound envelope* (sound wave shape)

- **pitch** – the speed of air pressure changes, measured in Hertz (cycles per second)

- **volume** – the force of air pressure changes

The average human is capable of detecting frequencies between 20 and 20,000 Hz. Sound stimuli (fluctuating waves of air pressure) are converted into electrical impulses for your brain to analyze via transduction, just as with the eyes. Here's how it works:

Like a pebble dropped into a pool sends ripples outward in expanding rings, sound causes a sphere of air pressure waves to expand outwardly. These air pressure fluctuations enter your *pinna* (outer ear) and ear canal, where pressure changes push your *tympanic membrane* (eardrum). The eardrum transmits vibrations to three tiny, linked middle ear bones – the *malleus, incus* and *stapes*. These are the tiniest bones in the human body, collectively called the *ossicles*, used to amplify sound. If the sound is extremely loud, feedback from your auditory cortex instantly tightens the muscles of these bones in response, protecting the delicate receptors of your inner ear. The *temporal bones*, just above and behind the jaw, are the hardest bony structures in the human body, further protecting these three delicate middle ear bones,

The *middle ear* contains the ossicles. It has a hollow, sealed space called the *tympanic cavity*, sealed off from the outer ear by the tympanic membrane, but a canal called the *Eustachian tube* branches down from it into the throat. The Eustachian tube allows air into the tympanic cavity, equalizing air pressure on both sides of the tympanic membrane, protecting it from extreme changes in air pressure, including extremely loud sounds.

The *inner ear* is comprised of the *labyrinth*, which resembles a chambered nautilus (pictured in purple below). Unlike the outer and middle ears, which are filled with air, the labyrinth is filled with a fluid called *perilymph*. As the tympanic membrane is pushed inward by a wave of air pressure, the *malleus, incus* and *stapes* shift in the middle ear, and the stapes, pushes inward, agitating perilymph fluid within the labyrinth. The coiled cochlea, which resembles a snail, converts this perilymph agitation into neural impulses. Compressing the inner liquid means the pressure must have "somewhere to go", instead of a completely closed space. Because of this, in addition to the oval window, through which the stapes pushes into the labyrinth, there is a membrane-covered *round window* below, which bulges outward to accommodate compression of the perilymph fluid within the labyrinth.

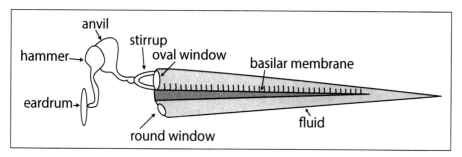

Within the coils of the cochlea, the *basilar membrane* separates fluid-filled chambers. On this basilar membrane is a specialized structure called the Organ of Corti. Cilia at the top of hair cells within the Organ of Corti bend as the membrane vibrates, pulling upon connections between them called *tiplinks*, and this opens potassium ion channels, causing depolarization and firing of the hair cells. The electrical signal travels down the auditory nerve to the brain. In the diagram above, the basilar membrane is uncoiled.

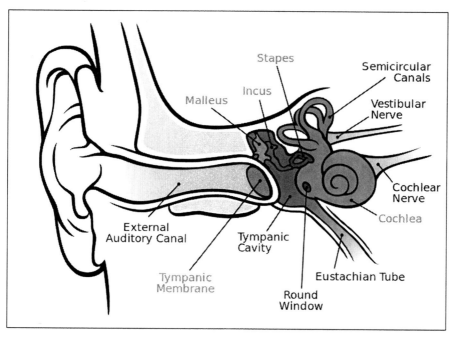

Hearing – fluctuating air pressure strikes a membrane stretched across the ear canal, transmitting vibrations to delicate amplifying bones in the ears. Anatomy of the Human Ear, Brockmann Chittka, 2009, Wikipedia Attribution 2.5

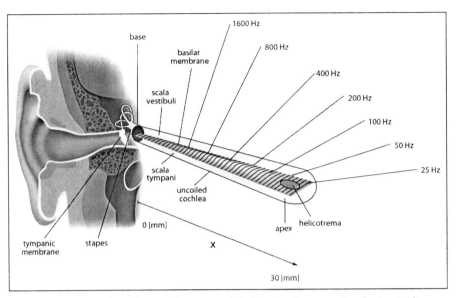

Kern A, Heid C, et al. Basilar membrane uncoiled. Creative Commons Attribution 2.5 license

The basilar membrane is arranged by *tonotopic organization*, which means that lower frequencies cause vibrations in the *apex* of the basilar membrane, while higher frequencies cause vibrations at the *base* of the basilar membrane. Thus, outer coils of the cochlea respond to high-pitched sounds, while inner coils respond to low-pitched sounds.

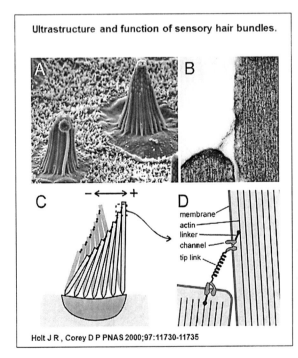

Ultrastructure and function of sensory hair bundles.

A B C D
membrane
actin
linker
channel
tip link

Holt J R , Corey D P PNAS 2000;97:11730-11735

*Sound vibrations are transferred to bristly **stereocilia bundles** that extend from the tops of hair cells in the cochlea of your ears. These stereocilia bundles are arranged in stair-step rows, climbing from lowest to highest. Tiny protein strands called **tip links** connect each adjacent stereocilium. Sound vibrations cause the stereocilia to tip to one side. As the stereocilia bend, this mechanically pulls open **mechanotransduction channels**, pore-like openings which permit potassium and calcium ions to flood into the hair cell and trigger a neural impulse. Image: Drs. Jeffrey R. Holt and David P. Corey, Two Mechanisms for Transducer Adaptation in Vertebrate Hair Cells. PNAS, October 24, 2000. Used with permission.*

Smell

Smell is triggered by *odorants*, airborne particles such as vanilla or eucalyptus, which bind to receptors on a special 1-inch wide, 2-inch long strip of tissue three inches up and inside your nasal cavity called the *epithelium*. These odorants lock onto protein odorant receptors, depolarizing the neurons, firing signals down the axons; these axons join others, converging upon *glomeruli cells* in your brain's *olfactory bulb*. Mitral cells in the olfactory bulb then relay these signals via Cranial Nerve One to several brain regions, such as the *anterior olfactory nucleus, piriform cortex*, medial amygdala, and entorhinal cortex. The entorhinal cortex assists in memory processing, linking odors with memories, while identifying odors seems to be chiefly the domain of the piriform cortex. The medial amygdala is involved in social interactions, including mating and recognition of animals within the same species.

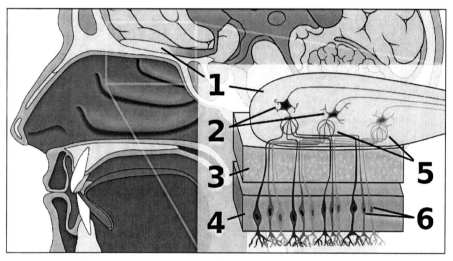

Human Olfactory System 1: Olfactory bulb 2: Mitral cells 3: Bone 4: Nasal epithelium 5: Glomerulus 6: Olfactory receptor cells; Patrick J. Lynch, 2007, Wikipedia Attribution 2.5

Your sense of smell, being vital to your survival, has one direct route to your olfactory cortex which bypasses your thalamus. The sense of smell is necessary, for example, in recognizing spoiled or poisonous foods, possibly in recognizing pheromones on an unconscious level (recent evidence indicates), and in warning of predators in the wild.

But while humans have highly advanced vision, bipedalism, a massive cortex and tremendously nimble hands, one evolutionary trade-off is that we lost a great deal of sensitivity in our sense of smell. Animals with less developed brains – for example dogs – still retain this primitive, sophisticated olfactory sense. This assists them in hunting, marking territory, and social recognition.

Still, 2004 Nobel-prizewinner Dr. Linda Buck says it's possible for you to distinguish anywhere from 10,000 to 100,000 different odorants; individual genetic differences will result in varying sensitivity from person to person, this sensitivity being dependent upon the density of receptors in your epithelium. The human genome, she says, encodes 347 different odorant receptors, each of which is capable of detecting a range of similar chemical structures. A combination of different receptors will simultaneously accept one type of odorant, and it's a *combination* of these receptors that encodes each individual smell.

You can classify smells the first time you encounter them with this flexible system – odorants activate multiple olfactory receptors, making the possible combinations of odors your olfactory system can distinguish quite huge: all the varied aromas you know are a mixture of responses from among a combination of 347 distinct odorant receptor types. Dr. Buck also notes that as much as five percent of the human genome may be devoted to encoding odorant receptors. In other words, in terms of DNA use, your sense of smell has been afforded an extremely large amount of genetic code, showing its great evolutionary importance.

A Sexy Stench

Non-human animals possess an olfactory system for *pheromones,* odorants which identify individuals, mark territory, trigger defensive behaviors, establish social rank, and communicate availability for reproduction. Because they need to float great distances in the air from their source, odorant molecules are small and lightweight. But pheromones, notes University of Maryland neuroscientist Dr. R. Douglas Fields, need not be small, as they can be transmitted during intimate contact, such as when kissing.

Most animals (except birds) process pheromones through the *vomeronasal organ (VNO),* a special olfactory processing center which is also seen in human fetuses, but has long been thought to atrophy upon maturation. However, in 2009, Dr. Fields published claims in Scientific American magazine that a 13th pair of human cranial nerves exists, apparently corresponding to the VNO pathways found in non-human animals.

Cranial nerves all enter your brain directly from your sense organs, all but two pairs connecting to your brainstem. All twelve pairs relay sensory data – sight, smell, hearing, touch and taste, as well as help control eye, jaw, tongue, throat and face muscles. They exit the bottom of your brain in pairs, the whole structure resembling a crab of sorts.

Since their discovery thousands of years ago, the cranial nerves have been classified and numbered starting from the *rostral* (front, behind the forehead) to the *caudal* (back, toward the brainstem). Starting with the olfactory nerve, they continue in sequence through pairs until the 12th cranial nerve, which connects your tongue and brain.

Recently, however an "extra" pair may have been discovered. Because this throws existing anatomical models out of sequence, for the time being, it's being called cranial nerve zero. Dr. Fields says it's found just in front of the olfactory nerves, but had been dismissed until recently, because it didn't have any immediately obvious functions. Some sceptics also argue this isn't a separate cranial nerve, but only a frayed strand of the olfactory nerve. Still, Dr. Fields expresses certainty a pheremone detection system exists in humans just as it does in other mammals.

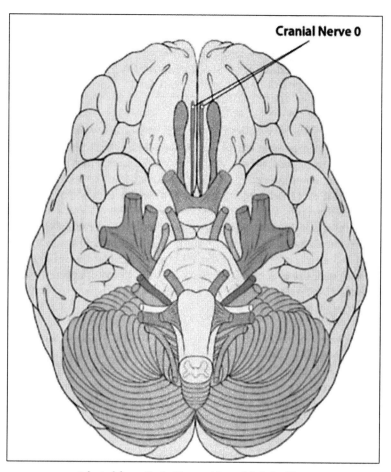

Cranial Nerve 0

Adapted from: Brain Human Normal Inferior View,
2009, Patrick J. Lynch, Creative Commons Attribution 2.5 Generic License

Nerve zero is, he says, unique in that it originates in the nasal cavity, but projects into brain regions which govern sexual behavior – the *septum* and the *medial pre-optic area* of the hypothalamus. Acetylcholine stimulation of the septum produces multiple orgasms, some lasting as long as thirty minutes, while the medial preoptic area of the hypothalamus controls pituitary gland sex hormone releases, governing sexual reproduction. Nerve zero, he adds, bypasses the olfactory bulb completely, connecting the nose directly with the brain's reproductive centers.

Aside from anatomically connecting the nose to the brain's sexual behavior centers of the brain, Dr. Fields says nerve zero has been shown to trigger release of a powerful sex hormone (*gonadotropin-releasing hormone or GnRH*) into the bloodstream. GnRH, released while babies are still in the womb, helps encode sexual identity; in adults, it controls ovulation and spermatogenesis.

Nobel laureate Dr. Linda Buck and colleague Stephen Liberles published research in 2006 identifying 15 new receptor proteins in the noses of mice, found on the surface of cells which specifically detect mouse pheromones. These receptors differ from normal olfactory receptors which bind to typical odorants; she also discovered humans possess genes which synthesize at least six of these same pheromone receptors.

Animals use their olfactory sense to determine reproductive suitability and status (ovulation status, age, general health, genetic compatibility, etc.) by detecting traces of hormones in urine and sweat. Among animal species which rely upon pheromones for sexual communication, the key sensory organ is the specialized region between the nose and mouth called the vomeronasal organ, which connects to an accessory olfactory bulb, next to the main olfactory bulb. When a snake flicks its tongue into the air, it's pulling odorants into its mouth to contact the vomeronasal organ for chemical analysis. In female prairie voles, exposure to males induces uterine growth and estrogen cycles; and the VNO appears to be central to the process; when it's removed, the effect no longer occurs. Additional literature confirms that adult humans also possess a VNO, though the authors claim they could not find axons projecting from it.

There is some experimental evidence to support Dr. Fields' claims of a human pheromone system, however: Biologist Claus Wedekind of the University of Bern in Switzerland discovered in the 1990s that people prefer the body odors of those with different immune-system genes than their own. A similar 1997 study by Dr. Carole Ober of the University of Chicago also demonstrated that people avoid mating with others whose immune-system genes are similar to their mothers.

From an evolutionary standpoint, this makes sense – having children with someone whose immune system differs increases the variety of diseases children are potentially able to resist, and incompatible partners can heighten the risk of death for offspring. Pheromone sexual compatibility messages are so powerful that the mere proximity of a potentially incompatible mate can trigger the spontaneous termination of pregnancy in mice.

Studies by Dr. Denise Chen at Rice University have shown that the scent of sweat from humans in different emotional states can have a marked impact on test performance, with volunteers performing better after smelling the sweat of those who had seen a scary movie. It seems to have generated a subconscious warning signal that heightens vigilance.

FMRI scans also show that odorless pheromones from pig sweat stimulate dopamine release in the same pathways of the human brain as the smell of roses. Dr. Benoist Schaal from the French National Center for Scientific Research has also discovered that pheromones are released from scent glands in the areolae (dark circles surrounding the nipples) of new mothers, helping newborns find the nipple and begin to suckle. Despite marketing claims to the contrary, however, no pheromonal perfumes or colognes currently available have yet been proven to attract members of the opposite sex.

Taste

Your olfactory and *gustatory* senses are interlinked – taste (gustation) relies upon your sense of smell to a great degree. When olfactory sense organs are damaged, it renders one incapable of tasting all but the coarsest of flavor categories: salty, sour or sweet.

If they're fully functional, however, your taste receptors can recognize a mixture of five basic human tastes – sweet, salty, bitter, sour, and the newest addition *umami* (glutamate) taste. Some argue for the inclusion of a sixth category called *piquancy*, the spiciness produced by chili peppers, ginger, mustard and other spices. In these cases, the chemicals *piperine* and *capsaicin* create burning sensations by binding to thermal- and chemical-sensitive heat and pain receptors, which send signals via the fifth cranial nerve, responsible for facial sensations.

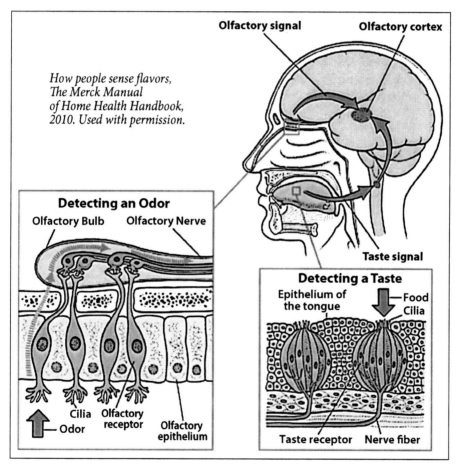

How people sense flavors,
The Merck Manual
of Home Health Handbook,
2010. Used with permission.

Taste receptors are found in categories which respond specifically to sweetness, bitterness, saltiness, umami or sourness, opening ion channels either directly or indirectly when the appropriate food molecules bind with them. The olfactory sense is much more complex than the gustatory sense, but sensitivity varies from person to person, based upon genetic expression of receptor proteins.

Touch

Your skin is your single largest organ, sensitive to changes in temperature, pain, and pressure through specialized receptors. The greater the density of these receptors, the greater the sensitivity of an area on your body. Each square inch of your hands has an estimated 600 touch sensors; those near the surface register feather-light touch sensations. Others buried deeper within your skin measure sustained pressure. Because your hands are so useful to you, they contain as many as 100 times the number of touch sensors as the backs of your legs. Heat sensors, on the other hand, are densest in your fingertips, nose, and elbows, while cold receptors are most densely concentrated in the upper lip, nose, chin, chest and fingers.

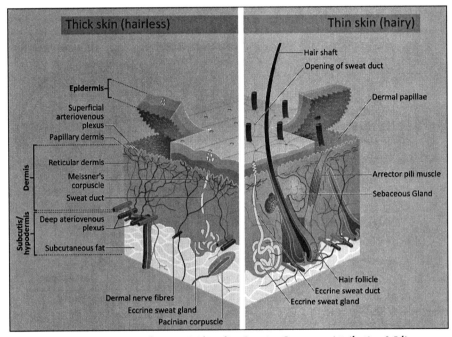

Skin Layers, M.Komorniczak, 2012, Wikipedia, Creative Commons Attribution 2.5 license.

Human skin is made up of three layers of tissue. The outermost is your *epidermis* (Latin for the words *over* and *skin*). It's a waterproof, protective layer of mostly dead skin cells which protects your body from exposure and infection, and contains the pigment *melanin*, that darkens to screen your skin from dangerous ultraviolet sunlight radiation. Below this is the *dermis*, the layer which contains hair follicles, sweat glands, *sebaceous* (oil) glands, blood vessels, nerve endings, and an estimated 5 million touch receptors, which route touch signals through an astounding 45 miles of nerve fibers throughout your body.

The dermis sustains and supports your epidermis by sending nutrients and forming new skin cells which are pushed up from below as the upper layer of the epidermis wears away. Waste from chemical processes within your dermal cells is excreted by oil and sweat glands, which open pores in the surface of your epidermis.

The deepest level of your skin is the *subcutaneous tissue,* made up of fat and connective tissue. The fat layer provides insulation to help you maintain optimal body temperatures and to cushion your underlying tissue from impact damage, while the connective tissue attaches your skin to your muscles and tendons.

Sensory receptors are located throughout your skin, muscles, bones, joints, and internal organs. Touch is considered a fifth sense, but it's actually a combination of four different types of neurons, grouped by function:

- *Mechanoreceptors* (responsive to pressure and vibration)

- *Thermoreceptors* (responsive to skin surface temperature changes)

- *Nocioreceptors* (which transmit pain-generating impulses).

- *Proprioceptors* (which report limb position)

Touch receptors respond to changes in external stimuli – changes in pressure, temperature and tissue damage – with neural impulses. The response is immediate, after which the response pulse slows and returns to its original passive state; the speed at which these pulses return to normal is called the *rate of adaptation.* In other words, touch sensors don't transmit information about resting objects, but about changes. You can't feel the roughness of something unless you press upon it or rub across it, and it's the change in state generating touch signals.

Mechanoreceptors sense pressure, texture and shape via tiny sacs called *corpuscles,* which, when pressed, change shape, opening sodium ion gates to allow ion flow and build up an action potential.

Thermoreceptors respond to temperature changes in your skin. They're found throughout your body in your skin's deeper dermis layer, and they are specialized to respond to changes in either heat or cold, but there are a greater number of cold receptors. The highest concentration of both appears in your face and hands (which is why your nose and hands always get colder faster than the rest of your body in winter).

Nocioreceptors (Latin for *injury receptors*) report skin and organ tissue damage. Over three million are found throughout your body, in your skin, muscles, bones, blood vessels, and some organs. They can detect mechanical, thermal, or chemical injuries, such as cuts, bruises, scrapes, burns, or insect stings. These receptors are located closest to your skin's surface to immediately alert you with sharp pain when there's tissue damage. This motivates you to quickly withdraw from harm.

Proprioceptors (proprius meaning *one's own* in Latin) sense the position of your body parts in relation to one another, and within your environment. They're located in your tendons, muscles, and joints, allowing your brain to detect changes in muscle length and tension. Your basal ganglia, cerebellum and somatosensory cortex use these place markers to coordinate movement.

Receptors vary according to the speed at which they adapt and return to normal rest states:

- **Fast Adaptation (Pacinian corpuscles)** – Pacinian corpuscles are mechano-receptors in the deeper skin layer which look like tiny onions. They're suited for detecting minute vibrations or roughness, as your fingertips move across a surface. They are the largest receptors, responding to changes in stimuli, but quickly adapting to the new state, returning to normal in less than one-tenth of second.

  These mechanoreceptors are found in deeper skin layers. Each corpuscle contains a nerve fiber ending within a capsule of connective tissue. When pressure is applied to the skin, the capsule changes shape, pressing on the nerve ending, triggering a neural impulse which travels to the spine, and up into the thalamus and sensorimotor region of your parietal lobe.

- **Moderate Adaptation (Meissner's corpuscles)** – these fine-touch mechanoreceptors are closer to your skin surface, such as in your fingertips. Meissner's corpuscles adapt to changes a little more slowly, continuing to send signals longer than fast adaptation receptors, so if you continue to touch a surface, these receptors will continue to register the feeling for a longer period of time. Hair follicle receptors also adapt at a moderate rate and respond to mechanical changes – the movement of hairs – useful for example in detecting the presence of potentially dangerous insects on the skin.

- **Slow Adaptation (Merkel's Discs, Ruffini corpuscles)** – Merkel's Discs are slow-adapting mechanoreceptors close to your skin surface that also respond to pressure and vibration. They're clustered in great numbers under your fingerprint ridges. These are extremely sensitive and more rigid, so the action potential response takes longer to fade. This also makes them useful for maintaining your grip on objects.

- **Ruffini corpuscles** are long and thin mechanoreceptors sensitive to stretching, helping contribute to control of movement and positioning of your limbs and fingers. Located deeper within the dermis and along joints, tendons, and muscles, these mechanoreceptors respond to vibrations travelling through your bones and tendons, rotational movement of your limbs, and stretching of your skin.

- **Temperature and pain receptors** are slowest to adapt, ensuring these vital warning signs continue to motivate you until you escape danger. They operate through special ion channel proteins called *Transient Receptor Potential channels* (TRP channels) on the membranes of the nerve endings, which open to allow ion flow in response to heat, cold, and pressure. Some TRP channels can be activated by the chemicals in spices such as garlic, chili pepper, wasabi, menthol, camphor, and peppermint, which is why these foods create sensations of heat and coolness – they're activating the same skin receptors.

There are two known cold receptor proteins, which start to activate and transmit sensations of cold when your skin surface falls below 95°F (35°C). Their stimulation peaks at a 77°F (25°C) skin surface temperature and they stop activating when skin surface temperature falls below 41°F (5°C). This neural shutdown is the reason your feet, hands and face start to feel numb in extreme cold. There are also four known heat receptor proteins, which begin to activate when skin surface temperatures rise above 86°F (30°C). Their stimulation peaks at 113°F (45°C). Beyond that point, pain receptors begin to activate, motivating you to protect your body from damage.

Working Up a Sweat – *Beneath your skin lie over a million sweat glands – providing you with an extremely efficient way to keep cool. Thermoreceptors in your skin detect heat above 98.3 degrees, and signal your hypothalamus, which triggers a cooldown response: your capillaries dilate – transferring heat through your bloodstream to your skin surface, where it can be quickly dissipated into the air. Sweat glands extract water from your blood and release it onto your skin; as sweat evaporates, it cools you, by transferring your body's kinetic molecular energy (heat) to water, which then evaporates into the air.*

You produce about two pints of sweat a day, but in extremes, as when running, you'll pump out a lot more. Four pints an hour is the maximum, and you'll need to replenish the supply – your body is comprised of 75% water, but your vital organs need their share to survive. If you reach critical dehydration, your brain shuts down sweating, and orders moisture back to your vital organs in an emergency.

Pain

Alongside heat sensors are pain sensors, which alert your brain to injury – tissue damage. This is your self-preserving alarm system. Without pain, humans wouldn't have survived as a species. Nocioreceptors have bare nerve endings which respond to physical damage or strong chemicals. When your skin is broken, your body responds by sending white blood cells to clean the wound; the surrounding tissue swells, (inflammation) irritating nociceptor nerve endings. But the response generally happens slowly enough to allow you sufficient time to escape before pain overwhelms you. In some extremes, your nervous system may not even register the sensations. The delayed pain of inflammation is a warning to protect and treat the injured body part.

Pain is processed in several brain regions, and the location varies somewhat from person to person, because it's a subjective interpretation of sensations based upon your unique emotional makeup, says University of California neurobiologist Dr. Alan Basbaum. But the conscious perception of pain is located in your brain, rather than your body, and this perception is strongly affected by seeing or hearing other data which allows you to judge the severity of damage, a sort of subconscious message like, *Ooh look at that blood – this must hurt!*

In extreme emergencies, the pain system shuts down in *stress induced analgesia (SIA).* This is when, for example, soldiers wounded in battle or athletes injured in sports events feel no pain during the battle or game; however, the pain returns after the crisis has ended. When the danger has passed and the body relaxes, pain sensations flood in.

What this means is that, if the situation warrants it, your nervous system can shut out pain – and studies are beginning to show you can learn to consciously manage it. Pain occurs in several brain regions, but it appears to be the *emotional responses to it* which can most easily be controlled.

Pain signals travel from nocioreceptors to your CNS, the signal conducted via your synapses. But the synaptic transmissions can be switched off with the release of endorphins from interneurons, blocking pain signal transmission. These natural opioids are stronger than morphine.

The Periaqueductal Gray in your midbrain orchestrates the process. Also coming into play is your insula, thought to help manage body awareness, anticipating pain and other unpleasant experiences before they occur, helping you judge the level of pain severity, and "reading" the physiological effects of emotions within your body.

Nocioreceptors and thermoreceptors in your body report tissue damage or intense temperatures, sending impulses up your spine to your PAG and thalamus. The PAG triggers serotonin release down your spine from the raphe nuclei. The serotonin excites interneurons which release endorphins. These endorphins bind to receptors and block substance P release, so pain signals are no longer transmitted to your brain.

From an evolutionary perspective, pain is extremely valuable for survival, lessening the likelihood of repeating dangerous behavior. It's also highly salient, meaning your amygdala "marks" painful events, making particularly vivid memories. Likewise, the prefrontal cortex, seat of your conscious thought, is triggered, because when faced with pain, one has a decision: while pain is generally seen as a form of suffering, it also serves the vital function of warning you when your body has received an injury, and your reaction is usually to retreat from the source of pain, but it's also possible to choose alternative responses such as fighting, shouting, cursing, or enduring pain for the sake of some anticipated reward.

UCSF Neuroscience Professor Dr. Howard Fields says that "...from a biological perspective, pain is best understood as a motivational state, a drive to escape, terminate and avoid the tissue-damaging process." At the point a creature feels pain, it's faced with a decision; often the dangerous situation occurs in the presence of motivations like hunger, or sexual attraction, which can conflict with the natural drive to escape pain. Dr. Fields' research shows enduring pain to satisfy a drive like hunger or sexual desire triggers systems which dampen pain transmission, while choosing to escape pain allows these pain perception systems to fully engage. What's more, adds Dr. Fields, "...through classical conditioning, initially neutral contextual cues can acquire the motivational power to elicit opioid-mediated analgesia." In plain English, this means you can train your mind to use cues as triggers to release natural painkillers in your body.

Sticks, Stones *and* Words

Because pain and emotion are so deeply interrelated, your brain doesn't make major distinctions between physical and emotional pain – heartache, disappointment and other emotional forms of pain are more than simply poetic language. Dr. Ethan Kross, assistant professor of psychology at the University of Michigan, used fMRI scans in 2011 to show the same neural circuitry activated by cutting your finger also lights up when you remember the loss of a loved one. 40 mentally and physically healthy volunteers who had recently been harshly rejected by their romantic partners were given fMRI scans as they performed two painful tasks. The first involved a heating device strapped to each volunteer's arm, which inflicted physical pain equivalent to holding a hot cup of coffee, while the second had the same volunteers look at photos of their lost lovers and recall moments they had shared. According to the study's authors:

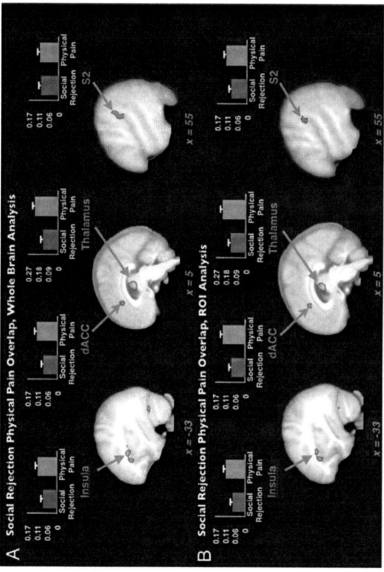

Social Rejection Shares Somatosensory Representations With Physical Pain,
Edward E. Smith, Ethan Kross, et al, 2011, Columbia University,
University of Michigan. Used with permission.

Both social rejection and physical pain are distressing, and both the ACC and insula respond broadly to stimuli that elicit negative affect....we propose that experiences of social rejection, when elicited powerfully enough, recruit brain regions involved in both the affective (mood) and sensory components of physical pain.

Social rejection and physical pain are similar not only in that they are both distressing, they share a common representation in somatosensory brain systems as well, highlighting the role that somatosensory processing may play in this process. They are also consistent with research on 'embodiment', which suggests that somatosensory processing is integral to the experience of emotion.

Says Kross, rejection and similar emotional trauma may even be the root cause of chronic pain disorders like *fibromyalgia*, the causes and mechanisms of which have largely remained a mystery to doctors. Koss believes treating the emotional pain may well relieve the physical pain, and vice versa.

Dr. Judith Scheman, who directs the Cleveland Clinic's chronic pain rehabilitation program, agrees, adding that emotional trauma can increase pain sensitivity, making people more susceptible to disorders like fibromyalgia, which includes chronic pain and fatigue. Her clinic tries to encourage patients to look for underlying emotional trauma and "psychological baggage" which can be resolved.

In other words, past traumatic events can increase pain sensitivity, and heartbreak really does hurt. In fact, as you'll see in book two, doctors have discovered it can even kill. Interestingly, it's also been found that *analgesics* (pain relieving medications like aspirin) appear to lessen emotional pain, such as after a breakup; the medications are thought to dampen signals from the insula, somatosensory cortex and thalamus, the same brain regions triggered by emotional pain.

The Blues Worsen Pain

Negative emotions like stress, fear and worry have been demonstrated to worsen and perhaps even cause pain. A 2005 study by Swedish obstetricians found higher reported levels of fear – the anticipation of pain – and higher levels of stress hormones such as cortisol in the saliva and urine of expectant mothers corresponded to increased levels of birthing pains.

Oxford University has also demonstrated that depression worsens pain: previously there had been two competing schools of thought about whether pain was "all in the head" or "all in the body", but the neural signals have been traced through a combination of two pathways, one physical and the other mental.

In 2010, Dr. Chantal Berna and colleagues scanned volunteers to see how their pain responses changed when they were made unhappy through depressing music or sad thinking. They found that being in an emotionally depressed state disables the ability to dampen negative emotional circuitry which are normally capable of decreasing physical sensations of pain.

Analgesia (pain relief) comes from activation of the periaqueductal gray area, sitting in your midbrain atop your brainstem. Stress, exercise and pleasurable activities can all activate this region. It, in turn, stimulates a zipperlike formation in the middle of your brainstem called the raphe nuclei, which release serotonin into neurons stretching down throughout the length of your spine as well as into your brain. Serotonin is a neuromodulator, controlling the effects of other neurotransmitters.

When triggered by the PAG, serotonin excites special interneurons along your spine which release endorphins (endogenous morphine, your body's natural opiate). These inhibit the release of the pain messenger neurotransmitter called substance P, so the pain messages that normally travel up your spine to your thalamus (sensation gateway) and somatosensory cortex (conscious pain interpreter and physical awareness center) never reach their destination.

A new related study has discovered that migraines are a progressive disease, centering around lesions (destroyed tissue) in white matter (axons or stems of your neurons) in the PAG - your pain shutdown center. Although they don't yet know the cause of these lesions or whether they are permanent or reversible, they also found a buildup of iron in the area, and so believe that poor iron homeostasis (ability to maintain chemical balance) may cause these lesions. They also suggest that progressive sensitization (increase in sensitivity from repeated firings of a neural circuit) may be a factor.

*They say it seems to be centered around progressive damage to the pain-modulating center in your brainstem, possibly because of an inability of the region to dispose of excess iron. They also mention abnormally high excitation of nociceptors (nerves which report tissue damage – the trigger for pain signals) in the **meninges**, the protective membranes surrounding your brain, in the medulla of your brainstem, and in the **trigeminal ganglion**, nerve clusters just above your palate which transmit information about conditions inside your skull. Abnormal serotonin control may also be a cause.*

What Did You Expect?

Oxford, Cambridge, Hamburg and Munchen University neuroscientists teamed up in 2011 to study the effects of patient expectations on their treatment, and found negative expectations are powerful enough to completely override potent painkillers. On the other hand, positive expectations can double painkiller effectiveness, according to patient reports and fMRI scans.

Everyone's heard of the placebo effect – where believing you've swallowed medicine causes measurable physical effects in your body, even when you've only taken sugar pills. A recent discovery proves there is also a *nocebo* effect, where pessimism can completely override the effects of the even the most powerful medications. Negative expectations can have a major impact on treatment, so patients who expect failure can actually cause the effects they expect.

To measure the effect of expectations on drug efficacy, twenty-two healthy adult volunteers were placed into fMRI scanners, and had painful heat applied to their legs, while a painkiller was fed to them intravenously. An average reported pain level of 70 on a scale of 1 to 100 was used to test responses to the painkiller and how that changed with expectations. As their brains were scanned, the volunteers reported the pain and pain relief they felt at different intervals. Without telling the volunteers, the researchers then turned on the painkiller, and, as expected, the patients reported much lower pain, and pain-associated brain activity decreased in the insula and the anterior cingulate cortex, both of which analyze and process pain. The average reported pain rating dropped from 66 to 55 when they were unknowingly given the painkiller.

In the second step, the researchers told their volunteers they were starting to inject painkiller – even though it had been administered the entire time. Pain ratings dropped further, showing the placebo effect at work – patient expectations created physical changes, resulting in significant pain reduction. Their reported pain ratings dropped to an average of 39, and fMRI scans showed similar drops in insula and ACC activity. Later, with no further change in drug administration, the volunteers were told the painkiller administration had been stopped and to expect an increase in pain. In response, reported pain intensity returned to nearly previous levels, at 64, and fMRI images matched reported increases in pain. This showed the volunteers really did experience significantly different pain levels when their expectations changed, although the painkilling medicine they received remained at constant levels throughout.

Belief Brings Relief – Filming The Placebo Effect At Work

In 2002, the University of British Columbia's Dr. Jon Stoessl and colleagues used fMRI scans to observe brains processing the placebo effect. They discovered the brain uses dopamine the same way when processing the placebo effect as when experiencing a positive reward. According to Dr. Stoessl, fMRI scans show the pain experience is comprised of two stages – expectation and experience. What's more, there isn't just a single placebo effect; there are, in fact, many.

His research shows the effects can significantly impact a wide range of mental and physical ailments, including Parkinson's disease and depression. The underlying mechanisms differ between each kind of placebo effect, but they all share a common component of expectation, believed to involve the prefrontal cortex and striatal dopamine.

The placebo effect state of expectation, driven by the prefrontal cortex and basal ganglia, appears to trigger a biochemical response specific to each condition – for Parkinson's patients, increasing dopamine in the striatum, and for pain sufferers, increasing endorphins via ACC, insula, and nucleus accumbens activity.

Placebo responses likely involve a combination of several neurochemicals, including serotonin and hormones, although this is yet unclear. It seems that the common element is that dopamine is released in the ventral striatum when a patient expects improvement, and that it thus constitutes a form of reward.

As a result of his groundbreaking studies on the placebo effect and Parkinson's disease, Dr. Stoessl has been awarded Canada's highest honor, the Order of Canada. In 2007, Dr. Stoessl teamed up with graduate student Sarah C. Christine Lidstone, using PET scans to track dopamine flow during the placebo effect. PET machines work by capturing images of radioactive tracers attached to specific chemicals (such as dopamine) as they flow through the brain. Stoessl and Lidstone scanned volunteers' brains as they reacted to hearing they were going to receive effective treatment.

Each of the volunteers was suffering from Parkinson's disease, a progressively degenerative motor control disease that results from insufficient nigrostriatal dopamine. Amazingly, PET scans revealed that simply believing they would receive effective treatment increased nigrostriatal dopamine, and their symptoms significantly improved.

Stoessl and Lidstone found the placebo effect originates from the frontal cortex, anterior cingulate cortex and striatum, with the ventral striatum activating in anticipation of reward (including the reward of pain relief). Dopamine neurons, as we've seen, participate in three major pathways. Each pathway is associated with different functions, such as memory, learning, motivation, addictive behaviors, reward processing, and voluntary movement. Disruption of dopamine function within these pathways can lead to Parkinson's disease, loss of *incentive salience* (motivation and willpower to do anything constructive), addictive behavior, and even psychosis.

The release of endorphins is also involved in placebo-induced analgesia: pain is processed across a number of regions, including the anterior cingulate cortex, prefrontal cortex, insula, amygdala, thalamus, and nucleus accumbens. When patients have been given a placebo and expect pain relief, researchers have observed a release of endogenous opioids in the ACC, prefrontal cortex, insula, and nucleus accumbens. Those with the greatest nucleus accumbens opioid transmission reported the greatest pain reduction.

In the prefrontal cortex, opioid release varied according to the expected pain relief, suggesting the region has inhibitory control of pain processing centers in the insula, ACC, thalamus, and PAG. When volunteers believed a topical placebo cream could reduce pain, it markedly reduced both their reported pain, and their insula, thalamus, ACC and PAG activity. Because the PAG is strongly linked to pain control and the endogenous opioid system, Stoessl and Lidstone concluded that expectations of pain relief in PFC regions triggered activation of PAG-controlled opioid systems. These are the same regions in the PFC and ACC involved in conscious emotional response regulation – restraint and the conscious choice of behave appropriately. In other words, the placebo effect seems controlled by the same areas responsible for exercising conscious will. For you, it means you can learn to shut down pain.

Your brain is capable of dampening or intensifying pain with both conscious and unconscious processing. So far, researchers have found at least four ways to naturally reduce both emotional and physical pain:

- mental distraction
- positive emotions such as joy or romantic love
- anticipating rewards such as rich foods and or an end to the pain
- exercise

In hopes that it might be possible to one day teach people how to "switch off" pain at will, researchers at Oxford University used fMRI scans to map neural responses to pain. Irene Tracey heads the studies, where volunteers agree to be subjected to various kinds of pain while their brains are scanned; pain infliction methods range from being stuck with pins to being burned, shocked, and having balloons shoved up their rectums and inflated (!).

Pain killers like codeine and morphine use an opioid made from the milk of opium seed pods, one of the oldest drugs known to man. These synthetic opioids block pain signal transmission, but are extremely addictive and not always effective. In search of safer pain relief which directly targets specific pain centers in the brain, Dr. Irene Tracey and other scientists are studying the mechanisms behind natural analgesia, such as when soldiers in the heat of battle are sometimes impervious to pain or people become distracted from their pain while intensely concentrating on tasks. What they've discovered is that pain isn't registered in a single, discrete brain region, but is spread over various locations in what lead researcher Dr. Tracey calls the *pain matrix*.

Pain travels twin nervous system pathways, an emotional and a physical channel. When you're injured, nocioreceptors in your skin, muscles, bones, tendons, joints and internal organs send signals to your spinal cord or the base of your brain. As damaged cells release their contents in an *inflammatory soup*, the area's nocioreceptors increase in sensitivity, and continue to respond more strongly to pain in the damaged region.

Meanwhile, deep within your limbic system, your amygdala processes emotional responses to the injury, while your insula, thought to be concerned with anticipation of pain and other unpleasant experiences, judges pain severity, and reads the physiological effects of your negative emotions within your body. Likewise, your prefrontal cortex, seat of your consciousness, is triggered, as at this point, you may be faced with a decision: the instinctive reaction is usually to retreat from the source of pain, but you can also choose fighting, shouting, or enduring pain for the sake of some anticipated reward.

Thus, your PFC can be recruited to consciously dampen the effects of pain, allowing you to consciously focus your awareness on another activity such as counting or reading. In fact, pain is modified by how much you pay attention to it, and pain-processing activity in the amygdala and ACC lessen as attention is focused away from the discomfort. Pleasant smells have also been demonstrated to uplift mood and reduce pain responses.

On the other hand, feeling depressed and thinking depressing thoughts can intensify pain, as shown by fMRI scans. And long-term pain, such as chronic backaches, has been shown to physically alter the brain, reducing grey matter and increasing activity in the prefrontal cortex, amplifying future pain – the more you give in to pain, the worse it's going to get, until the condition underlying it has been relieved.

Stanford University's Dr. Sean Mackey trains patients to significantly reduce their own pain at will, learning to control brain activity through *biofeedback*. Practicing visualization of the pain eventually enables pain control with the assistance of a biofeedback machine that displays brain activity. 34-year-old San Francisco event planner Laura Tibbitts, for example, had severe injuries to her arm, shoulder and back after being thrown from a horse. She learned to alleviate her chronic pain as much as 30 to 40%, by envisioning: "...The pain was literally being scooped out from me, taken away and carried off. Other times I used water imagery, like it was flowing through me and taking it away."

Dr. Mackey followed up with a related study in 2010, using fMRI scans to monitor volunteers who had recently entered romantic relationships as they were subjected to heat pain. As their brains were monitored for pain responses, they were either shown pictures of their loved ones, of attractive and familiar acquaintances, or they used distracting word-association games.

Dr. Mackey's team found that when volunteers looked at pictures of their loved ones, it activated dopamine release in the striatum and elsewhere, significantly reducing the pain they felt. The effects were just as strong as when holding their partner's hands.

The distracting word association games were to find out whether or not the pictures were just distractions from pain. Volunteers would, for example, be instructed to "think of sports that do not use a ball" and silently imagine as many responses as possible. This exercise also significantly reduced pain to the same degree, but through a different means, with most of the brain activity heightened in the prefrontal cortex – meaning attention was being diverted to distract them from their pain.

Let Fly! Keele University researchers found in 2011 that cursing is a pain reliever. 64 student volunteers immersed their hands in icy water, while researchers measured how long they could withstand the discomfort. The volunteers would curse while holding their hands in the ice water, and then repeat the experiment while saying neutral words.

Students were able to withstand the discomfort much longer while they were cursing, which, said Dr. Richard Stephens, raised heartbeat and appeared to trigger the fight or flight response, desensitizing them to pain perception.

Dr. Stephens and his team believe that this may be one of the reasons swearing has persisted across cultures and throughout history – it has evolutionary advantages.

For those not used to swearing, the effect was 400% stronger, while for those who curse regularly, the pain-relieving effects vanish. Among men prone to "catastrophizing" (anticipating and worrying over the worst), however, swearing had no effect on their abilities to withstand pain – one more reason to drop the worry addiction.

Additionally, women received stronger benefits than men in pain relief overall. In an episode which aired on April 28, 2010, the Discovery Channel's Mythbusters confirmed the experiment, finding an average 30% increase in tolerance time while swearing. They also found that among their 50 subjects, women significantly outlasted men: the average endurance of the 25 women was 100.4 seconds, while the men lasted an average of 84.3 seconds.

I've Got A Bad Feeling About This

Recent studies have also shown that you can mentally "brace yourself" to lessen the impact of traumatic or stressful events. In 2009, University of Alabama psychologists coupled *galvanic responses* (skin sweat electrical conductivity) with fMRI scans to find the extent to which loud noises disturbed volunteers.

This was the first time psychologists were able to see in detail how the brain responds to unexpected or traumatic events. Observing the fear, learning and memory centers as unexpected, loud static bursts were used to startle volunteers, and again when these volunteers knew in advance the noise would occur, researchers found foreknowledge significantly lessened frontal lobe activity and emotional response. According to Dr. David Knight, who led the study, "When participants are able to predict when they are going to hear the unpleasant static noise, you can see the regions of the brain quiet down so that a smaller emotional response is produced."

Needles And Pins

In 1996, I had stepped up my weight training regimen to a new level. I'd recently been training with two colleagues at the real estate firm I worked for and had cracked a 350-pound bench press for the first time. I was enthusiastic, and in the ensuing weeks overdid it, suffering my first and only sports injury on the pec-deck – the seated pectoral flyes machine.

Since the age of 25, I'd been able to easily use all the weight on the pec deck, but had upped the frequency of my upper-body workouts to three times a week. The nasty result was an overuse injury – I tore a ligament in my left rhomboid – the muscle connecting my shoulder blade and spine. I couldn't write or even sleep easily, and the pain was constant and severe.

As anyone who's seen Vancouver's skid row knows, opiates have some pretty scary consequences that I wasn't particularly interested in exploring, so I decided to try something novel and interesting, and asked my Chinese girlfriend to find an acupuncturist for me. The office she recommended was located in an upscale modern building at the corner of Burrard and Davie, and I went in not knowing what to expect.

When I arrived, the office was dark and silent, and a middle-aged, soft-spoken, elegantly professional woman stepped out from behind a door decorated by an unsettling chart of a human pincushion covered in hieroglyphics. She led me to a room with a wide soundproofed window overlooking the busy boulevard below, and had me remove my shirt and lie on my back upon a green table. The first step, she said, was to relax. She then pierced each of my wrists deeply with a pair of long, slender silver needles. The effect was completely painless and nearly immediate – stronger than a hospital anesthetic; within seconds, I was completely unconscious.

Approximately half an hour later I regained consciousness and she had me sit up, and she pushed pins deep into the muscles of my back. The pain did ease over time, not miraculously, but substantially. That's why I wasn't surprised to learn the US Military has begun to experiment with acupuncture to treat wounded soldiers in the field: http://www.youtube.com/watch?v=PmPJKO2Gxsg

fMRI scans conducted in 2010 at the University Hospital of Essen, Germany show that acupuncture significantly alters pain-related activity, primarily in the insula and somatosensory cortex.

The Inner Flame

Meditation is also becoming widely accepted as a means of easing pain – making substantial changes to both the brain and body – slowing heart rate, relaxing the muscles, resulting in less tension and anxiety. Doctors have begun using it to teach patients to lessen their emotional responses to pain – turning down the "reactive volume".

Focused attention meditation has been clinically demonstrated to reduce pain as much as 40 to 57 percent – 150% to 228% the effectiveness of even morphine or other painkillers. What's more, says Dr. Fadel Zeidan of North Carolina's Wake Forest Baptist Medical Center, the practice is so simple that a complete novice can learn it in under an hour and a half.

To clinically test its efficacy, 15 subjects were scanned before and after four 20-minute sessions using magnetic resonance imaging, as painful heat was applied to their legs for five minutes at a time. Post-meditation training brain scans showed pain decreased dramatically – from 11 to as much as 93 percent, with reduced activity primarily in the somatosensory cortex.

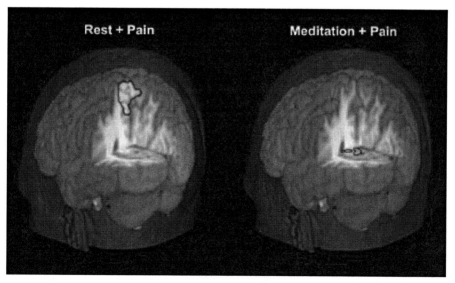

fMRI scan: Primary somatosensory cortex pain activation, with and without meditation, Fadel Zeidan, Ph.D, 2011. Used with permission.

Prior to meditation training, the volunteers had extremely high activity in their somatosensory cortices, but while meditating, no activity was detected in the region. However, Dr. Zeidan says meditation reduces pain throughout the brain, rather than in a single region, making it more effective than conventional painkillers.

Although the image of meditation is one of quietude, it actually increases activity across a wide range of areas, including the insula, which is involved in sensing heat, cold, pain and possibly *metacognition*, the awareness of and ability to observe your own thoughts. But the thalami grow quiet during the meditation, suggesting pain signals had been stopped before being transmitted to conscious-level brain processing areas.

Hypnosis – *In 1774, a theatrical German doctor by the name of* **Franz Mesmer** *began demonstrating the most astonishing feats of what he called "animal magnetism", treating patients for a number of disorders by staring deeply into their eyes and using special words and phrases to make them fall into trancelike states. A shoddy investigation was ordered by King Louis XVI, discrediting a colleague, and Mesmer was found guilty by association of engaging in sham science; this is probably at least partly the basis of hypnotism's shady reputation. However, in the 19th century, hypnosis was frequently used in place of anesthetics during surgery – until the discovery of ether, which was found to more consistently render all patients unconscious. The problem is that not everyone is susceptible to hypnosis, for reasons which are not yet fully understood. However, fMRI scans show there are very demonstrable effects within the brain.*

University of Oregon neuroscience professor Dr. Michael I. Posner received a 2009 Gold Medal Lifetime Achievement Award at the White House for pioneering work in neuroscience. He says hypnotism alters perception based upon expectations, and the neural mechanisms behind hypnosis are beginning to come clearly into focus: earlier experiments have already shown executive control and attention processes can alter memory, pain perception, and voluntary movement, but additional research in 2009 has uncovered how hypnotism-induced paralysis affects neural circuitry specifically involved in self-imagery and internal representation.

The University of Geneva's Dr. Yann Cojan studied motor and inhibitory neural circuits during hypnosis-induced paralysis. Using fMRI scans, his team found hypnosis produces changes to attention centers distributed throughout the prefrontal and parietal cortices, along with dramatic changes in motor cortex circuitry and its projections to other brain regions. They also found enhanced activity in the **precuneus**, *a parietal lobe region which deals with self-imagery and memory. Hypnosis, he says, induces changes here and to self-image centers in the cingulate cortex and disconnection of motor commands from normal voluntary executive control.*

Professor John Gruzelier at the University of London has also used fMRI scans of hypnotized patients to show substantial changes in the cingulate cortex and PFC. He says, counterintuitively, the imaging shows activity increase in both regions when patients are successfully hypnotized, and he believes it's because functional suppression requires these regions to work harder than a brain in its normal state.

San Diego dentist Ashley Goodman regularly uses clinical hypnosis instead of traditional anesthetics to shut off pain when he operates. As he notes in Discovery Channel's 2008 documentary The Human Body, "Pain is perception. Reality is perception. So what we can do is alter the perception of reality." Pain appears to register emotionally, and hypnosis can alter the perception of it, allowing it to be perceived differently, even as a pleasant sensation.

On The Horizon – A Safer Painkiller

On the more conventional side of medicine, it turns out that chronic pain can be shut down with a peptide that appears to be free of side effects, and is safer than addictive opioids or other current painkillers. Dr. Rajesh Khanna at Indiana University discovered a peptide called *CBD3* shuts down chronic pain by interfering with calcium channel signalling. Because calcium also regulates heartbeat and other vital functions, the fact that that CBD3 doesn't directly inhibit calcium influx (inward flow) is of great benefit.

Nocioreceptors have an abundance of calcium channels, key components in the pain signal pathway. A protein called CRMP-2 binds to these calcium channels, acting like a "remote control" in modulating transmission of excitatory pain signals, says Dr. Khanna.

The CBD3 peptide is a portion of this CRMP-2 protein. The molecule binds to calcium channels and reduces the number of excitatory signals without disrupting vital calcium flow. Since this doesn't directly stop calcium flow into neurons, it appears both safer and more effective than current pain relievers, he adds.

The Thinking Animal

"I Think I Am, Therefore, I Am... I Think"
– George Carlin, Napalm and Silly Putty, 2001

Thinking About Thinking

There is no one single "thought center" in the brain – it's an integration of massive parallel processing distributed throughout your brain, and engaging your body.

In general, your cortices analyze sensory data, your association areas integrate it into a coherent interpretation of reality, and your frontal cortex brings it all to your conscious awareness, where you judge, reason and decide, enacting behaviors required to attain your goals. For everything you encounter, your corticolimbic circuits shuffle through a complex web of memories in microseconds, to find memory matches that resemble each new encounter.

Values are attached to each of these memories – things you either like or dislike, so you're biased either for or against every piece of data your senses bring to your attention. These subconscious associations are triggered before you even fully, consciously identify what it is you're perceiving at any given moment.

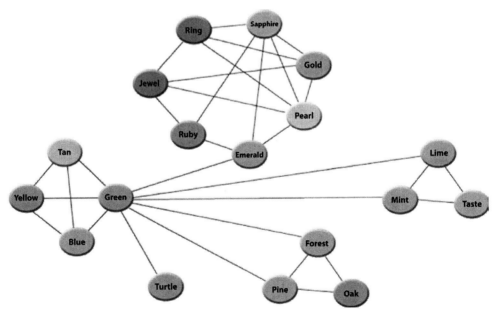

SCHEMATA - MEMORY MAPS

Information is organized in your memory according to webs of related information called schemata, such as concepts related to the word green. The closer the relationship between the concepts, the stronger the mental association will be. This is why it's effective to relate information you want to remember to things you already know.

Human thought is based upon the principle of association – a vast network of links. The way your brain learns quickly and efficiently is through organizing your understanding of the world into web-like clusters of these associations, networks of information called *schemata*.

The efficient linked structure of your schemata allows you to navigate through everyday life with little concentrated mental effort; all that is required is automatic processing. For example, your schema for *dog* allows you to instantly recognize one, even if it's a breed you've never seen before.

These clusters of interlinked impressions, beliefs and understandings can significantly influence your attention and perception – your brain is wired to notice things in the environment which match your existing mental schemata, and which confirm your expectations.

Your mind needs logical consistency, and is built to find it, allowing prediction, one of the human species' most powerful survival tools. But this need for consistency makes you prone to strongly rejecting things which don't fit your existing schemata, things that don't gibe with your subjective ideas of what is "right" or "true". Your schemata can even lead you to act in ways that cause your expectations of the world to come true.

Because of your brain's remarkable plasticity, your long-term memories are under constant adjustment, and your schemata evolve with experience. New information that matches your schemata is easily learned and added to your worldview. But if it doesn't match, or runs contrary to your schemata, you're likely to reject, or at best tentatively accept it as an "exception to the rule". Your preconceptions can interfere with your ability to learn, because you expect things to follow the logic of your schemata, even when the information it contains may be incorrect. Psychologists call this well-documented effect *confirmation bias*.

Confirmation bias is one of the reasons that, for example, prejudices are so difficult to purge. If you've been taught at an early age negative information about a certain social class, race or age range, you'll see things that confirm your bias – the information in your schemata – in every individual, even when others can clearly see your information is false.

Pattern Recognition

At the heart of your mental organization and ability to predict is an unrivalled, powerful aptitude for pattern recognition. This enables you to nearly instantly spot a predator lurking in the trees, for example, or recognize a dangerously thin patch of ice on a frozen lake.

Superior pattern recognition has served hominids well for an estimated 6 million years. Unfortunately, however, we're too good at it. This is why we often see patterns where none exist. For example, *apophenia* – also called *patternicity* – is the common experience of finding meaningful connections among random information. Humans tend to see patterns in natural occurrences all the time, in natural phenomena, gambling addictions, and even science, often ascribing supernatural forces to the patterns they see.

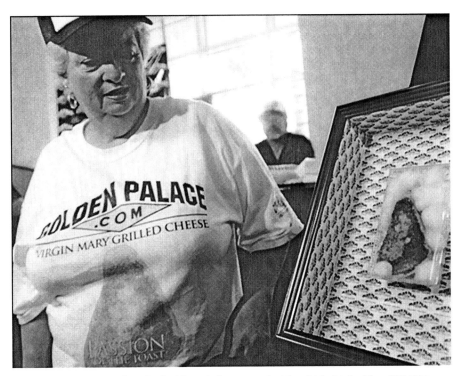

Diana Duyser poses beside the blessed cheese sandwich which fetched her $28,000 on Ebay in 1994. Image courtesy of the Associated Press, used with permission.

Frequently, for example, devout Christians find holy signs in everything from the shapes of trees to food items. Recently, such dubious relics have found a burgeoning online market, being auctioned to the highest bidder on sites like EBay. One of the most famous examples is a grilled cheese sandwich Diana Duyser claimed was imprinted with the face of the Mary Magdalene. The blessed toast sold – with a single bite taken out of the corner – for a bargain at $28,000. It's now enshrined at the headquarters of the Golden Palace online Casino in Kahnawake Mohawk Territory near Montreal, Canada.

Patternicity can also involve finding significance in vague or random phenomena, such as images or sounds –seeing images of animals or faces in the clouds, a face on the surface of the moon, or hearing secret messages on musical recordings played in reverse.

Reason

According to Yale University's Dr. Paul Bloom, human reason is built upon *rough and ready heuristics* – problem-solving using loose guidelines including *rules of thumb, educated guessing, intuition, stereotyping* and *common sense*. While the method is useful for fast decision-making, it's subject to error from four sources:

- **Framing effects** – People have natural *loss aversion*, meaning we hate the idea of losing anything. Because of this, the way something is *framed* (presented to us) can markedly change our perception of it.

This weakness in human logic is cynically exploited quite skillfully by politicians and advertisers: for example, says Dr. Bloom, you're much more likely to buy a hamburger that's advertised as "*80% fat free!*" as opposed to one that's "*20% fat!*"

- *Endowment effect* – Once you own something, that item's value increases in your own estimation. This is again related to loss aversion. You hate to give up something that's yours.

- *Availability bias* – The more often you hear something, the more frequently you'll think it occurs. For example, says Dr. Bloom, the odds of being killed by a shark are 1 in 5 million, while the odds of being killed by eating bad potato salad are 1 in 50,000. However, since you read more of shark attack stories, you're likely to perceive these events as a far more prevalent threat.

  Similarly, if a group of politicians talks repeatedly about "welfare cheats", or violent crime in your community, you'll start to believe there are many cases, when, in fact, there may be only be a single case.

- *Confirmation bias* – We form ideas about how situations work, then tend to more easily spot evidence to support these ideas. This is one of the reasons racism is so hard to erase once it takes root. For example, if your parents, friends and neighbors have told you that "…illegal immigrants just come to America and have lots of babies, then don't pay taxes and live off of the system", you may end up believing it, when in fact, illegal immigrants as a group pay at least $9 billion taxes annually in America, and cannot collect Social Security benefits, according to a 2008 AP news release.

You're a Prediction Machine

Says Cambridge neuroscientist Daniel Wolpert, your brain is essentially a prediction machine, which evolved to manage movement, your only means of output to the world. Your brain makes predictions, used in determining how you can best respond to your environment.

Your brain predicts based upon the principles of *Bayesian Inference*. Inferences are your beliefs about the world; your brain uses these beliefs and incoming sensory information to make predictions based on probabilities. If you say the range of probability is between 0 and 1, 0 means "I don't believe it at all", 1 means "I'm absolutely certain", and all the numbers in between are varying degrees of certainty.

Your brain calculates probability of results based upon two sources of input:

- Data – sensory input

- Memory – previous knowledge.

You then learn and improve by comparing your predictions with outcomes.

The Sure Bet

Gamblers differ in the reasons for their betting strategies, whether the game is roulette, kino, slot machines or craps. One player will choose his "lucky" number, because it's paid off in the past. This strategy is based on *reinforcement learning* – predicting the future based on previous events.

A second player may choose to watch a series of ball drops, numbers or dice rolls in hopes of discovering a pattern. Believing that a completely random event can be affected by a previous completely random event – the idea that something's "due" to occur – is the faulty logic behind the *gambler's fallacy*. And this, of course, is what the casinos rely upon to earn their keep.

These strategies are contradictory: in reinforcement-learning behavior, people choose something that has won a lot recently, believing it is "lucky" for them, and thus more likely to appear, while trusting the gambler's fallacy, prompts them to choose something that has lost a lot recently, believing it is more likely to appear. Both strategies are, of course, faulty. A random event is a random event – every time. As professional croupiers are taught to memorize, "the dice have no memory".

In 2011, researchers from Caltech and Ireland's Trinity College teamed up to study the specific brain regions at work as gamblers make these decisions based upon these two two different strategies.

In professor John O'Doherty's laboratory, games of chance – in this case roulette – were used with small payoffs to research how the brain operates as people made gambling decisions. While lying in an fMRI scanner 31 participants were asked to predict where a roulette ball would land a total of four times. For each round of play, they were charged half a euro, and for every correct guess, they were awarded two euros. The research team discovered that activity in the dorsal striatum changes depending upon the betting strategy people choose.

The dorsal striatum was more active in those who chose based upon reinforcement-learning (past winning) numbers compared to those who chose according to the gambler's fallacy (that it's a number's "turn" to appear, as if it had somehow decided it was ready). Out of 31 volunteers, only eight made logical predictions – choosing colors covering the largest area.

What's Your IQ?

Intelligence is the subject of much argument and debate. Psychologists don't yet agree on what it means, but for the time being, it's measured using the *Wechsler Adult Intelligence Scale*, a 90-minute series of tests first published in 1955 that measure comprehension, vocabulary and arithmetic to determine an overall IQ score.

IQ is a set of diverse problem-solving, information and memory-manipulating skills that underlie intelligence, most of which occurs in the prefrontal cortex. But skills comprising intelligence also such aspects as include working memory, rapid recognition, categorization, spatial navigation, and the ability to mentally "rotate" three-dimensional objects in the mind.

Because of concerns about limitations to standard IQ testing, Cambridge University, Discovery Channel and New Scientist Magazine have teamed up to create an online intelligence test based upon a newly-proposed model of intelligence called the *12 Pillars of Intelligence*. This draws upon 20 years of research by the UK Medical Research Council's Cognition and Brain Sciences Unit, and is an attempt to define all aspects intelligence, from memory to planning.

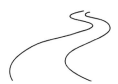

The Emotional Animal

"I just have one last thing: I urge all of you, all of you, to enjoy your life, the precious moments you have. To spend each day with some laughter and some thought, to get your emotions going." –
NCSU coach Jim Valvano, dying of cancer, acceptance speech, Arthur Ashe Courage and Humanitarian Award, March 4, 1993

How Do You Feel?

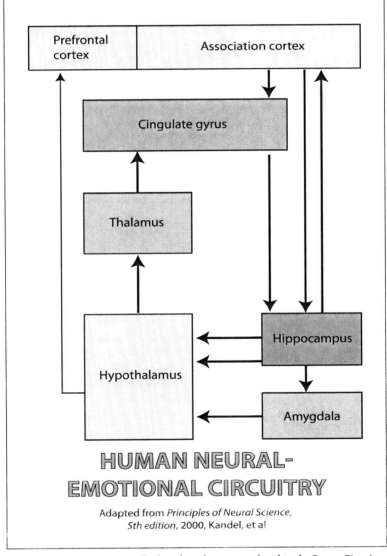

HUMAN NEURAL-EMOTIONAL CIRCUITRY

Adapted from *Principles of Neural Science,*
5th edition, 2000, Kandel, et al

*Your emotions were originally thought to be generated within the **Papez Circuit**.*
The original theory has been revised to include the limbic regions, as shown above.

Emotions, according to Yale Psychology Professor Dr. Paul Bloom, are what motivate you, compelling you to set goals and establish priorities. They direct your attention, and help you interpret the significance of what's going on around you:

> ...without them you wouldn't do anything, you couldn't do anything. Your desire to come to class to study, to go out with friends, to read a book, to raise a family, would be virtually nonexistent. Life would be impossible without those emotions.

Nobel winning neuroscientist Dr. Eric Kandel says they communicate emotional states to others and prepare the body for action. These built-in responses are biochemical changes and automatic reactions allowing you to, for example, instantly register potential danger and be physically ready to save yourself at lightning speed, or to instantly choose the most genetically beneficial mate, and send signals to stimulate mutual attraction without even being consciously aware of your own signalling; your emotions allow you to effortlessly and instantly link with others intuitively, your body physically experiencing their pain, joy, sorrow or anger simply through the act of observation.

All living creatures are motivated to maximize pleasant, rewarding stimuli and avoid unpleasant stimuli. Emotions such as fear, curiosity, joy and love thus guide behaviors, motivating you to do things that give you pleasure, such as eating and copulating, and avoid things that give you displeasure or pain such as injury. You want to repeat experiences that feel good, and avoid those that feel bad.

Emotions enhance communication – you have built-in facial expressions, body language and changes in your voice and body responses that convey to others what you're feeling without your conscious intent or thought. These expressions, may differ slightly from culture to culture, but appear to be built into your brain genetically, so that you can convey and recognize them without ever needing to be taught.

Overt emotional displays such as facial expressions or body language serve as a fast "shorthand" form of communication among animal species that live in social communities. This easy and powerful communication promotes species survival. Aside from facial expressions, you convey emotions through body language, muscular tension and perhaps even pheromones. What's more, emotions are also quite contagious, with profound effects, as you'll soon learn.

We share our fundamental emotions with other animal species, humans communicating them primarily through facial expressions. Among such facial expressions is the smile, a universal social signal also shared by monkeys.

Smiles are used to convey happiness, in which the eyes also narrow as the mouth forms a smile. They can also used for perfunctory greetings, in which the lips pull back, but the eyes don't change – what Professor Bloom calls the *Pan Am smile*.

Emotional display is controlled without voluntary thought by your paleomammalian brain through innate "programs" much like the motor programs used in complex actions.

However, humans are unique among animal species in being able to "fake it", e.g. simulating a false smile of pleasure. The process engages the prefrontal cortex – a false smile uses different brain regions to consciously control the underlying muscle movements. This ability to act deceptively, including lying, seems to be necessary in some modern communications. Japanese speak of two types of relating – using the *tatamae* ("public face") or the *honne* ("true face"). It's naturally assumed in Japanese society that there are times when a diplomatic show of emotion smooths social relations.

Of course, being too honest or blunt (*yes, those jeans DO make your ass look fat!*) can hurt others unnecessarily and disrupt smooth relationships. Ricky Gervais' comedy *The Invention of Lying* offers an entertaining look at the results of such complete honesty. But to return to the topic at hand, what exactly ARE emotions?

In the bestseller *Emotional Intelligence*, psychologist Daniel Goleman gives a working definition of emotions as "...a feeling and its distinctive thoughts, psychological and biological states, and range of propensities to act". He says psychologists generally suggest there's a huge spectrum of emotions (greed, ecstasy, gloom, resentment, fury, edginess, contentment, etc.), but they are all shades or variances of a group of "primary" emotions, just as the primary colors red, yellow and blue mix into all the visible hues.

Although the specifics aren't precisely agreed upon between scientists, Goleman provides a working list of eight: anger, sadness, fear, enjoyment, love, surprise, disgust and shame. Among these, studies have shown that the facial expressions of anger, enjoyment, fear and sadness are universal and can be correctly recognized by people from all over the world, even if they have never been exposed to people from other races, such as tribesmen who have never had contact with other civilizations, and who have lived in an unchanged culture since the stone age. These four universal primary emotions appear to be genetically encoded into human neural circuitry, so they are present without anyone's ever having to "learn" them.

In addition to the four so-called primary universal emotions, anger, sadness, fear, and joy, modern neuroscience has recently added three more: surprise, contempt, and disgust. Theoretically, the range of all your other emotions is a mixture of the se seven *primaries*. Among the secondary emotions are embarrassment, jealousy, guilt, envy, pride, trust, shame, and others.

Emotions come from four sources:

- the genetic traits of your ancestors
- the genetic traits of your parents
- the environments in which you've lived

542

- the experiences you've had

According to 2010 research at the University of Valencia, "Inducing emotions generates profound changes in the autonomous nervous system, which controls the cardiovascular response, and also in the endocrine system. In addition, changes in cerebral activity also occur, especially in the frontal and temporal lobes," according to lead author Dr. Neus Herrero.

Here is what happens biochemically when you experience them:

Anger triggers a release of epinephrine, norepinephrine and dopamine, releasing glucose for muscle use, while massively elevating your heartbeat and blood pressure in preparation for a fight. Anger arouses intense changes throughout the mind and body, including an increase in heart rate, arterial tension and testosterone, while the brain's left hemisphere becomes more stimulated. Interestingly, in the frontal lobes of the cortex, emotions trigger *asymmetric activation* – a greater amount of neural signalling in one hemisphere over another.

The model of "motivational direction" suggests that the left frontal cortex participates in positive emotions which motivate closeness, while the right participates in negative emotions which motivate withdrawal. Anger is unique among emotions, because it feels negative, but it evokes motivation for closeness - in this case, to try to eliminate the source of our anger.

Laughter decreases the stress hormones cortisol and epinephrine, and releases endorphins, your body's natural painkillers. It lowers your blood pressure and releases human growth hormone, which boosts your immunity.

Love – Oxytocin, vasopressin and massive amounts of dopamine are released in the presence of your loved ones. This is the *relaxation response*, the physiological opposite of the fight or flight response, where your parasympathetic nervous system calms your body, and these hormones foster bonding and cooperation. During obsessive love, however, mood-stabilizing serotonin drops, leading to obsessive thoughts and irrational behavior.

Lust begins in your limbic system, where your hypothalamus triggers your pituitary gland to release oxytocin/vasopressin and dopamine, flooding your body, enhancing feelings of affection and increasing bloodflow to your genitals.

Sadness – When you lose someone you love or experience a major disappointment, your brain triggers a sharp drop in dopamine, serotonin and endorphins, causing the same feelings a drug addict experiences during withdrawal. This brings a drop in energy and enthusiasm, and encourages the instinctive withdrawal that gives time to reflect, adjust to major life changes and to heal. This kind of "human hibernation" also allows you to gather your energy and mental resources to overcome a problem if you've failed in a previous attempt, but if the state persists, it becomes the debilitating (and health-jeopardizing) condition known as *depression*.

Brain Anatomy And Your Seven Primary Emotions

Washington State University Neuroscientist Dr. Jaak Panksepp essentially single-handedly pioneered the field of *Affective Neuroscience* – mapping the neural circuitry of emotions in the brain. By electrically stimulating various brain regions, he discovered seven specific emotional-behavioral systems within the brains of all mammals (including humans), governing emotional-behavioral responses that promote survival. *Affect* – from the title – refers to feelings, positive or negative – the range of emotions, feelings, cravings, needs and moods.

As he notes in *Affective Neuroscience: the Foundations of Human and Animal Emotions:*

> *Deep within your brain but well above the brainstem, neurons in your pituitary and hypothalamus evolved from cells that enabled your chordate ancestors to sense the chemical perfume of an unseen mate in a distant meadow and initiate a courtship. Now they sense and regulate the hormones in your blood.*

> *They lie deep in the subcortical, central region of the brain, which could be called the seat of your animal soul. This area, truly the heart of your brain, includes several important nuclei that produce and regulate your degree of arousal, the tone and depth of your feelings, and your emotionally directed behavior. The behavior produced in this middle portion of the brain is often labelled instinctual and unthinking because it is less easily modified than the more deliberately planned, finely turned responses generated in the newly acquired cerebral cortex above it.*

Aside from permanently putting to rest any doubt that animals possess "a rich emotional life", Dr. Panksepp's groundbreaking research shows the fundamental biochemical processes at work as these circuits coordinate electrochemical signals, progressively transmitting messages from one nerve cell to another until the specific organs are activated in a behavioral response.

The brain, he notes, is the only organ in the body in which evolutionary progression can be clearly seen – through comparative anatomy, you can clearly see how humans share the same deep-level, inner neural structures with other animals, from MacLean's primitive paleoreptilian brain to the paleomammalian brain; humans differ primarily in our comparatively massive outer layer – the cerebral cortex. Dr. Panksepp says we also demonstrably share the same ancient instinctive feelings with other sentient life forms. In fact, he contends, the very first mental processes must have been feelings – perhaps the reflexive shrinking away of a flatworm from a crab's claw-pinch.

He says the roots of affective neuroscience began in the 1930s, when University of Zürich physiologist Walter Rudolf Hess found that electrically stimulating a cat's hypothalamus caused it to arch its back and hiss in a defensive reaction. This led to the discovery of the fight-or-flight response, coordinated by neurons in the hypothalamus and brainstem, which trigger the adrenal glands to release the organ-controlling neurochemical epinephrine. Hess went on to share the 1949 Nobel Prize in Physiology or Medicine for his work in mapping out the brain regions responsible for controlling internal organs.

In *Affective Neuroscience,* Dr. Panksepp first proposed seven innate emotional-behavioral systems genetically "hard-wired" into the subcortical mammalian brain. These primal systems can be overridden to a certain extent however; for example, cats raised among other cats naturally hunt and kill mice or rats, but if they've been raised side-by-side with rodents since birth, they won't. Panksepp induces each of these seven systems by electrically stimulating specific neural circuits.

Says Dr. Panksepp, "We can turn on rage, fear, separation distress, and generalized seeking patterns of behavior.... Once an electrode is in the correct neuroanatomical location, essentially identical emotional tendencies can be evoked in all mammals, including humans."

Through hypothalamic control, neurotransmitters and hormones such as acetylcholine, norepinephrine, dopamine, ghrelin, melatonin and serotonin (among others) activate and modulate each of these systems, triggering behaviors that (ideally) ensure survival of an animal's genes. Dr. Panksepp says stimulation triggers an accompanying affect (mood) in addition to the behaviors.

Because the behaviors aren't triggered when stimulating the cortex, Dr. Panksepp concluded they arise specifically within the subcortical brain. In fact, says Dr. Panksepp, animals whose cortexes have been completely removed still display emotions. He notes, however, that the cortex is clearly involved in *inhibiting* emotional arousal and humans are also capable of evoking emotions by reflecting upon past experiences or current circumstances.

Dr. Panksepp's seven systems include:

- *Seeking*

- *Rage*

- *Fear*

- *Lust*

- *Care*

- *Grief*

- *Play*

In experiments where animals can electrically self-stimulate these seven circuits at will, they will repeatedly trigger *seeking* (dopamine release), *lust, nurturing,* and *play* circuits, and will avoid triggering *rage, fear* or *grief.*

1. Seeking

The Seeking emotional-behavioral system is guided by homeostatic imbalances, external cues, and past learning; it guides thirsty creatures to water, cold creatures to warmth, hungry creatures to food, and sexually aroused creatures to opportunities for orgasmic gratification. The neural circuitry that triggers seeking lies within the mesolimbic reward pathway – the dopamine circuit running from the VTA through the hypothalamus, nucleus accumbens and frontal cortex.

Dr. Panksepp says seeking can be triggered by stimulating the mesolimbic pathway:

> ...the area of the brain where local application of electrical stimulation will promptly evoke the most energized exploratory and search behaviors an animal is capable of exhibiting.... Stimulated rats move about excitedly, sniffing vigorously, pausing at times to investigate various nooks and crannies of their environment. If one presents the animal with a manipulandum, a lever that controls the onset of brain stimulation, it will readily learn to press the lever and will eagerly continue to 'self-stimulate' for extended periods, until physical exhaustion and collapse set in.

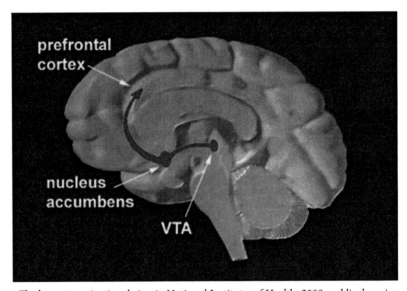

The human motivational circuit. National Institutes of Health, 2009, public domain

The mesolimbic pathway prompts intense interest in exploring the environment and excitement at the anticipation of fulfilling desires. This is the very heart of survival, prompting animals to seek out everything necessary for life – food, water, warmth, and sex. But it also seems the reason humans seek out interesting activities, being the fundamental basis of curiosity and the desire to learn and perfect skills.

When the area is stimulated in humans, volunteers report "...invigorated feelings that something very interesting and exciting is going on." When asked if they feel specifically *pleasure* during dopamine release, however, says Dr. Panksepp, volunteers report that it feels more like being "...really energized, excited, and interested about all kinds of stuff. Even really boring stuff becomes interesting."

Thus, says Dr. Panksepp, the term "dopamine reward system" is a bit misleading. Rather than specifically creating feelings of pleasure, increased dopamine levels create a state of *want*, *anticipation* of rewards such as food or sex. Once the want has been satisfied, however, dopamine levels immediately start to fall. Dopamine isn't specifically the pleasure chemical – in fact dopamine levels drop as the object of desire is being enjoyed.

Nor is dopamine, contrary to popular belief, specifically and always related to pleasure. Instead, it relates more to motivation and exploratory behavior aimed at securing a needed resource or escaping a perceived danger. It's also the basis of learning from *incentive salience*, where the mind links environmental cues (places, situations or people) with resources gauged to be of importance to survival.

Instead of a "pleasure or reinforcement system," the circuit promotes learning by inducing anticipatory eagerness, and creating links between events which allow prediction of future rewards or potential dangers. The system generates and sustains curiosity, promoting a sense of "engaged purpose" in both animals and humans:

> One of the important transmitters for addiction, dopamine, is a chemistry—but only one of the chemistries of this system—that kind of tunes it up. Whenever dopamine becomes active, the whole system becomes active. So, dopamine is an orchestral leader. It's like a command transmitter in the system.

> Animals able to self-stimulate the system with electrode implants trigger it enthusiastically, well past the point at which food is delivered to them.

> You cannot have an animal that does not like this subtle feeling. Well, I don't think it's subtle, I think it's intense, it's ecstatic; 'I'm living, I'm engaged, I want to find what I need, and I can do it.' It's that kind of can-do system. And, of course, animals are going to turn that on. But it's not a pleasure system; it's not a traditional reward system. This is the granddaddy of the positive systems. All the other positive systems in the brain, such as care, nurturance, lust, sexuality, and play, they use this system as a common substrate.

These circuits are inwardly triggered by hunger and other signals of homeostatic need, and outwardly triggered by reward cues. When the system activates, it prompts creatures to seek what they need, and the system then "turns down the volume" once the reward has been obtained. Dopaminergic neurons drive an animal to go after resources, but when those resources have been acquired, DA neurons stop firing.

Dopamine release signals the brain that resources exist in a certain location or can be obtained by engaging in a specific activity. This is the basis of learning; memories are encoded to allow a creature to locate resources reliably in the future. Through this system, creatures learn what will probably satisfy their desires. This is why seeing a favorite "watering hole" brings up overwhelming cravings in an alcoholic.

Dopamine is also the basis of *aversive* (avoidance) behavior, however. It's the chemical basis of motivation in general, so, surprisingly, if transmission to the nucleus accumbens has been artificially switched off, animals no longer even attempt to avoid painful or unpleasant situations.

As creatures move about the world, they are constantly bombarded with a tremendous amount of sensory data. After being relayed to the thalamus, this information is relayed to the appropriate cortical centers and to the amygdala, the brain's sentry and gateway to the emotion-regulating limbic system. By comparison with a creature's previous experience, the limbic system dictates how an animal will respond – with fear at the sight of a predator, lust at the sight of a potential lover, or relative indifference at the sight of something irrelevant to the creature's current needs.

The amygdala signals the rest of the limbic system, including the hypothalamus and autonomic nervous system, which prepare a creature for action. In the case of a threat, heart rate rises and glucose stores are freed for fast muscle activation. This arousal of the autonomic nervous system, in turn, feeds back from the body into the brain, which serves to amplify the emotional response.

Research shows events with the greatest emotional arousal (strongest neurochemical release) create the most vivid memories, a logical memory-based survival mechanism. Over a creature's lifetime, its amygdala and hippocampus work together to create a *salience landscape*, which maps out the emotional significance (survival value) of everything in that creature's environment.

Because of the dynamics of this system, every animal will associate its surroundings with the emotional state they previously experienced in those surroundings. Dr. Panksepp refers to the system as a *metabolic memory* for situations that generate brain opioids and other positive neurochemicals. Male rats, for example, prefer locations in which they have copulated, and salt-deprived animals will immediately seek out locations where they have previously found sodium; the memory of salt had been firmly recorded in their minds, so they retrieved the memory when desperately in need of it.

This incentive-salience-based learning system is precisely why recovering drug addicts are in grave danger of relapse when they encounter former "drug buddies" or find themselves in their former hangouts. The most powerful memories are activating, originating from the deepest centers of their brains, and it requires superhuman willpower from the (significantly drug-altered and likely damaged) frontal cortex to conquer the nearly overwhelming tidal wave of feelings.

Positive social interactions release opioids in the brain, the main source of pleasurable feelings that result. Playing, mutual grooming and sexual gratification are pleasurable due to opioid release. Many addictive drugs artificially induce the same gratifying feelings as endogenous opioids released by positive social interactions. Opiate drugs thus become a substitute means of inducing the positive mental states non-addicts normally get from social interactions.

Animals isolated in the lab readily turn to opiates to trigger these positive feelings and to offset separation distress; this explains the intense attachments – classical conditioning – drug addicts form with their habits. It also, unfortunately, explains why children who are victims of traumatic separation distress can be "programmed" both mentally and physically to suffer lifelong anxiety, depression and a stronger predisposition to addictions.

This system becomes impaired and underactive during chronic stress, withdrawal from addictive drugs, and in times of sickness, and is accompanied by feelings of depression, says Dr. Panksepp: "This is where one kind of depression occurs—when this system gets chronically low, and you can't get up the energy to do stuff. Life doesn't seem worth living; you don't have that kind of psychic energy. That's one kind of depression."

Conversely, when the system is overactive, it can lead to impulsive or excessive behaviors, psychotic delusions, extreme anxiety and manic thoughts. This is because the seeking system also encompasses *vigilance*, a constant, low-level attention to the immediate environment for any signs of a potential threat. If such a threat is found, it triggers the flight-or-fight response.

It's been theorized that people suffering from anxiety disorders are hypervigilant, with an extreme sensitivity to potential threats in the environment, always guarded and on the alert for potential trouble. Experiments point to a hyperactive amygdala, coupled with low levels of serotonin. Norepinephrine in the somatosensory cortex appears to promote the sensory aspects of hypervigilance, while dopamine in the basal ganglia appears to promote the motor aspects.

2) Rage

When seeking behavior is thwarted, this arouses a secondary instinctive behavior system – rage. Preventing an animal from receiving an expected reward, restricting its freedom to act or irritating its body surface activates rage circuitry. Dr. Panksepp notes that, for example, "a human baby typically becomes enraged if its freedom of action is restricted simply by holding its arms to its sides."

Your Bad Side – In 2009, University of Valencia scientists scanned human subjects as they become angry. During anger, the brain's left hemisphere becomes more active, and the amygdala, hypothalamus, pituitary and adrenal glands increase heart rate, testosterone production and arterial tension. Cortical changes occur particularly in the frontal and temporal lobes, according to Dr. Neus Herrero.

The left frontal lobe is more involved in positive emotions, while the right is more involved in negative ones. The left frontal lobe also engages during emotions related to closeness, while the right engages more in relation to withdrawal-provoking emotions. Typically, positive emotions like joy motivate closeness, while negative emotions like fear and sadness motivate withdrawal. Anger seems unique, however, running counter to this tendency. Anger seems to eleicit activity in the left frontal region, which typically associated with closeness-promoting emotions. Dr. Herrero suggests this is because anger prompts an instinctive approach to eliminate rivals.

Dr. Walter Hess won the 1949 Nobel Prize by first discovering in the 1930s that electrically stimulating specific certain brain regions can trigger animal rage. The effect has repeatedly been demonstrated in humans as well. Brain tumors which impinge upon the circuit have been shown to lead to uncontrollable rage, while impairment of the circuitry promotes serenity.

Rage arises from a circuit running primarily from the amygdala to the hypothalamus and down into the periaqueductal gray in the midbrain. Electrical stimulation results in sudden, intense anger without provocation. Two-way connections to the circuit also run to frontal cortex areas involved in reward evaluation, as well as two-way circuits to and from

- the *insula* – where somatosensory data converges, including pain perception

- the norepinephrine-producing *locus coeruleus* in the brainstem

- the serotonin-producing *raphe nuclei* in the brainstem

- the nucleus of the *solitary tract*, which gathers information from the vagus nerve related to bodily functions like heart rate and blood pressure

The rage system, says Dr. Panksepp, is near related fear circuitry and interacts closely with it – rage and fear are the two circuits governing fight or flight responses.

Activating the rage circuits causes hissing, growling, *piloerection* (hair raising), and ANS arousal, and animals will attack anything which poses a threat, including members of their own species. In humans, stimulating the same regions results in intense rage. Sympathetic nervous system arousal increases heart rate, blood pressure, body temperature and muscular blood flow. The experience is apparently unpleasant; animals which are cabable very quickly shut off rage circuit stimulation.

Dr. Panksepp found he could trigger three types of aggression by stimulating slightly different regions: *1) predatory aggression, 2) rage,* and *3) inter-male* or *dominance aggression.* Stimulating one region of the hypothalamus triggers predatory or "quiet-biting" attacks, while two others evoke rage-driven and dominance aggression.

As well as predation, rage, and dominance aggression, Dr. Panksepp says that animals have a type of defensive aggression based upon a mixture of both rage and fear. There are also a set of innate *appeasement* behaviors – defeated animals express surrender by exposing their bellies and necks – where their vital organs lie. These postures automatically trigger mercy – reduced aggression – in their opponents.

Dr. Panksepp also found prolonged social isolation and hunger increase aggression, while high serotonin levels reduce it.

The main neurotransmitters producing rage are substance P and glutamate, but endogenous opioids, GABA and especially serotonin inhibit the circuitry, calming enraged animals. In rodents (which share about 90% of human DNA), oxytocin also reduces all forms of aggression, and regular access to sex increases oxytocin levels up to 300% in males.

In other words, regular sex makes for kinder, gentler males. So while lab rats will normally kill all the young when invading new territory, if they've mated, offspring born from that point will be spared. This evolutionary adaptation promotes the survival of an individual's genes over a competitor who had previously impregnated a mate.

Stress and trauma have been found to lead to neuroadaptations that predispose animals to rage. In *Guilty by Reason of Insanity: A Psychiatrist Explores the Minds of Killers*, Dorothy Otnow Lewis writes:

> Brain concentrations of neurotransmitters like serotonin can vary, based upon experience. Thus, some stressors can reduce brain serotonin, creating significant behavioral changes. Isolating animals while they are young has been shown to trigger a drop in serotonin. Afterward, when released into the company of other animals, these isolated individuals become fiercely aggressive.
>
> Pain, hunger and fear have also been shown to decrease brain serotonin and promote aggression, which is why it's the method used to train pit bulls to fight. Environmental stressors such as heat, overcrowding, physical discomfort, and being raised by aggressive parent figures also increase animal aggressiveness in the same manner.

But selective breeding experiments have shown that aggressive tendencies can be inherited by both sexes.

The Deadliest Emotion – British general practitioner Dr. David Beales, who specializes in behavioral medicine, says that out of all the emotions **hostility** is the most toxic of all, raising adrenaline levels, which in turn increases cholesterol and suppresses the parasympathetic nervous system, making relaxation difficult. In fact, he says, elevated hostility levels dramatically increase the odds of dying for those 60 or under.

One study in the journal Health Psychology says hostility may in fact be a greater contributing factor to heart disease than high cholesterol, smoking or being overweight. Another says that hostile women are more likely to have hardened arteries.

Conversely, it's been demonstrated that optimism protects the heart: out of 1,000 patients studied over nine years, those rated as "highly optimistic" were 23% less likely to die of heart disease, irrespective of their smoking habits and blood pressure.

Happy people also have lower levels of the inflammatory stress hormone cortisol, which raises blood pressure, heart rate and cholesterol levels. Dr. Guarneri recommends in particular two traditional emotional remedies – gratitude and forgiveness, saying they are as just as significant for disease management as watching cholesterol levels.

---

3. Fear

"Fear is the mind-killer. Fear is the little-death that brings total obliteration. I will face my fear. I will permit it to pass over me and through me. And when it has gone past, I will turn the inner eye to see its path. Where the fear has gone, there will be nothing. Only I will remain."
– Frank Herbert, 1965, Dune

For a wild animal, survival is a fairly stark equation: outrun or kill your enemies, find food, and successfully mate to ensure your genes are passed on to future generations, or your lineage perishes with you.

The emotion that keeps animals out of danger long enough to survive and reproduce is fear, the brain-body signal that their safety is threatened. Pain, or the threat of injury or death elicits fear, triggering fighting, fleeing or freezing. This physiological reaction to fear – the fight or flight response – was first described by American physiologist Walter B. Cannon in 1929.

The *fear* pathway interacts with and runs parallel to the *rage* pathway, to create the dual fight or flight response, although fear and rage circuitry clearly activate different regions of the amygdala. The neurochemicals regulating fear are *neuropeptide Y* and *corticotrophin releasing factor* (CRF), and it's inhibited by GABA.

Central to the fear response is the amygdala, the brain's twin almond-shaped sentry, and it is also central to creating and solidifying memories of fearful situations. Fear is triggered by stimulating specific regions of the amygdala, hypothalamus and peri-aqueductal gray. Evoking the emotion makes the hypothalamus activate autonomic systems in the brainstem and spinal cord, triggering norepinephrine and epinephrine release from the locus coeruleus in the brainstem and from the adrenal glands atop the kidneys.

Fear responses include increased heart rate and blood pressure, elimination, and perspiration, with general feelings of "…apprehensive tension, with a tendency toward various autonomic symptoms such as *tachycardia* (rapid heartbeat often with palpitations), sweating, gastrointestinal symptoms, and increased muscle tension".

In moments of the most extreme terror, however, the body releases endogenous opioids and serotonin near the PAG, resulting in "fear-induced analgesia" – the numbness of terror.

Fearful animals respond with preprogrammed behaviors, either fleeing, if the danger seems avoidable, hiding or freezing, if the danger seems inescapable. In the lab, stimulating fear neurocircuitry makes animals flee in panic or freeze if they cannot escape, and forms strong memories of the event, so they subsequently avoid places associated with the fear. Human volunteers whose fear circuits have been stimulated report being "engulfed by an intense free-floating anxiety that appears to have no environmental cause."

A pair of Harvard Medical School researchers, Drs. Robert Greene and Donald Rainnie, found a single genetic change could shut down the fear response, resulting in maniacal mice. By genetically disrupting production of serotonin, they created a strain of fearless, superaggressive mutant mice.

Serotonin appears to be the end product of a series of chemical conversions requiring the *CAMKII enzyme* in the serotonin-producing neurons of the midbrain's raphe nucleus. The raphe system has major projections throughout the nervous system, modifying the entire nervous system's functioning.

Silencing the gene responsible for expressing CAMKII, Greene and Rainnie bred mice lacking serotonin's normal fear- and aggression-dampening neuromodulation. CAMKII normally comprises about one percent of total brain protein, a significant amount. Mice lacking the CAMKII gene suffered severe behavioral and cognitive abnormalities.

Suppressing this circuit by silencing a single gene, the team had created mice immune to fear. The results were disturbing, according to author Temple Grandin:

> *A normal mouse, with a normal amount of fear, does not fight to the death. He fights until he's beaten, or sees he's going to lose, and then he yields. Fear keeps him alive. The knockout mice were almost fearless, and they fought to the death.*

The team reported returning to the lab in the morning to find cages full of blood, fur, and violently slaughtered mice. Fearlessness is not a natural nor healthy state for most animals.

2010 research my Nobel-prizewinning molecular biologist Dr. Susumu Tonegawa shows that specific fear-conditioned memories are encoded by neurons in the *dentate gyrus* region of the hippocampus. A small group of specific hippocampal neurons bear such memory traces – also known as "engrams" – and they can be switched on and off to manipulate fear-based memories.

Fear can be divided into two types. The first is *conditioned fear*, by which an otherwise neutral stimulus like a blinking light or ringing bell becomes mentally linked to danger. This is the principle of classical conditioning, in which the stimulus (the light or bell) is repeatedly followed by a threat (like an electric shock), until the original stimulus arouses fear by itself.

The second type of fear is *innate*, an ancestral hand-me-down from ancient forebears, genetically programmed at birth. Innate fears are those which you're naturally born with; this includes snakes, spiders, storms and heights. Fear responses, however, can be controlled by the prefrontal cortex.

According to Carl Sagan, your instinctive fear of heights protects you from falling, even in infancy: a baby placed on a glass table will push out its hands in a reflexive motion to prevent itself from falling, even though it has never experienced falling. Sagan theorized that this instinctive response has been passed down from ancient ancestors who slept in trees, along with an instinctive fear of reptiles like snakes, and of insects and arachnids like spiders.

Fear is thought to be the most important emotion for survival, and thus plays a prominent, central role in the animal psyche. But chronic, unwarranted fear can underlie a number of disorders like anxiety, paranoia, phobias, and post-traumatic stress disorder.

In modern America, such problems are epidemic. Almost 20 percent of Americans suffer from anxiety, reports the National Institute of Health. Of those, 66% go untreated, with possibly serious progressions of such untreated symptoms.

Fear unfolds as follows:

You hear a sudden strange bang downstairs in the middle of the night. Your ears transform the sound waves into neural impulses. The neural circuit travels from your cochlea to your brainstem and up to your thalamus. The signals then travel down separate branches – one to the amygdala and hippocampus, the other, along a longer, slower circuit to your auditory cortex for analysis.

Your thalamus filters out other sensory data, amplifying your auditory sensitivity for better analysis of the mysterious noise. Your amygdala and hippocampus, which sort and file memories based on salience, shuffle through your memories to find similar experiences. Memories in your cortex are compared to the sound to see if you have any information to help identify it.

If your limbic system finds something reassuring, for example identifying the sound as the banging of a shutter, the alert doesn't escalate beyond this point. But if the sound is still alien to your brain, your amygdala sends an "alarm" signal that activates your hypothalamus and the locus coeruleus in your brainstem, arousing your ANS.

Your amygdala receives signals directly from your thalamus, olfactory bulb and viscera before they travel to your PFC, auditory and visual cortices. This means your amygdala is a first line of defense, constantly scanning and analyzing sensory input for salience, particularly in terms of danger.

Your amygdala, in turn, sends out projections to every major brain center, particularly your hypothalamus, which controls the emergency-response stress hormones that put your body in high alert status, and to your striatum, which helps govern voluntary motor control.

It also connects to your medulla, which can activate autonomic fight-or-flight responses in your cardiovascular system, muscles and digestive system without the need for higher cortical and subcortical input.

Fearless Rats Vs. The Rodent Terminator

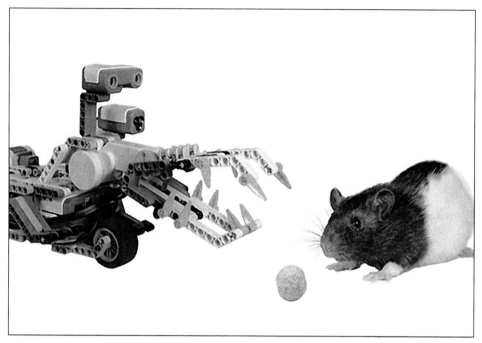

*Amygdala regulates risk of predation, Dr. Jeansok Kim, 2010, Kim Lab,
University of Washington. Used with permission*

In 2010, researchers at the University of Washington designed an experiment to simulate an encounter between a rat and a natural predator. Rats were placed at one end of a large rectangular space, equipped with a door to a separate nesting area. Dr. Jeansok Kim and his team placed food 25 to 76 cm away from the creatures' nests. At the other end, they placed a Lego Mindstorm robot designed to look like a dangerous predator, with eyes, a lunging motion, and snapping jaws.

Whenever a rat attempted to venture out of its nest for food, the robot would leap forward and snap its jaws. This would send the rats scurrying back into their nests, until hunger gradually compelled them to venture out again. The rats eventually grew the courage to quickly snatch the food closest to their nests and retreat again, but would not venture very close to the robot. Guessing that the amygdala underlay their fear, Dr. Kim injured the amygdalae of some rats and disinhibited the amygdalae of others.

The rats with amygdala lesions became fearless, and would snatch food immediately in front of the robot, while those whose amygdalae had been disinhibited were incapacitated by fright and lay huddled in their nests, clearly demonstrating the central role of the amygdala in regulating fear. The before and after videos can be seen online :

http://goo.gl/mNsrT
http://goo.gl/8xAdZ

The amygdala and hypothalamus give rise to opposing motivations: fear vs. desire. When faced with a reward accompanied by apparent danger, an animal performs several calculations on-the-fly, weighing potential risk vs. reward, estimating distance and velocity of a predator's approach, then comparing these estimates with its own speed and proximity to safety. Dr. Kim's experiment is a clear indication the amygdala is used in such calculations – weighing threats vs. the need for resources.

New Findings

Experiments conducted by Drs. Kevin A. Corcoran and Gregory Quirk of the Ponce School of Medicine in Puerto Rico show that a hyperactive prefrontal cortex plays a major role in pathological learned fear, as with PTSD, phobias and other anxiety disorders. The PFC appears to engage in learned but not innate fears.

The doctors induced a conditioned fear response in laboratory rats, teaching them to mentally link a 30-second tone with foot shocks. The next day, when hearing the tone again, these conditioned rats froze about 70 percent of the time while the tone sounded.

A second group of rats had a region of their PFCs called the *prelimbic cortex* chemically disabled. The prelimbic cortex is a part of the medial prefrontal cortex (mPFC), a region which helps oversee the regulation of emotions. The learning-impaired rats only froze 14 percent of the time in response to the sounding of the warning tone. Among these learning-impaired rats, however, natural, instinctive (innate) fears were apparently unaffected by blocking the region; these rats were just as likely to freeze at the sight of a cat or when placed into the open as normal rats. Tested the next day after restoration of their cortical function, they showed normal fear responses.

Drs. Corcoran and Quirk surmise that in modulating amygdala activity, the prelimbic cortex is critical for deciding which circumstances are appropriate for encoding fear responses into long-term memory. Innate fear responses seem to be automatic, requiring no cortical activation. This suggests the cortex can more easily control learned rather than innate fear.

The Panic Button – *In September of 2011, researchers at the Max Planck Institute of Psychiatry discovered twin functions of a single hormone that both generates and shuts down panic. Both fear circuits use the stress-response* **corticotropin-releasing hormone (CRH)** *and its type 1 receptor (CRHR1). The hormone binds to CHRH1 receptors on glutamatergic neurons in the limbic system, activating anxiety.*

But CRHR1 receptor activation **shuts down** *anxiety in dopaminergic neurons in the substantia nigra and ventral tegmental area. The team believes malfunctions of these CRH circuits may be central to mood disorders like panic attacks. Many sufferers of anxiety disorders and depression show atypical hormonal stress responses, with increased brain CRH. Recent, contradictory findings had showed this stress hormone somehow also reduces fear. This is because CRH has the opposite effect when it binds to CRH1 receptors on dopaminergic neurons, triggering a release of dopamine in the forebrain, which leads to a reduction in fear. The opposing panic-inducing and panic-inhibiting effect of the CRH/CRHR1 pair was illuminated for the first time by this study, offering new hope for sufferers of chemically-based mood disorders.*

The Fear Gene

Recent work by Dr. Gleb Shumyatsky and colleagues at Rutgers University led to the discovery of several genes involved in the amygdala's role in forming fearful memories. A protein called *stathmin* is now known to be central to creating fearful memories. Mice deficient in the stathmin-expressing gene cannot learn new fears or act appropriately to normally threatening situations.

They also show less anxiety when confronted with new environments or other potentially threatening situations. Memory formation requires new synapses, but mice lacking the stathmin gene don't have the synaptic plasticity of normal mice.

Researchers at Emory University also discovered in 2010 that *brain-derived neurotrophic factor* in the prelimbic cortex modulates learned fear. When the region is deficient in BDNF, mice forget their fear of electric shocks.

Dr. Kerry Ressler, who led the study, says BDNF is the brain's "fertilizer", a protein which bolsters a neuron's ability to create new synaptic connections. BDNF is vital for neuronal plasticity, learning and memory, according to Ressler, and interfering with BDNF's effects blocks fear memory formation.

Dr. Ressler says it's starting to become apparent that an overactive or under-regulated amygdala appears to underlie anxiety disorders, and individual variations in the BDNF-encoding gene are believed to be one of the bases for an increased risk of anxiety disorders, altering prelimbic cortex structure.

Using mice genetically-engineered without the prelimbic cortex BDNF gene, Ressler and his colleagues found that normal mice who received electrical shocks right after hearing a warning tone gradually learned to fear the noise, and would freeze upon hearing it, but BDNF-altered mice quickly and repeatedly forgot their fears.

4. Mating

The essence of natural selection is that genes which promote the best chance of survival have the greatest chance of being passed on to future generations, including genes that promote reproduction. The fundamental goal of genes – and thus the creatures that both host and are created by them – is to duplicate themselves.

In humans, this duplication is accomplished through sexual reproduction. Normally, humans branch into two distinct sexes. While this sounds incredibly obvious, it's not always true in the animal kingdom. For example, animals can have one or three sexes; one species of whiptail lizard produces only females, and bullfrogs have one female and two male genders. Some animals, like the clownfish (depicted in Pixar Studios' *Finding Nemo)*, even change sex (sometimes on multiple occasions) throughout their lifespans. But in humans, testosterone levels within the womb determine whether you will develop into a man or a woman.

Aside from the outward physical differences, there are also some differences in brain anatomy and function. While men and women share neurochemicals like oxytocin, different, gender-specific brain circuits and chemistries control sexual urges in males and females that foster reproduction.

We are (almost always) born either genetically female (with XX chromosomes) or male (with XY chromosomes). XX – female – chromosomes are the "default", meaning female development will continue to progress, unless some external source of testosterone intervenes. Masculinization actually occurs in the *second trimester* (four to six months) of human pregnancy as a result of fetal testosterone. The Y chromosome generates *testis determining factor* (TDF), which eventually results in the development of the male *gonadal* system that manufactures testosterone from *cholesterol*.

But, says Dr. Panksepp, sexual characteristics in the brain and body are developed independently, sometimes leading to individuals who are externally male, but with sexual urges typical among females of their species and, vice versa.

Sexual desire is triggered by two distinctly different biochemical processes in males and females; it's primarily regulated by testosterone and vasopressin in men and estrogen and oxytocin in women. This different biochemistry helps form behavioral tendencies specific to each sex, with oxytocin promoting a "receptive" sexual readiness in females (in addition to trust and confidence), and vasopressin promoting a "proactive" assertiveness (and possibly jealous competitiveness) in males. Dopamine-driven seeking behavior is also used to drive the search for sexual partners, just as with every other type of reward, including social-emotional rewards.

Paul MacLean, who first proposed the triune theory of brain evolution, also used electrical brain stimulation to map out functional neuroanatomy, and discovered that sexual arousal can be triggered by stimulating regions of the limbic system, primarily the *septum,* the neighboring *BNST (bed nucleus of the stria terminalis)*, and the *preoptic area of the hypothalamus*, which converge into the medial forebrain bundle – the motivational center.

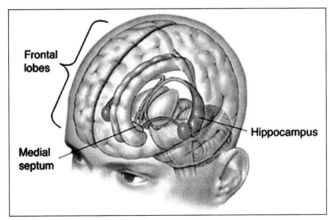

The Human Brain, Aaron M. White, 2004, National Institute on Alcohol Abuse and Alcoholism. Public domain

558

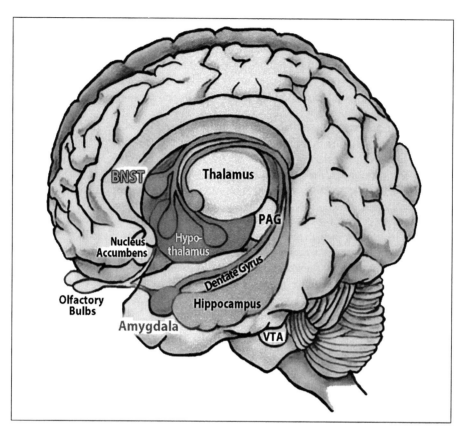

Human brain, including the amygdala (purple), bed nucleus of stria terminalis (BNST, orange), hypothalamus (purple), and hippocampus (aqua). The hippocampus attaches to the mamillary bodies (sky blue) via the fimbria-fornix. Olfactory input is received by the olfactory bulbs (yellow). Other structures include the nucleus accumbens, VTA, and periaqueductal gray (PAG). Adapted from Sokolowski and Corbin, 2012.

In mammals, two neurochemicals in particular combine with this neurocircuitry to trigger sexual (and parenting) behaviors: vasopressin and oxytocin, and both are present in men and in women. Vasopressin is more prevalent in male brains and appears to mainly induce male sexual and social behaviors like courtship, territorial marking, and male-to-male aggression, while testosterone triggers the search for sexual interactions. In females, vasopressin tends to induce aggressive maternal behaviors, such as protecting the young.

Sexual arousal and human male erection appear to be controlled by the hormone *vasoactive intestinal peptide* (VIP). In rats, this also controls cells in the hypothalamus that generate *lordosis*, a reflexive mount-ready position that signals receptiveness for sex in female animals. Sexual pleasure itself, however, appears to be derived from stimulation of the septum.

Randy Genes

Among rodents, when an aroused male touches a female's flanks, the hypothalamus controls whether or not that female will present her rump for mounting. In this manner, females control sexual reproduction. Female sexual eagerness arises from within the hypothalamus, and damage to this area impairs responsiveness.

Norepinephrine excites hypothalamic cells, preventing potassium ions from exiting them, and potassium ion buildup activates neurons in the ventromedial hypothalamus. The VM hypothalamus fires in bursts of electrical activity, resulting in sexual receptivity. The sex hormone *estradiol* activates genes which produce the VM hypothalamus receptors which respond to norepinephrine, strengthening the impulse to mate.

Oxytocin is more prevalent in female brains, and both opioid and oxytocin neurocircuitry is activated by pleasurable social activities like grooming, play, and sex. The sex hormones which prepare females for fertilization also significantly alter neurochemical sensitivity in the hypothalamus. During *estrus* (when a mammal is "in heat"), hormonal exposure called *priming* increases oxytocin receptors in the hypothalamus, and stimulates dendrite growth; these dendrites stretch out to complete the circuit which sensitizes the spinal cord's lordosis reflex.

5. Care

Dr. Panksepp says the drive to care for one's offspring arose from neurochemistry controlling reptile mating and egg-laying. The reptilian equivalent of oxytocin is *vasotocin*, which eventually evolved into oxytocin and vasopressin; these neurochemicals each differ by only a single amino acid.

Oxytocin, the neurochemical that triggers sexual receptivity in female mammals, also fosters nurturing behaviors in a mother's brain. Because of this neurohormone's presence, blood transfusion from a female which has recently given birth will trigger maternal behaviors in virgin females. Oxytocin has a similar effect upon men, promoting paternal instincts, reducing aggression and increasing familial bonding.

Hormonal changes peaking just before birth correspond with heightened maternal instincts; mothers start to engage in behaviors like nest-building. As childbirth approaches, estrogen, which remains at moderate levels throughout pregnancy, increases rapidly. At the same time *progesterone*, which supports *gestation* (the carrying of a fetus) remained at high levels throughout pregnancy, and begins to decline sharply just before birth.

There is also a sharp increase in *prolactin*, which triggers milk production and appears to play a central role in sustained maternal behaviors; injections have been found to induce nurturing behaviors. In the final days of pregnancy and the first days of lactation, oxytocin receptors throughout the brain and hypothalamic oxytocin-producing neurons increase markedly, primarily within the bed nucleus of the stria terminalis (BNST). Together with the hypothalamus, the BNST gives rise to maternal behaviors, and when the region is damaged, maternal behaviors completely cease. The ACC also appears to play a role in regulating these behaviors.

6. Grief

The *grief system* is vital to survival for newborns – human babies are particularly vulnerable, taking much longer than any other species to mature to the level of self-sufficiency necessary to live alone.

The grief system is an adaptive behavioral mechanism which causes babies to signal their needs to parents through *separation calls* (crying). Animal mothers, for their part, have built-in auditory circuitry (in the *inferior colliculi* and *medial geniculate nuclei* of the midbrain and thalamus) specifically attuned to their own children's distress calls.

Says Dr. Panksepp,

> *The life of a young sea otter is completely dependent on the care provided by its mother. After his sexual contribution, the father pays little heed to his young. It is the mother's job to be both caretaker and food provider, as often as not, on the open sea. The pup's life revolves around maternal devotion. When she dives beneath the dark surface of the water for food, being absent from her infant's side for many minutes at a stretch, the young otter begins to cry and swim about in an agitated state.*

> *If it were not for those calls of distress among the rising and falling waves, young otters might be lost forever. Their security and future are unequivocally linked to the audiovocal thread of attachment that joins them to their mothers. It is the same for all mammals. At the outset, we are utterly dependent creatures whose survival is founded on the quality of our social bonds—one of the remaining great mysteries, and gifts, of nature.*

Grief behavior motivates others to respond with nurturing, and this fosters social attachments. Social attachments activate serotonin and opioids, attenuating the grief circuits, calming the distressed animal. Experiments show that these opioids – which are also released in high levels when you're in love – powerfully reduce separation distress, and quiet anxiety.

Grief circuitry is found in the bed nucleus of the stria terminalis (BNST), a nerve bundle running from the amygdala to the hypothalamus between the thalami. These circuits are aroused by grief and sadness, feelings which result from low levels of endogenous brain opioids. Electrically stimulating the neurocircuitry produces separation calls in a number of species, including primates, rodents, and birds. A number of sites in the hypothalamus, BNST and septum give rise to these distress calls. These areas also play a major role in both sexual and maternal behaviors.

In human patients, stimulating this region elicits intense grief, including "...feelings of weakness and depressive lassitude, with autonomic symptoms of a parasympathetic nature, such as strong urges to cry, often accompanied by tightness in the chest and the feeling of having a lump in the throat."

Dr. Panksepp believes that separation distress neurocircuitry evolved from older, nearby pain mechanisms within the brain, because the neurocircuitry runs from the amygdala, hypothalamus, and BNST through the thalamus to the periaqueductal gray area – grief-related areas in the PAG are very close to regions which generate physical pain responses. The separation-anxiety/distress-call circuit is activated by glutamate and the stress hormone *CRH (corticotrophin releasing hormone)* and quieted by endogenous opioids, as well as oxytocin and prolactin. In other words, stress hormones excite grief circuitry, while attachment and bonding neurochemically inhibit it.

Grief circuitry is clearly different from fear circuitry, says Dr. Panksepp; it can trigger panic attacks, but primarily induces feelings of loneliness, grief, and distress at separation from companions. Thus, the grief system is related to loss of social attachments.

According to Dr. Panksepp, such social loss is the major environmental cause of depression. The initial grieving phase in response to social loss is protestation – separation calls or crying. The stress which accompanies this behavior depletes the brain's norepinephrine, serotonin, and dopamine reserves, leading to one form of depression.

He says the system is powerful enough so that early childhood loss can create a potentially *lifelong* vulnerability to depression and panic attacks, permanently modifying development of emotional systems responsible for quieting separation distress.

Glutamate, the most common excitatory neurotransmitter in the brain, is the primary neurochemical within the grief circuit, triggering separation calls. Activating glutamate receptors and releasing CRH into the region causes a dramatic increase in distress calls, even if other animals are nearby. CRH, if you recall, arises from the hypothalamus, and is central to triggering the fight-or-flight response. It's part of "virtually all emotions and many psychiatric disturbances, especially depression".

Blocking glutamate receptors causes a dramatic drop in distress calls, even when the grief circuit is directly stimulated. Opioids, oxytocin, prolactin and *tricyclic antidepressants* also decrease electrically-stimulated activation of the grief neurocircuitry.

7. Play

The drive to *play* is innate in a wide variety of animals. Dr. Gordon Burghardt of the University of Tennessee specializes in *ethology*, the study of behavior in evolution. He says animals that play include mammals, birds, and even reptiles and fish. To be considered play, he says, behavior has to meet five criteria:

- It differs from serious behavior in *structure* (how it's done), *context* (when and where it's done), or *ontogenetics* (what age range does it);
- It's repeated;
- It's not obviously useful at the time it's being done;

- It's rewarding;

- It's performed during relaxation or in low-stress environments;

Dr. Burghardt's *Surplus Resource Theory* is that animals with access to abundant food have surplus time and energy for play. Animals with abundant parental care are also more likely to play than animals born relatively ready to get around on their own. Reptiles don't have the energy reserves of mammals, so play is much less prevalent or obvious than in mammals; mammals take in oxygen for energy use and have an abundance of energy to expend on play, but reptiles are cold-blooded, so they quickly tire after engaging in motor activity. Their blood oxygen capacity is, on average, only 10 percent that of mammals. Aquatic turtles, however, are an exception. They move about in water, which requires much less energy, and thus have surplus energy to engage in play.

While on a superficial level, play doesn't seem essential for survival, Dr. Burghardt says it's essential, and a number of species (humans in particular) spend a great deal of time in collecting resources which allow play. You can see examples of play everywhere, among cats, dolphins, dogs, and even birds and fish. In videos available online at Radiolab.org and elsewhere, Dr. Panksepp even shows vivid examples of rats responding to play and to tickling with chirps of delight.

Play behavior seems to be primarily about learning skills, exercising emotional-behavioral systems, particularly social ones, within a relatively non-threatening environment. During play, animals may reach points where anger, fear, separation anxiety, maternal instinct or sexuality are evoked. This seems to help teach the young social, emotional and cognitive skills, including lessons about courting and parenting, cooperation, competition, social hierarchies, and one's place within them – integrating into a society requires that an animal understand who it can dominate, and who it be can dominated by. Play also helps in identifying individuals with whom it's possible to forge alliances and friendships, and individuals one needs to avoid.

Play teaches animals motor skills, enhancing fitness, dexterity, innovation and creative thinking. It also teaches critical survival skills – teaching hunting to predators, and avoidance or escape to prey animals. In humans, play may also teach deception, which allows us to, for example, create false impressions of our intentions if we wish.

To engage in play, animals must be free of stress and have their basic needs met. In a new environment, however, animals usually engage in strong exploratory activity, not engaging in play until they are familiar with their surroundings. Playfulness is also inhibited by hunger and negative emotions, such as loneliness, anger, and fear. Social isolation also has a major and lasting, destructive impact on the urge to play; this natural urge only re-emerges after social confidence levels return to normal, if ever.

In males, play seems to become more vigorous as the largest and strongest mature, compared with that of smaller peers; Dr. Panksepp believes this reflects the male drive toward dominance, and may explain the human public's love for rough professional sports. Interestingly, however, when an animal constantly acts domineering or bullying during play, less dominant animals begin to ignore the bully, offering fewer overtures for play and decreased interactions overall.

According to Dr. Panksepp, his own experiments have shown that play is not based upon prior experience, but is derived from a neural circuit which can be activated. This play neurocircuitry is linked to somatosensory processing in the midbrain, thalamus and cortex, he says; various regions of the thalamus help generate the motivation to play, and damage to thalamic play circuitry shuts down motivation to play, while keeping other complex behaviors intact, such as foraging for food.

The sense of touch seems central to instigating and sustaining play; Dr. Panksepp has found mammals, including rats, have skin regions which trigger play circuitry when touched. He calls these regions *tickle skin*, and believes specialized receptors in these regions signal playful intent between animals. But somatosensory input isn't necessary – the motivation for play appears even when the senses of vision, olfaction and *vibrissae* (whiskers which generate tactile information) are impaired. The auditory system seems to play a role in play motivation, however – deafened creatures play slightly less than others, and many animal species emit laughter-like noises while at play.

Laughter plays a special role in this innate circuitry, which seems to function as a social signal of both mood and bonding through a mutually-shared understanding. It's also innate – blind and deaf children also laugh. It's displayed at its height by an open mouth, which is a social cue in other animals, such as chimpanzees and dogs, of readiness to play. The neurocircuitry which generates laughter is located in the brainstem – we know this because the disease *amyotrophic lateral sclerosis (ALS)* destroys myelin sheaths which insulate brainstem axons, resulting in uncontrollable laughter.

Explorer Monkeys and the Genetic Basis of Sensitivity

Serotonergic neurons play a central role in regulating emotion and behavior. High serotonin levels produce greater emotional stability, but a reduced sensitivity to both risks and rewards. Conversely, low serotonin heightens emotional sensitivity, with both positive and negative consequences, says Dr. Panksepp. Low serotonin is a neurochemical state that can lead to impulsivity, or even such extremes as suicide – one of the most widely-supported findings in psychology is that casualties of suicide tend to have abnormally low brain serotonin.

Low serotonin levels also equate with high *vigilance* – an increased sensitivity to environmental cues, making such individuals ideally suited for the role of sentinels within their group. Low-serotonin monkeys, for example, serve as sentinels which detect predators, and may be the first of their group to find new food sources. While these behaviors may endanger the individual, they enhance the probability of close relatives surviving – and thus help propagate genes shared by the self-sacrificing individual.

Anxiety, a high sensitivity to environmental cues stemming from low brain serotonin, is equivalent to a constant, low-level activation of threat-coping mechanisms. For hypersensitive, anxious people, dangers may lurk around every corner, dangers which demand constant, increased vigilance, and they engage in an endless, generalized search for security in a world in constant flux. Obsessive-compulsive disorders are one form of such hypervigilance, an oversensitivity to environmental cues. Survival mechanisms have become *pathological* – altered by illness.

Stress Worsens The Problem

Persistent, uncontrollable stress, like that experienced by victims of ongoing domestic violence, people in noisy, overcrowded city environments or even dysfunctional work relationships, may well be a major cause of hypervigilance, and eventually manifest as obsessions and compulsions, particularly when there is no acceptable outlet to channel negative emotional energy, such as continuously-suppressed rage.

Catecholamines such as norepinephrine and epinephrine are released into the body from the adrenal glands in response to environmental stress. These neurohormones "turn up" heart and muscle function and "turn down" digestion in preparation for fight-or-flight responses, to prepare animals for eliminating or escaping the stress which gave rise to them.

But chronic or traumatic stress results in neurochemical changes which can eventually impede PFC function, hampering self-control and the ability to suppress destructive impulses.

According to Dr. Amy F.T. Arnstem, founder of the Arnstem Lab at Yale Medical School, catecholamines impair working memory and strengthen the amygdala's emotional responsiveness. In other words, chronic stress gradually weakens behavioral control from your conscious, logical PFC, giving greater power to your more primitive, fear-conditioned amygdala.

In addition to behavioral control, your PFC is critical for the use of *working memory*, a sort of temporary, conscious holding area required for guiding appropriate behavior, inhibiting inappropriate behavior, planning, performing day-to-day calculations, and a number of other higher mental processes. Traumatic injury to the region results in reduced attention management, and disorganized, hyperactive and impulsive behavior.

Emotions Engage Your Entire Brain And Body

It would be a mistake to believe that emotions only involve limited, specific circuits. A team of psychologists from Harvard, Yale, Columbia, Northeastern and the Universities of Colorado and California say emotions can't be completely localized. Emotional formation is, they contend, a complex process involving at least four separate cognitive processes, as demonstrated by hundreds of neuroimaging experiments.

There are two theories about emotions – *locationists* say emotions like fear can be localized to a specific region like your amygdala, while *constructionists* say emotions are created by the interaction of distributed neural networks functioning together.

Each region may have a number of basic, low-level functions, but these functions are merged to create the emotions you experience, and no single region functions in isolation to create emotions.

According to constructionists, emotions are only actually formed when you define your mood based upon related past experiences and personal interpretation of what "anger", "fear", "joy", etc. mean to you, and information from your body and your surroundings contributes to the process.

Four Components of Emotion:

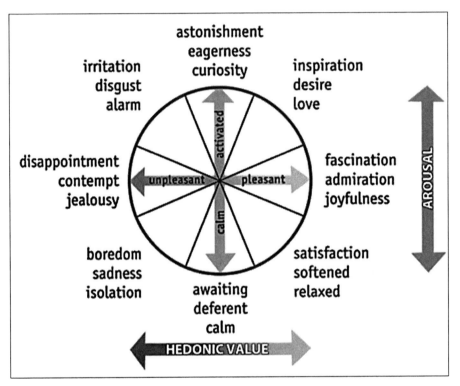

Adapted from "Framework of Product Experience", Desmet, P.M.A. and Hekkert, P., 2007, International Journal of Design, 1 (1) 57-66.

1. *Core Affect* – Emotions are said to be a combination of *arousal* (a scale running from *calm* to *excited*) and *hedonic valence* (a scale running from *pleasant* to *unpleasant*). Your *core affect* (emotional state among these two variable scales of feeling) influences all your mental and physical states, coloring your thoughts, perception and behavior: if you're feeling "blue" for example, things around you seem dreary, and you act and feel accordingly; when you're "pumped", you have energy to spare, the world seems full of possibility, and you act decisively, with an enthusiastic and optimistic anticipation of positive results.

    Reading your core affect primarily engages your amygdala, insula, basal ganglia, and frontal cortex. In short, core affect is the mental reading of body cues based on your degree of arousal and your levels of pleasure/displeasure.

Your core affect is the mental and physical state that helps you navigate the world – coloring how you interpret sensory perception of your environment, helping you decide how to act; helping you decide if you've just encountered a potential friend or enemy, and whether a situation holds a reward or a threat.

Your core affect can also be independent of external events, based upon your *temperament* (long-term) or *mood* (short-term), or it can be altered by external events which lead to an *emotional episode*. The amount of such external influence is subject to change, depending upon your circumstances, and whether you've developed an internal or an external locus of control – the extent to which you blame outer events for your lot in life, vs. believing your fate is in your own hands.

2. **Categorization** – You interpret sensory information from your body and environment by comparing it with stored memories of similar situations. Using *episodic memories* – memories of your experiences – to help you understand what you're experiencing in the present allows you to make predictions about others' thoughts, motives and feelings, to interpret what their actions and facial expressions mean, and to predict future possibilities. This engages your PFC, temporal lobe, hippocampus, and cingulate cortex.

3. **Language** – categorization (interpreting what you're experiencing in the present based upon comparisons with past memories) requires interpretive labels such as *anger, disgust* or *joy* to help you "compartmentalize" and define your sensations as emotions you can consciously describe and communicate. This engages your *ventrolateral (front and sides)* PFC, and anterior temporal lobe.

We tend to think of and label colors as discrete categories like red, blue, green and so forth, when in fact light (and colors) are a continuous, unbroken spectrum of wavelengths ranging from the infrared to the ultraviolet. In the same way, we label and think of emotions as distinct, discrete categories like joy, fear, and sadness, when in fact core affect is also a continuous spectrum of states. It's believed that we categorize and apply labels to our core affective states just as we do with colors, and so part of experiencing an emotion involves verbally sorting out exactly what our feelings are.

For example, someone smiling at his children's laughter while they play would experience sensations, subconsciously categorize them based on stored knowledge, and then recognize the state as "joy". In the past, it was believed that this experience simply triggered a dedicated neural "happiness circuit".

4. **Executive Attention** – the previous three "emotional ingredients" are combined into an emotion by *executive attention* processes, the selection of which cognitive or perceptual elements to heighten, maintain, or suppress. Such selective attention engages your *dorsolateral* (rear and sides) PFC and *ventrolateral* (front and sides) PFC.

Dopamine Hath Charms

"Musick has Charms to sooth a savage Breast,
To soften Rocks, or bend a knotted Oak.
I've read, that things inanimate have mov'd,
And, as with living Souls, have been inform'd,
By Magick Numbers and persuasive Sound."
– William Congreve, The Mourning Bride, 1697

Composer Frederick Delius called music an "outburst of the soul". Confucius said it was capable of producing "a kind of pleasure which human nature cannot do without". One of the reasons it – as with all the arts – has flourished for at least 750 centuries, is that it evokes very deep and powerful brain activity related to wellbeing.

Every form of art, including music, dance, painting and even comedy triggers a dopamine release. For example, Dr. Semir Zeki, founder of the Institute of Neuroesthetics at University College London, has used fMRI scans to show how viewing beautiful paintings results in the same chemical release as romantic love.

And according to 2011 research at McGill University, your favorite music also stimulates dopamine release in your striatum. Reading brain activity with MRI scans, researchers found peak moments of dopamine release during the moments subjects said "gave them chills". These chills aren't just subjective feelings – they're a clear pattern of arousal of the autonomic nervous system, which controls such things as heartbeat, breathing and hormonal releases. It also may explain why, as Oscar Wilde suggested, we experience bursts of pleasant recollection while listening to music we enjoy: studies of smokers show nicotine triggers this same dopamine release, in turn stimulating the recall of episodic memories.

If you're curious, a list of the most stimulating passages in the study can be found online here: http://www.plosone.org/article/fetchSingleRepresentation. action?uri=info:doi/10.1371/journal.pone.0007487.s001

According to the University of Groningen's Professor Jacob Jolij, conscious perception comes from a constant comparison. Information gathered from all of your senses is compared with your beliefs and knowledge about the world. The results of this comparison are what each person decides is "reality". But your brain can build up expectations based upon past experiences and current mood.

You use memories and expectations about the world (schemata) to interpret visual, auditory, tactile and other input; but your perception is also deeply influenced by your emotional state, which strongly affects both what you notice and how you interpret it. In other words, your worldview doesn't just depend upon your knowledge of "how things work", or even your expectations and biases; it also very much depends upon how you *feel* from moment to moment.

So music does more than just temporarily make you feel good. In Dr. Jacob's 2011 study of music's effects upon moods and perception, his team demonstrated that mood significantly alters perception, and because music so strongly influences mood, it can be used to reliably alter mood so its effects upon perception can be studied.

Even more amazingly, music really *can* put people "on the same wavelength": a fascinating 2009 study in Austria found that when guitarists play together, their brain waves synchronize, the frequency of neural firing occurring in harmony. This synchronicity occurs both before the actual playing of notes and afterwards, suggesting that "interpersonally-coordinated actions" bring our minds together on a more fundamental level than previously realized. Dr. Ulman Lindenberger, who led the study, believes this synchronization may occur in a wide range of shared activities, including team sports, dancing, and even child-parent bonding.

The Social Animal

Discoveries on the frontiers of science are permanently, radically changing what it means to be human. We're answering some of the most fundamental, age-old questions about human nature for the first time in history. For example, are human beings basically good or basically evil at heart?

Studies have conclusively shown your behaviors, beliefs and attitudes are habitual – acting evil is indeed a slippery slope, and the more you lie or engage in morally weak or criminal behaviors, the easier it becomes, and the harder it is to act in a more morally upstanding manner. The latest research shows we're all basically wired to tell the truth – but we can override that natural tendency, and the more often we do, the easier it becomes to lie. According to a 2010 cooperative study between the Netherlands and Belgium:

> Brain imaging studies suggest that truth telling constitutes the default of the human brain and that lying involves intentional suppression of the predominant truth response.... Results showed that frequent truth telling made lying more difficult, and that frequent lying made lying easier... habitual lying makes the lie response more dominant.

This, as we'll see, applies to a wide range of human behavior. Being good is the healthy, default human state – kindness, honesty, compassion, the drive to cooperate come to us naturally. But at any point, we're able to deviate from this path, and research seems to indicate that the more you practice being good, the more natural and ingrained the behavior becomes, and the more you practice being evil, the worse you will become.

You can choose to override your inherent propensity for goodwill – allowing your baser nature to predominate, degenerating like Gollum in *The Lord of the Rings*; or ultimately reclaiming your better nature like Scrooge in *A Christmas Carol*. The choice is always yours, but the more frequently you act either good or evil, the more it starts to become your default state, eventually defining you. And, given time and practice, the harder it will become for you to go against the path you've chosen for yourself.

Your Brain's Output

There is ultimately only one form of data input in your brain – action potentials transmitted across your neural network. All information delivered to your brain, no matter how it's acquired, is converted into a series of ionic charges, through transduction. All thoughts, memories, sensations, and emotions are encoded in exactly the same way

– ion flow through neurons. There is also ultimately only one form of output from your brain. All output – your actions upon the world, including speech – is through action potentials activating muscle contractions. Every single effect you have upon the world is through identical electrical signals activating your muscles – from delivering a speech to playing a complex piano concerto to simply breathing.

Action!

Every muscle in your body contracts in response to your CNS's excitatory impulses, sent through the spinal cord to stretch receptors buried in your muscles. When a muscle is triggered, the tendon pulls on it, and it contracts. And each muscle has its opposite, providing control in the form of resistance, and used to move a body part in the opposite direction.

Any action, from simply walking to swinging a golf club, is accomplished through a learned or instinctual motor pattern, coordinated by your motor cortices, cerebellum, basal ganglia and a bundle of spinal cord neurons called *central pattern generators*. Such motor patterns guide Tiger Woods as he visualizes and executes a perfect swing.

Because of the brain's incredible adaptability, motor patterns can be shifted to different groups of muscles. For example, signing your name on a contract and writing it in large letters on a chalkboard accomplish the same end result – a recognizable individual signature – but for a piece of paper, the motor program operates mostly your forearm and hand muscles, whereas for a chalkboard, the same motor program operates your shoulder and upper arm.

Being able to translate motor patterns into coordinated movements requires tracking each of your body parts in space and in relation to one another. Your parietal lobe, hippocampus, premotor and motor cortices all cooperate in generating and maintaining mental coordinate systems which map out space around you. One map is centered upon your location within your environment, the other upon objects on which your attention is focused. As you move, your brain refers to these mental maps, comparing where you intended to move with where your body parts actually ended up.

Input from your sensory cortices is integrated in the association areas and sent to your prefrontal cortex. Your premotor and secondary motor areas organize the desired behavior, and, at commands initiated by your prefrontal cortex and basal ganglia, your primary motor cortex executes the desired movement. Your basal ganglia provide corrective feedback to the motor areas, while your cerebellum also receives cortical input, providing the primary motor cortex with feasibility and status feedback on the movements, relying on proprioceptors to report the position and angle of your body parts in space.

Interestingly, imagining a movement (motor pattern) and actually executing this movement activate the same brain pathways, which is why mental practice is sometimes nearly as beneficial as physical practice when mastering complex skills.

571

fMRI studies show that performing, imagining and even just watching physical actions activates the exact same brain centers in which relevent motor patterns are stored.

Of course, muscles physically adapt and grow in response to training, and their potential strength can be retained for many years, even if they fall into disuse. Danish researchers reported in 2010 that muscles retain long-lasting "memory" of former fitness even if they *atrophy* (weaken) from disuse. These "muscle memories" are stored as DNA-containing nuclei, which increase in response to exercise. During muscle atrophy, a number of unused cells die off in the process called *apoptosis*, but these additional nuclei remain, allowing muscles to quickly return to former strength levels. This is yet one more compelling reason for people to begin exercising at an early age.

Motor training and other forms of learning also require sleep. Sheer repetition, mnemonic devices and the logical breakdown of complex ideas or actions into manageable pieces are traditional learning aids, but sleep also appears to be critical, particularly when it occurs within 12 hours or less after learning.

In fact, learners need only watch others perform physical actions and then sleep to see some benefits – test subjects who slept within twelve hours of merely watching others perform finger-tapping sequences were 22% faster and had 42% fewer performance errors than their non-sleeping peers.

The Carrot And The Stick – Motivational Paths

All sentient creatures are motivated to seek their own well-being by two opposing instinctual drives – maximizing pleasure and avoiding pain. Animals seek out and approach things that look rewarding, and avoid things that past experiences suggest cause discomfort. These twin motivations have enabled life to adapt and survive in a variety of environments, from the comfortable to the extreme.

Pleasure-seeking is thought to be the primary motivating system, but the negative (*aversive*) system complements this positive (*appetitive*) reward system. Appetitive motivation directs creatures toward goals that produce pleasurable sensations such as eating food or engaging in sex, while aversive motivation entails escaping from an unpleasant condition, such as pain or cold.

Two brain circuits give rise to these drives: the reward circuit and the punishment circuit. The reward circuit motivates using a *desire-action-satisfaction cycle*, while the punishment circuit (*periventricular system*, or *PVS*) activates the *fight or flight response*. Ideally, the end result ensures a creature's further survival, and restores its body's homeostasis.

These principles underlie *operant conditioning*, which uses three methods to guide training: positive reinforcement, negative reinforcement, and punishment.

- *Positive reinforcements* are stimuli (e.g., food) which increase the probability of a desired behavior;

- *Negative reinforcements* are circumstances in which *stopping* a negative stimulus (e.g., escaping an electric shock) increases the probability of a behavior;

- *Punishments* are negative stimuli (e.g., electric shocks) which *decrease* the probability of a behavior.

Generally, positive reinforcement is linked to pleasant experiences (rewards). It produces *approach behavior*, while negative reinforcement and punishment are generally linked to unpleasant experiences and produce *avoidance behavior*.

The appetitive and aversive circuits can also be directly stimulated, as James Olds and Peter Milner demonstrated in 1954, electrically stimulating certain brain regions to elicit specific behavior; their lab animals could be induced to press a lever over 100 times a minute to trigger electrical pulses to neural pleasure centers.

Motivation from this direct electrical activation proved even stronger than such normal rewards as food and water. Animals chose to starve in favor of stimulating these pleasure pathways. Additionally, their desire to stimulate didn't wane, as they chose to press the levers continuously until they dropped from exhaustion. Although other brain regions also produce pleasurable effects, the medial forebrain bundle is associated with the strongest effects.

Electrically stimulating these reward pathways in both humans and animals has shown the stimulation is intensely pleasurable for both; some human volunteers have likened the effects to intense orgasms, and these volunteers have been known to develop strong romantic attractions to the scientists performing the experiments. Such direct brain and vagus nerve stimulation is also currently being used to treat Parkinson's disease and depression, with the potential to offer relief from diseases long thought incurable.

Drugs are also used to study brain reward mechanisms. In such experiments, animals press levers to release drugs into their brains or bodies. These studies have shown the drugs that are addictive for humans are also addictive for laboratory animals, the most potent among them stimulants like amphetamine or cocaine and opiates like heroin and morphine.

The Reward Circuit

For a species to survive, its members must carry out such vital functions as eating, reproducing, and responding to aggression. In humans, evolution has developed certain brain regions whose role is to provide a pleasurable sensation as a "reward" for carrying out these vital functions. These areas are interconnected to form the reward circuit, the medial forebrain bundle. Here, the ventral tegmental area (VTA) and hypothalamus receive information from several other regions that tell how well fundamental needs are being satisfied.

First described in the early 1960s, the MFB is a bundle of axons that connects your limbic system and brainstem. It plays a central role in your most pleasurable moments, such as savoring victory or experiencing orgasm. It originates in the reticular formation of the brainstem, crosses the VTA, passes through the hypothalamus, and continues into the nucleus accumbens, amygdala, septum, parts of the thalamus and prefrontal cortex. All of these regions are interconnected, converging upon the hypothalamus, informing it of the presence of rewards. The hypothalamus then acts reciprocally upon the VTA, and, via the pituitary gland, upon the autonomic and endocrine systems of your entire body.

When the cortex has received a sensory stimulus that points to a reward, it sends an announcement to the VTA, whose activity increases. The VTA then forwards this information to the nucleus accumbens, using the chemical messenger dopamine. In addition to the nucleus accumbens, the VTA secretes dopamine into the septum, amygdala, and prefrontal cortex. This dopamine increase, particularly in the nucleus accumbens, reinforces the behaviors by which humans satisfy fundamental needs. Thus, the nucleus accumbens promotes behaviors (motor activity), while the prefrontal cortex directs the focus of attention.

In this way, the medial forebrain bundle (MFB), leads to repetition of gratifying actions. The reward circuit is the first of two major dopaminergic pathways, known as the *Mesolimbic Pathway* (ancient brain). The second major dopamine circuit is the *Mesocortical Pathway*, running from the VTA to the frontal cortex. Its major function is to help your frontal cortex suppress inappropriate impulses, emotions and reactions. In addition to dopamine, the circuit also uses serotonin, endorphins, and GABA to help shape behavior.

The Pain Circuit

Aversive stimuli (painful or frightening events) activate your brain's punishment circuit (the periventricular system, or PVS). Acetylcholine stimulates the secretion of *adrenal corticotrophic hormone* (ACTH). ACTH in turn prompts the adrenal glands to release adrenaline, preparing your body for defensive activity, coping mechanisms which mainly involve your amygdala, thalamus, hippocampus and hypothalamus.

The MFB and the PVS are twin, opposing mechanisms which appear to cancel one another out: when the punishment circuit is engaged, its effects inhibit the reward circuit – it's difficult to feel pleasure in the presence of pain or fear. Conversely, when the reward circuit is engaged, it inhibits activity in the pain circuit. In other words, pleasure soothes anxiety and pain.

The Surrender Circuit

The situation is quite different for the third circuit, the *behavioral inhibition system* (BIS), associated with the septum, hippocampus, amygdala, and basal nuclei. The BIS receives input from your PFC and outputs to your brainstem, activating the release of norepinephrine from your locus coeruleus and serotonin from your Raphe nuclei.

Instinctive Behavior Modes

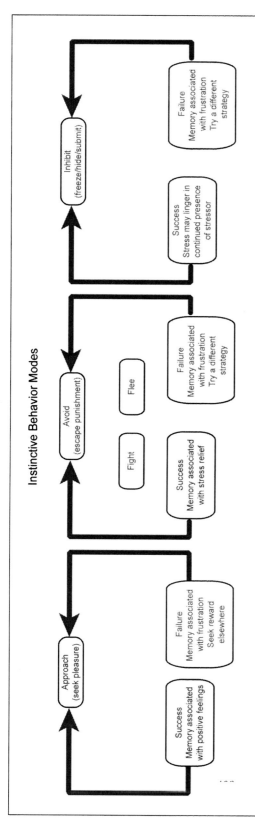

All healthy living creatures instinctually seek their own mental and physical well-being, approaching new resources, hoping to find rewards. This is our "default program", upon which we act on a moment-by-moment basis.

Occasionally, however, past experiences may teach us that seeking a reward in the current context might lead to punishment, such as pain, injury or social stigma. In the face of such threats, we have two other behavioral programs our brains can automatically launch - the fight or flight behavior pattern (two options for overcoming danger) or inhibiting our behaviour to avoid confrontation, by submitting or escaping notice.

The above chart shows how our default behaviour patterns interact and are reinforced, as we associate positive or negative values with the memories of those experiences. These emotionally-charged memories allow us to adapt and correct our future behavior based on what we remember. (original source: McGill.ca, copyright Polyglot Studios, KK 2011)

BEHAVIORAL MODELS

The BIS is activated when both fight and flight seem impossible. It's the instinctual drive to surrender or display a complete lack of aggression when no other survival options are available. The PFC activates the Behavioral Inhibition System when the only available options appear to be giving up, playing dead or even freezing in the face of danger.

This system can even be triggered by an overactive imagination, excessive worry over potential outcomes preventing any action at all. In the long term, repeatedly activating this behavioral inhibition can be extremely destructive to the health. The brain actively suppresses other instincts, and this mental stifling comes at a price – over time, weary resignation or a chronic belief in one's own helplessness leads to a toxic buildup of stress hormones that wear down the body and impair its normal functioning, eventually leading to serious illness. For example, a fearful wife who constantly, defeatedly gives in to a domineering husband may well be hastening her approach to an early grave.

Four Behavior Systems

Human behavior is built upon a limited repertoire of preprogrammed, fundamental instinctual behaviors built through natural selection to keep creatures alive and spread their genes. Healthy living creatures instinctually seek their own mental and physical well-being, approaching new resources, hoping to find rewards. This is the default program upon which humans and other animals act on a moment-by-moment basis.

However, this doesn't quite satisfactorily explain all the intricacies of human behavior, such as altruism – if all motivations are selfish, how can someone like Mother Teresa ever come to exist? At least four types of behavior systems are at work, providing humans with a complex wealth of responses to the environment.

The chart on the following shows how default human behavior patterns interact and are reinforced, as we associate positive or negative values with memories of past experiences. These emotionally-charged memories allow humans to adapt and correct future behavior.

Old School

Freud suggested personality had three aspects, which work together to produce all behavior: the *Id*, *Ego* and *Superego*. Picture a prudish catholic schoolmarm (the Superego) dragging a kicking, biting and cursing student (the Id) by his ear into the office of the dispassionate, clinically logical old headmaster (the Ego).

It was Freud's belief that these three aspects of personality had to be in balance for mental health and energy. The Ego, he said wrestles with competing demands from the Id and Superego, and the struggle to balance their demands and ultimately find happiness is the basis of everyone's primary life challenge. The strategies one uses to resolve this inner conflict slowly shape the personality.

HABITUAL BEHAVIOR

Consciousness Level: Subconscious

Uses: Learned behaviors that have become so familiar as to become habits, requiring little to no thought to accomplish (e.g. riding a bicycle)

Options evaluated by: A "cached value system" tapping into previously learned skills

Advantages: Fast; allows attention to be focused elsewhere.

Disadvantages: Largely inflexible; requiring effort to train or retrain

Relevent Brain Regions: Striatum; influenced by dopamine and serotonin

STRIATUM

GOAL-DIRECTED BEHAVIOR

Consciousness Level: Mostly conscious

Uses: Logical decision-making based on available info

Options evaluated by: Comparing alternatives using available information, from the objective (environment) or subjective (memory)

Advantages: Rational and extremely sophisticated

Disadvantages: Slow, and requires adequate, high-quality data

Main Relevent Brain Regions: Prefrontal Cortex, striatum

PFC

CONDITIONED RESPONSES

Consciousness Level: Subconscious

Uses: Everyday instincts, conditioned responses – learned, semi-permanent responses to specific stimuli

Options evaluated by: Instinctive evolutionary behavior mechanisms

Advantages: Fast and effective for promoting survival

Disadvantages: Very inflexible

Relevent Brain Regions: Many; primarily the striatum and periaqueductal grey region of the brainstem. Dopamine and serotonin play a major role

PAG

EPISODIC-MEMORY TRIGGERED BEHAVIORS

Consciousness Level: Conscious

Uses: Earliest stages of learning, where the situation is familiar but there is little available information to evaluate

Options evaluated by: Memories of what proved effective in previous, similar circumstances

Advantages: Fast, and compensates for a lack of available knowledge

Disadvantages: Does not integrate information

Relevent Brain Regions: Primarily the hippocampus

HIPPOCAMPUS

The Id: The emotional, irrational part of your mind; anatomically, this would correspond with the primitive impulses of your hypothalamus. At birth, a baby's mind is entirely occupied by Id – a state of perpetual want. And throughout life, like an eternal, spoiled child, the Id wants all its dreams fulfilled, immediately. This is the seat of your libido (sexual energy) and other desires. If your Id is overly dominant, you'll be selfishly and completely absorbed in feeding your endless need for instant gratification, satisfying hunger, thirst, physical comforts, aggression, and sexual desires.

The Ego: The rational part of your mind, corresponding to your prefrontal cortex, which grows from maturation and the awareness that you can't have every desire fulfilled. Your Ego relates with the outside, real world, realizing the value and need of compromise. It mediates between your Id and Superego, negotiating a workable compromise between instant gratification and long-term consequences. Fulfilling your Id's desires within reason, and calculating the long-term consequences, your Ego denies both instant gratification and stoic denial, seeking a middle road.

The Superego: The final stage of your mind to develop, your superego is your "moral compass", an embodiment of parental and societal values, which might be said to anatomically arise from your dorsolateral prefrontal cortex.

Your superego remembers the rules you're taught by society, your parents and peers, and imposes them upon your impulses. It's a demanding taskmaster, settling for no less than perfection, and producing anxiety when your Id and Ego fail to meet its lofty standards. If your Superego is too strong, you may be plagued by constant guilt, and may act insufferably holier-than-thou, a perpetual "goody two shoes".

Freud theorized that there were two subdivisions of the superego – the *Ego Ideal* and the *Conscience*. The Ego Ideal consists of rules of good conduct and standards of perfection for the Ego to aim at – often acting like the voices of one's parents in one's mind, the Ego Ideal is what one's parents valued or approved of. The conscience, on the other hand, embodies bad behavior – all those things of which one's parents disapproved. Both the Id and Superego, said Freud, are essentially mindless, and constantly at war, and this war is mediated by the Ego.

To Freud, most human motivations, preferences and behaviors are driven by aspects of the personality of which one is unaware – ideas, attitudes and preferences shaped during infancy, or otherwise outside one's awareness. Some of these drives and impulses, he believed, are personally unacceptable or repugnant, and so one hides them from one's own conscious mind through what he called *defense mechanisms*. Among these defense mechanisms are:

- *Projection* – Desires or impulses so unacceptable one accuses others of having them. One example would be the recent rabid public homophobes among American conservative politicians who, Freud would say, are hiding their own homosexual impulses from themselves.

- *Rationalization* – Explaining behaviors in terms one finds acceptable, such as a mother who enjoys hitting her little boy, but says, "I'm a good parent, so I'm doing this for his own good!"

- *Sublimation* – Acting out impulses in alternative ways, such as the bully, who, beaten by his father, is unable to fight back or lash out in hatred, so instead picks on other, smaller kids or defenseless animals.

- *Regression* – Reverting back to a childlike or infantile state.

Who Are You?

This sounds like a simple question with an easy answer, but it actually has many answers. Philosophers and psychologists have been arguing over the meaning of self and identity for thousands of years and they still haven't reached a consensus. But there are, generally speaking, two "selves" in each of us. The first is fluid, changing from moment to moment, the ongoing stream of consciousness that is one's thoughts, emotions, and perceptions. This is the result of neural *activation*.

The second self is more stable, collected memories which form an *identity*. These are physical *connections* between neurons in a human brain. The combination of these connections among 100 billion neurons is staggeringly complex and unique for each of us. Neuroscientists refer to this network as a *connectome*, and say that this is where identity resides.

Neurons *reweight*, constantly strengthening or weakening synaptic connections, creating and eliminating synapses, rewiring by growing or retracting branches, and even, in limited regions, generating new cells. This constant rewiring is the result of experiences – the actions we take, the events we encounter, the thoughts, emotions and perceptions we experience.

On the other hand, the physical dimensions of brain tissue provide the potential which can be exploited through use. According to MIT neuroscientist Dr. Sebastian Seung, if one imagines human consciousness as a river of flowing water, the sum of the brain's physical connections – its connectome – is its riverbed. The riverbed dictates where and how the river flows, but, over time, the flow itself will in turn gradually reshape the riverbed.

Thus as one grows from childhood through adulthood, one's identity – connectome – changes. Just like trees, nerves grow new branches, and lose old ones. Synapses are created or eliminated, and grow larger or smaller. Genes program this, but neural activity can activate these genes, changing these connections – thus, the mere act of thinking alters one's connectome.

So, in general, identity implies that you are, and have always been, "you", but it's also an adaptive, fluid state, one that changes in relation to life exploration and the personal and social commitments you make. Along with these experiences, your genes also help determine who you will become, helping to make you unique. Identity is also your day-to-day, ongoing self – your beliefs, morality, memories, collected experience and knowledge, ethnicity, social status, gender, age, general temperament, uniqueness, and social associations. Sadly, there are many people who even choose to identify themselves by what they own.

You publicly convey your identity through what sociologists call *markers* (language, dress, behavior and choice of space), which you display for the benefit of others. These markers set *boundaries* – similarities or differences between the displayer and perceiver, and the effectiveness of these social markers depends upon mutual understanding of their meaning.

Think about the different markers that define, for example a jock, a yuppy or a skater punk – the group's slang or professional jargon, the clothes, the gestures, shared values, preferences and outlooks in life. If you're familiar with the subcultures, you'll understand the values attached to these markers. If it's the first time you're encountering them, however, they can be mystifying.

2012 research bears Dr. Seung's theories out – personality differences stem from variations in the brain's neural connections. These differences are greatest in cortical association areas – regions which integrate information – and in regions dedicated to attention and control; but much less so in areas which process perception. Differences appear to stem primarily from cortical folding (sulci depth) and long-range neural connections, particularly in areas of high connectivity.

Massachusetts General Hospital's Dr. Hesheng Liu led a team which ran fMRI scans on 23 volunteers five times during a six-month study, comparing results with a meta-analysis of 15 studies which found links between functional connectivity and individual differences in cognition and behavior.

The team compared seven primary neural networks, and found variability ranged from highest to lowest in the following order: frontoparietal control network (FPN), ventral and dorsal attention networks (vATN, dATN), default network (DN), limbic (LMB), sensory-motor (Mot), and visual (Vis) networks.

Currently, the US National Institutes of Health is funding Massachusetts General Hospital, UCLA, Washington University and other partners in the *Human Connectome Project*, an initiative which dwarfs the Human Genome Project in scale. Researchers are attempting to map out the most complex structure in the known universe, in hopes of finally cracking open specifically what makes each of us unique, and why the system sometimes goes awry.

Your Personality Profile – Test Yourself

Psychologists currently use the *Five Factor Model* (FFM) for describing personality. The system was first developed in 1933 by Chicago psychologist Dr. Louis Leon Thurstone, using empirical (observed) data from a huge number of studies; it's come to be accepted as the general standard by professionals. The system consists of five personality aspects ranging on a scale from low to high, as follows:

Openness – People scoring high in this trait are eager to consider new or unusual concepts. They tend to have a high appreciation of the arts, science, emotions, and possess a sense of adventure. They generally possess strong imaginations, are driven by curiosity, and have a deep appreciation of beauty. Open individuals are typically more creative and attuned to their feelings than closed individuals, and may hold unorthodox beliefs.

Those who score *low* for openness are more "down-to-earth", practical and conventional. They generally have more traditional interests, and prefer clear and direct matters instead of abstract, ambiguous, complex or subtle matters. They tend to be conservative, and are likely to view art and science as dull, even looking upon them with suspicion.

Conscientiousness – Conscientious people tend to be self-disciplined, with a strong sense of duty and goal-oriented behavior. They are efficient and organized, as opposed to careless or easy-going people. Those scoring high in this trait prefer planned activities over spontaneous behavior. Conscientiousness influences how one manages and directs inner impulses. It also involves the *Need for Achievement* (NAch) drive.

Extraversion – Extraverts have positive personalities, seeking stimulation and the company of others. Those high in extraversion prefer to engage the world, and they find the opinions and thoughts of others stimulating. They tend to be energetic and outgoing, as opposed to introverts (low scorers), who are more reserved or shy. They enjoy the company of others, and are usually quite energetic, enthusiastic, and dynamic, relishing excitement. In groups, they tend to talk a lot and to draw attention to themselves.

Conversely, introverts aren't driven by the need for external stimulation, and tend to lack the social exuberance and energy of extraverts. They tend to be quieter, more deliberating, and less socially engaged. Their lack of social involvement is sometimes misinterpreted as aloofness, shyness or depression, but introverts simply need less stimulation and prefer more solitude than extroverts. Outside of social situations, they may possess a lot of energy.

Agreeableness – Agreeable individuals tend to act friendly, cooperative and compassionate, as opposed to competitive, antagonistic or sceptical. They prefer to preserve social harmony – what the Japanese call *wa*. This personality dimension reflects the extent to which one is willing to consider the interests of others over oneself. Agreeable individuals are willing to suppress their true feelings in the interest of preserving the peace or avoiding offending others – strategies which may not always be healthy.

People who score high in agreeableness tend to be optimistic about human nature, believing people are honest, decent, and trustworthy at heart. Because of this, they are thought of as considerate, friendly, generous, and helpful, because of their willingness to sacrifice their own interests in favor of other people. They also tend to have a great degree of *empathy* – the ability to understand the feelings of others – which motivates them to want to make others feel better.

On the opposite end of the scale, overly outspoken individuals tend to consider "honestly expressing themselves" as more important than diplomacy. They tend to care more about "being true to themselves" than about any discomfort they may cause others. Because of this, they tend to be unwilling to tell little white lies to lubricate social situations, and are often blunt, or even tactless. They tend to care little about getting along with others or making their peers happy. This, however, shouldn't be interpreted as an uncaring nature – these individuals just believe that directly expressing opinions is the best way to behave.

The tendency can cause social friction at home and work, but such individuals believe it's better to air out any problems than to cover up issues in the interest of smooth relations. Because they don't care overmuch about being liked or appreciated, these people are less likely to extend themselves for the sake of others, and thus may appear selfish. However, they prefer to extend favors more anonymously; scepticism about the motives of others tends to make them suspicious and uncooperative.

Neuroticism – (also called emotional instability) This aspect of personality runs along a scale from nervous/sensitive at the high end, to confident/secure at the low end. Neuroticism is the tendency toward negative emotions like anger, anxiety, or depression. Those scoring high in neuroticism are highly reactive emotionally and tend to be vulnerable to stress, to interpret minor frustrations as hopeless or mundane circumstances as threatening. Their negative emotional reactions generally persist for extended periods, so these individuals can often be in dark moods. Such difficulties in regulating their emotions diminishes their ability to think clearly, to decide, or to cope effectively with their own unhappiness.

On the other end of the scale, those scoring *low* in neuroticism tend not to get upset easily and react less emotionally. They're generally calm, emotionally stable, and are free from lingering negative emotions. This relative absence of negative emotions doesn't mean low neuroticism scorers are full of positive emotions; they just tend to experience fewer extreme lows.

Low	Medium	High
Openness		
Conscientiousness		
Extroversion		
Agreeableness		
Neuroticism		

My Five Factor Personality Score results, 2011, BBC Online

To find out more about your own personality, please take the free Five Factor Personality Test at BBC Online: https://www.bbc.co.uk/labuk/ experiments/personality/

THE FIVE FACTOR PERSONALITY MODEL

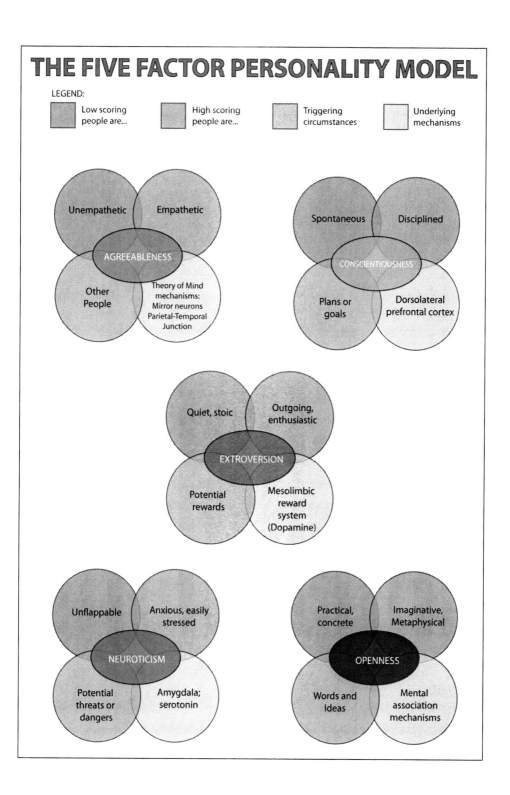

LEGEND:

Low scoring people are...

High scoring people are...

Triggering circumstances

Underlying mechanisms

AGREEABLENESS
- Unempathetic
- Empathetic
- Other People
- Theory of Mind mechanisms: Mirror neurons Parietal-Temporal Junction

CONSCIENTIOUSNESS
- Spontaneous
- Disciplined
- Plans or goals
- Dorsolateral prefrontal cortex

EXTROVERSION
- Quiet, stoic
- Outgoing, enthusiastic
- Potential rewards
- Mesolimbic reward system (Dopamine)

NEUROTICISM
- Unflappable
- Anxious, easily stressed
- Potential threats or dangers
- Amygdala; serotonin

OPENNESS
- Practical, concrete
- Imaginative, Metaphysical
- Words and Ideas
- Mental association mechanisms

583

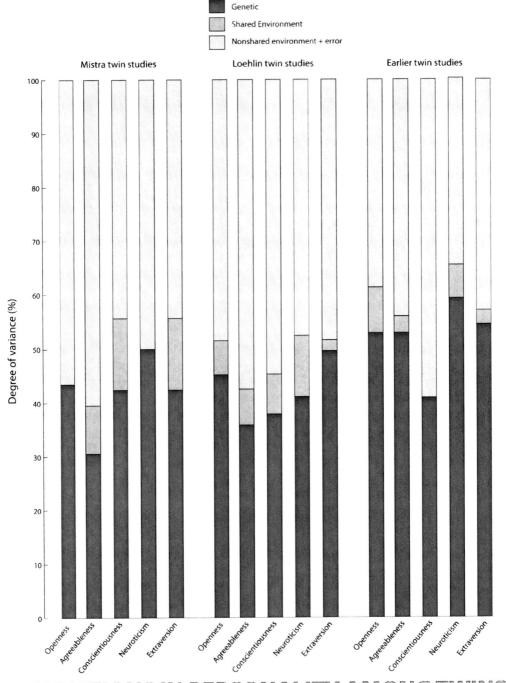

VARIATIONS IN PERSONALITY AMONG TWINS

By studying identical twins – who share the same DNA – and comparing those who have been raised in the same environment with those who have been raised in different environments, it's possible to measure the relative influence of genetics vs. environments in personality formation. Multiple studies are fairly consistent – showing a roughly 50% influence from each factor. Adapted from **Principles of Neural Science**, *4th Edition, Eric R. Kandel, et al, 2000, McGraw-Hill*

Are Parasites Controlling Your Brain (?!) Intestinal bacteria have been shown to markedly influence brain chemistry and behavior. Several common gastrointestinal diseases had previously been linked to anxiety and depression, but research conducted in 2011 at McMaster University in Hamilton, Ontario, has shown that when antibiotics disrupt normal intestinal bacterial content, it can lead to marked behavioral changes and an increase in **brain derived neurotrophic factor** (BDNF) linked to depression and anxiety.

About 500 species of bacteria are known to live in the human intestinal tract, in levels estimated as high as 1 quadrillion microorganisms, many times the number of cells in your body. The relationship between these bacteria and their human hosts is symbiotic, meaning both host and parasite benefit: bacteria have access to plentiful food, and humans receive energy, vitamin and hormonal synthesis, as well as protection from more harmful bacteria.

Dr. Stephen Collins led a series of experiments in which completely intestinal bacteria-free mice were produced, and then seeded with intestinal bacteria from either "brave" mice or "cowardly" mice. Within two weeks, the recipients' exploratory behaviors changed to match that of the mice from which their bacteria had come: passive germ-free mice bred from passive stock were given intestinal bacteria from mice with higher exploratory natures, and became more daring and active, while normally active germ-free mice became passive after being given bacteria from passive mice.

Using antibiotics to disrupt the bacteria also produced marked changes in behavior and BDNF levels, which returned to normal after antibiotic administration was discontinued. The research appears to clearly indicate that intestinal bacteria variety and stability influence behavior and that disruptions to these bacteria (for example, from antibiotics or infection) can result in profound behavioral changes.

In *The UltraMind Solution*, Dr. Mark Hyman says such a gut-brain connection and its influence on mood and cognitive function is obvious in his own patients. He says treating the gut is a key part of relieving the symptoms of ADHD, depression and anxiety.

Nature vs. Nurture: Settling the Debate

In 1869, Charles Darwin's half-cousin Dr. Francis Galton was the first to study the interplay of inheritance (nature) and environment (nurture) in the development of human personality traits. Since then, twins are commonly used for such studies. *Identical twins* are *monozygotic*, meaning they grow from a single fertilized egg which separates into two. Because of this, they have identical genes. *Fraternal twins*, however, are *dizygotic*, meaning they grow from two separate fertilized eggs. Dizygotic twins therefore share about half of their DNA, just like non-twin siblings.

By testing the personalities of identical and of fraternal twins, it's possible to measure how much genes contribute to the development of specific personality traits; if identical twins have a greater *concordance* (similarity) in a personlaity trait than fraternal twins, that personality trait is due, at least to some degree, to genes.

The effects can be further deduced by studying identical twins that have been separated at a young age and have grown up in different households. Although such separated identical twins grow up in significantly different environments, they share a surprising number of what are normally thought of as distinctive, individualistic personality characteristics, such as religious, intellectual, and academic interests. The similarities in characteristics between identical twins who were separated from birth are partly due to genes, though environmental factors also play a role.

The environmental contribution to behavioral traits is often divided into shared and nonshared components. Shared environmental influences, such as child-rearing practices or income, may underlie observed phenotypic similarities among family members. In contrast, nonshared influences, such as interactions with peers in school, can create differences among members of the same family.

It's still not known how many and precisely which genes influence behavior, but as science progresses, the specific genes at work in shaping personality will become clearer.

The Moral Animal

"Injustice anywhere is a threat to justice everywhere. To ignore evil is to become an accomplice to it." – Dr. Martin Luther King, Jr., Letter from Birmingham Jail, 1963

"The law, in its majestic equality, forbids the rich as well as the poor from sleeping under bridges, begging in the streets, and stealing bread."
– Anatole France, Le Lys rouge (The Red Lily), 1894

"We must indeed all hang together, or, most assuredly, we shall all hang separately."
– Benjamin Franklin, address to the Continental Congress, before signing the Declaration of Independence, 1776.

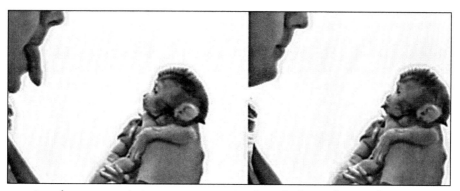

A newborn macaque imitates tongue protrusion, 2006, Evolution of Neonatal imitation, Public Library of Science, public domain.

Hard-Wired For Harmony – Monkey See, Monkey Do

On a sunny 1989 afternoon, a tiny macaque monkey sat in a university lab cage in Parma, Italy, electrodes protruding from its motor cortex. As the monkey moved about, its motor neuron activity registered on a nearby monitor. A graduate student had just returned from lunch, and was enjoying an ice cream cone near the monkey, when he noticed something astonishing: as the monkey watched him raise the ice cream to his mouth, its motor cortex fired, activating the monitor – even though the monkey had not moved a muscle.

The same motor neurons were firing as if the monkey were feeding itself, while it was simply watching the student eat. The lab's research team, under the direction of Dr. Giacomo Rizzolatti, began to study this phenomenon, which occured every time macaques watched or even just heard others eating peanuts, raisins and other items.

Dr. Rizzolatti's team came to the conclusion that specialized *mirror neurons* were allowing their monkeys to mentally mimic actions without moving.

"Mirror neurons", says Dr. Rizzolatti, allow us "...to grasp the minds of others, not through conceptual reasoning but through direct simulation. By feeling, not by thinking." His team's accidental discovery would throw open the doors to a new understanding of primate learning. Since the find, a number of the world's leading scientists have concluded these special neural centers are not only central to learning, but they may even be the basis of modern civilization.

You learn primarily on the basis of imitation, but mirror neurons allow you to mentally experience another's actions without even executing the movements. This means you can almost instantly learn many complex behaviors simply by watching. Modern psychology suggests that mirror neurons have allowed you to learn everything from your first baby steps to dancing the watuzi. You watch and learn, then perfect and consolidate motor memories through *physical rehearsal*. Children in particular learn by imitation from birth; according to the University of Washington's Dr. Andrew Meltzoff, within a few minutes of birth, babies will stick out their tongues in imitation of adults who are doing it.

The mirror neuron system may well be the fundamental driving force behind human culture and morality. Two and a half million years ago, mirror neurons allowed one of our Australopithecine ancestors to watch another bash a hand chopper out of a river stone and immediately understand to perform the action without having to be taught. In effect, his motor neurons had already accomplished the deed for him, activating the same neural traces as if he were making the tools himself.

This ability to learn instantly is an evolutionary leap over the painfully slow trial-and-error learning practiced by most other animal species, and almost certainly helped propel the human animal into a technologically-advanced future.

Through this capacity, says Dr. Rizzolatti, humans are able to instantly, intuitively and vicariously experience the same sensations and emotions of others. In terms of evolution, this puts us light years ahead of all the competition: just by watching, it seems, we're able to almost instantly learn anything from practical skills – how to forage, fish, hunt and skin, build shelter and fires – to the intentions of other creatures.

Renowned neuroscientist V. S. Ramachandran believes "...mirror neurons will do for psychology what DNA did for biology: they will provide a unifying framework and help explain a host of mental abilities that have hitherto remained mysterious and inaccessible to experiments." He contends that the evolutionary development of motor neurons about 50,000 years ago is what enabled our early ancestors in East Africa to begin organizing into societies, using tools and developing languages.

A great deal of follow-up research around the world over the last two decades appears to have confirmed the existence of these special neurons in humans; researchers have identified several clusters that fire in sympathy with the actions and emotions of others. fMRI scans have repeatedly monitored neural activity reflecting observed motor system activity; motor planning neurons echo movements, and somatosensory cortex neurons transmit the sensations of executing those movements. Even watching someone carry a heavy load triggers sympathetic sensations.

According to University of California neuroscientist Dr. Marco Iacoboni the effects are profound:

> When you see me perform an action – such as picking up a baseball – you automatically simulate the action in your own brain. ...you understand my action because you have in your brain a template for that action based on your own movements. When you see me pull my arm back, as if to throw the ball, you also have in your brain a copy of what I am doing and it helps you understand my goal. Because of mirror neurons, you can read my intentions. You know what I am going to do next.
>
> And if you see me choke up, in emotional distress from striking out at home plate, mirror neurons in your brain simulate my distress. You automatically have empathy for me. You know how I feel because you literally feel what I am feeling.

This explains the appeal of watching dance, sports and other public performances, but it also appears to work with facial expressions – fMRI scans and film footage of sympathetic facial muscle micro movements show that mirror neurons cause you to mentally mimic – subconsciously and automatically – the facial expressions of others in your mind – and doing so triggers the same feelings they're expressing. Mirror neurons also send signals to your limbic system, so you share the pain, joy, sadness and frustration of others – just by watching.

In other words, mirror neurons seem to allow you to simulate the actions, intentions and emotions of others. For example, when someone else smiles, your mirror neurons fire, and you experience the sensation of smiling. Your own brain fires in sympathy, mirroring pain when you see a friend wince in agony, and, without moving a muscle, you seem to mentally rehearse the same motor patterns as the soccer player racing downfield for a goal. People become so engrossed in professional sports because their neural circuitry appears to simulate actual participation in the game.

Your mirror neurons allow you to vicariously experience actions, feeling the rush of joy when watching a mother share a smile with her baby, or the thrill of a game-winning touchdown. Scientists say this constitutes an innate mechanism for understanding motivations and actions: studies link mirror neurons to intuitive understanding of intentions and behavior prediction.

When motor cortex neurons are artificially stimulated, patients report feeling strong urges to perform certain physical actions. But a special neural gate seems to block us from actually carrying out these actions. Says neuroscientist Christian Keysers, who heads the Social Brain Lab at the Royal Netherlands Academy of Arts and Sciences, this part of the motor cortex constitutes the "stronghold of our freewill".

Thus, while your mirror neurons let you feel the physical thrills as you watch Olympian Julia Mancuso hurtle down the slopes, your conscious will prevents you from doing this, presumably through behavioral control circuits in the prefrontal cortex.

589

In a sense, mirror neurons allow us to engage in a constant, low-level form of mind control; as others watch you perform an action, they automatically perform it themselves. Your acts become theirs, and theirs become yours, an mental exchange of physical sensations.

Through the same mechanism, emotions are contagious; our brains trigger hormonal releases that cause us to feel the emotions we read on the faces of others. And since mirror neurons also make us experience the pains and joys of others, they give us a "default program" for moral behavior – we're compelled to share, to help those in need, and to make others happy, by what Dr. Keysers calls *intuitive altruism*, more commonly known as the *Golden Rule*. Our brain is, he says, ethical by design, although we can override our inner better natures, performing a low-level cost-benefit analysis on the fly, and allowing our own self-interests to override our empathy.

Language acquisition is also thought to be based upon mirror neuron activity. USC neuroscientist Dr. Michael Arbib says Broca's area contains circuitry for both spoken and sign language, the same circuitry controlling both the complex hand gestures of sign language and complex motor activity which produces speech.

Reading Intent – The connection between your visual cortex and amygdala is critical to your ability to read emotions; specialized circuitry in your visual cortex only responds to specific facial expressions and gestures, which seems to clearly indicate humans (and other primates) are genetically built to automatically read facial expressions.

In other words, you're born to empathize. From an evolutionary standpoint, this circuitry helps you instantly determine whether an approaching creature intends to attack, make friendly overtures, or try to mate. But this amygdala-cortical circuit appears to not just govern emotion interpretation, but also to assist in formulating appropriate responses. When the connection is severed, victims become unable to read emotions or to respond appropriately.

Throughout The Cortex

Mirror neurons have been found within the premotor cortex, parietal lobe, temporal sulcus and insula, and rudimentary mirror systems also appear to exist in non-human apes, in monkeys, and possibly in elephants, dogs and dolphins. They exist in sets, including a basic set which observes movement, and supporting sets which help read the intent of movement. Thus, mirror neuron systems perform several functions, including helpting to generate empathy – the ability to intuitively grasp the mental states of others.

In 2010, UCLA Medical Center's Dr. Mukamel found neural mirroring in response to facial expressions and grasping in 1,177 neurons within the supplementary motor area and medial temporal cortex. Several additional experiments using fMRI, electro-encephalography (EEG) and *magnetoencephalography* (MEG) have found regions in the insula, cingulate cortex, and inferior frontal cortex which activate when people feel emotions like joy, pain and disgust, and when they observe others experiencing the same emotions. This explains how the greatest actors can move you to tears, or make your heart pound with excitement. The very existence of this biological mirroring system suggests that human beings have evolved to be social creatures. In other words, we're built to get along; if there were no need to relate with others, such a system of empathic neural mirroring would be unnecessary.

UCLA neuroscientist Dr. Marco Iacoboni believes mirror neuron and limbic system communication allows you to tune into others' feelings, as a unifying mechanism allowing people to deeply and instantly connect. Negative social emotions such as pride, disgust, embarrassment, guilt, lust and shame all seem to engage the insula, used in processing both physical and emotional pain. Feeling disgust or just seeing it expressed on another's face triggers the same insula mirror neuron activity.

According to Dr. Christian Keysers of the University of Groningen (author of *The Empathic Brain*), fMRI scans show that when you see a hand caress someone, and another push it away rudely, your insula activates, and you vicariously experience the social pain of rejection; humiliation, it seems, is also derived from the physical pain-processing neural circuitry.

Problems with this system may be at the heart of autism. According to UCLA's Dr. Mirella Dapretto, autistics can identify and even imitate facial expressions of emotions like anger, but don't feel the emotions when they observe or imitate them.

Autism spectrum disorder patients tend to be very poor at reading non-verbal emotional signals and other social cues, though once they're otherwise made aware of another's feelings, they can share those emotions intensely.

I Feel Your Pain

Empathy is your capacity to understand and share, to varying degrees, the feelings and emotions of others. It's a sophisticated imaginative process, which involves the ability to imagine yourself as that other person or animal.

There are both *cognitive* (logical thought) and *affective* (emotional) aspects to empathy: the cognitive component involves putting yourself in someone else's shoes, using *theory of mind* – combining observation, knowledge, reasoning and experience to infer the thoughts and feelings of others. The affective component is your ability to respond with appropriate emotion to those perceived thoughts and feelings.

Recognizing others' mental states is related to mental simulation, based upon an innate ability to link observed movements and facial expressions with their associated sensations. But you're also born with the ability to read emotions from tone of voice, muscle tension, body language and possibly pheromone signaling (though this is still controversial).

The Empathy Deficit

In 2011, University of Chicago neuroscientist Dr. Peggy Mason teamed up with Drs. Jean Decety and Inbal Ben-Ami Bartal to test for altruism in rats. What she found was that, not only will rats will very quickly release their peers from confinement, they will repeat the behavior even if it's remote, and they are denied the reward of being reunited. Even more surprisingly, if presented with a cache of chocolate, rats voluntarily free their peers to share it. Said the researchers, the creatures unambiguously show empathy and altruism. According to Dr. Mason, the only reward they receive is feelings from helping another individual. Similar findings worldwide show that humans aren't the only animals which have evolved instincts to help others, even at a cost to themselves. Says Dr. Mason, "The bottom line is that helping an individual in distress is part of our biology."

When we empathize, according to modern-day neuroscientists and social psychologists, we experience the distress of others and, unless we suffer from brain damage or abnormal development, we feel an emotional compulsion to alleviate their suffering. As a result, like trust and altruism, empathy is a "social glue" thought to be at the heart of the evolution of human cooperation.

American psychology pioneer Edward B Titchener first coined the term in 1909, inspired by the German word Einfühlung, which means "feeling into". He said empathy was a process in which an art object evoked mental or actual motor movements and emotions in a viewer.

Mirror neurons are thought to lie at the heart of the mental process, but only make up part of the "empathy circuit", which includes the amygdala, central to emotional learning and reading emotional expressions, the anterior cingulate cortex, which activates when one experiences pain or observes it in others, and the insula, which activates in response to one's own pain or that of a loved one, as well as such emotional triggers as disgusting sights, smells, and tastes.

Most important, however, appears to be the medial prefrontal cortex, a region in the middle of the frontal lobe which essentially performs lightning-fast cost-benefit analyses and other higher-order evaluations. These include weighing alternatives, behavioral error-handling and processing social interactions.

Damage to this region makes it extremely difficult for patients to learn from previous emotional experiences or to use emotions in guiding decision-making, so each alternative weighs equally in the balance of the decision. Patients with damage to the medial PFC show a markedly lower sympathetic nervous system response to normally emotionally upsetting images, such as scenes of wartime carnage. Their lack of elevated heartbeat and other stress responses echoes the responses of psychopaths, and dispassionate killers.

Psychopaths can be expert at reading the emotions of others, while remaining emotionally unperturbed. Violent adolescents diagnosed with "conduct disorder" show similar responses, and can even get a dopamine rush of pleasure at the sight of others in pain. This is known as *schadenfreude*, pleasure derived from the misfortune of others, a dopamine rush in the nucleus accumbens of the mesocortical limbic pathway – the brain's pleasure/reward center.

Empathy can also be deliberately suppressed: After shooting 69 defenseless strangers bathing in a lake, Norwegian mass murderer Anders Behring Breivik declared at his 2011 trial that he felt empathy but used a "meditation technique" to override those feelings, after years of practice.

Dr. Ute Frevert, Co-Director of the Max Planck Institute for Human Development, says, "The fact that human beings are naturally equipped to feel what others feel does not mean that they always do so. They might just turn away and act indifferent."

We can see this reflected in the rash of heartless cuts to America's social benefits that protect the poor, even as the ranks of America's homeless swell to historical proportions – by far the majority among them children and single mothers.

In the wake of a rash of horrific shootings that sent shock waves rippling through the country in late 2012, US President Barack Obama said America's *empathy deficit* constituted a graver problem for America than even its mountain of federal debt. Implicit in his speech was the notion that this deficit can be altered – that empathy can be "learned".

So is it possible to increase empathy? Most psychologists suggest it can be done through encouraging greater perspective-taking – we're kinder to those whose humanity we recognize, much less so to those we view as "subhuman", a finding the Pentagon and Intelligence divisions worldwide have exploited to great effect in centuries of brutal warfare. When we expend the energy to mentally "walk a mile in the shoes of another" and see things from their perspective, it becomes much harder to ignore their suffering.

Mass media are also powerful tools for fostering greater empathy by exposing people to mental perspectives of those we could not normally encounter. Says Harvard psychologist Steven Pinker, this fostering of a wider worldview, coupled with "humanitarian reason" is responsible for a steady decline in societal violence since the Age of Enlightenment.

Unfortunately, such empathy is all too often fleeting, as our minds have been trained to quickly seek new sources of stimulation. Empathy can also often lead us astray, rather than serving as a moral compass, as in judges giving lenient sentences to white-collar criminals sharing the same social background. That's not to suggest that we should abandon attempts to increase it.

Experiments show that empathy – the ability to accurately "read" mental and emotional states – can be dramatically improved through special meditation, as shown by both behavioral testing and fMRI brain scans. fMRI scans of Buddhists who train in daily meditations on compassion show increased activity in regions of the brain responsible for generating empathy.

Cognitively-Based Compassion Training, or CBCT, is a special type of meditation developed at Emory University by Dr. Lobsang Tenzin Negi. Derived from ancient Tibetan Buddhism, the CBCT program is secular in content, training people to analyze and reinterpret their relationships.

Twenty-one randomly selected healthy subjects without previous meditative experience were divided into two groups. Half were scanned with fMRI while undertaking a *Reading the Mind in the Eyes Test* (RMET) test of empathic accuracy, both before and after completing CBCT training, while the other half were a control group scanned after a simple health discussion among subjects such as the effects of exercise and stress upon well-being.

The Reading the Mind in the Eyes Test (RMET) consists of black-and-white photographs that show just the eyes of people making various expressions, and test subjects must decide what the person in the photograph is thinking or feeling.

After eight weeks of once-weekly training followed by at-home practice, CBCT participants showed significant increases in their abilities to accurately read the mental states of others according to RMET scores, and they showed greatly increased activity in the dorsomedial prefrontal cortex (dmPFC) and inferior frontal gyrus (IFG), both central to empathy.

Participants in the CBCT group improved RMET scores an average of 4.6 percent, while control group participants showed, in the majority of cases, a decrease in RMET scores. Similar studies at Emory had demonstrated that CBCT meditation reduces emotional distress and enhances physical resilience to stress in healthy adults and high-risk foster care adolescents.

According to Dr. Negi, "CBCT aims to condition one's mind to recognize how we are all interdependent, and that everybody desires to be happy and free from suffering at a deep level."

From An Early Age

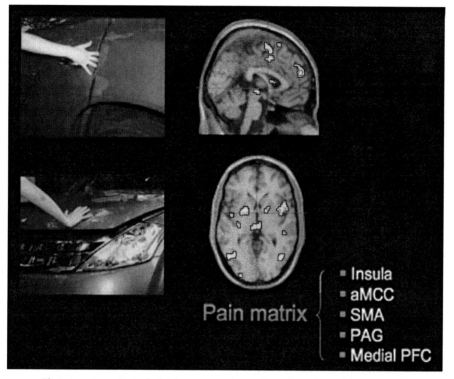

The pain matrix activates both when you experience pain and you observe it in someone else.
Dr. Jean Decety, 2009, University of Chicago. Used with permission

You're built to care from an early age: fMRI scans show when 7- to 12-year-olds see images of people in pain, their brains register it as if they were experiencing the pain themselves, and when they see a person intentionally hurt, it activates special moral reasoning centers.

Dr. Jean Decety is one of the world's leading authorities on neural correlates of empathy. An internationally-recognized cognitive neuroscientist, he studies empathy with fMRI and PET scans. According to his research, when we see others experience pain, the same neural circuitry activates within us.

This sympathetic activation, which he calls *somatic sensorimotor resonance*, is the basis of empathy, an innate function that children as young as 2 display. By the age of seven, children begin to develop empathy responses on a level of sophistication on par with adults. The capacity is innate, rather than specifically the result of parental guidance or nurturing, he says.

Dr. Decety uses fMRI scans on subjects from different sample groups, while present-ing films and pictures of people who suffer harm either accidentally or intentionally. Watching others in pain activates the same neural circuits which report one's own:

the insula, somatosensory cortex, cingulate cortex, periaqueductal gray, PFC and sup-plementary motor area.

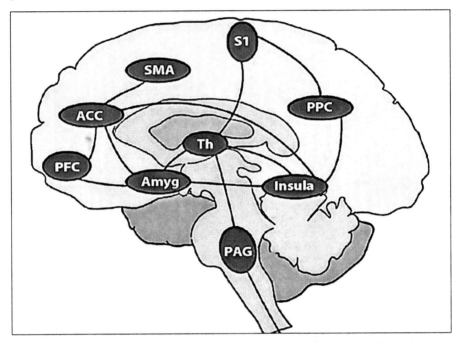

The pain matrix is generated by the thalamus (Th), amygdala (Amyg), insular cortex (Insula), supplementary motor area (SMA), posterior parietal cortex (PPC), prefrontal cortex (PFC), cingulate cortex (ACC), periaq-ueductal grey (PAG), basal ganglia and cerebellar cortex (not shown) and the primary (S1) and secondary (S2, not shown) sensory cortices. Adapted from Arne May, MD, Universitäts-Krankenhaus Eppendorf.

Children and adults both respond in the same manner to seeing someone intention-ally harm another, and in addition to the sympathetic emotional response, witnessing intentional harm activates regions used for social interaction and moral reasoning in the temporoparietal junction, orbitomedial frontal cortices, and amygdala.

But the capacity for empathy can vary: recent research suggests you're naturally more willing and able to empathize with those you find most similar to yourself, culturally, socioeconomically and in terms of identity.

Studies show moral reasoning originates in distinct neural networks which include the temporal-parietal junction (which generates the body-sensation-based sense of "self" and helps us evaluate the actions of others), as well as the amygdala and ventro-medial prefrontal cortex, which supports communication between systems underly-ing affective states, cognition, and motivation. The data seems to show that evaluat-ing intent is the first step in moral computation, with emotion acting as a "volume control" for moral judgment, signalling the viewer of the moral salience (importance and personal relevance) of a situation. It also shows the pervasive role of emotions in moral sensitivity and reasoning.

People can determine within a split second whether a harmful action they're witnessing is intentional or not, according to Decety's research. His study shows the brain is naturally hard-wired to recognize intentional harm, and he is currently trying to shed light on how emotion and morality guide and affect this recognition.

Dr. Decety and his assistant Stephanie Cacioppo tested adults as they watched videos of people suffering unintentional and intentional harm. As the subjects watched, their brain activity was monitored with a system which accurately maps responses over different brain regions and records the timing between them. This system is called *high-density, event-related potentials technology*, and it offers an advantage over the "snapshot" nature of fMRI scans.

Determining intent appears to be the first step in any moral computation, according to Decety and Cacioppo. Watching acts of intentional harm creates almost instant responses in the brain: within 62 milliseconds, the temporal-parietal junction (TPJ) activates, distinguishing intentional vs. accidental actions. If the harm was intentional, this is quickly followed by activation of the amygdala within 122 ms, and the ventromedial prefrontal cortex in 182 ms. The vmPFC is the brain region central to moral evaluations and decisions.

The entire process takes just over 180 milliseconds. If the harm is unintentional, only the temporal-parietal junction activates, without the amygdala or ventromedial prefrontal cortex, and the process occurs in about a thrid of the time.

Additional fMRI studies by Decety's team have repeatedly shown these same brain regions activate whenever people see others deliberately harmed, though this is the first time the specific activation sequence and timing have been worked out.

This capacity to recognize and emotionally respond to intentional harm is the central source of morality universal among humanity, says Decety. "It is part of humans' evolutionary heritage. The long history of mammalian evolution has shaped our brains to be sensitive to signs of suffering of others. And this constitutes a natural foundation for morality and sensitivity to justice."

His research suggests that emotion and the perception of harmful intent, rather than logical reasoning, give rise to moral responses, which stem from caring about others. This research is expected to help other areas of neuroscience research, including studies on moral responses in psychopaths and children who lack empathy for others, displaying so-called *callous-unemotional traits.*

Sensitivity – how accurately one can infer other people's thoughts and feelings, and the strength of the emotional responses they evoke – varies from person to person, but psychologists say that in healthy people empathy can be fostered. It's a skill which is gradually developed throughout life, growing in proportion with the frequency of contact between individuals. In other words, you get better at caring, and the more often you see someone, the more likely you are to care about them.

Foreign language Professor Jean-Pol Martin has devised a way to help students naturally develop empathy, through his *Learning by Teaching* method, now taught throughout Germany. With his method, students learn new content, and then teach it to their fellow students. In this manner, not only do they more fully absorb the material, but students develop empathy naturally – to teach effectively, they have to constantly gauge the mental processes of their fellow students as they learn.

Martyr Squirrels And The Evolutionary Basis Of Altruism

Empathy, says Yale psychology professor Dr. Paul Bloom, is when the pain of another matters to you. But on the face of it, caring and willingness to help others seems counter to natural selection: it seems more logical that selfish creatures would have a greater chance of survival – yet only some of us are selfish in temperament.

From 1974 to 1977, Berkeley zoologist Dr. Paul Sherman spent three years clocking over 3,082 hours of observation in the Sierra Nevada mountains of California, studying Belding ground squirrels, trying to determine why some would sacrifice themselves to issue warning cries at the approach of a predator, something that seems to contradict evolutionary common sense. The population he studied was marked with dyes to allow them to be identified at a distance, so individuals, exact ages and familial relationships could be identified. His conclusion was that the behavior evolved to protect the entire *phenotype* – the genes shared by a *family* rather than a single *individual*. Sacrificing one's life for the safety of many is an advantageous adaptive behavior he calls *nepotism*.

Similarly, the willingness to die for another seems to be a trait unlikely to promote long-term genetic survival, but it's also widely found in humans. In terms of pure evolutionary biology, it seems individual survival is much less important than gene duplication. By being willing to sacrifice themselves, individuals significantly increase the chances of survival of their kin, who share a large amount of their DNA. This seems to be the genetic basis of *altruism*, the willingness to selflessly help others.

Martyrdom has also been found among prairie dogs. Dr. Ron Chesser's work on genetics and prairie dogs has shown *consanguinity* – the degree of relatedness among organisms – is linked to self-sacrifice. The more closely-related creatures are, the more likely they are to sacrifice themselves.

But in humans, the matter goes beyond a simple willingness to "take a bullet" for another; we also physically experience sympathetic pain at the sight of another's injury, and even babies are known to cry in sympathy when they hear the distress of others. In a word, we're wired to care. Through natural selection, human beings have evolved a capacity for love and compassion, and this has helped us to survive as a species.

Of course, those who are incapable of caring – weapons merchants, mortgage-busting billionaires, environment-destroying magnates – are doing their utmost to destroy humankind, and take down as many other species as they can in the name of personal gain, but it is hoped that their kind will eventually be weeded out of existence by natural selection.

People that engage in acts of altruism know it feels great, and for good reasons. There's truth to the adage your parents may have taught you: in terms of endocrine responses, physical sensations, self-esteem and overall health, it really IS better for you to give than to receive.

As Jonah Lehrer points out, fMRI scans have shown that giving away money activates stronger neural activity in the dopaminergic neural circuits than simply keeping it. Selflessness is really good for you, mentally, spiritually, and – as we shall see shortly – physically.

Selfless By Nature

Researchers at the University of California Berkeley are challenging the long-held belief that humans are wired for selfishness. In a wide range of studies, social scientists are amassing a growing body of evidence to show we evolved to become ever more compassionate and collaborative in our quest to survive and thrive.

In contrast to *every man for himself* interpretations of Charles Darwin's theories of evolution by natural selection, Dacher Keltner, a UC Berkeley psychologist and author of *Born to be Good: The Science of a Meaningful Life*, is building the case that humans are successful as a species precisely because of our nurturing, altruistic and compassionate traits. Keltner calls this *survival of the kindest*:

> *Because of our very vulnerable offspring, the fundamental task for human survival and gene replication is to take care of others. Human beings have survived as a species because we have evolved the capacities to care for those in need and to cooperate. As Darwin long ago surmised, sympathy is our strongest instinct.*

The More You Give, The More (Respect) You Get

Studies show that bonding and social connections make for a healthier, more meaningful life, but UC Berkeley researchers are also asking, "How do these traits help ensure survival?" One answer, according to social psychologist Dr. Robb Willer is that the more generous you are, the more respect and influence you wield.

In a recent experiment, Dr. Willer and his team gave volunteers a modest amount of cash and directed them to play games that would benefit the public good. The results showed that participants who acted more generously received more gifts, respect and cooperation from their peers and wielded more influence over them.

> *The findings suggest that anyone who acts only in his or her narrow self-interest will be shunned, disrespected, even hated. But those who behave generously with others are held in high esteem by their peers and thus rise in status....*

> *Given how much is to be gained through generosity, social scientists increasingly wonder less why people are ever generous and more why they are ever selfish.*

Science Of The Greater Good

These results validate findings of such *positive psychology* pioneers as Martin Seligman, a University of Pennsylvania professor whose research in the early 1990s shifted away from mental illness and dysfunction toward the mysteries of human resilience and optimism. While much of positive psychology studies focus on personal fulfilment and happiness, UC Berkeley researchers have narrowed their investigation into how psychology can contribute to the greater societal good.

One outcome is the campus's *Greater Good Science Center,* a West Coast magnet for research on gratitude, compassion, altruism, awe and positive parenting. Christine Carter, executive director, is creator of the *Science for Raising Happy Kids* Web site, whose goal, among other things, is to assist in and promote the rearing of *emotionally literate* children. Carter translates research into practical parenting advice. She says many parents are turning away from materialistic or competitive activities, and rethinking what will bring their families true happiness and well-being.

"I've found that parents who start consciously cultivating gratitude and generosity in their children quickly see how much happier and more resilient their children become," said Carter, author of *Raising Happiness: 10 Simple Steps for More Joyful Kids and Happier Parents.* "What is often surprising to parents is how much happier they themselves also become."

> *Good at Heart – How do we know people are basically good? One clue among many is what psychologists call the* **linguistic positivity bias.** *Scientists at Washington University and the University of Arizona have analyzed the 10,000 most-frequently used words in the English language, in studies of both written and spoken English, and found that people overwhelmingly use positive adjectives, verbs and nouns over negative ones. We tend to prefer saying words like "love" much more frequently than we do equally familiar negative words like "hate". This tendency varies somewhat depending upon gender – women tend to use even more positive words than men – and personality, with those scoring highly in the personality traits of extraversion and agreeableness using the most positive words. In other words, we unquestionably prefer to talk about the brighter side of life.*

A Sympathetic Touch

Meanwhile, in searching for biological bases of positive emotions, Keltner and his team are zeroing in on the vagus nerve (Cranial Nerve X), part of a uniquely mammalian circuit which ennervates all your organs and regulates your heart rate and breathing. Both the vagus nerve and oxytocin play a role in communicating and calming.

In one study, two people separated by a barrier took turns trying to communicate emotion though touching via a hole in the barrier. For the most part, says Dr. Keltner, participants were able to successfully communicate sympathy, love, gratitude and calm. Researchers saw activity in threat response regions of the limbic system, indicating many of the female participants grew anxious while waiting to be touched. However, as soon as they felt a sympathetic touch, their vagus nerves activated and oxytocin was released, calming them immediately.

"Sympathy is indeed wired into our brains and bodies; and it spreads from one person to another through touch," Keltner said.

The principle also applies to other mammals. UC Berkeley psychologist Darlene Francis and McGill professor Michael Meaney found that rat pups whose mothers nurtured them showed reduced stress hormones, including cortisol, and had generally more robust immune systems. Overall, these and other findings challenge the assumption that nice guys finish last, and instead support the hypothesis that humans, if adequately nurtured and supported, tend to err on the side of compassion. Says Keltner:

> This new science of altruism and the physiological underpinnings of compassion is finally catching up with Darwin's observations nearly 130 years ago, that sympathy is our strongest instinct.

The Root Of All Good: The Basis Of Human Morality

In the King James New Testament, 1 Timothy 6:10 says *The love of money is a root of all kinds of evil*. But more broadly, that should be revised to say *greed is the root of all evil*. Greed corrupts. Greed kills. Greed destroys.

But you wouldn't know it to look at our economic institutions: in Oliver Stone's brilliant *Wall Street*, the ruthlessly self-serving Gordon Gecko lays out what is has become the central tenet of modern capitalism, in a speech summed up by his introductory phrase *Greed is good*.

In the 1700s, when settlement of the American colonies was – for better or worse – driven by a pioneer spirit, economist Adam Smith first laid out his theories in the groundbreaking *Wealth of Nations*. The central premise of *laissez-faire capitalism* – a hands-off style of economic governance – is that simple human desire is the engine that will drive economies. People gather wealth simply to make their lives better, and, in this way, the economic system is self-regulating. Since it's theoretically a level playing field, everyone has a "shot at the top".

While laissez-faire capitalism certainly helped drive America to unprecedented economic, industrial and technological dominance, in time it's become apparent that, to paraphrase George Orwell's *Animal Farm*, "some people are more equal than others".

No one in Adam Smith's day could have predicted a future where the American President would push for a war against a country which both the Secretary of Defense and of State had publicly announced "posed no threat to its neighbors" let alone the US; nor that he would award exclusive wartime contracts to a company in which his Vice President owned significant stock; or that deregulation would allow banks, with complete impunity, to drive millions of Americans out of their homes through misrepresentation and reckless fiscal mismanagement.

That said, recent experiments indicate that, while self-interest may indeed drive a lot of human behavior, such selfish, greedy bastards are – fortunately – in the distinct minority. Heartless sociopaths, while often high profile, are thought to only number about one in a hundred at most.

At heart, the vast majority of us are built to care. Most of us are shocked and appalled at the thought that international corporations receive billions in incentives, then pay no taxes on billions in profits, while ruthlessly slashing domestic jobs, only to export them overseas, hiring third-world starvees for pennies an hour while raking in historically record-breaking, obscene profits.

Most of us inwardly wince at the knowledge that education, health, research, food and public safety, and the protection of treasured natural parks are all being sacrificed in the name of fattening defense budgets.

The American military now eats over half of America's discretionary spending, while hundreds of thousands of men, women and even children live in the streets, with inadequate food, healthcare, education, and no hope for the future. Estimates are about 1 in every 200 Americans – a shocking statistic.

The truth is, healthy human beings are built specifically to cooperate, share, and care about those we see in distress. Dire economic hardship can dull that natural goodness, but, for most of us, the core is still there – it's not easy to completely ignore a man sleeping in the gutter without some twinge of sadness – and that, my friend, is the greatest part of you, the very heart of what it means to be human. Stifle it at your own peril; lose the ability to care about the suffering of others, and you lose a core part of your capacity to feel, to love, and to fully engage in life.

Cheating Makes You Anxious

Norms are socially accepted rules of behavior, such as wearing clothes in public and speaking politely to others. Such unwritten codes, along with laws and private rules ensure safety and stability among a large populace. On a subjective level, emotions such as guilt, fear, excitement, loyalty and love appear to be the motivation behind choosing to follow *mores* – culturally-accepted standards of right and wrong.

As you mature, you develop extremely strong feelings about what you believe to be right or wrong; when you live up to the moral code you ascribe to, it activates your endogenous reward system, and you feel good. When you don't live up to this moral code, however, you feel bad - shame, guilt and regret.

This moral code is derived from the culture in which you live by your *orbitofrontal cortex* – this area of your brain begins observing, deducing and encoding these rules of social interaction from birth, just as specific areas of your brain encode language. We can see this through fMRI scans as subjects are asked to make decisions about hypothetical moral dilemmas (e.g. *"Would you push someone in front of a bus if you knew it would save the lives of 12 passengers?"*)

A 2011 study at the University of Toronto tested moral forecasting and actions among three groups of students. Each was given a 15-question test and told they would receive five dollars if they answered right on ten or more questions. The first group was told the software was buggy, and that hitting the computer's space bar would make the correct answer appear onscreen, although nobody else would know.

The second group was told of this situation and each was asked whether or not they would cheat. The third group took the test without being told of the "spacebar cheat". During the test, blood pressure, heart rate respiration and sweating were measured to see when their anxiety levels rose. Those with the opportunity to cheat had the highest anxiety, even as they resisted cheating. The control groups had normal emotional responses.

Compelling You to Play Fair – *Human societies are built upon expectations that members will cooperate, act trustworthy, and follow accepted codes of conduct, ranging from common courtesies such as giving up a seat on the bus for the elderly, to complex legal agreements between corporations or even countries.*

Guilt works to foster obedience to these norms. Guilt is believed to arise when one feels he or she has failed to live up to the expectations of others. Wanting to avoid unpleasant guilty feelings is thought to motivate this cooperation; one cooperate because it feels good, activating the brain's reward pathways, but people also do it because they don't want to feel bad – guilt aversion.

In a 2011 study at the University of Arizona, volunteers played a money-awarding game while their brains were scanned with fMRI. Investors would award money to trustees, with certain expectations about how much they would get back. As the trustees decided how much money to return, their brains were scanned. The experiment showed that trustees felt guilty whenever they gave less than expected. Different brain areas activated when choosing to be generous than when choosing to be selfish.

Neural systems which process expectations play a critical role in moral decisions, helping sustain cooperation, even in the face of temptations toward selfishness. In situations such as the experiment, there are competing motivations for minimizing guilt and maximizing reward as a person chooses between selfishness and fair play.

Minimizing guilt is associated with the **aversive circuits** – *insula, anterior cingulate cortex and supplementary motor area, while maximizing personal gain is associated with the* **appetitive circuits** – *striatum and prefrontal cortex.*

Of Morals And Magnets

A joint 2010 MIT-Harvard study demonstrated that moral judgment is primarily derived from activity in the right temporoparietal junction (RTPJ), located just behind the right ear. Disrupt its function, and moral judgment breaks down. The TPJ shows increased activity when people evaluate the motivations of others, such as when a jurist considers criminal intent in a murder case. The region appears to be central to sizing up people's intentions, a critical part of the moral decision-making process.

In the MIT-Harvard study, volunteers were given various hypothetical scenarios; in one example, a woman named Grace is touring a chemical plant with a friend. They stop for coffee, and when her friend asks for sugar in her coffee, Grace pours in white powder from a container marked "toxic". The central question is, did Grace think the powder was sugar or some kind of poison, and, if her friend died, given either situation, what is her *culpability* – how guilty is she?

Grace and her friend are taking a tour of a chemical plant. Grace goes over to the coffee machine to pour some coffee.

Her friend asks for some sugar in hers. The white powder by the coffee is in a container marked 'toxic'. Grace puts the substance in her friend's coffee, and her friend drinks it.

Outcome

Belief		Neutral	Negative
	Negative	Grace believes the powder Is sugar, and it is, so her friend is fine.	Grace believes the powder is sugar, but it's toxic and her friend dies.
	Neutral	Grace believes the powder is toxic. but it's only sugar and her friend is fine.	Grace believes the powder is toxic, and it is, so her friend dies.

Adapted from The Neural Correlates of Moral Sensitivity: A Functional Magnetic Resonance Imaging Investigation, 2002, Harvard University.

The researchers found that applying a magnetic field to the region – a process called *transcranial magnetic stimulation* – disrupted right TPJ function, impairing the ability of volunteers to gauge the intent behind certain behaviors. This, in turn, markedly influenced their moral judgments: under normal circumstances, people judge criminal culpability based upon whether or not the crime is intentional.

In this scenario, even if Grace knowingly fed poison to her friend, when the right TPJ was impaired, volunteers thought her intentions didn't matter, as long as the friend was okay. In other words, even if Grace was trying to kill her friend, because she didn't succeed, she hadn't done anything wrong in the magnetized minds of these volunteers. The researchers believe the impairment affected assessment of the circumstances, rather than the ability to make a moral judgment itself.

On the other hand, a related 2007 joint experiment by Harvard and the Universities of Southern California and Iowa found that injury of the ventromedial prefrontal cortex (vmPFC), which lies just below the forehead, leads to an inability to feel empathy and compassion; this in turn leads to *utilitarian* (treating people as objects to be used), dispassionate moral decisions. So while the amygdala, hypothalamus and other areas of the limbic system may be responsible for giving rise to emotions, the vmPFC appears to regulate them, particularly emotions in response to others.

Under normal circumstances, say the authors, "...we forgive unintentional or accidental harms and condemn failed attempts to harm." But skin conductance and fMRI scans show an impaired vmPFC leads to a lack of emotion when making morally difficult judgments. Normal people typically feel strong aversive emotions when they perceive someone's deliberate intent to harm someone else, but those with vmPFC injuries don't; nor do they judge failed attempts to harm others as immoral. The vmPFC appears to weigh the emotional impact of events such as harmful actions:

> *Specifically, the vmPFC was robustly recruited when subjects evaluated emotionally salient harms to an individual that were intended as a means to maximize aggregate welfare, for example, pushing a person into the path of a trolley in order that his body stops the trolley from hitting five other people.*

So while people with this disability may still have typical intelligence, logic and an understanding of normal social behavior and rules, they fail to choose appropriately in daily life situations which require moral judgment calls, unable to process social emotions like empathy and embarrassment or feel emotional responses like guilt and regret.

Coauthor and Harvard Professor Marc Hauser says normal emotional qualms are part of a *universal moral grammar* – a commonly-shared, genetically-encoded, subconsciously-programmed sense of right and wrong. Choosing to harm or even kill someone for the greater good usually leaves people feeling emotionally torn, but not among those with vmPFC impairment. Feelings of aversion usually prevent people from hurting one another, a drive co-author Antonio Damasio describes as "...a combination of rejection of the act, combined with the social emotion of compassion for that particular person."

Morality also evolves as one matures, with physical changes to the neural circuitry as sensitivity grows, according to Dr. Decety, who uses a combination of fMRI scanning, eye-tracking and behavioral measures to track differences in moral judgment as people age. Interestingly, he says that children tend to judge those who harm others or property much more severely than adults, even when the harm is unintentional. It seems we mellow with age, becoming more tolerant and less automatically assumptive of guilt.

> *What Would You Do? Imagine someone close to you had AIDS and planned to deliberately infect as many people as possible, and you had to choose between allowing it to happen or killing that person, what would you do? Considering the possibility triggers slight anxiety in most people, but for those with impaired vmPFC function, there is a detachment – emotional feelings aren't stirred at all by such a dilemma.*

Your Moral Compass

Morality can be completely overpowering at times. Jonah Lehrer relates how, even in the heart of battle, soldiers are known to suffer complete paralysis when faced with killing. This is why the military trains troops with exhausting repetition – endless weapons training and combat drilling, until eventually the motor programs for killing become habitual, activating before the cortex has time to fully engage. The idea is to override the programming, to turn soldiers into killing machines.

This is certainly not the norm. Humans appear to be born with an inner moral compass, an innate sense of fairness underpinning all social interactions and evaluations. This underlies everything from daily personal decisions to the workings of legal, political, and social systems. Emotion plays a critical role in this automatic moral judgment system, guiding us by assigning moral values to situations, objects and behaviors.

Psychologists say there are standard emotions and so-called "moral emotions" which are linked to the benefit of people outside of ourselves. These emotions come in response to witnessing behaviors or situations with a moral component, whether good or bad. Both words and images can evoke these moral emotions – verbal descriptions or pictures of moral violations (physical assaults, poor street children or war scenes).

We evaluate these situations with moral labels such as *commendable, regrettable, fair* or *unfair, right* or *wrong, good* or *evil*, and interpret situations as conveying, for example "…a sense of friendship, betrayal, pity or care for others, humiliation, gratitude, or indignation."

"What's In It For Me?"

Harvard psychologists Amitai Shenhav and Joshua D. Greene believe, however, that moral choices aren't derived so much from an innate, high-minded sense of what is right. They say you use the same brain circuitry for making difficult moral choices as you do for making commonplace decisions such as what to eat or where to shop.

The same circuits, also present in other animal species, are used to evaluate based upon predictions, a process more commonly known as a *cost-benefit analysis*. Specifically, one uses these neural centers to consider *how rewarding or punishing are the possible consequences of this action?* and *What are the odds of each happening?*

According to Shenhav, one's ability to make both simple choices and complex life-and-death decisions depends upon neural centers that first evolved for making low-level survival decisions about such things as obtaining food. fMRI scans show many of the same brain regions activate when making major moral choices and when people or other animals make choices about mundane items like money and food. Specific circuits track the probability and magnitude of various outcomes, integrating the information into decisions, according to Dr. Green.

The same regions that merge this evaluation of outcome probability and magnitude into decisions are used to make everyday food and spending choices. Using fMRI scans, Drs. Shenhav and Greene had 34 volunteers choose between definitely saving one life or the more remote possibility of saving several lives, with no guarantee of success. The number of lives and odds of success varied. The ventromedial prefrontal cortex (vmPFC) was primarily activated when gauging the moral value of the less certain option, integrating the probability of saving lives with the number of lives potentially saved.

Such choices can sometimes affect thousands of lives, as, for example, the decision to delay pumping cooling seawater into the nuclear power plants at Fukushima, Japan after they'd been struck by a tsunami. It's been suggested that this single company decision to save expensive equipment at the risk of human lives was directly responsible for displacing half a million residents and making large regions of Japan uninhabitable, essentially for the rest of human history.

Say Shenhav and Greene, your mind uses the same basic mechanisms for judging whether an extended warranty is worth a few dollars extra, as for whose lives to save during a disaster. As callous as it sounds, *triage* – the moral decision as to who to save and who to let die in wartime or disaster – appears to use the same neural circuitry as that used for choosing which brand of shampoo to buy.

> ***The Empathy Gene*** – *A recent study has found compelling evidence that some people are genetically predisposed for greater empathy: "The tendency to be more empathetic may be influenced by a single gene," says Oregon State University's Dr. Sarina Rodrigues. She and UC Berkeley graduate student Laura Saslow have found people with a particular* **oxytocin gene receptor variant** *are more adept at reading emotional states and become less stressed by difficult circumstances.*
>
> *Informally called the cuddle hormone, oxytocin is secreted into your bloodstream and brain, where it promotes social interaction, nurturing and romantic love, among other functions.*

Shut Down

People with injuries to specific regions of their frontal lobes can be crippled by an inability to care, even while otherwise able to think logically. This can also cripple them morally and socially, leading them to act in inappropriate ways, suggesting the frontal lobes play a central role in moral appraisals, an automatic "tagging" of moral values to behaviors and situations. fMRI scans show the region, called the orbitofrontal cortex (OFC) is a major guide of social–emotional appraisals and social behavioral responses; the region is involved in empathic and moral judgments, and reward and punishment decision-making.

In concert with your OFC and *superior temporal sulcus* (STS), two additional regions also participate in moral and negative emotions – your midbrain and limbic system (thalamus, amygdala, insula). Their emotion-generating functions are critical for social behavior and perception, enabling you to use emotions as a guide in making moral appraisals. The OFC, STS and limbic regions seem to work in conjunction to allow rapid and automatic appraisal of social–emotional events, integrating cognitive, emotional, and motivational systems for moral judgment and behavior choices.

Political Morality

Scientists are reaching a new consensus on the origin and principles of morality, and believe that behavior and moral choices are shaped by one's values: if you're a conservative, you're more likely to care about social hierarchies and respect, while if you're a liberal, you're more likely to care about fairness and compassion.

University of Virginia psychology professor Johnathon Haidt says moral decision-making is based upon three principles:

- *Intuitive primacy* – human emotions and gut feelings

- *Moral thinking if for social doing* – we engage in moral reasoning to persuade others of our "rightness", and to try to win their support

- *Morality binds and builds* – morality and gossip (!) are critical for living in large, highly-cooperative societies.

Studies, he says, have shown that people tend to follow their gut instincts, and then justify their actions upon moral grounds after the fact.

> *Unfortunately, [most] of us behave more like lawyers, using any arguments we can find to make our case, rather than like judges or scientists searching for the truth. This doesn't mean we are doomed to be immoral; it just means that we should look for the roots of our considerable virtue elsewhere – in the emotions and intuitions that make us so generally decent and cooperative, yet also sometimes willing to hurt or kill in defense of a principle, a person or a place.*

His studies show that liberals make moral judgments based upon harm and fair play, while conservatives make moral judgments based upon hierarchies: authority, social status, in-group boundaries, and ideals of spiritual purity.

> *We often end up demonizing people with different political ideologies because of our inability to appreciate the moral motives operating on the other side of a conflict.... An understanding of moral psychology can also point to some new ways to bridge these divides, to appeal to hearts and minds on both sides of a conflict.*

Take a brief test of your own moral values at http://www.yourmorals.org

---

A Rousing Tale – *Want to persuade someone to behave better? Try telling them a heroic story. USC neuroscientist Dr. Mary Helen Immordino-Yang led studies which show the brain stimulates physical sensations in response to stories with strong emotional content.*

This, in turn, promotes introspection, leading to moral behavior. These mentally-induced physical twinges of emotion are detectable with fMRI scans, and Dr. Immordino-Yang says the moral behavior to which they give rise promotes species survival. The physical-emotional reactions lead to reflection, promoting moral choices and motivating people to emulate altruistic behavior by helping others. This finding, she says, holds the power to fundamentally change lives.

In her experiments, volunteers were told true, emotionally-charged stories during private, recorded interviews, and then asked to describe how they feel. Her team told emotional stories, recorded volunteer reactions, and used fMRI scans to record physiological responses.

One volunteer, hearing of a young boy acting selflessly toward his mother, reported feeling a sensation like a balloon inflating under his sternum. Reflecting upon this physical sensation led him to consider his own relationship with his parents, and he made a promise to himself to express greater gratitude to them.

Dr. Immordino-Yang found similar reactions among other volunteers, to varying degrees. Her group has conducted approximately 50 similar analyses at USC and in Beijing, China. Her experiments, she says, indicate contemplating the behavior and emotions of others leads to introspection and a conscious self-evaluation of one's own emotionally-induced physical sensations. Feeling empathy for another's distress, or admiration for someone's virtuous behavior are thus important components of morality, helping us decide how we should treat others.

We analyze the mental and emotional states of others using theory of mind, which is based upon our own experiences, and the self-reflective comparison invokes empathy, leading to the desire to act in similarly positive ways.

Dr. Immordino-Yang says humans are naturally intensely social, and thus story-telling is a very natural means of evoking positive emotions. These are the gut feelings so often described in response to stories, being clinically measured for the first time.

Vampire Bats Spreading Joy

Yale Professor Paul Bloom's lectures are fascinating and insightful, particularly his talk on the evolutionary development of emotions. He points out that if it's universally shared, a trait must logically confer some survival benefit, so with this in mind we can ask: what is the benefit this particular trait confers?

In the case of altruism – the drive to help others – the question's a puzzling one. A number of species engage in altruism. For example, says Dr. Bloom, animals will give off warning cries if a predator is sighted. If a mountain lion is about to pounce, the deer that sounds a warning is losing precious time it could use to escape, as well as making itself stand out from the group, markedly increasing the chance it will be attacked. So it stands to reason that such social animals act in this manner to protect others within their group.

Animals are also known to help in caring for others' offspring. Says Dr. Bloom, from an evolutionary standpoint, this seems illogical. In terms of pure "survival of the fittest" behavior, the most "logical" (albeit repugnant) course of action would be to eat the young for their protein. But they don't. In fact, animals share food. Why does such selflessness exist? If you consider it, self-sacrifice and sharing don't seem particularly good strategies for individual survival. Being selfish seems more beneficial in terms of survival and reproduction, and thus a behavior more likely to be passed on to future generations. So why aren't all animals selfish?

Dr. Bloom points to studies on vampire bats, one species known to share food. He says that when bats leave their homes in search of food, when one "strikes it rich" and finds, for example a horse, it will bite, lap up a huge amount of blood, then fly back to the cave. At this point it will proceed to share the food it's found, regurgitating it into the mouths of others in its community, so that everyone benefits from this one bat's good fortune.

In terms of evolutionary psychology, how is this behavior enforced or encouraged? It seems the logical course of action would be for a bat to gorge itself and let others fend for themselves.

When vampire bats share, says Dr. Bloom, it demonstrates the principle of *reciprocal altruism* – "you scratch my back, I'll scratch yours". There is greater benefit for a community of animals to work together than for individuals to try to survive on their own.

Good behavior between social animals is based upon the assumption of reciprocation, a silent and perhaps unconscious understanding that – in one form or another – "I'll benefit from you in return later". These benefits can range from the simple pleasures of shared companionship, to outright expectations of repayment. Reciprocal altruism seems to be enforced across species by *ostracism: cheaters* and *freeloaders* who take without giving back to the community are punished by social isolation.

Scientists experimented with individual vampire bats by giving them food and then restricting their ability to share. What they found was that the community would respond by excluding those individuals who didn't share. They would be "marked" as cheaters, and passed by when others returned to the cave with food. In other words, in the wild, selfish bats get starved out, and don't live to pass on their genes.

In this way, cooperation evolves as an *evolutionarily stable strategy*, according to Dr. Bloom; animals are neurally wired to punish cheaters, which, of course, means they must have the mental capacity to recognize, remember and be motivated to punish cheaters.

In the case of humans, Dr. Bloom gives an illustrative example of the freeloader at the bar. If everyone at the bar takes turns buying a round except for one person, he gets marked as a cheapskate, and people's innate sense of fair play gets aroused, they feel resentment, and eventually nobody wants to buy a round for the moocher. This sensitivity to fair play, says Dr. Bloom, plays a major role in the evolution of social behavior and social emotions.

The Prisoner's Dilemma

A classic way in which psychologists test reciprocal altruism is through variations of a challenge called *The Prisoner's Dilemma*, invented in 1950 by RAND Corporation psychologists Merrill Flood and Melvin Dresher. In this hypothetical scenario, two friends have committed a crime, such as robbing a bank. They're caught and brought into the police station for questioning, where they're isolated and each is offered the same deal: "Tell the police everything, and you can go free, but your friend will go to jail for twenty years".

Both suspects know they've each been offered the deal, but they're held in separate interrogation rooms. Given the conditions, if one suspect decides to talk, he goes free, but his friend goes to jail for twenty years. If both suspects cooperate and confess, they each serve a five-year sentence. But if both refuse to cooperate with police and just stay silent, they each receive only a light sentence (one year instead of twenty), and then get to go free.

The crucial point of The Prisoner's Dilemma is that, from a selfish standpoint, the "best" course of action is to betray your accomplice. If suspect A confesses and subject B stays silent, subject A walks away free. If suspect A confesses AND suspect B confesses, both go to jail, but only for five years. Finally, if suspect A stays silent, but B squeals, suspect A serves a full 20-year sentence.

A competition was held to invent a computer program that plays The Prisoner's Dilemma. The problem was to be made more abstract and put through several repetitions, and the computers would run the programs to play against one another. The program with the most wins emerged victorious. Logically, the strategy options were: play nice, play mean, cooperate, take advantage or punish. Out of 63 entries, the winner was a program with only four lines of code called *Tit for Tat*. Its strategy was simple – play nice on the first round, and just imitate the behavior of the rival on every round thereafter. This, says Dr. Bloom, is precisely the strategy that social animals adapt.

Computer scientist Robert Axelrod, who devised the competition, used the results to deduce that this is how human cooperation evolved: we imitate what we see, reward cooperation, and punish selfishness. Just like the computer program Tit-for-Tat, the default behavioral strategy for social animals is to be nice the first time they meet, and to respond in the same manner they're treated in the future.

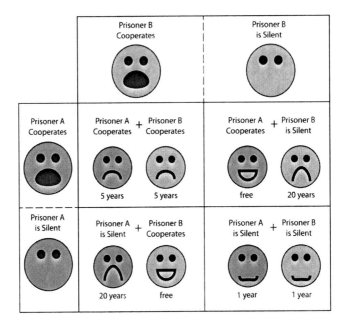

THE PRISONER'S DILEMMA

Says Dr. Bloom, human social behavior is modelled upon principles of the Prisoner's Dilemma: we like people who cooperate with us, and are motivated to be nice in return. Conversely, if someone betrays our trust, we mistrust them and feel resentment, motivating us to betray or avoid them in the future. And we feel guilt if we betray someone who's been kind or cooperative with us, motivating us to behave better in the future.

An Eye For An Eye

"An eye for eye, and soon the whole world is blind." – Mahatma Gandhi,
Indian political and spiritual leader (1869 – 1948)

"Hello. My name is Inigo Montoya. You killed my father. Prepare to die."
– The Princess Bride, William Golding, 1973

In the wake of Bin Laden's assassination, a number of Americans gleefully celebrated. Although Bin Laden – his CIA-funded roots aside – was certainly a despicable man, the effect his assassination had on Americans raises an interesting question: what makes us crave vengeance?

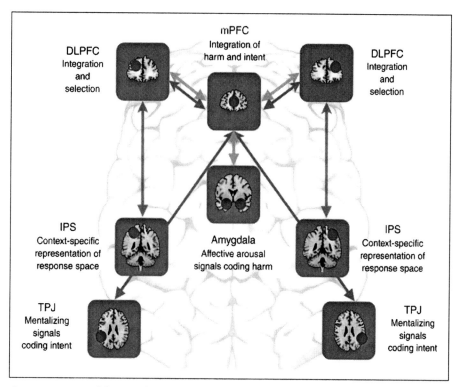

*Core components of the neural "**justice circuit**": According to Dr. Joshua W Buckholtz of Harvard University and Dr. René Marois of Vanderbilt, the **temporoparietal junction** calculates criminal intent and culpability, based upon assessments of an alleged wrongdoer's state of mind. The **amygdala** generates an emotional arousal signal equivalent to the severity of the transgression; this arousal signal is thought to be used as a **heuristic**, or rough guide, in deciding appropriate punishment severity levels.*

*The **medial prefrontal cortex** is believed to integrate the intent formulated in the TPJ with amygdalar harm magnitude signals, and this integrated data is conveyed to the **dorsolateral prefrontal cortex**. Drs. Buckholtz and Marois believe the DLPFC and **intraparietal sulcus** then integrate this intent/harm signal with possible context-specific responses to decide appropriate punishment severity.*

The interplay between these circuits is thought to guide selection from among a variety of punishment options maintained in the DLPFC. This model is based upon the assumption that punishment is motivated by a desire to give wrongdoers their "just desserts", which, says the authors, is supported by studies. Image: Buckholtz and Marois, 2012. Used with permission.

University College London's Dr. Tania Singer used the Prisoner's Dilemma to explore vengeance-craving in human nature. In the Prisoner's Dilemma, two suspects have been captured by the police and are being separately interrogated; each is offered a deal: If one confesses (incriminating his partner) — while the partner chooses to remain silent — then the confessor will go free, while the uncooperative partner has to serve a full sentence. However, if both remain silent, each receives a very mild sentence, since the police lack the evidence to convict both members of the full charges. The last option is where both parties confess, both receiving a somewhat stiffer sentence.

When the scenario was played out in front of experimental subjects, people formed strong opinions of each of the game's "suspects." Many of the volunteers grew to strongly dislike those who "squealed", seeming them as "cheaters".

Next, participants were placed into an fMRI scanner and watched as painful shocks were given to other volunteers. Those in the scanner showed empathic pain responses (in the insula, somatosensory cortex, cingulate cortex, periaqueductal gray, and supplementary motor area), but these responses were significantly reduced when "cheaters" were punished. "Disloyalty" reduced observer sympathy, making them less emotionally involved while watching "bad suspects" in pain.

In men though, there was an additional effect: each time a "cheater" got punished, it activated the mesolimbic reward pathway – the men (but none of the women) got a buzz of pleasure from watching "betrayers" get punished. This seems to uphold the theory that men feel satisfaction at seeing "justice served" when social wrongdoers are punished.

Straight Shooters

In the early 1980s, economists devised a similar experiment to shed light on human motivation. *The Ultimatum Game* is a variation of the Prisoners Dilemma, consisting of a simple set of rules: people are paired, and one is given ten dollars to distribute. The cash recipient – the *proposer* – is allowed to decide how the money will be divided. His partner – the *responder* – can choose to accept or reject the offer. If the offer is accepted, both partners keep the cash, but if it's refused, both walk away empty-handed.

It was assumed that the outcome would always be the same: the proposer would offer the smallest amount possible – perhaps a dollar – and the responder would accept. This constant result would, of course, clearly show the innate selfishness of human beings. What researchers found, however, surprised them – proposers almost always offered about half, and it was almost always accepted. Over the years, variations of the experiment have been repeated around the world, with the same results. From the standpoint of sheer self-interest, it makes little sense – aren't we all inherently greedy?

It would seem not. According to Jonah Lehrer, players in Japan, Russia, Germany, France, Indonesia and everywhere else almost always play fair with one another, offering to share the money equally. We are innately generous, he says, because of our neural empathy circuitry.

A 2011 Sweden study has further illuminated this human propensity for fair play: when you see someone acting unfairly, it arouses your amygdalae, and you instinctively seek to punish the cheater for his behavior. In this study, 35 volunteers were asked to play the Ultimatum Game, with one player proposing how to share 100 kroners (about 16 US dollars) between each pair of volunteers. The partner had the option of accepting the offer, or declining it, in which case neither received any money.

While volunteers discussed how to share the money, their brains were scanned with fMRI machines. Whenever subjects made unfair offers (such as 80-20 splits), their partners punished them, even if it meant neither would receive any money. Previous studies have pointed to the prefrontal cortex and insula as the areas governing analysis and choice in financial decisions, but in this case the desire to punish was governed by the amygdala.

This punishing, aggressive response to "unfair" offers was higher in men, a result possibly driven by testosterone, which is thought to increase aggressiveness. After being given an amygdala-inhibiting tranquillizer called *Oxazepam*, however, subjects were more willing to accept unfair offers, even if they had specifically said they thought these offers were unfair.

An Impaired Sense Of Justice

In conjunction with University of Southern California's Dr. Antonio Damasio, MIT neurologist Dr. Liane Young studied nine patients with aneurisms or tumors in the ventromedial prefrontal cortex (vmPFC), an area roughly the size of a plum found behind and over the eyes. Patients with such injuries have difficulty processing social emotions like empathy or embarrassment, although their ability to use logic and other higher-level mental functions is unimpaired, according to Young.

The vmPFC, used for regulating emotions, appears to mediate amygdala-driven outrage to unfairness, according to Dr. Young. Patients with damaged vmPFCs don't feel typical outrage at scenarios such as unsuccessful murder attempts, judging the events based only upon end results, without holding anyone responsible for the attempted killings.

Subjects were presented with 24 fictitious scenarios, which included botched murder attempts and accidental killings. Those with vmPFC damage had no difficulty in logically understanding the thought processes and intentions of would-be assassins, but they failed to assign moral responsibility for the crimes, even judging failed attempts as less serious than accidental harm – the reverse of how most (uninjured) people would respond. Like Star Trek's *Spock*, people with vmPFC injuries understand logic, but cannot ascribe emotional meaning to events. Murder attempts seem perfectly fine, if no one has actually suffered harm.

This study provides a look at the underlying mechanisms whereby emotion helps determine morality. The researchers say there are two components to making moral judgments – a logical appraisal of intentions, and an emotional reaction to such intentions. This research suggests the emotional component of such moral judgments is regulated by the vmPFC.

Institutionalized Greed

Although Adam Smith's *Wealth of Nations* is often dredged up in modern-day defenses of such moral crimes as CEO compensation 1,000 times that of "lesser" employees, or of bloody mass firings during times of historically record-breaking profits, Smith also wrote *The Theory of Moral Sentiments*, which dealt with the psychological basis of morality. Smith believed – and modern science has since borne his theories out – that our innate emotional compass usually steers us toward altruistic moral decisions. We're not all coldly calculating accounting machines. Said Smith, morality stems from imagination, allowing us to "mirror the minds" of others: "...By conceiving what we ourselves should feel in the like situation," we feel an instinctive sympathy for those around us.

We now know that Adam Smith was absolutely right – the reason we're compelled to seek fair dealings is because we're able to guess (and internally experience) how others will feel if we cheat them. We know they'll be angry, hurt or insulted, and so we're compelled to "do the right thing"; this instinctive capacity to feel the pain of others also drives acts of heroic altruism, such as the drive to rescue others from danger or to volunteer to help the less fortunate.

Scientists at Duke University have used brain scans to pinpoint the seat of theory of mind – the ability to guess at, imagine and neurologically experience the thought processes and motivations of others, saying it primarily engages the *superior temporal sulcus*. They've found subjects with the greatest brain activity in regions correlating with sympathy also reported more interest in the emotions of others, and a greater capacity to accurately deduce and experience it within themselves. People with such heightened empathic sensitivity also tend to be the most altruistic – willing to help others for selfless reasons.

Of course, personalities are shaped by experience just as well as genetics, so if you're beaten, ignored, starved or exploited, particularly as a child, your personality can become warped, turning you into a selfish, hostile or coldhearted "misdirection" of the ultimate human potential for good.

Most of us are naturally deeply disturbed by the pain or distress of others. We can be desensitized, but it usually takes substantial time and energy to bypass our natural inclinations toward kindness and empathy. Repetitive cruelty or deprivation can shut down our innate capacity for empathy and love, but it isn't easy, fast or even necessarily permanent.

Good And Evil

What makes someone "good" – compassionate, generous and altruistic – or "evil" – self-absorbed, violent, deceptive or cruel? First, it's important to realize that norms, moral codes of acceptable behavior, vary from culture to culture – in contemporary America, many consider killing innocent civilians in an aerial strike *acceptable collateral damage* during wartime. In strict Muslim societies, severing the hands of a thief or stoning a woman (but not her male partner) to death for unwed sex is considered by many to constitute justice.

According to Georgetown University's Dr. Abigail Marsh, genetic variations (*alleles*) for the serotonin transporter gene *SLC6A4* correlate with personal ideas of what is right and wrong. In her study, volunteers responded to justice-related dilemmas with varying outcomes, and Dr. Marsh's team found people with a short allele generally find allowing innocents to be harmed in the interest of saving a great number of people to be unacceptable. Those with long alleles were more likely to believe harming innocents for the "greater good" is acceptable.

As for deception, Harvard's Dr. Joshua Greene conducted a 2011 fMRI study in which subjects had the chance to lie about coin flipping results. Dr. Green categorized participants into *dishonest, honest* and *ambiguous* categories, and found that dishonest participants had distinct PFC activation when they lied, while honest volunteers did not. He believes this is because people struggle with temptation when given an opportunity to lie.

Wealth And Desensitization

The latest research seems to indicate that people of different economic classes think about the world in fundamentally different ways. University of California psychologists Dacher Keltner, Michael W. Kraus and Paul K. Piff say, contrary to the popular belief that class doesn't matter, it profoundly shapes your identity. A 2011 study found that people in the highest economic brackets have difficulty in recognizing emotions in others, while those in lower-class brackets are much more adept at emotional recognition.

This variation in empathic sensitivity appears to be learned, a product of the cultural environment, rather than innate; in general, say the team, as people rise in economic status, their empathy declines. Dr. Keltner suggests that low-income people have greater empathy out of a frequent need to cooperate for survival. For example, someone who can't afford daycare will often look to relatives and neighbors to watch the kids.

With fewer resources and less education, turning to others becomes critical for adapting to difficult circumstances, he says.

> People who grow up in lower-class neighborhoods, as I did, will say, 'There's always someone there who will take you somewhere, or watch your kid. You've just got to lean on people.'

Social class is more than just accumulated wealth: economic status shapes behavior and perception in ways which signal social class and reinforce economic-based cultural identities. In turn, these identities shape perception, thought, emotion and behavior.

According to the team, lower economic-status people tend to explain events in terms of their outer environment. As a result, they're more attuned to the emotions of others, and better at judging these emotions. Across three separate studies, lower-status subjects received higher test scores for empathic accuracy than higher-status subjects, judging the emotions of their test partners more accurately, and reading emotions from images of eye movement more accurately. Says Dr. Keltner,

> What I think is really interesting about that is, it kind of shows there's all this strength to the lower class identity: greater empathy, more altruism, and finer attunement to other people. One clear policy implication is, the idea of noblesse oblige or trickle-down economics, certain versions of it, is bull. Our data say you cannot rely on the wealthy to give back. The thousand points of light – this rise of compassion in the wealthy to fix all the problems of society – is improbable, psychologically.

In fact, he says, the wealthiest among us tend to hoard resources and generally be anything but charitable.

The Shocking Truth Or Confirmation Of An Assumption?

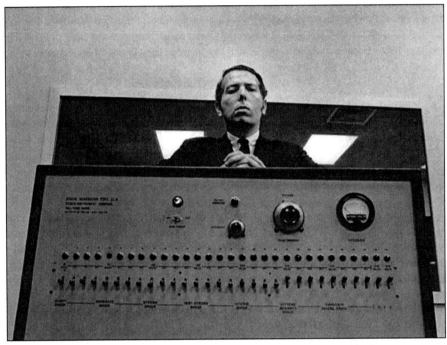

Dr. Stanley Milgram and his "shock box", 1963, Yale University, public domain

Dr. Stanley Milgram's Obedience to Authority experiments are often cited as proof that the majority of ordinary people will torture or even kill if ordered to do so by an authority figure, but perhaps this blanket judgment of the human species is based on somewhat flawed experimentation.

In 1961, the Yale professor set out to test how willing ordinary people are to act against their morality if an authority figure orders it. He was trying to discover why Nazi soldiers participated in the brutal crimes of the Holocaust. Volunteers were led to believe they were teaching a series of word-pair memorization exercises to a "learner" volunteer, and that they were to shock the learner for every wrong answer. In some of the experiments, the learners also mentioned having a "heart condition". Unbeknownst to the "teacher" volunteers, however, both the "scientist" directing them and the "learner" they were supposed to shock were paid actors, and no real shocks were given.

The volunteer teacher and fake scientist were placed into one room, separated from the fake learner. The teacher (volunteer) was seated at a machine labeled with progressively higher voltages, up to a (presumably deadly) 450 volts. Teachers and learners communicated via microphones and speakers.

The teacher was instructed to inflict an increasingly higher voltage shock for each wrong answer the learner gave. These voltages were labeled from "slight shock" to "severe shock", and a series of triple XXX's for the last switches, said to deliver 450 volts. As the experiment progressed, a recording was played of the learner shouting in pain, protesting, demanding to leave, and finally silence. If the teacher protested, or tried to stop delivering shocks, the scientist (actor) would tell them repeatedly that they had to continue, and "had no choice".

According to Dr. Milgram, 65% of the volunteers delivered 450-volt "shocks" three times each. This, he said, was proof that even ordinary people will act without mercy when ordered to do so by an authority figure. Milgram himself says the volunteers aren't sadistic, but that his experiment "...raises the possibility that human nature cannot be counted on to insulate men from brutality and inhumane treatment at the direction of malevolent authority".

The experiment has been repeated around the world many times since, with generally consistent results of 61% to 66%. But does it really prove that two out of every three ordinary people are willing to murder simply because an authority figure told them to?

If so, you have good reason to constantly be on your guard; after all, the majority of people you pass in the street are happy to kill you simply because someone in a uniform tells them they must. But perhaps this conclusion isn't quite so clear:

When people see a "scientist" in a lab coat or another uniformed authority figure, the natural assumption is that the person in charge is trained to prevent mishaps, and that he or she will intervene if there is any real danger. There's an element of natural trust involved.

Additionally, as far Milgram's volunteers knew, the "learners" in the experiment had signed the same waiver as they themselves had, and the volunteers thought they stood an equal chance of being made the "learners". The volunteers were fully aware the "learners" wouldn't die or even be badly injured; they were specifically told there would be no "permanent tissue damage".

In 2009, the BBC restaged the experiment, and one volunteer who complied all the way to the end specifically stated she continued only after she'd been reassured by the "scientist" that there would be no long-term harm to the "learner".

A good portion of compliant volunteers surely must have believed the same. And in Milgram's own video of the experiment the "scientist" actor clearly tells an objecting volunteer, "As I said before, the shocks may be painful, but they're not dangerous". You also see a volunteer repeatedly insisting that the "professor" go in and check to make sure the "learner" is all right.

Finally, the volunteers were under the impression that the "learners" were volunteering in the name of advancing science, and, presumably, allowing themselves to be subjected to this for the betterment of mankind.

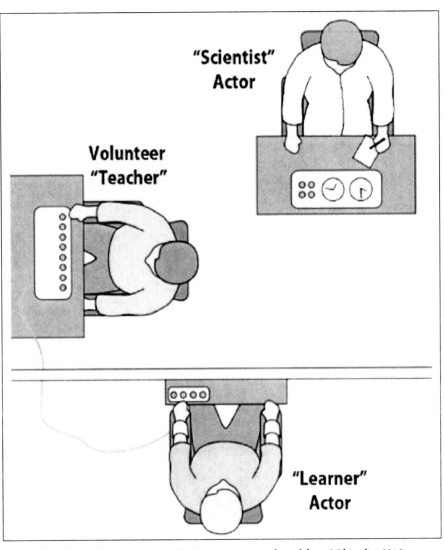

"Scientist"
Actor

Volunteer
"Teacher"

"Learner"
Actor

The Milgram Obedience to Authority Experiment, adapted from Wikipedia, 2010.

Fighting Nazis – *Many military historians say that in World War Two most Germans either didn't support or secretly helped oppose the Third Reich. Out of over 70 million citizens, only about 12% – 8.5 million – were listed as members of the Nazi party by the war's end in 1945.*

This was at a time when crossing the Nazis was an extremely dangerous proposition: between 1933 and 1945, some 77,000 Germans were executed for engaging in subversion and conspiracy. The **Gestapo** *(secret state police) tightly controlled the civilian population, with an estimated 100,000 spies and informants. Anti-Nazi criticism or attempts to rescue Jews or others from the Nazis was met with public execution by hanging or being shot on the spot.*

Even so, throughout World War II, ordinary Germans like the hero of Steven Spielberg's brilliant **Schindler's List** *helped thousands of Jews escape the Nazi death camps at great risk to their own lives and families, sharing scarce food and other resources, hiding and protected Jews and thousands of others until the defeat of the Nazis.*

Laying an Urban Legend To Rest:
38 Heartless Witnesses

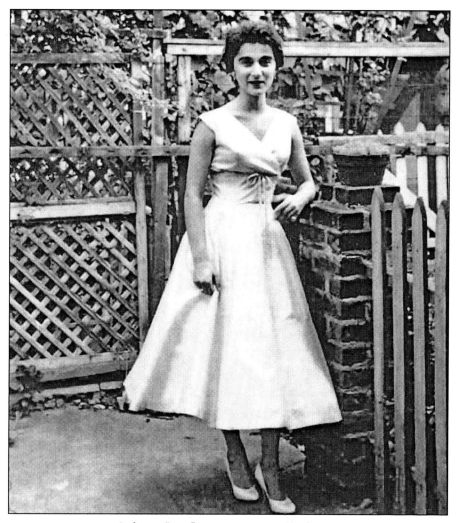

Catherine "Kitty" Genovese, 1963, public domain.

The neighborhood was cold, dark and quiet as 28-year-old Catherine "Kitty" Genovese pulled her red Fiat into the parking lot adjacent to her Queens apartment. It was 3:20 in the morning on March 13, 1964. She had just finished a late shift at Ev's 11th Hour Sports Bar, where she worked as a night manager. She had no idea she was being followed.

Genovese climbed out of her car, and began walking to the apartment she shared with her lover, Mary Ann Zeilonko. As she headed toward the rear entrance, she spotted a stranger striding silently toward her in the darkness. The menacing figure was approaching quickly, with murderous intent;

Genovese turned to run, but her attacker quickly closed the distance, stabbing her twice in the back with a large hunting knife. Each of her lungs had been punctured, but she still managed to cry out, *Oh my God, he's stabbed me! Please help me!* before crumpling to the ground.

Several of her neighbors awakened at the sound, and came half-asleep to their windows. According to Queens County District Attorney Charles E. Sullivan, the majority were quite elderly, in their sixties and seventies. Among them, however, directly cross the street in the 10-story Mowbray Apartment House, was assistant superintendent Joseph Fink, on duty as the night elevator operator.

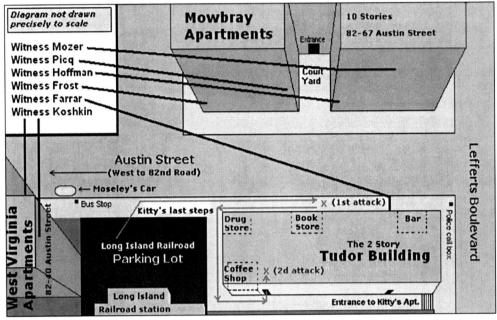

The Catherine Genovese murder site, Joseph De May, HomicideSquad.com, (retired New York City Police Department detectives), 2007. Used with permission.

Prosecutor Charles E. Skoller would later express horror at Fink's callousness, Fink being the only witness with a clear view of the first stabbing from his chair overlooking the Mowbray Apartment bay windows. Incredibly, Fink admitted to the police that he clearly saw the attack and had "briefly considered going to get his baseball bat", but instead did nothing, choosing in the end to go downstairs and sleep. Upstairs on the seventh floor, however, senior Robert Mozer flung open his window and shouted "Let that girl alone!"

It worked, or so he and the other eyewitnesses thought. The attacker ran at the noise, and Genovese wordlessly rose to her feet, and then staggered silently off to the back of her apartment building's stairwell. She'd been knifed just a few feet from the entrance of the Old Bailey, a bar known for rowdy, late night disturbances. Although the Bailey usually stayed open until 4 am, that night it had closed early because of a fight which had broken out. This was nothing new; neighbors had previously complained about the bar's noisy early-morning patrons.

Thus, it was hardly surprising when 15-year-old Michael Hoffman thought he was seeing the aftermath of a drunken quarrel. He had originally flung open his window in anger, as he explained to police, to shout *Shut the Fuck up!*, but after seeing the woman on the sidewalk, and her attacker fleeing, he urged his father to call the 102nd Precinct to report a beating he believed he'd witnessed outside the bar.

A 1995 Newsday article recounts this as just one of several unfortunately vague telephone reports that came in immediately to report the incident. But none of the witnesses were quite sure of what had occurred. French immigrant Andree Picq, for example, saw what she thought was a man crouched over a woman on the pavement, but when the man was frightened off, the woman staggered off silently, presumably to safety, and her attacker got into his car and drove away.

Another unnamed witness said her husband awoke, thinking he had heard a scream, "but when he looked out the window, no one was there". "We thought it was a lovers' quarrel," said a third witness. "I went back to bed."

At the time, an anonymous 911 emergency service didn't exist, and it's likely that the multiple eyewitnesses who monoamine oxidase A had called immediately after the initial attack were reluctant to divulge their identities, instead electing to hang up. The police were, for their part, used to receiving constant "crank calls" and false alarms, and were thus hesitant to act upon vague, anonymous reports of a lover's quarrel which had apparently already ended outside a well-known "rough" bar.

Meanwhile, Genovese's assailant had backed his car around the corner, parked one block over, and then cut the engine, waiting and listening in the darkness. After hearing nothing but silence for 10 minutes, he returned to find the lights from the surrounding apartment windows had once again gone out. Most of the witnesses had returned to bed, while Genovese had silently hobbled away, reportedly leaving the impression she had stumbled drunkenly home.

Seeing he was apparently safe, the attacker returned on foot, a fedora now disguising his face. He hunted the back alley from door-to-door for Genovese, hoping to finish her off, and found her lying bleeding on the hallway floor in the rear of her building, out of sight of witnesses. Genovese managed what NY Chief of Detectives Albert A. Seedman described as "...a low cry, too weak for a scream, as the door closed".

Her attacker stabbed her in the throat to silence her, then raped and robbed her of $49 as she lay dying. Of all the witnesses who emerged from the investigation, only one saw the horrific brutality of the crime at this point: reclusive artist Karl Ross opened his door and saw a man knifing Genovese on the floor below. Ross was allegedly drunk on vodka, so he called neighbor Sophie Farrar, who reported the murder to the police, then rushed to Genovese's side, as the killer fled. Farrar then cradled the dying girl in her arms until the ambulance arrived. Genovese died of asphyxiation en route to the hospital.

Six days after Genovese's murder, 28-year-old Winston Moseley was picked up on suspicion of burglary. He was a married father of two, working as an office machine operator. He also happened to be a serial killer, rapist and necrophiliac, who soon confessed to murdering 15-year-old Barbara Kralik two months earlier in her home while her parents were in the house.

NY Times reporter Martin Gansberg took 127 short lines from the police blotter and went on to paint an elaborate, lurid picture of 38 inhuman witnesses casually watching 35 minutes of screaming, bloody violence with blasé indifference. His story revised nearly every detail with breathtaking creative abandon, but nonetheless ran on the front page of The New York Times.

Gansberg claimed three dozen neighbors watched the brutal murder unfold over the course of half an hour and couldn't be bothered to call the police as the murderer looked up, shrugged and walked away. Their apathy, said Gansberg, had shocked even the world-weary police inspector. Unfortunately, none of the claims were accurate, but the myth of the icy-veined New Yorkers who sat by their windows watching a grisly, half-hour-long knifing had been born, and has persisted, even appearing in countless introductory psychology textbooks, which have only served to perpetuate the urban legend.

It's probably a stretch to consider a dozen New Yorkers within separate apartments and buildings to be a "group", but the Genovese murder did spur studies which led to a deeper understanding of what's come to be known as the *Bystander Effect*: psychologists Bibb Latané and John Darley found that the more witnesses present at an emergency, the less likely anyone will be willing to help. In emergencies, individuals in a group instinctively look for others more qualified than themselves to take charge and accept responsibility. But the motives aren't malice or indifference. The Bystander Effect, they say, arises from two lines of reasoning:

1. *Pluralistic Ignorance* – each witness is unsure of the seriousness, and seeks confirmation from others, thinking, "No one else is helping; is this person really in need of my assistance?" They doubt their own ability to help, believing others must be more qualified, and will know what to do.

The first step in deciding to help someone is realizing they actually need help. A witness first needs to know he's seeing an actual emergency and that the victim needs help. Because of this, eyewitnesses often fail to intervene because they don't even realize they're witnessing a crime.

In an ambiguous situation, when we're unsure as to whether or not an emergency exists, we look around to see how others are reacting, assuming they know something we don't, and gauging their reactions before deciding how to respond. If everyone around is acting like there's an emergency, we'll act accordingly. But if everyone around is acting calm, we may fail to recognize the urgency of a situation and refuse to get involved. Witnesses look to each other to decide if they're seeing a crime, and if no one reacts, then they all can mistakenly conclude a situation is not an emergency, and no one steps forward to help.

Darley and Latane recreated the phenomenon in the lab: as volunteers filled out forms, smoke was emitted into the room from underneath a door in the back. A pair of lab assistants posing as volunteers was instructed to remain calm no matter what happened.

When test subjects were alone as smoke poured into the room, they immediately left to report it 75% of the time, but when the fake "participants" were also in the room acting casual, only 10% of the test subjects raised the alarm, even when the smoke got so thick they could barely read their questionnaires.

2. Diffusion of Responsibility – each witness thinks, "Someone must have already called the police." Even when witnesses realize they're seeing a crime, they may still fail to help: the more witnesses present, the less responsibility each one feels.

If you're the only eyewitness, you are 100% responsible for providing help (or not). But if there are five bystanders, you're likely to feel only 20% of the responsibility is yours – responsibility has been diffused among the group. In such circumstances, people tend to assume someone else is more qualified to help. Unfortunately, if everyone makes the same assumption, no one intervenes.

Drs. Darley and Latane studied this phenomenon in the lab as well: they asked volunteers to join a discussion over an intercom system. Some volunteers spoke one-on-one with another person via the intercom, while others talked among a group of six. In the middle of the discussion, one of the "people" (actually a recording) shouted over the intercom that they were having a seizure, and cried out for help. Among those who were speaking "one-on-one", 85% sought help for the alleged victim, while only 31% of those among the group of six participants sought help.

The volunteers who believed they overheard a seizure but chose not to help were interviewed after the experiment to find out why. They were obviously distraught, many with shaking hands, and many asked if the victim was alright. In other words, they weren't unconcerned or heartless; they had just assumed someone more qualified would take the initiative to help.

What this means for you personally is that, if you find yourself witnessing an emergency among several other bystanders, you need to overcome your initial instincts to evade responsibility for helping. *Be aware that you – along with every one of the other onlookers is each 100% responsible for providing assistance when someone is in danger.* To get others in a crowd to help when someone else is a victim, you should point to one person and charge them with a specific task: "You! Call an ambulance!" "You! Get these people out of the street!" "You! Direct traffic until help arrives!" etc. This cuts through the fog of groupthink, and counteracts diffusion of responsibility.

If you're personally in danger, you need to make one of the bystanders feel personally responsible for your well-being. EMT and self-defense training both teach that you should choose one member of the crowd, look them directly in the eyes, point to them and then tell them specifically that you need their help. Making a specific individual feel personally responsible for your safety increases the odds they'll assist you.

Self-defense instructors also often advise women to yell *fire!* instead of *help!* if they're being attacked, because *help* is used in non-life-threatening situations, and thus does not necessarily constitute an emergency, but in yelling *fire,* you immediately make those around aware that an emergency exists.

In the end, if any good can be said to have emerged from Kitty Genovese's tragic end, perhaps it's that, as a cautionary tale, it reminds us to watch out for each other. An instructive modern myth, like the story of the boy who cried wolf, it serves as a moral lesson to make each of us more likely to intervene when precious seconds count.

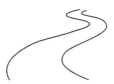

The Violent Animal

"I begin by taking. I shall find scholars afterwards to demonstrate my perfect right."
– Frederick the Great, King of Prussia 1772–1786

Picture the cliché movie bully: Biff Tannen, dim-bulb teen thug in the Spielberg hit *Back to the Future*; Regina George, the nasty but beautiful alpha female in the Lindsay Lohan vehicle *Mean Girls*. These stereotypical bullies share certain traits:

- high status within a closed group – generally maintained through fear

- strong tendencies toward jealousy

- a distorted sense of self-worth and importance (either extremely high or extremely low)

- an external locus of control (caring a great deal about the opinions of others)

- sadism – deriving pleasure in watching others suffer.

So if human beings are generally wired by default to share and to care about the wellbeing of others, why do people like this exist, and what causes them to engage in their nasty, antisocial behaviors?

Henpecked

The great majority of human behavior is driven by the subcortical brain, which encodes instincts to dominate and protect territory – primitive drives inherited from our reptilian forebears. As social, predatory animals, humans are driven to establish and maintain social hierarchies. People – like other animal species – feel a need to have our lives governed by a sense of order and predictability, including the security of knowing "who's in charge".

Maintaining such social hierarchies means a constant, ongoing assessment of member status and perpetual jockeying for position, both covertly and overtly. If you've ever heard the term *pecking order*, it refers to the behavior of chickens in a flock; there are always a few that are missing feathers and have bleeding red marks upon them. They're constantly pecked by other hens, marking them as the lowest-status members of the group.

The same core reptilian brain we share with birds drives humans to also instinctively seek to establish a social order, treating others with "low status" in a manner similar to hens physically tormenting one of their own. Social animals will always have an alpha member – one feared, respected and/or given the best treatment by peers, and these peers look to their leader for cues as to the "right" way to behave.

> *The Costs of Violence – An April 2012 study by the Institute for Economics and Peace says that in the US, violence and violence containment costs the average taxpayer $3,257 every year, and that the total cost of violence in the US, including lost productivity, is well over $460 billion (incarceration, medical bills, policing, repairs, insurance, etc.)*

Frontier Rules

Yale's Dr. Paul Bloom says that in cultures perpetually at war or fraught with violence, one's capacity to engage in violence is considered a "manly virtue". In such circumstances, turning the other cheek isn't thought to be morally enlightened, but contemptibly weak and stupid. Non-violent responses to challenges mark one as a target, so swift aggression is the accepted response to signs of disrespect or dirty looks.

This, says Bloom, seems irrational in civilized societies, but in environments where people constantly interact with little protection from law enforcement, establishing a reputation as "someone you don't want to mess with" becomes important, sometimes even vital for survival. In this way, culture can shape emotional responses, particularly in societies referred to as *cultures of honor*.

Such cultures share certain common features, such as resources that can be easily taken by force, coupled with an inability to rely upon law enforcement. These conditions, it's been theorized, require men to establish reputations for violent retaliation, as in the historic Scottish highlands, cowboy-era American frontier, and among the Masai warriors and Bedouin tradesmen, where resources like cattle are vulnerable to theft, with no readily available help from the law.

Honor, loyalty, courage and self-reliance are character traits of high value in such societies, and the capacity to violently defend oneself and one's "territory" is considered necessary. Similarly, says Bloom, the American South is said to be one such modern-day culture of honor. Originally settled by herdsmen, with a less central legal system, its culture of honor has persisted, in contrast with the cultures in the American north.

Bloom notes that, for example, southern gun laws are more permissive, approval of the military, and of corporal and capital punishment are higher, and people tend to be more forgiving of retaliatory violence, all social mores that are typical of cultures of honor. Reacting to threats or insults with violence is seen as more acceptable, for example punching someone in the face for insulting your girlfriend, or shooting and killing a trespasser.

Drs. Richard E. Nisbett and Timothy Wilson conducted an experiment upon University of Michigan white, male undergraduates, in which volunteers were invited to the psychology building to participate in an experiment. As they walked down the hallway, a graduate student who was secretly part of the experiment would bump into them, look them in the eyes, mutter, *Asshole*, then continue walking.

Although no fights broke out, the volunteers next arrived in the psychology lab, where their stress responses were tested. Significant differences in stress responses were found, with American southern men showing greater stress hormone levels in their bloodstreams, and answers in a follow-up survey suggested they'd become extremely angry.

For example, in responding to the fill-in-the-blank question "John went to the store and bought a 'blank'", northern students would reply with benign answers like "an apple", while southerners would respond with answers like "a gun", says Bloom.

People in the American South were not overall more violent than in the American North, but they were more sensitive to provocations of honor.

Dr. Nisbett, (himself an American southerner), reported his first experiences in the northern US were astonishing, as people seemed so rude. Bloom says this is because the American north is not particularly concerned with honor – and since there is no fear of violent retaliation, people are less concerned about having to be polite toward strangers.

The Violent Animal

The most recent estimates by the World Health Organization say there are 1.6 million deaths from violence worldwide every year, and violence is the leading cause of death in 15- to 44-year-olds worldwide. Although we've evolved as a species to the point where we can erect cathedrals, send machines to other planets and cure diseases like the plague and malaria, for some reason, we still act like unreasoning animals when it comes to violence and killing. Why?

Aggression is an action intended to inflict physical harm, either upon others or, more rarely, oneself. In terms of evolution, it's important for winning mates, protecting territory, establishing status and gathering food.

Psychologists regularly conduct experiments on *maternal aggression* and *resident-intruder models*, where mice defend their territory against newcomers. These same primitive behaviors have been preserved in humans, who appear to enjoy aggression: it can result in a dopamine release, functioning as a rewarding behavior just like sex or eating.

In modern societies, socially healthy people sublimate aggression, channeling it into less destructive behaviors, such as working in a competitive field, or watching and playing competitive sports.

But a 2007 University of Michigan study showed that people with high testosterone levels enjoy aggressing, finding angry facial expressions so rewarding they actively and even "vigorously" try to elicit them. That is, people who tease or bully appear to get positive mental stimulation – MFB dopamine release – from looks of annoyance, and repeatedly attempt to draw such unhappy or irritated looks from others.

Dr. Michelle Wirth, the study's lead author, says the human brain's built-in mechanisms for reading and responding to facial expressions uses them as signals to help guide behavior, even on a subconscious level.

Her experiment, however, indicates that people with low testosterone seek to avoid provoking negative facial expressions, while people with high amounts actively seek to elicit them; testosterone has previously been linked with the drive to dominate.

All Kinds Of Nasty

Aggression toward others may be from the desire to dominate, to take something by force, or by fear of a loss of control, while self-injury or property destruction are usually motivated by a wish for attention – even angry attention is still a positive form of reinforcement from a parent or caregiver.

Aggression can be either *premeditated* or *impulsive*. Impulsive aggression – exaggerated aggressive responses to comparatively normal situations – is said to be common among the mentally disabled and drug addicts – 44% engage in violence at least once in their lives. There are also less direct forms of aggression:

- *Passive aggression* – one person ignores another or refuses to do something as punishment or to control by causing frustration, guilt or other negative feelings.

- *Social aggression* – hostile social acts – for example, teenage girls spreading rumors

- *Affective aggression* – animal hissing, bellowing, *piloerection* (hair- raising), or other signals designed to scare off enemies or other threats.

Your PFC has the ability to inhibit aggressive impulses, through release of the mood-stabilizing neuromodulator serotonin. In contrast, striatal dopamine is excitatory – bolstering aggression. Blocking dopamine receptors reduces aggression, not to mention other behaviors like general movement and daily functions. So during animal encounters and fights, dopamine level increases and serotonin levels drop. The effects also persist long after aggressive behavior has ended.

Humans and other animals become more impulsively aggressive after ingesting alcohol, because it binds to inhibitory GABA receptors, undermining cortical self-control. Alcohol acts upon both the GABA and dopamine systems to create the loss of control seen among drinkers.

Ethanol, the active ingredient in alcohol, inhibits the action of the monoamine oxidase enzyme, which normally breaks down dopamine in the synapse. This allows dopamine to act upon the post-synaptic neuron for longer than normal, causing enhanced sensations of pleasure. Ethanol also enhances inhibitory GABA's effects within the prefrontal cortex, inhibiting the release of other neurotransmitters in impulse-control regions of the PFC.

Ethanol also binds to GABA receptors, causing chloride ion channels to remain open longer. This renders post-synaptic neurons incapable of normal functioning. Unable to release signals, neurons in prefrontal cortex which normally inhibit socially unacceptable behavior and assist in decision-making have impaired function.

Varied reasons for aggression appear to include:

- High levels of testosterone may contribute to sadistic tendencies, and a personality that derives pleasure from others' discomfort

- Fear of a loss of social status, territory, mate selection or survival resources

- Injured or underdeveloped PFC impulse control centers

- Injured or otherwise impaired amygdala, hypothalamus or other limbic areas

- Impaired empathy, due to genetics or to amygdala or PFC damage

- A desire for attention from a parent or other caregiver

- A combination of genetic defects, environmental stressors and/or hormonal releases

- Alcohol or substance abuse problems

- Primitive pleasure responses to conflict

The Warrior Gene

Rational Choice Theory suggests that individual animals, including humans, operate purely out of self-interest. However, as we've seen, humans also act altruistically, and try to secure and ensure fair play. It appears that individual aggression also affects levels of the will to punish or to inflict violence in response to provocations.

Aggressiveness has been linked to *Monoamine Oxidase A* (*MAOA*) and the so-called warrior gene. MAOA is an enzyme which catabolizes (breaks down) monoamines like serotonin, dopamine and norepinephrine in the synapses. Those who produce less MAOA number about one-third of modern western populations. Historically warring populations, on the other hand, have twice the population with the low-activity allele.

People with inefficient MAOA genes are up to 700% more likely to be violent if they've been exposed to violence or other major environmental stressors. A 2008 international collaboration between Princeton, Brown, Berkeley, Santa Barbara, Edinburgh, London universities, and Italian and Indian national science institutes found that those with short alleles of the Monoamine Oxidase A gene (which underproduces MAOA), respond with greater aggression to provocation than those with typical MAOA genes.

Researchers at the University of South Carolina have discovered a genetic predisposition for severe aggression in both humans and mice: low levels of MAOA. Those born with the enzyme deficiency respond violently to stress. "The same type of mutation that we study in mice is associated with criminal, very violent behavior in humans," said Dr. Marco Bortolato, who led the study.

"Low levels of MAOA are one basis of the predisposition to aggression in humans. The other is an encounter with maltreatment, and the combination of the two factors appears to be deadly: It results consistently in violence in adults," says Dr. Bortolato. Bortolato and his team replicated human pathological aggression in mice, by inducing low enzyme levels as well as creating early stressful events, such as childhood trauma and neglect.

In overly hostile mice, this appears to be due to a malfunctioning neural receptor; the team discovered this rage can be blocked by deactivating the target NMDA receptor, pointing to potential new treatments for severe aggression, a personality trait characterized by impulsive, violent outbursts and hostile overreactions to stressful situations. These findings show great promise for new drug targets to alleviate pathological aggression, a component of Alzheimer's disease, autism, bipolar disorder and schizophrenia, among other common pathologies.

Blocking the "aggression receptor" moderates the behavior. The receptor also appears to play a central role in helping sort through multiple, parallel streams of sensory data, however, suggesting there may be negative side effects. The team is currently testing "antagonists" – drugs which reduce the NMDA receptor's activity.

Testosterone, vasopressin, oxytocin and serotonin all seem to modulate aggression, with high levels of testosterone and vasopressin appearing to increase the likelihood of aggression; oxytocin and serotonin decrease its likelihood.

Territorial defense and other types of aggressive behavior have been elicited in laboratory animals and studied with fMRI scans, showing aggression is regulated by the PFC, and originates from the limbic system and midbrain:

- *Amygdala* – fMRI scans show threatening stimuli increase amygdala activity, while injuries to the amtgdala reduce dominance-related aggression.

- *Hypothalamus* – Stimulating certain regions of the hypothalamus triggers affective aggression (physical displays of aggression in response to real or imagined threats).

- *Thalamus* – Irritating sensory stimulation (rubbing a cat the wrong way or restraining a baby for example) is modulated by the thalamus, and can trigger hostility. Thalamic activation of the amygdala triggers this rage.

- *Midbrain* – Electrically stimulating the periaqueductal gray matter triggers aggression. When the PAG is damaged, it results in passivity.

Rampaging Mice

Optogenetics – brain stimulation using beams of light –has revolutionized biological research. In 2011, using light pulses on transplanted photosensitive ion channels, New York University researchers were able to activate mouse neurons that trigger violence. Dr. Dayu Lin says a small region of the *ventromedial hypothalamus* (VMHvl) can trigger both violent and sexual behavior. Normally, the hypothalamus is the body's main regulator, controlling appetite, thirst, sleep cycles, body temperature and balancing blood chemistry.

However, some VMHvl neurons can trigger aggression, and others sexual behaviors. Interestingly, they appear to compete as well: violence-inducing neurons suppress sexual activity and vice versa – during sex, the violence-linked neurons are held in check.

Stimulating rhodopsin-activated ion channels (light-sensitive proteins like those in your retinas) on hypothalamus neurons made the mice indiscriminately violent – attacking male or female mice, and even inanimate objects. The only way to suppress the violence was through sex; if the animals were in the midst of copulation, the aggressive behavior could not be triggered. Post-coitus, however, the induced rage behavior returned.

Genetic manipulation can also increase aggression. In 1999, Nobel Prize-winning biologist Dr. Susumu Tonnegawa developed a gene suppression technique to target and inhibit the expression of specific individual genes. Together with colleagues Drs. Chong Chen, Robert Greene and Donald Rannie at Harvard Medical School, he used the technique to suppress a single gene in mice and thus created crazed, fearless mice that would fight to the death, massacring any rivals.

This is highly unusual, to say the least; mice typically never fight to the death; they fight until they see they cannot win and then retreat – it's fear keeping them alive. But researchers would reportedly arrive at their labs in the morning to find a mouse apocalypse, with dead mice, backs broken, and blood splattered everywhere.

Knocking out the gene created a deficiency of an enzyme (alpha-calcium-calmodulin-dependent kinase II or α-CaMKII), which only comprises about one percent of total brain protein, but disrupts serotonin release from the raphe nuclei. Since the raphe nucleus projects throughout the CNS, it modifies nervous system function profoundly. Serotonin, as we've seen, helps regulate aggression.

This single genetic change wreaks chemical chaos in the brain and almost certainly underlies a predisposition to psychiatric disorders like borderline personality disorder, a pattern of intense, inappropriate anger and increased risk-taking.

Ohio State Professor Randy J. Nelson, and University of Sao Paulo Professor Silvana Chiavegatto also point to serotonin as the central mediator of inter-male aggression. In mice, inter-male aggression has been linked to testosterone levels. By using forced isolation, they were able to raise aggressiveness, and introduce "intruder mice" to trigger territorial aggression.

Human violence, they point out, is primarily inflicted by men. In fact, males in almost all vertebrate animals are significantly more aggressive than females. Mice share approximately 90% of the same genes as humans, but, while human males often inflict violence upon women, male mice rarely attack females. Unlike in mice as well, this testosterone-aggression link has not yet been proven in humans.

Aggression Circuits

There are several types of aggression in humans and other animals, including:

- Anti-predator aggression

- Fear-induced (defensive) aggression

- Predatory aggression

- Dominance aggression (inter-male)

- Maternal aggression

- Sex-related aggression

- Territorial aggression (resident-intruder)

- Irritable aggression (induced by stressors like shock)

Brain regions associated with aggression and its regulation, as shown by Dr. Panksepp, include the PFC, amygdala, cingulate cortex, hypothalamus and periaqueductal gray (PAG), which appear to form an integrated network involved in regulating aggression. Damage or other impairment in one or more of these areas can increase the propensity for impulsive aggression and violence.

In rats, attack behavior can be elicited by electrically stimulating a region of the hypothalamus, called the *attack area*, which has two-way connections with the amygdala, PFC, septum, thalamus, VTA, and PAG. Neurons in these areas are thick with steroid hormone and serotonin receptors. Several types of steroid hormones influence aggression, and castration (the surgical removal of the testes to shut down hormone production) has been used throughout history to stop reproduction and eliminate aggression.

Androgens are steroid hormones such as testosterone, which guide male fetal development. They bind to androgen receptors, guiding cell production. Androgens tend to facilitate aggression, whereas serotonin tends to inhibit aggression, and exposure to androgens early in life affects the expression and distribution of serotonin receptors, probably strongly influencing the likelihood of aggression.

Although recent studies have dramatically increased the catalogue of signalling molecules known to influence aggression, serotonin has consistently been shown to dampen aggression and violence in humans and other animals. Serotonin "...remains the primary molecular determinant of inter-male aggression, whereas other molecules appear to act indirectly through 5-HT signalling".

In nonhuman animals, the causal link between testosterone and aggression is well-established, but such a link has yet to be fully proven in humans, except among anabolic steroid abusers. Post-puberty, testosterone stimulates neural circuits, possibly increasing sensitivity to aggression-inducing stimuli by making them more salient.

Estrogens are the primary female sex hormones, which direct the development of female physical, mental and sexual preference characteristics in the womb. Studies indicate estrogen is also important for regulating social behavior in both males and females, and disrupting the estrogen receptor gene reduces aggression in male mice.

Cranky When You're Hungry – *Hunger and other forms of stress can deplete your brain of serotonin, affecting concentration, memory, arousal and emotional regulation. Brain serotonin production declines when you haven't eaten or are stressed, and this can impair your ability to exercise self-control, according to a 2011 study at the University of Cambridge.*

Low levels of serotonin weaken the communication between your amygdala and frontal lobes, making it difficult for your PFC to control anger generated by your amygdala. Being sensitive to this serotonin depletion also makes you more prone to aggression.

Co-author Dr. Luca Passamonti said: "Although these results came from healthy volunteers, they are also relevant for a broad range of psychiatric disorders in which violence is a common problem. For example, these results may help to explain the brain mechanisms of a psychiatric disorder known as intermittent explosive disorder (IED). Individuals with IED typically show intense, extreme and uncontrollable outbursts of violence which may be triggered by cues of provocation such as a facial expression of anger. We are hopeful that our research will lead to improved diagnostics as well as better treatments for this and other conditions."

Born Mean

Behavioral geneticists use twin and adoption studies to examine hereditability of aggression, antisocial disorders and psychopathy. One 2010 study has zeroed in on genes involved in serotonergic and dopaminergic pathways, particularly serotonin transporter (5HTT) and Monoamine oxidase (MAOA) genes believed to play a major role in the onset of antisocial spectrum disorders and psychopathy.

Although a number of signalling molecules including vasopressin and histamine affect aggression, most seem to have indirect influence, by interacting with serotonin function. Meta-analyses suggest 56% of the development of antisocial personality and related behaviors is due to genetic factors, with 31% due to unique environmental and 11% due to shared environmental effects, although some studies rate the genetic contribution as high as 80%.

Antisocial personality disorder is predominantly male, while borderline personality disorder is predominantly female. The genetic risk of violent behavior such as antisocial personality disorder appears to be mainly influenced by dopamine, serotonin and androgen receptors and transporters.

Epigenetic factors also play a role, appearing to alter genetic expression. For example, tobacco and alcohol use appear to strongly alter methylation and thus genetic protein expression, including expression of the dopamine transporter gene. Childhood and even fetal stress and abuse may also increase the risk of adult antisocial behavior through epigenetic mechanisms.

The Curious Case of M. Larribus – *A chilling example of the limbic system's direct role in aggression is the story of Mark Larribus, who in the mid 1990s began to behave progressively more and more aggressively to those around him, until one day he flew into a mad, blind rage, assaulting and nearly killing his girlfriend's two-year-old daughter.*

Upon Larribus' arrest, he was taken to the University of California Davis Medical Center, where Drs. Joe Tupin and Alia Karim conducted CAT scans and discovered a tumor in the form of a cyst (fluid sac), putting increasing pressure on his hypothalamus and amygdala. After doctors surgically removed the tumor, Larribus returned to normal, once again capable of anger control. Found not guilty of assault due to insanity, he returned to normalcy, and his girlfriend's daughter fully recovered.

Bullies In Training

Psychologists and neuroscientists believe empathy inhibits aggression and that the tendency to act aggressive is primarily a deficiency in empathy for the suffering of others, as well as an abnormal processing of fear and guilt, which normally inhibit violent impulses. People who exhibit social cognitive disorders such as antisocial personality disorder or conduct disorder are often empathy- and guilt-impaired.

In 2009, Dr. Jean Decety conducted studies on the empathy in children between the ages of 16 and 18 with aggressive conduct disorders, youth who repeatedly started fights, used weapons and stole in confrontational ways. His findings show bullies function quite differently from others:

Empathy, he says, is connected to brain regions which process personal pain. When you perceive people in pain, it activates the same network in your brain – the insula, medial prefrontal cortex, and periaqueductal gray – involved in experiencing pain yourself. In healthy people, witnessing others' pain activates this pain circuitry, and it's an aversive, unpleasant experience – you're compelled to help them so you both can relieve these unpleasant feelings.

This empathic pain response triggers only the emotional aspects of pain, not the actual sensory components (in other words, seeing someone accidentally hit his hand with a hammer induces a wincing emotional response and you may feel a sympathetic tingling, but your hand doesn't actually send your brain neural signals of tissue damage).

Personal history can significantly affect, and even distort the emotions one reads in others. Aggressive, bullying children have been found to have a reduced capacity to recognize the facial expressions of emotion. They misread disgust as anger, projecting their own inner hostility onto others. They also have a reduced capacity to read fear, and thus may not realize when their actions are frightening other children.

A test of empathic accuracy – the ability to accurately guess at and respond with appropriate emotions to another person – was developed by Dr. William Ickes in 1997. The video-based test measures empathic accuracy, and has been used to study the empathic inaccuracy of aggressive and abusive spouses, among other topics.

Enjoying the Pain of Others

Empathic impairment and abnormal reward processing are probably the basis of schadenfreude, the enjoyment of others' misfortune, and of sadism, the enjoyment of inflicting pain or humiliation on others.

For bullies, watching others in pain doesn't appear to be aversive; when 16 to 18-year-old boys with a history of violence and sadistic behavior are scanned while watching videos of people being hurt, their pain recognition brain circuits activate, but so do their amygdalae and ventral striata – regions of the limbic system and medial forebrain bundle which register rewards, or pleasurable stimuli. In other words, teenage boys with a history of bullying recognize pain in others, but instead of finding the experience unpleasant, they appear to enjoy it. Additionally, unlike teens in the control group, the aggressive boys showed no activation of social interaction and moral reasoning centers in the TPJ, OMPFC, and cingulate cortex.

Conduct disorder is a syndrome characterized by repeatedly violating rules or the rights of others, including verbal or physical aggression, cruelty toward animals or people, destructiveness, lying, skipping school, vandalism, and theft. It tends to be much more prevalent among boys than girls. Depressive conduct disorder is an additional combination of conduct disorder with persistent depressed moods, appetite and sleep pattern disturbances, hopelessness and a general loss of interest.

Most children and teenagers act out destructively or aggressively at least once as a means of coping with stress, but healthy children outgrow the behavior, finding more constructive coping strategies. Only when the behavior persists is it considered a conduct disorder, and such children may need psychological help.

Psychologists have found that those who resort to violence are overwhelmingly young men driven by feelings of powerlessness. Misdirected attempts at gaining feelings of empowerment motivate their violence.

Causes of conduct disorders can include inherited temperament, ineffective parenting, or living in an environment where violence is commonplace. Conduct disorder will continue and even worsen if the behavior is reinforced, "rewarded" by the environment.

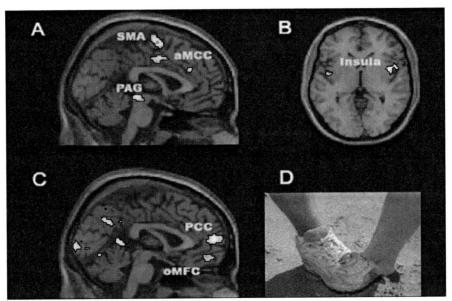

A: When children see an image of someone in pain, their brains process the pain in a sympathetic response as if they were experiencing it. B: Nonaggressive children who see someone intentionally hurt also have activation in brain regions associated with moral reasoning.

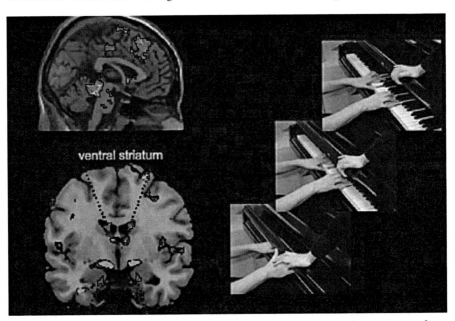

Among aggressive children, these regions remain quiet. Instead, their ventral striata – site of processing rewards – activates. When they watch someone intentionally hurting another (like slamming a piano lid on their hands), they appear to enjoy it. In addition to pleasure center activation, fMRI scans show brain regions which regulate emotion are inactive in bullies. In other words, they lack control mechanisms to keep their behavior in check when, for example, someone accidentally bumps into them. Dr. Jean Decety, 2009, University of Chicago, used with permission.

These rewards (reinforcements) contribute to a greater frequency of unacceptable thoughts and behaviors.

Behavior therapies are recently being used to teach alternative approaches to people with conduct disorders, suggesting new and more effective behaviors, and blocking the influence of unhealthy "rewards". More information is available online at the Society for Clinical Child and Adolescent Psychology online here: http://www.clinical-childpsychology.org

Scarred For Life – Childhood Trauma Permanently Alters The Brain

Children subjected to violence have brain responses like those of battle-hardened soldiers, according to the latest studies. These kids' brains have been trained to anticipate pain and to be hypersensitive to possible threats. Such adaptations are helpful in surviving abusive environments, but result in lifelong susceptibility to pathological stress, anxiety, diminished health, and shortened lifespans.

As abused children become adults, they're plagued by high levels of aggression, anxiety, depression and other behavioral problems. University College London's Dr. Eamon McCrory's team is the first to use fMRI to study the specific adaptive neural changes.

"For them to detect early cues that might signal danger is adaptive. It allows them to react, to try and avoid the danger," said Dr. McCrory; however, "a very similar neural signature characterizes quite a few anxiety disorders."

In abused children, angry faces intensely activate the insula and amygdala, brain regions involved in processing threats and pain – their response patterns match those of soldiers who have experienced combat.

There are also marked and lasting physical effects. A 2011 joint study between Yale and Vanderbilt Universities showed that children aged 12 to 17 who had been subject to mistreatment had reduced cerebral gray matter linked to behavioral difficulties, with reductions in the mass of the PFC, striatum, amygdala, sensory association cortices and cerebellum. According to the report, which appeared in *Archives of Pediatrics and Adolescent Medicine:*

> *An estimated 3.7 million children are assessed for childhood maltreatment (CM) each year in the United States; because many cases do not come to professional attention, this likely is an underestimate of the number of children experiencing maltreatment....*

> *...exploratory analyses support prominent reductions in prefrontal cortex volume common across physical abuse, physical neglect, and emotional neglect CM subtypes, as well as patterns of additional regional gray matter volume decreases in the CM subtypes. Findings in girls were in regions associated with emotion regulation, whereas findings in boys were in regions subserving impulse control.*

Long-Buried Memories

Early childhood memories – even those created at a very young age, before consciousness has fully emerged – can exist buried, and exert a lifelong, powerful influence on behavior. Abuse and neglect in particular can profoundly influence behavior, cognition and emotions throughout one's lifespan. The influence goes back as far as one's earliest moments of life.

How much attention newborns receive the first week after birth has a powerful impact on mammals: those receiving the most nurturing grow up better equipped to handle both stress and memory-dependent tasks. Studies have shown that genes encoding the glucocorticoid receptor – found in nearly every cell in the brain and body – are chemically modified during the first week after birth, and how much nurturing a newborn receives can have a major influence.

The modification – methylation – locks cells into their roles, so a liver cell, for example, remains a liver cell. Less maternal care during this critical formative week results in greater methylation, with results that last for a lifetime.

Because of this change in methylation, GR receptor production is reduced for life throughout the hippocampus – where memories are consolidated. GR receptors play a key role in the central nervous system, particularly in your brain's responses to stress, and in regulating mood. It's thought that GR receptor function may be a major part of serious psychological disorders, including depression, playing a part in norepinephrine and serotonin transmission.

Meanwhile, trauma also reduces production of NMDA receptors – which control the strength of neural connections (and thus the strength of memories). This results in a significant loss of plasticity in the hippocampus – the ability to encode events into long-term memory. These epigenetic effects of childhood neglect appear to be hereditary as well, passed down, profoundly affecting behavior through generations.

Precisely The Wrong Prescription

Research shows that a child's risks for learning and behavioral problems as well as obesity rise in proportion with psychological trauma, according to Stanford University and Lucile Packard Children's Hospital psychiatrist Dr. Victor Carrion. These findings suggest that children being treated for attention deficit/hyperactivity disorder (ADHD) would often be better served by treatment for post-traumatic stress disorder (PTSD). Symptoms of both conditions are similar, but the treatments are significantly different.

Dr. Carrion's team studied children from violent, low-income neighborhoods, and found a surprisingly strong correlation between abuse, neglect and trauma, and the mental and physical health of the study's young subjects. Among the findings was that children who were exposed to trauma had a 3000% greater likelihood of behavioral and learning problems than those who had never experienced trauma.

Neighborhoods where children witness shootings and other violence pose "a constant environmental threat," according to Dr. Carrion. Contrary to popular wisdom, rather than getting used to the trauma, children continue to experience compounding, chronic stress in response to such events, with a profound impact upon their physiology and psychology. Dr. Carrion says this means pediatricians should regularly screen children for exposure to trauma. Pediatricians often misdiagnose PTSD as ADHD, a serious problem which could be solved by simply asking a few questions, he says.

His team studied the medical records of 701 children treated at a clinic in the Bayview-Hunter's Point area of San Francisco, known for high levels of poverty and violence. Approximately half of the subjects were African- American, with the rest from a variety of ethnic backgrounds. Each child's traumatic exposure was rated on a scale from 0 to 9, and one point was given for each type of adverse experience. The team also studied the children's records for obesity and learning or behavioral difficulties.

About 66% of the children had been exposed to at least one type of trauma, and 12 percent had been exposed to four or more categories. Adversity scores of 4 or more made children 3000% more likely to have learning and behavior difficulties, and twice as likely as children with scores of 0 to be obese; and even those children with an adversity score of just 1 were 1000% more likely to have learning and behavioral difficulties when compared with those who had not been exposed to trauma.

Earlier studies had linked worsening adult health to exposure to adverse childhood events, such as being a victim of abuse or neglect, having a substance-abuser in the household, family members who were jailed or mentally ill, a mother who was a victim of violence, or living in a single-parent household. Middle-class men who had been exposed to these events in childhood had increasingly greater numbers of chronic diseases as adults. These studies show a need for early identification and intervention in such cases of trauma-derived health problems.

Research has also demonstrated that approximately 30 percent of children from violent neighborhoods have PTSD symptoms, including learning and behavioral problems such as those found in the current study, Carrion said. But if a pediatrician is unaware of a child's trauma exposure, and finds the child to be hyperactive and suffering from cognitive difficulties, the diagnosis will likely be ADHD instead of PTSD.

Says Carrion, the disorders require opposite treatments; children suffering from PTSD need therapy, not the stimulants prescribed for ADHD, which will worsen their problems. Untreated trauma, he adds, is extremely costly for both the individual and society in general.

Abandoned and Doomed

Studies of orphaned Romanian children in 2010 and 2011 found a correlation between lower IQs, behavioral problems and time spent in social deprivation and neglect. Researchers at Children's Hospital Boston and Tulane University found such conditions even affect a child's DNA – prematurely shortening *telomeres*, the protective tips of chromosome strands that gradually wear down with time and appear to predict longevity.

Because telomeres protect chromosomes, their premature shortening is associated with health risks and shortened lifespans, according to Dr. Charles Nelson, director of the Laboratories of Cognitive Neuroscience at Children's Hospital. Studies among adults have associated shorter telomeres with cognitive defects and increased incidences of cardiovascular disease and cancer. Dr. Elizabeth Blackburn (awarded a Nobel prize in 2009 for co-discovering telomeres), and Elisa Epel of the University of California, have published a report that women who look after children with chronic illnesses have shorter telomeres, equal to 9 to 17 lost years of life.

Historically, Romanian orphanages which housed abandoned children were notorious for severe child neglect. Government regulations now ban institutionalization of children under the age of two in Romania, unless they suffer from profound handicaps. They have also fortunately built a network of foster care families. DNA samples collected from mouth swabs among 62 Romanian boys and 47 girls showed that the longer children had been exposed to institutional care before the age of 5, the shorter their comparative telomere length when they reached the ages of 6-10.

Previous studies also found shortened telomeres in adults who had experienced childhood trauma, hardship or serious illness. It's not yet clear whether the condition reverses after living in a more caring, stable environment, or whether such shortening is permanent.

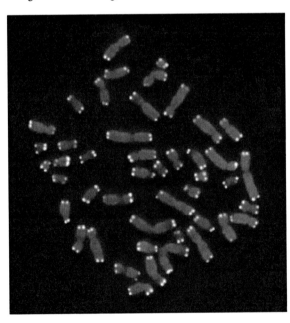

Telomeres—the tips shown highlighted in white, capping the ends of chromosomes. National Institutes of Health, 2009, public domain

Teaching Babies To Abuse

In the 1980s, Berkeley professors Mary Main and Carol George examined twenty toddlers from stressful homes. Half had been victims of severe physical abuse, and the other half were from broken homes—many living with foster families—but hadn't been abused. Comparing how these babies responded to crying classmates, Main and George discovered that, while the nonabused children showed instinctive concern and tried to console their upset peers, toddlers who had been abused seemed unaware of how to respond – some made sympathetic gestures, but these degenerated into aggressive threats when the other children didn't stop crying. Soothing words and caresses eventually turned into hitting or shouting if their peers continued to cry.

Apparently, the abused toddlers lacked an education in feeling. Denied normal, tender sympathy, they had been permanently and seriously damaged. They weren't deliberately cruel or callous, but appeared to completely lack fundamental knowledge of normal human comforting behaviors. Because of this, they reacted to crying classmates just as their own abusive parents would: with threats and violence.

This, however, is far from the norm. Humans are programmed to instinctively feel the pain of others, and experience extreme distress when hurting another or committing moral transgressions. Sympathy is one of our most fundamental instincts. If we grow up with reasonably loving parenting and don't suffer from genetic disorders, we're instinctively wired to abhor violence and injustice, and to care about the discomfort of our fellows, predisposed from birth to play fair and try to comfort those in distress. It even extends to our primate brethren: experiments with rhesus monkeys show they prefer starvation nearly to death over subjecting their fellows to painful shocks – even when it's the only way to obtain food.

Violence Begets Violence

The more violence children are exposed to, the more it becomes "normal" to them, according to a 2011 study published in the Social Psychological and Personality Science Journal. And the more normal children believe violence to be, the more often they will act aggressively.

A group of 777 eight- to twleve-year-olds were surveyed about violence at school, in their neighborhoods, homes, and on television. The survey also measured whether the children found aggression to be appropriate, asking their agreement with statements such as, "Sometimes you have to hit others because they deserve it." The children were also asked if, for example, they had ever been victims of domestic violence. Finally, each child was rated for aggression, based on his own reports and what his peers reported about him.

A follow-up survey was conducted six months later, using the same questions, showing if witnessing or being a victim of violence resulted in higher aggression levels. Schoolchildren who witnessed violence showed more aggression, with a delayed effect. Witnessing violence at the time of the first survey predicted higher levels of aggression six months later, above and in addition to the aggression these children had initially possessed. The same effect was found in victims of violence – victimization led to increased aggression six months later.

The increased aggression appeared to stem from how each child's perception of the acceptability of violence changed. Being a victim of violence or witnessing it at home, school, or on TV, seemed to make it appear common, normal, and acceptable, which, in turn led to more acts of aggression. According to the authors of the study, when people are exposed to a steady, heavy stream of violence, they begin to see aggression as an appropriate means for solving conflicts and getting what they want. Such beliefs, in turn, say the authors, lower natural human inhibitions against committing violence toward others.

Misinterpretation

A major reason delinquent kids have problems is they misread facial cues, and project their own inner anger onto others. Having been traumatized by violence, often they're hypersensitive to threats or see threats more frequently, even where none exist. It's a maladapted survival mechanism.

A 2009 study in the journal Child and Adolescent Psychiatry and Mental Health shows that juvenile delinquent boys, for example, often misread the expression of disgust and believe it to be anger, one possible explanation for their aggression. Japanese university professors Wataru Sato and Naomi Matsuura led a team in comparing emotional state recognition abilities of 24 delinquent boys with their more well-adjusted peers. The boys were all shown 48 photographs of faces displaying six basic emotions, and were asked to match each face with an emotion. Delinquents were far more likely to misread disgust as anger. The researchers believe this faulty reading of anger may be the reason delinquents perceive situations as hostile; delinquents might be projecting their own inner heightened anger onto others.

From an Early Age

A 2010 study at the University of Haifa in Israel has found some preschool children have unusual patterns of fearlessness and aggression. These kids are social, but overly aggressive and lacking in empathy, regret and guilt. They have trouble particularly in recognizing fear in the facial expressions of classmates. These aggressive children have no difficulties in identifying anger, surprise, happiness or sadness, but they tend to engage in such antisocial behaviors as taking advantage of their friends, and show a marked lack of emotional depth; and, while friendly and able to connect, they lack the ability to easily identify a friend's distress, and show a lack of interest in helping such distressed companions.

A 2010 study conducted at Cambridge University demonstrated that children who often act violently toward others often misread facial expressions of their peers. Facial expressions are, of course, the means by which humans communicate emotional states. Maladjusted children have difficulty in recognizing these states, particularly expressions of anger and disgust. They also tend to see hostility in their peers which doesn't exist, or misinterpret mild annoyance as a threat, lashing out in what they see as "self-defense".

Because of this perceptual bias, even neutral events can become confirmation of vendettas, and antisocial children attack in response, for reasons they believe are justified. There's a heightened sense of the need to defend themselves from a hostile world (which often exists completely in their own minds). In response, other children understandably avoid the company of such aggressors. These aggressive children then become more isolated, and see themselves as victims, maintaining internal lists of their unfair treatment.

The University of Cambridge's Dr. Graeme Fairchild and colleagues have measured teen girls' ability to recognize the six primary facial expressions – anger, disgust, fear, happiness and sadness, and come to the conclusion that antisocial behavior or *conduct disorder* isn't simply a matter of poor choices, but more the consequence of brain function that differs from those who are better adapted socially. This difference, says Dr. Fairchild, means they may not realize when they've aroused anger, and may not learn from punishment. Thus, the brains of antisocial people apparently operate differently than those who are more socially well-adjusted.

About five percent of children in the UK are said to meet the diagnostic criteria for conduct disorder. These teenagers seem unable to control their anger, and frequently lash out, destroy things at home and elsewhere, and get in fights or commit violent offences that rise to the level of assault convictions or worse.

For reasons not yet understood, these difficulties in reading emotions seem to emerge later in girls than in boys, but boys are three to four times as likely to exhibit conduct disorder. Among girls, rather than violence, early pregnancy seems to be the typical long-term result. Various factors underlie it, from domestic abuse to ADHD. Currently, a promising new type of treatment called *multi-systemic therapy* is being explored in Britain.

Similar results have been found in United States boys labelled by their peers and adults as bullies. These boys are shown videos of situations where, for example, one child bumps into another, spilling schoolbooks onto the floor. The child whose books fall then punches the boy who bumped into him. When asked after watching, bullies claim the child who bumped into the other had malicious intent and deserved to be struck. Well-adjusted children see no such hostility or justification for violence in the videos.

This is true when such antisocial children grow into adults as well – antisocial people of all ages carry a perceptual bias, automatically reading and assuming hostility all about them, and they're quick to lash out in response to the "unfairness" inflicted upon them.

The more this mode of behavior is chosen, the more habitual it becomes, and the neurochemical and neural bases of alternative behaviors becomes gradually more difficult to activate instead of their strongly habituated, automatic, quick and overwhelmingly powerful angry responses.

The ability to think rationally – to question one's own interpretations of events, to make a tension-relieving joke, to excuse events – becomes increasingly further out of reach every time aggression is chosen. And, of course, this warped interpretive system and range of behavioral responses leads to trouble throughout life – incarceration, unemployment, substance abuse, violence, suicide and murder.

Bringing Bullies Around

Part of the problem with antisocial people is the assumptions they make. Before finding out all the details in a situation, they assume the worst, and, before stopping to consider alternative courses of action, they fall back upon what they've always done, and engage in aggression.

As we've seen, the more often a thought (or emotion) pattern is used, the deeper it becomes ingrained – repeat a mental experience, and you engage the same neural circuit, strengthening its connections. The thoughts, emotions and behaviors it encodes become more powerful, easier to access in moments of frustration, hurt, or anxiety.

The key to reform, says Daniel Goleman, lies in teaching antisocial people to watch for sensations of rising anger, and to take these as a "warning bell" that they need to stop and think about the situation and their responses. If the habitually aggressive are then able to consider alternative interpretations for the behavior of others, or to see how they look to others around them, it can completely change their lives. "Counting to ten", walking away, and other aggression delaying strategies have also been shown to work.

Gloomy Gus And The Wallflowers

Some children are isolated because they're depressed and don't quite know how to interact with their peers. Children who are depressed may be too shy to accept attempts at friendship or be unapproachable. As a result, they end up rejected and isolated, and begin to see themselves as unworthy or inherently unpleasant, and begin to act in ways that reinforce these beliefs, neglecting their hygiene or wearing unattractive clothing. It's a vicious circle that leads to spiralling loneliness in life.

And, since depression kills motivation and impairs memory and attention, poor performance can lead to failing grades. So these depressed children sit alone, flunking out of school, not making any social ties or learning any positive social skills, and their self-worth continues to erode.

Kids learn lifelong social skills by imitation, and if they're constantly alone during this critical development period, they may grow into adulthood never learning rudimentary social skills.

Studies have shown that one of the major defenses against this downward spiral of depression lies in *self-efficacy* – believing one has control over a situation. For example, the optimistic, *No matter how tough things get, I'll pull through!* or *If I pull up my socks, I'll get better grades next time* can lead to positive change instead of *I'm just stupid and ugly*, which, of course, leads to worsening despair.

Believing bad events stem from personal flaws one is helpless to change is central to the problem. If a depressed child believes he can bring things around through his own efforts, there is greater a chance of positive results. Once again, self-talk – specifically optimistic rather than pessimistic self-talk – has profound effects, even leading into and out of the pit of depression. As Goleman puts it:

> Children who develop a pessimistic outlook – attributing the setbacks in their lives to some dire flaw in themselves – begin to fall prey to depressed moods in reaction to setbacks. What's more, the experience of depression itself seems to reinforce these pessimistic ways of thinking, so that even after the depression lifts, the child is left with what amounts to an emotional scar, a set of convictions fed by depression and solidified in the mind: that he can't do well in school, is unlikeable, and can do nothing to escape his brooding moods. These fixed ideas can make the child all the more vulnerable to another depression down the road.

He points out that medication which may be effective for adults is metabolized differently by children, and not just ineffective, but at times possibly fatal (he specifically mentions *desipramine*, under scrutiny by the FDA as a possible cause of child fatalities).

Stepping In

Goleman says weekly intervention classes for ten- to thirteen-year-olds with signs of depression have shown promise, with a 50% decrease in depression rates. In these classes, developed by Dr. Martin Seligman, children are taught that anger, anxiety and sadness aren't just uncontrollable forces that descend upon them, but that it's possible to change the way they feel by changing what they think. Teaching these children how to handle disputes, how to think before launching into action, and how to question their pessimistic self-talk can nip depression in the bud. For example, if a child fails on an exam, instead of thinking *I'm just too stupid*, they're taught to say, *Wait a minute – if I study harder, I can do better next time!* Eventually, positive results reinforce this behavior until it becomes habit.

This kind of cognitive therapy has also proven effective for obsessive-compulsive disorder, where someone is unable to stop worrying, and tries to banish worry through ritualistic behavior. Stopping and questioning the behavior before engaging in it becomes gradually easier and easier to do, as the brain's synapses undergo adaptive physical changes.

Roots Of Racism

Categorizing is essential to your survival – you need to very quickly be able to recognize things. Your brain categorizes through broad generalizations – heuristic evaluations based upon comparisons with your past experiences and existing beliefs. This is the basis of stereotypes.

When one applies this to entire groups of people, however, making snap judgments and applying inaccurate labels, it can unfairly denigrate an entire range of people and shape all your future impressions of any individuals who match the category (e.g. believing all Muslims are dangerous, or black men are dishonest). This is the basis of racism.

Remember too, that because humans try to protect their schemata (worldviews), we remember things which support what we already believe, and dismiss or forget examples which contradict our biases, because it's critical and comforting to have a consistent world view. However, this can be misleading and unfair. We can also be misled by popular media, with isolated cases distorting our ideas about how frequently something actually occurs.

Scarcity Alienates – *Whether you're on the job or at home, in school or enjoying the outdoors, one central component of your social life involves determining who "fits in" and who doesn't. This means that, unbenownst to you, your biases guide you to favor those within your own social ingroup.*

Researchers believe these universal ingroup biases provide a competitive advantage against other groups, particularly when resources are scarce. Dr. Christopher Rodeheffer and a team at Texas Christian University studied whether such scarcity influences judgments about who belongs to one's own social group.

In-group membership is often determined by outward appearances, so Rodeheffer and his team theorized that people exposed to deprivation might narrow their definition of who "fits in", and show less likelihood of including people with racially ambiguous faces into their racial in-group.

The first experiment had 71 white university students examine captioned photos showing situations where resources were alternately scarce (e.g., pictures of empty offices with captions describing job shortages) or abundant (e.g., pictures of thriving offices with captions describing an abundance of good jobs).

The researchers then created a series of images of "biracial" faces, averaging a black and white face with facial-averaging software. They then had participants examine the images and categorize whether each face was black or white.

What they found was that subjects who viewed pictures depicting scenes of scarcity tended to categorize more faces as black than did subjects who had viewed pictures of abundancy.

The results were confirmed with a second experiment, in which students were verbally primed to ponder resource scarcity or abundance with analogy problems. Further studies are planned to see if the results extend to groups from other races.

When Fear Trumps Humanity

You're built to instinctively respond to danger – risks of injury, death and disease – with fear and avoidance: looking over the edge of a steep cliff makes you nervous, and you instinctively leap away from spiders and snakes. These are adaptive emotional and behavioral responses which promote your survival, and they alter both individual thought and emotional processes, and culturally-shared beliefs in a number of ways, on a very deep level.

Your danger-avoidance instincts trigger psychological fear responses, reducing perceived threats to your well-being. But these innate fear responses overgeneralize: you're built to react with fear even when there's no real danger, and these reactions can instantly and automatically arise.

In our ancient ancestry, certain cues predicted danger, such as a growling animal, or the shape of a spider. Quickly detecting and responding to these cues provided a survival advantage, so the responses were passed down through hundreds of millions of years of evolution. While some of these fears, as we've seen, are innate, others are learned, where, like Pavlov's dogs, a certain cue comes to elicit a certain response – in this case fear. In situations where one is more vulnerable (alone at night in a dark alley, for example), these danger-avoidance responses will be amplified, and hypersensitive.

This protective behavioral avoidance system errs on the side of caution, meaning it's very error-prone, and gives a lot of false positives, perceiving danger where none exists. After all, it's much more dangerous to miss a genuine threat than to perceive that something harmless is dangerous.

Interactions with people can also hold the potential danger of physical assault, transmission of diseases, robbery, etc., so just as danger-avoidance mechanisms evolved to promote detection and avoidance of spiders, other danger-avoidance mechanisms seem to have evolved to detect and avoid specific kinds of people who might pose threats to one's safety.

During much of human history, people lived in small tribal groups. Unexpected encounters with strangers may have aroused violence, representing a health and survival threat. Thus, danger-avoidance mechanisms probably evolved to help in detecting and responding to cues identifying tribal outsiders, arousing emotions such as fear and persistent impressions and beliefs – stereotypes associating other tribe members with dangerous traits.

Like natural hazards, people can also be occasionally dangerous, and so one may instinctively react with fear and avoidance when encountering them. But often these fears are irrational, not based on any real threat. Some people may make you anxious and you may avoid them or react negatively simply because they match some heuristically-broad inner profile of danger. Because of this inner danger-avoidance system, your perceptions of an entire group of people may be distorted, evoking negative stereotypes which reflect your concerns about hostility, trustworthiness, health and cleanliness. This is the believed to be the personal and cultural basis of person stereotyping and prejudices.

You may judge some people negatively simply because they have superficial features (such as skin color) which irrationally trigger your personal danger-avoidance responses. Not only does this potentially do entire human populations a grave injustice, it also limits your personal potential for growth and knowledge. What's worse, it spreads, and, like a cancerous growth, is poisonous and exceedingly hard to remove once it takes root.

Although modern environments are completely different from those in our evolutionary past, in theory any group of people which fits a "tribal" profile could trigger innate danger-avoidance responses. Experiments seem to bear this theory out; interactions with members of other ethnic groups elicit self-reported fear and anxiety, sympathetic nervous system arousal and activation of brain structures linked to warning emotions like fear.

Central to every social interaction is an assessment of others' intentions, primarily through reading facial expressions. The human brain is particularly quick at detecting emotional expressions of anger, which most clearly signal an impending threat. This sensitivity to anger varies from person to person, based on genetics and history; for example, children who have been victims of physical abuse, have heightened limbic sensitivity to hostility and are therefore particularly accurate at anger-detection.

To test the theory that danger-avoidance instincts – specifically anger detection – may underlie negative racial stereotyping, an experiment was conducted in 2004 upon white American men and women, using photographs of black and white men and women with neutral facial expressions.

The volunteers were told that the people in the photographs were trying to mask their true emotions, and were asked to detect "hidden" anger, fear, happiness and other emotions. Before taking the test, the volunteers had each been shown one of a variety of short movie clips. One clip had been previously demonstrated to arouse fearful, vulnerable, self-protective emotional states in its viewers. A control group watched emotionally neutral movie clips.

The tests showed that after feelings of vulnerability (leading to fear) had been induced, volunteers read more anger in the faces of black men, and black men only; nor were greater levels of emotions such as fear or happiness perceived in the faces of black men. The participants appeared to have projected their expectations onto the men in the photographs; their feelings of vulnerability led them to perceive anger – a warning sign of danger.

Later that year, the experiment was repeated, with white American men and women viewing pictures of white Americans or Arab men and women. Before the experiment, each volunteer took a test which measured any stereotypes they held of Arabs. Since it was a period in which US-Arab relations were greatly strained, and there were frequent media portrayals of Arabs in hostile roles, no priming movie was presented beforehand.

As might be expected, those who self-reported holding the highest negative stereotypes of Arabs saw the most anger (but not other emotions) in Arab faces (but not white ones); this bias didn't emerge at all in those who held no negative stereotypes. The fear was projected into the faces in the photographs – presenting signs of danger where none existed. This projection varied from person to person, depending upon the types and strengths of stereotypes each one held.

The same dynamics are at play when people make judgments about entire ethnic groups as opposed to individuals. In a related 2003 experiment at a Canadian university, student volunteers each took a *Belief in a Dangerous World* (BDW) self-reporting test, which measures ongoing personal concerns about vulnerability to danger.

Each was asked to rate men from Canada and men from Iraq in terms of four personality traits: hostility, untrustworthiness, ignorance and open-mindedness Prior to their ratings, in the experimental group the lighting was shut off, so volunteers in one group completed their ratings in complete darkness, while a second control group gave their ratings in fully-lit conditions. In this way, it was possible to test both the individual and the combined effects of states of chronic vulnerability (high BDW scores) and states of temporary vulnerability (darkness), neither of which had direct bearings upon ethnic groups.

Those who reported believing the world is dangerous showed no particular bias in rating Iraqi men as a threat – until the lights were shut off. In darkness, those with high BDW scores strongly rated Iraqi men as hostile and untrustworthy, and Canadian men as especially non-hostile and trustworthy. There were no such effects on those who did not normally view the world as threatening (low BDW scorers). In other words, feeling vulnerable exaggerates and distorts racial stereotypes of both individuals and entire populations. Follow-up studies on other ethnic groups have duplicated these findings.

Most of the experiments found stronger stereotyping among men than among women, particularly among those with increased vulnerability. Although women are physically more vulnerable than men (because of typically smaller physical size and comparatively less upper-body muscle mass), from an evolutionary point of view, ancient men were more frequently apt to have unexpected encounters with strangers; in primates closely related to humans, males range more widely than females and tend to spend more time at territorial boundaries. Additionally, tribal battles typically involve males much more frequently than females. Because of this, from an adaptive standpoint, it makes sense for men to have evolved a greater wariness of outsiders than women.

Passing It On

Experiments indicate that people talk about – and remember – traits that appear to indicate danger – with the possibility of generating persistent stereotypes based upon race, culture, sexual preference, visible handicaps or deformities, dietary or hygienic practices and even weight. Threat of contamination is at the heart of social rejection of people sick with contagious diseases.

This is understandable; disease and parasites were a great concern in more primitive eras. But less rational negative reactions to physically healthy people also result from broad cues suggesting contagious disease – tremors, physical deformities, etc. Studies again show these reactions are strongest among people who feel highly vulnerable to disease or who are sensitive to feelings of disgust.

Danger of disease may be heuristically signalled not only by unusual features but also by cultural unfamiliarity, particularly by evidence that others don't follow local standards governing behavior relevant to disease control (e.g., food preparation, personal hygiene).

Born Immune To Racism

Further support for the "fear gives rise to stereotyping" theory comes from a fascinating new finding. Children with a rare neurodevelopmental disorder called *Williams Syndrome* (WS), are overly friendly and have no fear of strangers. They also never develop negative stereotypes about other ethnic groups (although they still tend to share the gender stereotyping of other children).

Williams Syndrome patients show abnormally low amygdala activity, indicating differences in processing potential social threats – and in triggering unconscious negative emotional reactions to other races.

In assigning positive and negative attributes to pictures of people from various ethnic backgrounds, WS patients, unlike non-WS volunteers, show no particular bias, although they do assign typical gender stereotypes. According to Dr. Andreas Meyer-Lindenberg, director of Mannheim, Germany's Central Institute of Mental Health, who led the 2011 study, this is because fear is not an aspect of gender stereotyping.

Stamping Out Ignorance

Says Daniel Goleman in *Emotional Intelligence*, prejudices and stereotypes are a deep-seated emotional form of learning, passed down through families, cultural teachings, or social circles, and are thus not easily rooted out, the powerful associations being directed by limbic regions which deal with emotion instead of logic. But, says Goleman, stereotypes change very slowly, so it's much more effective for work and government institutions to suppress stereotyping behavior through clear policies of what will and will not be tolerated, rather than trying to eliminate attitudes.

Among students, cross-racial and cross-ethnic friendships improve social and academic experiences. UC Berkeley psychologist Rodolfo Mendoza-Denton has found that cortisol in both white and latino students drops as they gradually become acquainted through one-on-one get-togethers. Having diverse groups cooperate to achieve a common goal has also been found to help break down racism.

We Really *Are* All Brothers And Sisters

When you meet someone who spouts racist nonsense, take pity on them – it shows that they're fearful, profoundly lacking in education, and suffering from a tragically limited future of life-enriching experience and mental, physical and spiritual growth. Here's the truth about race:

Genetic diversity increases a species' chance of survival, making children more environmentally and behaviorally adaptable, with a wider range of disease immunity. On the other hand, children born within a smaller gene pool, such as those in a family trying to preserve a bloodline, are at a tremendously greater risk of genetic defects such as *hemophilia*, a disease where blood doesn't clot properly, and the slightest bruise or cut can spell death.

Genetic anthropology has shown conclusively that you, along with every living human being today, share DNA passed down from a common ancestor born 200,000 years ago in eastern Africa, somewhere around the region now known as Ethiopia.

Our ancient ancestors began to migrate approximately 85,000 years later, to southern Asia, China, Java, and eventually Europe. From there, evolutionary adaptations to climate and diet resulted in the distinct physical variations of people that are seen as modern races.

Genetic studies have shown the oldest human DNA lineage is the Sandawe, the "click"-language-speaking tribe from Tanzania, Africa. DNA in cellular mitochondria – energy-production organelles in animal cells – is only passed down through maternal lines, and the purer the DNA (fewer variations), the longer a population has existed. In this way, it can be conclusively demonstrated that Africans from the Ethiopia-Tanzania region were the first humans in existence, their DNA now shared by every living human being today. Meet your brothers and sisters.

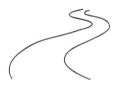

About the Author

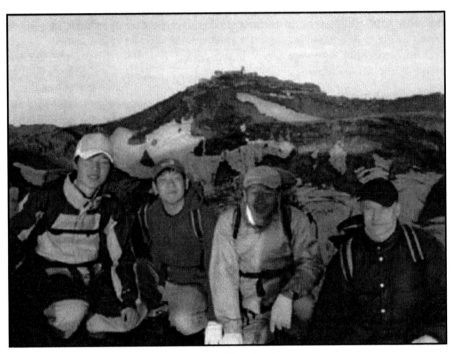

Summit of Fuji, 2010

Eric A. Smith is a freelance journalist, currently studying for a PhD in cognitive neuroscience in Tokyo, Japan. A graduate of the University of North Carolina, he was a science reporter and photographer for The Beacon newspaper in Research Triangle Park before moving to Canada and opening his first company.

As owner of Hot Damn! Design, he taught IT and graphics at La Salle, Capilano and Dorsett Colleges, and trained the design staff of Pacific Press, the largest newspaper publisher in western Canada. He was also an associate editor of world-acclaimed Adbusters magazine.

Since arriving in Tokyo, he has earned JLPT certification in Japanese and established Polyglot Studios, KK. In his spare time, he sings and writes original rock and folk songs, plays guitar and drums, and trains in weight lifting and Brazilian jiu jitsu. His cats are named Onion and Beebee.

Continue the Path in Book II: Destinies

CPSIA information can be obtained at www.ICGtesting.com
Printed in the USA
LVOW11s2008310713

345419LV00005B/44/P

9 780983 443407